Manual of
Medical Therapeutics

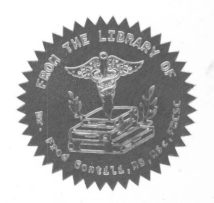

Manual of
Medical Therapeutics

NINETEENTH EDITION

Department of Medicine
Washington University School of Medicine
St. Louis, Missouri

JAY W. SMITH, M.D.
EDITOR

LITTLE, BROWN AND COMPANY
BOSTON

Library of Congress Catalog Card No. 64-22714

NINETEENTH EDITION

Sixth Printing

Published in Great Britain by J. & A. Churchill Ltd., London
British Standard Book No. 7000 0147 6

PRINTED IN THE UNITED STATES OF AMERICA

Preface

Over the past 25 years the *Manual of Medical Therapeutics* has been a useful guide to medical therapy for students and house officers at Washington University School of Medicine and Barnes Hospital. It has been compiled from material used by medical residents in teaching therapeutics to senior medical students. Because increased demands made private printing and distribution from the Department's office impractical, Little, Brown and Company has published and distributed the Manual during the past five years.

The national popularity of the Manual is evident from its frequent presence on medical wards throughout the country. It is particularly useful to students and house officers because it is written by them for them. We are encouraged that other physicians find it useful.

Revision for this nineteenth edition was undertaken by numerous current and recent house officers. The names of the physicians who supervised the revision of the chapters are listed in the table of contents. Because a generation of house officers has now contributed to the Manual through 19 editions, space does not permit us to give credit in this edition to all previous contributors.

The approach taken by the numerous contributors has not been identical, but an attempt has been made to keep the style consistent. Each chapter has been brought up to date, incorporating new drugs and therapeutic principles. No attempt has been made to make this Manual an encyclopedic textbook of therapeutics. The emphasis has been to compile frequently used therapeutic information in a concise manner. The approach taken to therapeutic problems is the approach taken by most of the physicians practicing medicine in the Washington University–Barnes Hospital Medical Center.

The editor is indebted to all the house officers, past and present, who contributed, to members of the Department of Medicine for critical review, and to Dr. Carl V. Moore for his gentlemanly patience and generous supervision.

Jay W. Smith, M.D.

Contents

NOTICE

The indications and dosages of all drugs in this Manual have been recommended in the medical literature and conform to the practices of the general medical community at Washington University. The medications described do not necessarily have specific approval by the Food and Drug Administration for use in the diseases and dosages for which they are recommended. The package insert for each drug should be consulted for use and dosage as approved by the FDA. Because standards for usage change, it is advisable to keep abreast of revised recommendations, particularly those concerning new drugs.

I. ORDERS FOR PATIENTS

A. Hospital orders

1. Orders should be written promptly, completely, clearly, and in terms that cannot be misinterpreted. Each order must be signed and dated (preferably with the time of day also) by the physician.

2. Previous orders should be canceled specifically before new orders are written.

3. PRN orders are generally unwise, especially orders for narcotics. Most patients sick enough to receive a narcotic are sick enough to be seen each time the drug is given. If a PRN narcotic order is written, a definite time limit (maximum of 48 hours) should be specified.

4. Writing orders: A routine for writing orders should be established so that important therapeutic measures are not overlooked. Immediate and later measures should be included under each of the following headings:

    a) General observations and precautions—e.g., nurses' notes, isolation technique, vital signs, as T-P-R and blood pressures, etc.

    b) General measures: rest and activity, diet, fluids, intake and output, bowel care.

    c) Treatment of symptoms (e.g., pain, fever, distention): physical measures and drugs.

    d) Specific therapeutic agents—e.g., antibiotics, diuretics, cardiac drugs, hormones, etc.

    e) Prevention and treatment of complications—e.g., wrapping or elevation of legs, skin care, frequent turning and padding to prevent decubitus ulcers, etc.

B. Orders written for drugs to be taken at home should be written in terms that can be completely understood by the patient or his family.

C. Prescriptions should include name of patient, date, name of drug, dosage, amount dispensed, an explicit explanation of how the medication is to be taken, number of times prescription is to be refilled, whether it is to be labeled, and the signature of the physician. The following points are important:

1. The generic rather than the trade name should be recorded whenever possible.

2. Dosage should be written in metric units.

3. Instructions for administering the drug should be explicit. If the directions are complicated they should be written in detail, not given verbally, and the SIG inscribed: Take as directed.

4. The name of the medicine and the tablet or capsule size should be recorded on the label in most instances, and the prescription should be marked: Label as such.

5. No prescription should be refilled ad libitum.

6. As a rule patients should bring all their medicines when visiting the physician. By knowing the amount previously dispensed the physician will have an idea as to how regularly the patient has taken his medications.

II. **ADVERSE DRUG REACTIONS** are a major problem in medical therapeutics. Recent studies have shown that 10–20% of hospitalized patients have drug reactions. Any undesired and unintended effect caused by a drug should be considered an adverse reaction. The rate of drug reactions increases as the number of drugs dispensed increases. Most drug reactions are toxic or side reactions (not allergic reactions), are pharmacologically mediated, and are in large part dose-related. Therefore, to reduce the number of drug reactions:

A. Use as few drugs as possible.

B. Pay careful attention to drug dosage.

C. Know how the drugs you use are metabolized and excreted.

D. Learn the major adverse effects of the drugs you prescribe.

E. Always consider a drug reaction as a possible etiological factor in a patient's illness.

F. Take a careful history of previous drug reactions and record both in the patient's chart and on the order sheet.

G. Report drug reactions which you suspect to the F.D.A. or A.M.A.

III. **FLUIDS** Fluid intake should be specified on all patients. Fluid balance and electrolyte and acid-base problems are discussed in Chapter 2.

A. When neither fluid restriction nor administration of extra fluids is necessary, leave an order for fluids ad lib.

B. In case of dehydration, 3000–5000 ml of fluids should be given each 24 hours until dehydration is corrected. The responsibility for adequate fluid ingestion may be delegated to the nurse.

C. If sodium intake is restricted and large quantities of water are allowed, dilutional hyponatremia may result. Water restriction and not hypertonic salt administration is the usual treatment of choice.

D. Fluids must be given parenterally if the patient cannot take them orally. The rate of intravenous infusion should be slow when cardiac reserve is compromised. Preferably intravenous fluids should be monitored by central venous pressure in patients with expanded extracellular fluid volumes.

E. Careful input and output records should be charted on patients with congestive heart failure, renal failure, liver failure, or dehydration, and on patients with severe vomiting or diarrhea.

F. Thiamine deficiency may be precipitated during refeeding of starved patients. The minimum thiamine requirement is 1 mg/1000 calories. If actual thiamine depletion has occurred, several times this amount should be given. Severely debilitated patients should receive about 5 mg/day. Ascorbic acid in doses of 100–300 mg/day should also be given. Preparations of B complex vitamins with vitamin C for administration in intravenous fluids include Folbesyn, Solu-B with C, and Vi-Cert.

IV. **HOSPITAL DIETS** provide adequate nutrition for the patient, but selection of an appropriate diet, so important in many disease states, is often neglected. Sick people frequently have poor appetites and often select inadequate diets. Dietary manuals (e.g., the Barnes Hospital Dietary Manual) that describe routine and special diets should be consulted. A dietitian may tailor a diet to meet specific needs.

A. **Liquid diet**

1. **A clear liquid diet** contains water, sugar, and salt; only such foods as broth, tea, coffee, strained fruit juice, and carbonated beverages are allowed. It is inadequate in protein, vitamins, and minerals. It is usually the first diet ordered after surgical procedures and after oral feedings have been withheld for gastrointestinal disease.

2. **A full liquid diet** requires no chewing, but does require normal gastrointestinal function for digestion and assimilation. It allows the foods listed above plus milk, eggnog, ice cream, cereal, gelatin, and strained cream soups. It is inadequate in protein, thiamine, niacin, iron, and phosphorus. Larger servings are usually given at mealtimes, and between-meal supplementary feedings can be ordered.

3. Liquid diets are indicated for:

   a) Acutely ill patients for whom the effort of eating may be exhausting.

   b) Patients with constricting lesions of the esophagus or pylorus.

   c) Patients in whom intestinal bulk must be kept at a minimum (e.g., those recovering from abdominal operations or severe gastroenteritis, etc.).

   d) Vitamin supplements must be given to patients on liquid diets.

B. **Soft diet** contains foods of low residue; easily assimilated proteins and carbohydrates are given. Such foods include refined cereals, white bread, crackers, well-cooked vegetables, cooked fruits, minced meats, eggs, cottage cheese, starch desserts, spongecake, bananas, applesauce, and the foods listed under Liquid Diet. This diet is useful for patients unable or unwilling to chew. It is recommended as a transition from liquid to regular diet, and in those situations in which easily digested foods are required. Fried foods, raw fruit, and highly seasoned foods are excluded. Caloric, vitamin, and protein requirements are fulfilled.

C. **Regular diet** has no restrictions except for foods requiring a long time for digestion, such as fried foods and some raw vegetables.

D. Special diets such as diabetic, ulcer, and low-salt diets require a specific order to the dietitian.

E. Tube feedings may be given to patients who cannot or will not take feedings orally. Their use in selected debilitated or malnourished patients allows the administration of high-calorie, high-protein mixtures. Precise diets can be given, and fluid and caloric intake maintained. Small, flexible plastic tubes may be left in place for prolonged periods of time with essentially no danger of irritation to the mucous membranes or ulceration of the esophagus. When ordering tube feedings, one should specify the protein and salt content, number of calories, and volume to be administered each 24-hour period. The mixture is then prepared basically from milk solids and Dextri-Maltose, to which have been added vitamins and minerals. Remember:

1. **Aspiration** of gastric contents is an ever-present danger; in comatose patients with absent gag reflex, for example, the high incidence of this complication may preclude use of a feeding tube. Risks may be reduced by elevating the patient's head during, and for a short time after, administration of the feeding, by suctioning the stomach prior to each feeding (to ensure that gastric distention and retention have not developed), and by limiting the volume of feeding to 300 ml (e.g., 250 ml formula followed by 50 ml water) every 3 hours.

2. **Diarrhea** may occur. Preventive measures include frequent rinsing of the feeding cylinder, irrigation of the feeding tube, and avoidance of excess volumes of water in the feeding mixture. Therapeutic measures for diarrhea are outlined in the section on treatment of diarrhea. Addition of 30–60 ml Kaopectate and/or 4 ml paregoric to each feeding will frequently control the diarrhea.

3. **Dehydration, azotemia, and hypernatremia** may develop following administration of an excessive solute load and inadequate water. This complication is most common in obtunded patients receiving high-protein (or high-carbohydrate and high-salt) feedings who are unable to express their sensation of thirst. The hyperosmolarity may appear rapidly, especially if renal function is compromised, and reflects the discrepancy between fluid intake and obligatory solute excretion by the kidney. Large volumes of urine of high specific gravity may be excreted as the dehydration worsens. To preclude such developments adequate amounts of water must be given, the amount depending on the protein and salt content of the feeding, degree of protein catabolism, insensible water loss, and state of renal function. Generally speaking, 2000–2500 ml of fluid daily (including the volume of tube feeding plus additional water) will provide sufficient water if the feeding mixture contains less than 100 gm protein, 10 gm salt, and 2500 calories.

V. TREATMENT OF CONSTIPATION

A. General comments

1. Physiologic bowel action should always be encouraged. The simplest approach is stimulation of the gastrocolic reflex by administration of a glass of warm water or cup of coffee each morning upon arising, and feeding a breakfast of fruit and bulk cereal. Bedside commodes rather than bedpans should be used whenever possible.

2. If these measures are not effective, mild cathartics and/or enemas may be useful, but their chronic use must be discouraged. Prolonged use of strong laxatives may lead to hypokalemic alkalosis and to a clinical picture that has been mistaken for ulcerative colitis. In some patients, particularly the elderly, it is difficult to empty the rectum when the stool is not formed. Laxatives act by stimulating motility, by adding moisture to the stool, lubricating it, or by increasing its bulk. An appropriate preparation may be chosen when one decides which type of action will be most beneficial.

B. **Laxatives** are useful for:

1. Bedridden patients, especially elderly patients, who frequently become constipated when not ambulatory.

2. Patients for whom straining at stool may be dangerous.

3. Patients in whom it is especially desirable to prevent desiccation of fecal material, e.g., patients with hemorrhoids, diverticulitis, etc.

4. Patients who have had barium for gastrointestinal examination or who are taking drugs that produce constipation.

C. **Contraindications** include undiagnosed abdominal pain, chronic constipation, and intestinal obstruction. It is undesirable to write orders for laxatives routinely for all hospitalized patients.

D. **Preparations**

1. **Mineral oil** lubricates the feces and causes few toxic effects, since it is essentially unabsorbed. It may inhibit the absorption of carotene and fat-soluble vitamins, and if it gains access to the lungs may cause lipid pneumonia. Dose: 15–45 ml, usually given at bedtime.

2. **Cascara** (fluid extract of cascara sagrada) acts by stimulating the colon and usually causes a single bowel movement 8–12 hours after administration. It is frequently given at bedtime. Dose: 4–12 ml. A satisfactory combination is 4 ml cascara plus 30 ml of milk of magnesia.

3. **Castor oil** is usually given when the bowel is being prepared for special examinations. It stimulates the small intestine and causes prompt evacuation. It is not used routinely. Dose: 15–30 ml.

4. **Extract of senna (Senokot),** like cascara, stimulates the colon only. It may be useful in the treatment of patients with chronic laxative habit. Dose: 1 teaspoon of granules or 1 tablet once or twice daily.

5. **Bisacodyl (Dulcolax),** an analog of phenolphthalein, stimulates peristalsis primarily in the large bowel, probably by direct contact with the mucosa. Dose: 2 or 3 5-mg tablets. A 10-mg rectal suppository usually acts within 1 hour.

6. **Dioctyl sodium sulfosuccinate (Colace** and **Doxinate)** is a surface-active dispersing agent which permits water to penetrate the stool. The drug is useful for patients who should not strain during defecation. It should not be given with mineral oil, since absorption of the oil may be promoted. Dose: 240 mg Doxinate or 50–200 mg Colace daily.

7. **Bulk-forming agents** provide indigestible residue to the feces which stimulate peristalsis by a reflex mechanism. Effective preparations

include psyllium (Metamucil) and methylcellulose. Dose: psyllium, 1–2 teaspoons in glass of water BID–TID; and methylcellulose, 1–1.5 gm BID–QID.

8. **Saline cathartics** are solutions of relatively nonabsorbable hypertonic ions which increase osmotic pressure within the colon and therefore increase its fluid content.

   a) **Milk of magnesia**   Dose: 15–30 ml at bedtime.

   b) **Magnesium sulfate**   Dose: 15–30 ml of a 50% solution.

   c) **Magnesium citrate solution**   Dose: 200 ml of standard solution.

   The latter two are rather violent cathartics, and their use, aside from preparing patients for special examinations, is rarely indicated. Since 20% of the magnesium ions may be absorbed, **magnesium cathartics must not be used in patients with renal failure.**

E. **Enemas** should be used when immediate evacuation of the bowel is indicated, e.g., in preparing patients for certain surgical procedures, sigmoidoscopic examinations, x-ray studies, etc., and in preventing or combating paralytic ileus. Enemas will often be necessary for chronically ill patients. Types of enemas include:

1. Tap water or saline: 1000–2000 ml. An effective enema for removal of desiccated stool may be made by adding 10 ml of 1% solution of dioctyl sodium sulfosuccinate to 90 ml tap water.

2. Oil retention: 200 ml olive oil.

3. Magnesium sulfate, glycerin, and water: 60 ml of each.

4. Soapsuds enema.

5. Fleet disposable enemas induce complete and prompt emptying of the left colon, and are useful in preparing patients for sigmoidoscopic examinations, etc.

VI.   TREATMENT OF DIARRHEA

A. General considerations

1. Attempts should be made to establish the precise etiology, especially in those situations in which diarrhea is more than a transient self-limited episode. A discussion of differential diagnosis, diagnostic measures, and therapy of prolonged diarrheas is beyond the scope of this Manual; ulcerative colitis is discussed in Chapter 11. The electrolyte abnormalities which may occur in acute and chronic diarrheas, and their correction, are discussed in Chapter 2. Symptomatic therapy of diarrhea is discussed below.

2. Put the gastrointestinal tract at rest by administering only liquids and foods low in bulk. It may be necessary to withhold oral feeding entirely. Some observers question the efficacy of preparations other than opiates in the treatment of acute self-limited diarrhea of bacterial or viral origin.

B. Antidiarrheal agents

1. **Kaopectate** (kaolin with pectin): 60–90 ml QID.

2. **Paregoric** (camphorated tincture of opium): 4–8 ml after each liquid stool or QID.

3. **Opium and belladonna:** 30 mg powdered opium and 15 mg belladonna in capsule TID or QID.

4. **Codeine:** 16–64 mg BID or QID.

5. **Morphine** should be reserved for selected patients who have severe diarrhea that fails to respond to conservative measures. Small doses which would not provide significant analgesia are usually effective. It should not be used in chronic diarrheal states.

6. **Diphenoxylate hydrochloride (Lomotil)** is a synthetic drug structurally related to meperidine. It effectively inhibits excess gastrointestinal propulsion; 2.5 mg are approximately equivalent in antidiarrheal efficacy to 4 ml paregoric. Although its effects on the bowel are similar to those of morphine, diphenoxylate possesses low analgesic activity and is free of parasympatholytic actions and addiction potential when used in the dosage range described below. It is narcotic exempt. Side effects are uncommon (nausea, dizziness, vomiting, and rarely pruritus and skin rashes). The drug is contraindicated in patients with advanced liver disease. Each Lomotil tablet or 5 ml liquid contains 2.5 mg diphenoxylate and 0.025 mg atropine sulfate (a subtherapeutic amount added to discourage deliberate overdosage). Dose: 5 mg TID or QID until initial control of diarrhea is effected, then maintenance dosage of 2.5 mg BID or TID.

VII. TREATMENT OF FEVER

A. General comments

1. The cause of fever should be established as rapidly as possible. Acute infections may be readily apparent as the cause of elevated temperatures, but numerous diagnostic problems are engendered by those fevers due to chronic granulomatous disease, malignant disease, collagen-vascular disease, drug sensitivity, etc.

2. Complications of marked temperature elevation include increased tissue catabolism, dehydration, acute brain syndromes, and convulsions (rare in adults). Tachycardia may be deleterious to patients with heart disease, especially tight mitral stenosis.

3. The type and severity of fever may provide important clues in establishing the diagnosis or in assessing the efficacy of antibiotic therapy. The routine administration of salicylates or other antipyretics is to be discouraged when the cause of the fever is obscure, unless it is imperative that the temperature be lowered. It is often difficult to decide when to treat a fever. There are certain situations, especially in very acutely ill febrile patients, when it is better medical practice to give antibiotics after appropriate bacterial cultures have been obtained. (See Chapter 9, Antibiotics and Infectious Diseases.)

B. **Treatment** A hypothermic blanket may be effective; however, rectal temperatures must be monitored closely, and shivering may be a problem. Tepid sponge baths with water-alcohol mixtures are less effective in adults than in children. Phenothiazines have been recommended, especially for treatment of fever due to heatstroke or thyroid storm. Salicylates are the drug of choice, however.

Analgesic-antipyretic drugs may be divided into three classes:

1. Salicylates.

2. Para-aminophenol derivatives: phenacetin, acetaminophen.
3. Pyrazolon derivatives: antipyrine, aminopyrine, phenylbutazone.

All of the above are effective antipyretic agents and are discussed in the following section. Salicylates may be given orally, intravenously, or rectally. Patients with Hodgkin's disease and other lymphomas are occasionally very sensitive to salicylates and develop hypothermia and hypotension after small doses. Although this complication is rare, it is wiser to use other antipyretic agents in patients experiencing a marked fall in temperature after administration of small doses of aspirin. Since salicylates cause a prolongation of prothrombin time, patients taking coumarin drugs should be given acetaminophen rather than aspirin.

VIII. RELIEF OF PAIN

A. General comments Numerous drugs are available; all are effective within defined limits. The drug or combination of drugs to administer will depend on many factors, especially the nature of the pain, its severity, chronicity, and etiology, and the personality of the patient. Nonnarcotic preparations should be used whenever possible.

B. Nonnarcotic preparations

1. **Salicylates** Aspirin is the most commonly used analgesic-antipyretic drug. Its mechanism of action is unknown, but it is useful in relieving the discomfort of myalgias, neuralgias, arthralgias, headache, dysmenorrhea, sore throat, etc. It is the mainstay of treatment in acute rheumatic fever, rheumatoid arthritis, and degenerative joint disease. Uricosuric effects may be marked in dosages of 5–6 gm daily, but with smaller doses urate retention and hyperuricemia occur. Aspirin should not be given concurrently with coumarin because it prolongs the prothrombin time.

   a) Preparation and dosage Acetylsalicylic acid (aspirin) is the preparation of choice. Sodium salicylate, buffered preparations, and enteric-coated tablets (which are often poorly absorbed) do not reduce gastric irritation significantly. Usual dosages of aspirin for relieving pain or reducing fever are listed below; dosage of aspirin for treatment of rheumatic fever and arthritis is discussed in those respective chapters.

   Orally 0.3–1.0 gm (5–15 grains) every 3–4 hours.

   Rectally One or two 0.3-gm suppositories every 3–4 hours.

   Intravenously Sodium salicylate 0.5 gm may be added to fluids and infused intravenously over 4–8 hours; generally, the dosage should not exceed 1.0 gm/24 hours. Rapid infusions may cause thrombophlebitis, and extravasation may lead to soft-tissue sloughs.

   b) Toxic effects The toxicity of aspirin when given in high dosage is significant; the major problems are upper gastrointestinal distress, tinnitus, and decrease in auditory acuity. Idiosyncratic reactions are very rare and the symptoms usually mild, but severe and fatal reactions may occur.

   i) Salicylism is characterized by dizziness, tinnitus, decreased auditory and visual acuity, sweating, thirst, nausea and vomiting (due to CNS effects as well as local gastric irritation), confusion, and, rarely, by an erythematous skin rash. Symptoms subside when dosage is reduced.

ii) Irritation of the gastric mucosa is common, and in the majority of patients small amounts of blood are regularly lost into the intestinal tract. Peptic ulceration, blood loss sufficient to cause iron-deficiency anemia, and even massive bleeding may occur. Although antacids are frequently given to patients receiving sustained doses of aspirin, there is no clear-cut evidence that they will prevent these complications.

iii) Severe toxic symptoms include central nervous system manifestations (restlessness, incoherent speech, anorexia, diplopia, hallucinations, stupor, convulsions, coma) and bleeding (due to hypoprothrombinemia, and corrected by administration of vitamin K_1). Although individual sensitivity varies greatly, CNS manifestations are uncommon at serum salicylate levels below 20 mg/100 ml.

Protein and formed elements (white blood cells, red blood cells, casts) may appear in the urine and then disappear when salicylates are discontinued. Since approximately half of salicylate excretion is renal, severe toxic symptoms may develop when renal function is impaired. Recent reports have suggested that aspirin administration may induce bone marrow failure.

Acute salicylate poisoning is discussed in Chapter 17.

2. Para-aminophenol derivatives

a) Preparations

i) **Phenacetin** is a common constituent of a number of proprietary analgesic mixtures. Although the drug does not have anti-inflammatory properties, its antipyretic and analgesic actions are essentially the same as those of aspirin. Prothrombin is not affected.

ii) **Acetaminophen** is the major metabolite of phenacetin, and its pharmacologic actions are essentially identical. The usual dosage is 325–650 mg every 4–6 hours; preparations include Tylenol or Tempra tablets (325 mg) (5 gr.), and Tylenol elixir or Tempra syrup (120 mg/5 ml).

b) Side effects and toxic reactions   Most side effects are rare. Methemoglobinemia, hemolytic anemias (particularly in patients with glucose-6-phosphate dehydrogenase deficiency), skin rash, and drug fever may occur.

An increasing number of reports have pointed out an association between "analgesic abuse" and renal disease. Circumstantial and epidemiologic evidence seems sufficient to relate chronic ingestion of large amounts of analgesic compounds to chronic interstitial nephritis, to renal papillary necrosis, and to a unique susceptibility to pyelonephritis.

Most reports suggest phenacetin as the offending agent, but whether nephrotoxicity is due to phenacetin per se, to metabolites of phenacetin, or to certain impurities occasionally present is not known. Clinically, analgesic nephropathy occurs in patients ingesting large amounts of the drug over a number of years—at least 1–3 gm daily for a total intake of 5 kg or more.

Azotemia and polyuria (due to decreased concentrating ability) are the major manifestations; pyuria, bacteriuria, and acidosis associated with progressive renal insufficiency may occur.

3. **Pyrazolon derivatives** Antipyrine and aminopyrine are not recommended as routine analgesics because agranulocytosis and even aplastic anemia may follow their administration. Phenylbutazone is generally not employed as an analgesic except for pain associated with inflammatory diseases; the same hematologic complications may occur. Its use is discussed in Chapter 16.

4. **Propoxyphene (Darvon)** is a nonnarcotic analgesic structurally related to methadone, with potency similar to codeine. It is better tolerated than codeine, and side effects (nausea, vomiting, epigastric distress, dizziness, drowsiness, pruritus, skin rashes) are minimal. It has recently been associated with hypoglycemia. Oral dosage is 32–65 mg every 4–6 hours. Combinations of propoxyphene and salicylates are more effective than is either agent alone.

5. **Pentazocine (Talwin)** is a new nonnarcotic analgesic which produces significant analgesia 15–20 minutes after intramuscular injection. Thirty mg is usually as effective as 10 mg of morphine; drug addiction does not occur, although mild withdrawal symptoms may occur. Because it is a narcotic-antagonist, it must be given with caution to patients receiving narcotics. Adverse effects include over-sedation, dizziness, nausea, vomiting, euphoria, and respiratory depression. Dosage is 30 mg IM, IV, or subcutaneously. Its primary clinical usefulness is in those patients who require chronic administration of analgesics.

C. Narcotics

1. **General comments** These drugs are used for the treatment of severe pain and for the control of severe cough and diarrhea. Dyspnea caused by acute left ventricular failure is frequently relieved by morphine. About a dozen narcotics are commonly employed. Morphine is the most active and is considered the standard against which the efficacy of other analgesics is measured.

2. **Pharmacologic actions,** in addition to analgesia, include respiratory and circulatory depression, sedation, alteration of mood, bronchospasm, increase in sphincter tone, atony of the bowel, nausea, vomiting, antidiuresis, addiction, and rarely true allergic reactions. Tachyphylaxis usually occurs. There are probably no major differences in adverse effects when given in equianalgesic doses, but patients will usually tolerate one drug better than another.

3. **Clinical use and precautions**
    a) Narcotics should not be used when other drugs or physical measures will provide relief of pain. They should not be prescribed for longer than 24–48 hours at a time except in patients with far-advanced malignancy. They are most effective parenterally. They should be used cautiously in patients who develop euphoria with relief of pain, for these individuals may be particularly susceptible to habituation or addiction. More stable individuals do not develop physiologic dependence until the drug has been given for two weeks or longer, but habituation may occur more quickly. Hazards of addiction should not preclude long-term administration of narcotics to patients with terminal malignancy.

b) Narcotics should not be used in certain acute disease states (e.g., suspected surgical abdomen) in which the pattern and degree of pain are important diagnostic signs. Patients with suspected acute head injuries should not be given narcotics, for their administration will prevent accurate assessment of neurologic changes.

c) Narcotic-induced vomiting may be frequently circumvented by giving a small dose (to depress the vomiting center) before the planned therapeutic dose. Side effects may also be reduced by keeping the patient recumbent.

d) Narcotics depress the respiratory center, the effect being directly proportional to the dose. Therapeutic doses diminish the tidal volume; larger doses decrease the respiratory rate. Bronchospasm may occur. The response to hypercapnia, but not to hypoxia, is depressed. When narcotic-induced respiratory depression has occurred, hypoxia is usually the stimulus for respiration, and oxygen, therefore, should be given with caution. Narcotics should be used cautiously in patients with pulmonary insufficiency.

e) Narcotics increase the sphincter tone in the gastrointestinal tract, biliary tree, ureters, and urinary bladder. They should be given with great care to patients with biliary colic, fulminant ulcerative colitis, and prostatic hypertrophy. Transient elevation of serum amylase may follow the administration of morphine.

f) Narcotics impair reflex activity from receptors in the aortic arch, carotid sinus, and pulmonary vessels, and may occasionally produce orthostatic hypotension, syncope, and circulatory collapse.

g) Narcotics should be used with extreme caution in patients with hypothyroidism, Addison's disease, hypopituitarism, anemia, and severe malnutrition or debilitation. In patients with increased intracranial pressure narcotics may further elevate the CSF pressure. Since narcotics are metabolized in the liver, patients with liver disease may be inordinately sensitive to the usual dosage. Phenothiazine drugs (and occasionally monoamine oxidase inhibitors) may markedly potentiate the effects of narcotics. In all these situations it is wise to reduce the usual narcotic dosage by approximately one-half until the patient's response to the drug can be evaluated.

4. Preparations and dosage

a) Morphine sulfate The usual effective dose is 10–15 mg IM, but occasionally as little as 5 mg affords excellent relief of pain. A 15-mg dose provides maximum analgesia, and larger doses should not be given at first, although it may be necessary to increase subsequent doses as tolerance develops. Intravenous administration may be helpful when an immediate effect is desirable, such as in a patient with acute myocardial infarction and pulmonary edema. The duration of action of a 10–15 mg dose is 4–7 hours; the peak action is achieved in 60 minutes. Some patients will show slight withdrawal signs after receiving as little as 15 mg QID for 2–3 days.

b) **Codeine,** the methyl ester of morphine, is dispensed as water-soluble sulfate and phosphate salts. Its analgesic action is about one-fourth that of morphine. It is less addicting and produces fewer gastrointestinal complications than morphine. It is often used to depress cough, but is only one-third as effective as morphine. Effective control of cough may be achieved with 15–30 mg every 4–6 hours. Codeine is much more effective parenterally than orally in equivalent dosage. Dosage is 15–60 mg IM every 3–4 hours; 30–60 mg may be given orally. The duration of analgesia is 3–5 hours, with a peak at 90 minutes. Headache is a common side effect.

c) **Dihydromorphinone (Dilaudid)** is a morphine derivative of shorter duration of action. It may be given orally, parenterally, or rectally. It is useful for relieving pain without producing sedation. It is five times more potent in producing analgesia than morphine. The usual dose is 2–4 mg. Its adverse effects are similar to those of morphine, with addiction and tolerance appearing more rapidly.

d) **Methyldihydromorphinone (Metopon)** is twice as potent an analgesic as morphine. Tolerance develops less rapidly. Nausea, vomiting, and drowsiness probably occur more frequently. The dose is 5–15 mg orally. It is the narcotic of choice for treatment of severe chronic pain.

e) **Meperidine (Demerol)** is a synthetic drug producing rapid, short-duration analgesia with less respiratory depression than morphine, and little sedation or smooth-muscle spasm. It causes little constipation. Its chief use is in relief of severe, intermittent pain produced by smooth-muscle spasm. The usual dose is 50–100 mg; it may be given orally, IM, and occasionally IV. Subcutaneous administration is irritating. Dizziness occurs frequently. Large doses may produce sweating, syncope, tremor, incoordination, or convulsions. Nausea, vomiting, and tachycardia are common. Tolerance and addiction develop rapidly, making the drug unsuitable in the control of chronic pain.

f) **Anileridine (Leritine)** is a synthetic compound similar to meperidine in its respiratory depressant and subjective side effects, but its analgesic potency is slightly greater. It may be given orally, IV, IM, or subcutaneously every 3–4 hours in doses of 25–50 mg. It is quite effective when given orally.

D. **Narcotic antagonists   Nalorphine (Nalline)** is a semisynthetic congener of morphine used for counteracting the symptoms (particularly respiratory depression and hypotension) of excess dosage of morphine, codeine, or the synthetic morphine substitutes such as meperidine. It is ineffective in counteracting the effects of nonnarcotic alkaloids of opium and the barbiturates. If administered to patients who have not received narcotics, its actions are similar to those of morphine and it may cause respiratory depression. **Dosage in the treatment of respiratory depression:** 5–10 mg IV, repeated every 10–15 minutes if respirations remain depressed, but total dose not to exceed 40 mg. Nalorphine is also useful in the diagnosis of narcotic addiction: **Dosage in diagnosis of narcotic addiction:** 3 mg subcutaneously; if no withdrawal symptoms develop after 20–30 minutes inject 5 mg and wait another 20–30 minutes; if no withdrawal symptoms appear, inject 8 mg. If withdrawal symptoms have not appeared after the third dose the patient probably has not recently taken addictive amounts of narcotic.

IX.   SEDATIVE-HYPNOTIC DRUGS

A. **General comments**   Sedative-hypnotic drugs are useful in a wide variety of situations, and are particularly useful in treating mild anxiety. There is little propensity to addiction. A large number of drugs is available; the situations in which each may be useful are listed below. The drugs should be given orally if possible, and with care to elderly patients (who are occasionally very sensitive to their effects) and to patients with anemia, high fever, heart failure, renal failure, hepatic insufficiency, myxedema, hypoxia, or hypotension. Patients with renal, hepatic, or pulmonary disease should be given drugs that are not primarily detoxified or excreted by the diseased organ system. Idiosyncrasies are rare. Urticaria, fever, or other allergic manifestation, "hangover," excitement, and other CNS symptoms may occur.

B. **Barbiturates**

1. Barbiturate preparations of either long or short duration of action are available. Long-acting barbiturates are excreted chiefly by the kidneys, while the short-acting preparations are metabolized in the liver. Most preparations may be given orally or parenterally, but phenobarbital and amobarbital are the most frequently used parenterally. They should be given intravenously only in emergency situations such as status epilepticus. As a rule, the oral and the parenteral dosage is the same. Phenobarbital is more of a cerebral depressant than are other barbiturates and may cause confusion, excitement, and disorientation.

2. Barbiturate addiction is a danger when large doses (e.g., 5–10 times the usual therapeutic dose) are given for protracted periods of time (3–6 months). Patients who become addicted often show serious mental and physical deterioration. When drugs are withdrawn from such patients, the daily decrement in dosage should be 100 mg/day or less in order to avoid such serious physiologic reactions as disorientation, hallucinations, and convulsions.

3. Acute barbiturate poisoning accounts for a significant percentage of suicides. From 80% to 90% of these patients will recover if treated promptly; their management is outlined in Chapter 17.

4. Several of the preparations commonly used as hypnotics are listed below:

   a) **Long-acting**   Effects are noticeable in 30–45 minutes and last 4–8 hours. "Hangovers" are frequent. Dosage of phenobarbital (Luminal) is 100–200 mg at bedtime; for daytime sedation 15–30 mg QID.

   b) **Short- to intermediate-acting**   Effects last 2–4 hours, and hangovers are uncommon.
   Smaller doses may be effective in the elderly.
   Pentobarbital (Nembutal): 100–200 mg.
   Amobarbital (Amytal): 100–300 mg.
   Secobarbital (Seconal): 100–200 mg.

C. Chloral hydrate is a rapidly effective hypnotic which seldom produces excitement or hangover. Sleep usually begins in 15–30 minutes and lasts 5–8 hours. It can be given safely to patients of all ages, but since it is detoxified chiefly by the liver it should be used cautiously in patients with severe hepatic insufficiency. The incidence of skin reactions is low, so chloral hydrate is a valuable sedative or hypnotic for patients with skin disorders. Complications occasionally encountered are a burning sensation of the mucous membranes of the mouth and gastric irritation. A reduction product, trichloroethanol, may give positive results for urine sugar with Clinitest tablets.

Sedative dose is 250–500 mg. The **hypnotic dose** is 1–2 gm, the larger dose usually required for adequate effects. The drug may be given orally as 250- or 500-mg capsules, or dispensed in syrup of wild cherry or orange in a concentration of 500 mg/5 ml. Suppositories or retention enemas (1–2 gm chloral hydrate in olive oil) may be used. Beta-Chlor, a complex of chloral hydrate and betaine, hydrolyzes or decomposes slowly in the gastric contents, yielding chloral hydrate; gastric irritation is said to be less, but there are no other advantages. Each 870-mg tablet yields 500 mg of chloral hydrate.

D. Paraldehyde has a rapid, smooth hypnotic action (within 10–15 minutes), and is relatively safe, making it a very valuable drug when a quick hypnotic effect is desirable. It is frequently used in the treatment of tremulousness following alcohol withdrawal. Unfortunately it has a burning, disagreeable taste, a pungent odor, and significant irritant effects on the mucous membranes, making its use undesirable in the presence of nausea, vomiting, esophagitis, gastritis, etc. Excretion is chiefly by the liver and lungs; the drug should be given cautiously to patients with severe liver disease. It may be given in the presence of renal insufficiency.

The drug should be given orally whenever possible. Profound metabolic acidosis may follow chronic ingestion of large doses of paraldehyde or the use of solutions that have been stored for long periods of time. Paraldehyde is unstable and decomposes to acetaldehyde and acetic acid. Chronic paraldehyde intoxication results in tolerance and dependence; withdrawal symptoms include delirium tremens and hallucinations. **Doses are listed below:**

1. **Oral:** Usually 8–10 ml, but varies from 3–20 ml. Cracked ice and orange juice, tea, milk, or wine will help mask the taste.

2. **Rectal:** Olive-oil or mineral-oil enemas in which the drug is suspended may be given. The usual rectal dose is 10–20 ml. Fresh solutions should be used in order to avoid serious rectal burns. It is often necessary to anesthetize the mucous membranes of the anus in order to prevent local irritation which may lead to expulsion.

3. **Intramuscular:** The usual dose is 4–8 ml, but quantities greater than 4 ml should not be given in one injection site. The solution used should be fresh but need not be sterilized. Injections are irritating and should not be given in the vicinity of nerves (to avoid a neuritis) or into subcutaneous tissues (to prevent a slough).

E. Antihistamines Diphenhydramine (Benadryl) in doses of 50–100 mg may provide excellent sedation for patients with severe hepatic or renal insufficiency.

F. Other commonly used preparations include:

1. **Chlordiazepoxide (Librium)** Sedative dose is 30 mg/day; 10–20 mg is recommended for geriatric patients; 200–300 mg/day may be used in treating alcohol withdrawal. Adverse effects are those primarily of CNS depression; delirium, ataxia, and vertigo may occur. Skin rashes are rare. Agranulocytosis, menstrual irregularity, and marked stimulation of appetite have been reported. Plasma levels of the drug fall slowly over several days when the drug is discontinued.

2. **Ethchlorvynol (Placidyl)** Sedative dose is 100–200 mg TID; hypnotic dose is 500 mg. It works quickly and has a short duration of action; blood levels are not detectable 3 hours after an oral dose. Mental confusion, hangover, ataxia, and nausea have been reported. Excessive reactions occur when taken with alcohol.

3. **Glutethimide (Doriden)** Sedative dose is 125–250 mg TID; hypnotic dose is 500 mg. Onset of action is usually rapid (within 30 minutes), but absorption tends to be somewhat irregular because of the limited solubility of the drug in water; effects last 4–6 hours. Adverse effects include addiction, CNS depression, and symptoms from prominent anticholinergic activity (mydriasis, paralytic ileus, atony of the urinary bladder, etc.). Acute intoxication, usually with doses over 5.0 gm, may cause hypotension and respiratory depression. Hemodialysis may be required.

4. **Meprobamate (Equanil, Miltown)** Sedative dose is 400 mg QID; hypnotic dose is 800 mg. Toxic effects include excessive drowsiness, ataxia, allergic reactions, and (rarely) blood dyscrasia. It may be used as a muscle relaxant.

X. PHENOTHIAZINE DERIVATIVES

A. General comments The phenothiazines, of which chlorpromazine is the prototype, are valuable, widely used drugs. Substitutions on the basic structure have resulted in more than two dozen congeners with different properties; ethopropazine (Parsidol) has primarily anticholinergic actions and is used for the treatment of parkinsonism; trimeprazine (Temaril) and methdilazine (Tacaryl) antagonize the actions of histamine and serotonin and are used primarily as antipruritic agents; promethazine (Phenergan) has prominent antihistaminic properties and is most commonly used as a sedative or as an adjunct to anesthetics or narcotics. The other preparations, used primarily for the treatment of nausea and vomiting or psychiatric disorders, are discussed below; although they have many similarities, there are significant differences in their potency and actions.

B. Pharmacologic properties

1. The exact mechanism of action is unknown. Phenothiazines have anticholinergic and antihistaminic actions; they block the action of serotonin, cause peripheral adrenergic blockade, produce sedation, depress brain-stem function (in large doses), and stimulate the extrapyramidal system; slight skeletal muscle relaxation and diuretic actions may occur.

2. Absorption from the gastrointestinal tract is rapid; action begins within 30 minutes and continues for about 4 hours. Between 60%

and 70% is excreted by the liver after conjugation with glucuronic acid, and small amounts are excreted in the urine. Although most patients with renal insufficiency tolerate large doses, some evidence suggests that high dosage should be reduced by half if there is a marked decrease in glomerular filtration rate. The drugs should be given cautiously to patients with liver disease.

C. Clinical use In moderate to large dosage phenothiazines have been effective in the treatment of anxiety, agitation, and psychoses. In average dosage they are useful in the following situations:

1. To suppress the nausea and vomiting that occur with uremia, generalized neoplastic disease, acute infections, viral gastroenteritis, hyperemesis gravidarum, alcoholism, irradiation therapy, or the administration of narcotics and nitrogen mustard or similar drugs. They are not effective in controlling the nausea and vomiting of digitalis intoxication or motion sickness.

2. To control intractable hiccups, especially those occurring in uremia.

3. To control pruritus, especially that due to neurodermatitis. They are not very effective for relieving pruritus associated with jaundice, lymphomas, or polycythemia vera.

4. To lower body temperature when there is hyperthermia associated with heatstroke or thyroid storm.

5. To facilitate drug withdrawal in narcotic addicts.

6. To potentiate the effects of the sedative and analgesic drugs. When a patient who is receiving narcotics is given a phenothiazine, it is advisable to reduce the narcotic dosage by 25–50%.

D. Preparations, dosage, and administration

1. Phenothiazines may be divided into three subgroups, depending on their chemical structure. Table 1-1 lists the pharmacologic name, trade name, and selected properties of certain preparations.

2. Most preparations may be given orally, rectally, or intramuscularly in the same doses; IV dosage is usually less. The usual dose of Thorazine is 25–50 mg TID–QID, of Compazine 5–10 mg TID–QID, and of Sparine 25–50 mg TID–QID.

    The dosage range of phenothiazines is exceedingly variable and is determined by the indications for their administration and the effects desired. Because of the wide range, it is difficult to suggest an "average" dose except for the examples cited.

3. The piperazine compounds have the most potent antipsychotic and antiemetic actions. They cause a significant incidence of extrapyramidal effects, but little hypotension or drowsiness. Compazine is the preparation most frequently used for the treatment of nausea and vomiting.

4. Sparine is often beneficial in the treatment of alcohol-withdrawal symptoms, especially delirium tremens.

5. The two preparations used for the treatment of pruritus are Temaril 2.5–5 mg TID–QID or Tacaryl 8 mg BID–QID.

TABLE 1-1. Phenothiazines

Subgroup	Generic Name	Trade Name	Size of Tablets (mg)	Extrapyramidal Effects	Antiemetic Effects	Sedative Effects	Hypotensive Effects
Dimethyl-aminopropyl	Chlorpromazine	Thorazine	10, 25, 50, 100, 200	Moderate	Moderate	High	Moderate
	Promazine	Sparine	10, 25, 50, 100, 200	Moderate	Moderate	Moderate	High
	Triflupromazine	Vesprin	10, 25, 50	High	High	High	Low
Piperidyl	Thioridazine	Mellaril	10, 25, 50, 100, 200	Very low	Low	Moderate	Moderate
Piperazine	Prochlorperazine	Compazine	5, 10, 25	High	High	Moderate	Low
	Fluphenazine	Permitil, Prolixin	0.25, 1, 2.5, 5, 10	High	High	Moderate	Low
	Trifluoperazine	Stelazine	1, 2, 5, 10	High	High	Moderate	Low
	Thiopropazate	Dartal	5, 10	High	High	Moderate	Low
	Perphenazine	Trilafon	2, 4, 8, 16	High	High	Low	Low

Other preparations include: promethazine (Phenergan), thiethylperazine (Torecan), thioperazine (Vontil), etc.

Adapted from L. Goodman and A. Gilman: *The Pharmacological Basis of Therapeutics* (3rd ed.). New York: Macmillan, 1965.

E. Adverse reactions Phenothiazines are remarkably safe drugs with few serious adverse reactions; nonetheless, many side effects may occur.

1. Conventional doses may cause faintness, palpitations, drowsiness, weakness, hypo- or hyperthermia, dry mouth, nasal stuffiness, constipation, somnolence, lethargy, depression, hallucinations, excitement, insomnia, galactorrhea, gynecomastia, menstrual irregularities (including amenorrhea), false-positive pregnancy tests, inhibition of ejaculation, myalgias, arthralgias, tachycardia, and ECG abnormalities (similar to those seen after quinidine administration; rarely ST segment and T wave changes may occur). Very rarely, seizures or sudden death have been described.

2. Hypotension due to peripheral adrenergic blockade and inhibition of centrally mediated pressor reflexes may occur; rarely, syncope or profound shock may follow parenteral administration of large doses. Hypotensive effects are most common with Thorazine, Sparine, and Mellaril. Mild hypotension usually disappears after the first few days of continued treatment.

3. **Extrapyramidal reactions,** other than the dystonia and dyskinesia occurring after prochlorperazine administration, are usually related to dosage and length of therapy. They are fairly common at high doses, and include a parkinsonian syndrome and akathisia (motor restlessness). Dystonia and dyskinesia are characterized by torticollis, opisthotonos, tics, grimacing, dysarthria, and various involuntary muscle movements, a striking example of which is the oculogyric crisis.

   a) Parkinsonism and akathisia occur more frequently in women, usually after several weeks of therapy, and most often with the piperazine derivatives; the reported incidence varies from 15% to 45%. Symptoms usually disappear with reduction in dosage, but treatment may require administration of sedatives, antihistamines, and antiparkinson drugs.

   b) Dystonic reactions occur in 2–3% of patients and are usually of sudden onset early in the course of treatment; Compazine is most frequently implicated. Signs and symptoms usually cease after withdrawal of the drug, but additional treatment is occasionally required; diphenhydramine and barbiturates control the clinical manifestations well. A recent report suggests that rarely extrapyramidal side effects may be irreversible.

4. **Skin reactions,** which occur in about 5% of patients, include hypersensitivity reactions (urticarial, maculopapular, petechial) and photosensitivity, resembling severe sunburn or eczema.
   Abnormal skin pigmentation (slate-blue to purplish-brown discoloration of the exposed areas) may occur in patients receiving high doses of phenothiazines, particularly Thorazine, for longer than 1–2 years. The pigmentation is due to accumulation of melanin deposits (and questionable chlorpromazine or its metabolites in addition) in the skin.

5. **Ocular abnormalities** rarely occur in patients given high dosages of phenothiazines for longer than a year. These include hazy brown pigmentation of the exposed sclera, and corneal and lens opacities. Retinitis pigmentosa has occurred in patients receiving long-term high doses of Mellaril.

6. **Hypersensitivity reactions** are unrelated to dosage.

   a) Cholestatic jaundice, which occurs in less than 1% of patients, is most common after Thorazine; it usually appears within the first four weeks of treatment and generally subsides without residual after withdrawal of the drug.

   b) Blood dyscrasias (leukopenia, eosinophilia, leukocytosis) are not rare; pancytopenia and agranulocytosis are uncommon.

   c) Skin manifestations are described above.

XI. **ANTIDEPRESSANTS** A number of drugs are available for the treatment of depression; the most commonly used fall into two major pharmacologic groups, the monoamine oxidase (MAO) inhibitors and the iminodibenzyl derivatives. Very little is known about the relationship between their pharmacologic actions and their therapeutic effects. It is difficult to assess their efficacy in the treatment of depression and to compare their value with that of electroshock therapy. Because the antidepressants are widely used in general medical practice and are potent drugs with many adverse (occasionally fatal) side effects, their actions and toxicity are reviewed in the following paragraphs. It is beyond the scope of the Manual, however, to discuss classification of depression, indications for treatment, types of treatment, and selection of appropriate drugs.

   A. **Monoamine oxidase (MAO) inhibitors** These drugs inhibit the enzyme monoamine oxidase, which is necessary for the metabolic degradation of naturally occurring amines, such as tyramine, dopamine, norepinephrine, epinephrine, tryptamine, and serotonin. They inhibit many other enzymes as well, and exhibit actions unrelated to enzyme inhibition.

      1. Effects include elevation of the mood, increase in psychomotor activity, autonomic nervous system blockade (with varying degree of inhibition of both sympathetic and parasympathetic activity), and increase in threshold for pain.

      2. Currently available preparations include the hydrazines, nialamide (Niamid) 75–100 mg/day, phenelzine (Nardil) 45 mg/day, and isocarboxazid (Marplan) 30 mg/day, and the nonhydrazine, tranylcypromine (Parnate) 20 mg/day. The hydrazines are slower-acting and more likely to cause side effects; toxicity parallels potency and effectiveness. **Remember:** A latent period of days to weeks may exist before effects of these drugs become apparent. Dosage should be gradually reduced after a beneficial effect is produced. Effects are cumulative, and undesirable reactions may appear suddenly.

      3. **Adverse reactions**

         a) Severe headache, dizziness, postural hypotension, blurred vision, constipation, urinary hesitancy, inhibition of ejaculation, impotence, weakness, restlessness, muscle tremor, hyperpyrexia, sweating, hallucinations, confusion, insomnia, peripheral neuropathy, edema, and skin rashes may occur. The type, frequency, and severity of these side effects are related in part to the drug used and its dosage, but individual sensitivity is probably the most important factor. Anemia, leukopenia, and seizures are uncommon, but do occur.

b) Severe hypertension is the most serious side effect; sudden and striking elevation of the blood pressure may be associated with clinical manifestations similar to those seen in patients with pheochromocytoma. Excruciating headache occurs suddenly, often associated with fever. Fatal intracranial hemorrhage or acute heart failure may ensue.

Such reactions occur in less than 0.5% of patients and are often associated with the ingestion of certain foods (particularly aged cheese, but possibly wines, beers, and yogurt as well) which contain substantial quantities of tyramine. Presumably MAO inhibition prevents the oxidative deamination of tyramine, which then causes release of norepinephrine from its usual storage sites. Similar reactions may occur after ingestion of broad beans (which contain dopa), methyldopa, or sympathomimetic amines.

Treatment requires immediate administration of an adrenergic blocking agent, such as phentolamine (Regitine), 5 mg IV, injected slowly; dosage may be repeated in 4–6 hours, if needed. Levarterenol should be immediately available in case an exaggerated hypotensive response occurs.

c) Hepatocellular damage with jaundice and other abnormal liver function tests, though not common with currently available preparations, may occur; hepatotoxicity does not seem related to dosage or duration of therapy, and probably represents hypersensitivity.

d) Numerous adverse reactions may occur when other drugs are administered concurrently with MAO inhibitors. **Note the following precautions.**

i) Iminodibenzyl derivatives Imipramine, amitriptyline, and their derivatives must not be given concurrently with, or within two weeks of administration of, MAO inhibitors, for severe, occasionally fatal reactions (characterized by hyperpyrexia, marked atropinism-like effects, hypertension, and seizures) may occur.

ii) Antihypertensives Effects of thiazides and ganglionic blocking agents are potentiated; severe hypotension may occur. Reduce their dosage when MAO drugs are given concurrently. Paradoxical hypertension may follow methyldopa administration.

iii) Phenothiazines Increase in incidence and severity of extrapyramidal effects and hypotension are reported. Give these drugs cautiously.

iv) Narcotics Exaggerated responses to usual therapeutic doses of meperidine are not uncommon, and may include marked CNS and respiratory depression, hyperpyrexia, agitation, and severe hypotension; several deaths have been reported. Other narcotics are occasionally implicated. Do not give large doses.

v) Sympathomimetic drugs Amphetamines, ephedrine, phenylephrine, metaraminol, and phenylpropanolamine may cause severe headache, hypertension, and cardiac arrhythmias. Intracranial bleeding and circulatory failure may occur.

Avoid use of these drugs, if possible; when they are required, administer cautiously in reduced dosage.

Numerous proprietary cold remedies, available without prescription, contain sympathetic amines, and patients should be cautioned against taking such preparations while they are taking MAO drugs.

vi) Actions of the following drugs may also be potentiated: insulin (hypoglycemia), antiparkinson compounds, barbiturates, procaine, and general anesthetics.

B. Iminodibenzyl derivatives (of which imipramine and amitriptyline are the prototypes) possess marked anticholinergic activity; they also enhance the action of epinephrine and norepinephrine at peripheral sympathetic receptor sites. Imipramine is identical with the phenothiazine, promazine, except for the linkage between the two benzene rings; the chemical structure of amitriptyline is closely related to that of the antihistamine, cyproheptadine.

Iminodibenzyl derivatives are the drugs most widely used for the treatment of depression. In comparison with MAO inhibitors, their onset of action is more rapid; they are short-acting and not cumulative; and they seldom, if ever, potentiate other commonly prescribed drugs.

1. Effects include elevation of the mood (occasionally aggravation of anxiety and tension), cholinergic blockade, inhibition of certain cardiovascular reflexes, and sedation (rather than the euphoria often produced by MAO inhibitors).

2. Currently available preparations include imipramine (Tofranil) 50–150 mg daily, and its demethylated derivative, desipramine (Pertofrane, Norpramin) 75–200 mg daily; and amitriptyline (Elavil) 50–150 mg daily, and its derivative, nortriptyline (Aventyl) 30–100 mg daily. The derivatives of the parent compounds are alleged to act more rapidly and induce fewer autonomic side effects.

3. **Side effects and toxic reactions**

a) Side effects primarily reflect the atropine-like actions of the drugs, and include dry mouth, constipation, blurred vision, urinary retention, dizziness, and tachycardia. Other untoward effects, which are not uncommon, include excessive sweating, anorexia, bad taste in the mouth, epigastric distress, nausea, vomiting, drowsiness or agitation, fatigue, weakness, persistent fine tremor, myoclonia, numbness and tingling of the extremities, and headache. Patients receiving large dosage may experience sudden, severe tremors, a parkinsonian syndrome, and, very rarely, marked agitation or convulsions.

b) Orthostatic hypotension may be severe; administration of imipramine is occasionally followed by edema, congestive heart failure, and myocardial infarction, possibly secondary to rapid tachycardias or cardiac arrhythmias.

c) Hypersensitivity reactions: Skin rashes, eosinophilia, leukopenia, and rarely agranulocytosis have been reported. Jaundice, when it occurs, is usually cholestatic, in contrast to the hepatocellular damage induced by MAO inhibitors.

d) Note the following precautions:

 i) Iminodibenzyl derivatives should not be given concurrently with, or within two weeks of administration of, MAO inhibitors.

 ii) The drugs should be given cautiously, if at all, to patients with glaucoma, benign prostatic hypertrophy, pyloric stenosis, severe heart disease, or agitation.

XII. ANTIHISTAMINES When given orally or parenterally, these drugs inhibit hypotension, bronchospasm, wheals, and other manifestations of histamine. They may be very effective in relieving minor allergic phenomena associated with immediate hypersensitivity; they are most widely used in treatment of allergic rhinitis, urticaria, pruritus, and asthma. They are administered frequently before transfusion of blood to minimize minor allergic reactions. Occasionally antihistamines are effective sedatives, especially in elderly patients. Diphenhydramine (Benadryl) controls the dystonic reactions of phenothiazines. **Side effects** occur in 10–20% of patients and include drowsiness, dizziness, disturbed coordination, inability to concentrate, muscular weakness, gastrointestinal irritation, and rarely excitation. Individual response to the antihistamines varies widely; if the side effects of one preparation are particularly annoying, another should be tried instead. More than forty preparations are available and are discussed in standard pharmacology texts.

TOPICAL THERAPY OF THE SKIN

I.   GENERAL COMMENTS The following objectives are to be kept in mind in prescribing topical therapy for the skin:

A. Eradication of causative agents with specific therapy such as antibiotics.

B. Destruction of abnormal cellular proliferations (tumors, etc.).

C. Alleviation of symptoms.

D. Reduction of inflammation.

E. Cleansing and debridement.

F. Protection.

G. Restoration of hydration (oil and water content).

H. Reduction of scaling and callus.

The successful treatment of a particular skin lesion may require the achievement of some or all of these objectives, and any one form of therapy may achieve one or several of these goals. Many of the therapeutic agents to be described here require vehicles for topical application. The choice of proper vehicle is important (see III. Vehicles, farther on in this chapter). If an eruption does not respond in the expected period of time, the physician must consider the possibility of another diagnosis or the existence of a complication such as contact sensitivity to one of the ingredients of the topical preparation, sweat retention, or secondary bacterial infection. All therapy should be aimed at returning the skin to its physiologic state; its regenerative powers are remarkable.

II. **METHODS** of achieving the above objectives are outlined below:

A. Eradication of causative agents with specific therapy

1. **Antibiotics and chemotherapeutic agents** Neomycin sulfate, 5.0 mg/ gm of base; bacitracin, 400–500 units/gm; polymyxin B, 5,000 to 10,000 units/gm; gramicidin, 0.25 mg/gm; gentamycin sulfate, 1.7 mg/gm. Combinations of these antibacterial agents are found in commercial preparations such as Neosporin and Neo-Polycin. Penicillin and sulfonamides should not be applied topically because of their propensity for skin sensitization and also because of frequent systemic use.

2. **Ammoniated mercury** 2–5% in acid medium is mildly antibacterial.

3. **Halogenated quinolones** Vioform (iodochlorhydroxyquin) in 3% concentration is mildly antibacterial and antifungal.

4. **Sulfur** (precipitated) 2–5% is mildly antibacterial and antifungal.

5. **Anticandidal agents** Nystatin, 100,000 units/gm base; Amphotericin B, 3%; gentian violet 1% in water or 70% alcohol.

6. **Tolnaftate** (Tinactin) 10 mg/gm base is an antidermatophyte.

The above agents are applied sparingly 2–4 times a day.

7. **For infestations:** Lindane 1% (Kwell) (scabies, lice); crotamiton (Eurax) 10% (scabies, lice); benzyl benzoate 12.5% (scabies, lice); DDT 10% (lice). Antiscabietic therapy is applied to the patient and his contacts at bedtime after bath, and is washed off in a bath the next morning. All clothing and bed linens are thoroughly washed before reuse. The use of delousing agents should cover the period of hatching the nits.

B. Destruction of abnormal cellular proliferations

1. Histologic confirmation of the clinical diagnosis of tumors and pigmented lesions is essential (punch or excision biopsy). Surgical excision, desiccation and curettage, radiotherapy, and cryotherapy should be left to those experienced in their use.

2. **Podophyllin** 20%–25% in tincture of benzoin compound is applicable to condylomata acuminata. It should be applied by the physician, *avoiding normal skin*, and washed off in bath 2–6 hours later.

3. **Cantharidin** 0.7% is applicable to warts and molluscum contagiosum. It should be applied by the physician, *avoiding normal skin*, and covered with tape for 24 hours.

4. **5-fluorouracil** 1–2% is the best drug available for treatment of extensive actinic keratoses. It is applied topically to involved areas BID for 3–4 weeks. The drug causes marked inflammation and erosion of all lesions, and therapy must be carried out under close supervision. Avoid sunlight during therapy and after to prevent solar damage.

C. Control of symptoms of itching, burning, and pain

1. **Camphor** 0.5%–1.0% provides cooling through evaporation as well as creating a counterirritant effect.

2. **Menthol** 0.1%–0.25% provides sensation of coolness by action on cold receptors.

3. Phenol 1% anesthetizes nerve endings.

For example, these could be compounded in Nivea oil. Avoid these agents in weeping, raw, or ulcerated areas because of danger of excessive systemic absorption.

Antihistamines and local anesthetics (Novocain, etc.) are preferably not used topically because of their tendency for skin sensitization with cross-sensitization to systemically administered drugs such as sulfonamides, thiazides, and oral hypoglycemic agents.

D. Reduction of inflammation with consequent reduction in symptoms such as itching

The fluorinated corticosteroids are significantly more effective on a milligram-for-milligram basis in chronic dermatoses than are the non-fluorinated corticosteroids such as hydrocortisone. Occlusion under plastic wrap significantly enhances penetration into the skin. One must be aware of the complications of occlusion therapy, including sweat retention, maceration, microbial overgrowth, and suppression of the pituitary-adrenal axis (*New Eng. J. Med.* 273:831, 1965). Tar preparations were used for this purpose with some success prior to the steroid era and are still useful.

1. Most commonly used corticosteroids

a) Hydrocortisone   0.25–2.5%
b) Betamethasone 17-valerate 0.1% (Valisone)
c) Triamcinolone acetonide   0.025–0.5% (Kenalog) (Aristocort)
d) Fluocinolone acetonide   0.01–0.2% (Synalar)
e) Flurandrenolone   0.025–0.05% (Cordran)

These preparations are applied sparingly 3–4 times a day. The patient may be instructed to cover the treated areas with plastic gloves or plastic wrap during the day and, most commonly, during the sleeping hours.

Bacterial, viral, and fungus infections of the skin are not absolute contraindications to addition of corticosteroids to topical therapy. The anti-inflammatory effect often hastens recovery without aggravating the infectious component. Many combinations of antibiotics and steroids are available in commercial preparations.

2. Tars

a) Crude coal tar   5%
b) Coal-tar distillate   1.0–3.0%
c) LCD (liquor carbonis detergens)   3.0–10.0%
d) Ichthammol   3%

Folliculitis is a possible complication of prolonged tar therapy; it should never be applied under occlusive dressings.

3. Halogenated quinolones These drugs have nonspecific anti-inflammatory properties as well as antimicrobial effects and have been used extensively in treating inflammatory dermatoses. They should be applied 3–4 times a day. Iodochlorhydroxyquin (Vioform) 3% is often combined with a corticosteroid in topical preparations for enhanced effect.

E. Cleansing and debridement

1. **Cleansing, cooling, and soothing wet compresses** are particularly useful in weeping, vesiculobullous, pustular, and ulcerated lesions. What is added to the water is of less importance than the technique of application. One teaspoonful of salt per pint of water is the most universally available and useful solution. Besides cleansing and debriding qualities, this form of therapy affords temporary but significant relief of pruritus and reduction of inflammation. **Technique of application:** As a general rule the solution should be at room temperature; for furuncles and cellulitis a warm solution is better. For small areas of involvement, which can be treated at home, a clean, soft, white cloth such as a diaper or old linen cloth is immersed in the solution, gently squeezed, and applied to the affected skin. The cloth is reimmersed in the solution every 2–3 minutes to enhance debridement, to maintain the desired temperature, and to allow for evaporation. This process is continued for 20–30 minutes and repeated as often as every 2 hours, depending on the requirements and response of the lesion. For larger areas of involvement such detailed care may not be possible. In such cases the wet cloths or bandages can be left on the involved area for ½ to 2 hours. As wet compresses have a drying effect, the patient should be warned to discontinue them before xerosis and fissuring occur. The following are some of the solutions, other than saline, that can be used:

   a) **Aluminum acetate** (mildly bacteriostatic, astringent, and coagulant).

      i) Burow's solution (aluminum subacetate): Dilute 30 ml USP stock solution in a pint or quart of water.

      ii) Commercial preparations now readily available are Domeboro or Bur-Veen powder: Dissolve one packet of powder in a pint of water.

   b) **Magnesium sulfate (Epsom salts)** (bacteriostatic): One tablespoonful per quart of water. Inexpensive.

   c) **Potassium permanganate** (excellent for infected, malodorous processes; staining is main drawback; *must be completely dissolved* because particles may cause burns): 1:4000 solution prepared by adding 0.3 gm tablet to 1½ quarts water. 1:9000 solution prepared by adding 0.06 gm tablet to pint of water.

   d) **Silver nitrate** (good bacteriostatic; staining is main drawback) 0.5% solution made up from stock 10% or 25% solutions. When used for burns, it is applied as continuous dressing covered by bandages to minimize evaporation and protein denaturation.

2. **Colloidal baths** Used in weeping, vesiculobullous, ulcerated, and exfoliative erythrodermic processes when they are too generalized to be managed with wet compresses. The patient is instructed to soak in the bath for 20–30 minutes and to pat himself dry instead of rubbing with a towel. Can be repeated 2–6 times a day depending on the acuteness of the process.

   a) **Oatmeal or Aveeno:** Mix 1 cupful in 2 cups of water, then add to tub of water.

b) Oilated Aveeno: Use as with Aveeno when the soothing effects are desired without excessive drying.

F. Protection from irritants, contact allergens, and trauma

1. Thin, white, **cotton gloves** under rubber gloves. The cotton gloves can be washed and thoroughly rinsed frequently.

2. **Unna Boot** (bandages impregnated with zinc oxide paste) available commercially as Dome-Paste or Gelocast. Provides protection and support. Useful in the management of stasis ulcers and self-inflicted neurotic excoriations. Apply like plaster cast up to the knee, being careful that it is not as tight in the vicinity of the knee as it is at the ankle and foot.

3. **Sunscreens**   In dermatoses that are exacerbated by exposure to ultraviolet light, these agents are useful adjuncts to long sleeves, wide-brimmed hats, and a warning to the patient that there is considerable radiation outdoors even on cloudy days. It should be noted that certain light-sensitive eruptions (e.g., porphyria, phytophotodermatoses) are responsive to wavelengths above 3200 A and will not be prevented by some nonopaque sunscreens.

   a) Para-aminobenzoic acid derivative PABA 10% or 15% (in Ruggles' cream) absorbs ultraviolet light only in the erythema-producing range (2800 to 3200 A).

   b) Benzophenone derivative 2-hydroxy-4-methoxybenzophenone-5-sulfonic acid 10% (Uval) absorbs ultraviolet light between 3200 and 6500 A wavelengths.

   c) Titanium dioxide 5% (A-Fil) (Solar) and zinc oxide 2.5% are opaque, absorb throughout the spectrum, and would be ideal except for cosmetic unacceptability.

G. Restoration of hydration (oil and water balance)   Skin that is described as xerotic, ichthyotic, or asteatotic should be bathed less frequently; and soap should be used only on the face, axillae, crural areas, and feet. Oil should be added to the bath water. Lubricating ointments and oils should be used as needed. Attention should be given to *humidification* of the indoor environment during the winter.

1. **Bath oils** (Patients should be warned to get in and out of the tub cautiously because of slippery surfaces when using these oils.)

   a) Many commercial preparations available, such as Alpha KERI and Mellobath.

   b) Corn oil, 1 tablespoon, and Calgon powder, 4 tablespoons.

   c) With added tar: Balnetar or Polytar bath oils.

2. **Lubricating ointments**   It is not necessarily true that the greasiest preparations are the most lubricating. Aquaphor, Eucerine, Nivea, lanolin, hydrophilic ointment USP, vas alba (white petrolatum), or mineral oil can be applied as needed for dry skin.

3. **Excess water** is the problem in intertriginous skin where maceration results from water retention in a warm, closed area. Drying and ventilation are required. Powders may be used to reduce moisture and friction.

   a) ZeaSORB powder

b) Talcum powder

c) Bentonite   10.0
Starch   10.0
Talc   qs   100.0

d) Magnesium carbonate   4.0
ZBT powder   qs   100.0

Camphor 0.5% can be added to any of the above powders for anti-pruritic effect. These powders can be dusted onto affected areas as often as necessary after cleansing with clear water and patting dry. They need not be used at night, when loose-fitting garments can allow for ventilation, and should not be used on weeping, raw eruptions in order to avoid "caking" and fissuring.

H. Reduction of scaling and callus   Although there are a few exceptions (e.g., ichthyosis vulgaris) scaling and callus are usually the result of rapid proliferation of epidermal cells. Scaling and callus can, then, be reduced with various combinations of keratolytics and suppression of epidermal proliferation. The agents listed in this section (except for corticosteroids) are *not* used on weeping or ulcerated areas.

1. Keratolytics

a) Salicylic acid 2–3% for scaly processes. Up to 20% can be used for callus-like hyperkeratoses and applied 2–4 times daily; 40% salicylic acid plasters cut to fit the lesion exactly are applied for 4–5 days under adhesive tape occlusion in treating warts and dense calluses.

b) The following can be used in the same manner:

Salicylic acid   2.0   ⎧ 1.0
Lactic acid   2.0   For children   ⎨ 1.0
Flexible collodion   qs   20.0   ⎩ 20.0

2. Suppressors of epidermal proliferation   The pharmacologic effect of most of these agents is through suppression of nucleic acid and protein synthesis (*J. Invest. Derm.* 45:529, 539, 1965).

a) Sulfur (precipitated) 3–5%

b) Ammoniated mercury 3–5%

c) Tars especially effective in combination with ultraviolet light. (See Goekerman regimen in Some Specific Therapeutic Regimens on page 29.)

d) Anthralin 0.1–1.0%. This is an old form of therapy which is being revived. To be used with caution because of irritative effects.

III.   **VEHICLES**   The choice of vehicle depends on whether the lesion is of the acute eczematous type, the dry scaly type, or a variation of these. In general the number of ingredients incorporated into a vehicle should be kept down to reduce the risks of sensitization and incompatibility. Topical preparations should be applied sparingly for economic as well as cosmetic reasons. A thick layer of vanishing cream applied with a tongue blade is no longer "vanishing." It should be applied with the fingers and massaged in (inuncted) gently.

A. Lotions and liniments   For lesions on the acute, eczematous side of the spectrum, shake lotions are appropriate. These are suspensions of powder in water or alcohol. As the liquid evaporates from the skin with resultant cooling, soothing, and drying, a thin layer of protective powder remains. The residual powder is not good for weeping, raw, or ulcerated lesions.

Liniments are mixtures of lotions with oils; they are used when excessive drying is to be avoided.

As vehicles for pharmacologically active ingredients, lotions and liniments generally provide less percutaneous absorption than creams and ointments, and they should be applied 2–6 times a day, depending on the acuteness of the eruption. The following lotions and liniments are listed in decreasing order of drying effect.

1. Wise's shake lotion (shuttle lotion)

Aluminum acetate		12.5
Glycerin		20.0
Talcum powder		25.0
Zinc oxide		25.0
Calcium hydroxide solution (lime water)	qs	100.0

2. Calamine lotion

Calamine		8.0
Zinc oxide		8.0
Glycerin		2.0
Bentonite		25.0
Calcium hydroxide solution	qs	100.0

3. PMZ lotion (Schamberg's lotion)

Phenol		1.0
Menthol		0.25
Peanut oil		45.0
Calcium hydroxide solution		45.0
Zinc oxide powder		8.0
Water	qs	100.0

4. Starch liniment

Zinc oxide		10.0
Starch		10.0
Glycerin		10.0
Olive oil ⎱ Calcium hydroxide solution ⎰	aa˙ qs	100.0

5. Calamine liniment

Calamine		8.0
Zinc oxide		8.0
Olive oil ⎱ Lime water ⎰	aa qs	100.0

B. Pastes Mixtures of 20–50% powder in ointment. Indications for pastes are few. They have a protective quality while allowing evaporation of sweat or transudate. This protective quality is useful in herpes zoster, ulcers, and radiation dermatitis. Pastes are more useful than ointments in eruptions in which acute and chronic characteristics coexist. Percutaneous absorption from this base is less efficient than from creams and ointments. Pastes are applied with some difficulty, using a tongue blade to smooth a thin layer onto the lesion or the inner surface of a dressing before applying it to the skin. The paste should be reapplied every 24 hours, after wiping off the old layer with a cotton cloth impregnated with mineral oil.

Lassar's paste

Zinc oxide	25
Starch	25
White petrolatum	50

C. **Creams** (oil-in-water bases)   Oil droplets dispersed in a continuous phase of water make these bases water-washable, nongreasy, and very acceptable cosmetically. These bases allow excellent percutaneous absorption of incorporated ingredients. Useful in a wide range of eruptions, including weeping, acute eczematous processes, and subacute inflammatory and infiltrative lesions. If used in dry eruptions, a lubricating agent should be used after each application. Several commercial preparations are available: Dermabase, Neobase, Acid Mantle cream, Lubriderm, etc.

D. **Ointments** (water-in-oil bases)   Water droplets dispersed in a continuous phase of oil provide lubrication, barrier function, and good percutaneous absorption of added ingredients. Not used in weeping processes or intertriginous areas because of occlusive nature. Very good for dry scaly eruptions.

1. Hydrophilic ointment USP

2. Lanolin

3. Several commercially available products: Eucerine, Nivea, Hydrosorb, Aquaphor, and Qualatum

E. **Inert oils**   Mixtures of hydrocarbons that are protective and greasy but not necessarily lubricating. Their occlusiveness promotes retention of body heat and debris. Although percutaneous absorption is not very good from these vehicles, lipid-soluble antimicrobials are often incorporated into them because of stability and constant, even contact with the skin. Preparations include yellow petrolatum, white petrolatum (vas alba, petroleum jelly), and mineral oil.

F. **Propylene glycol**   A stable vehicle with good spreading property, particularly for use on the scalp; it allows good percutaneous absorption of added drugs. It tends to have a drying effect.

G. **Adherent dressings** are bases which dry quickly and adhere to a confined area such as a wart. Quick drying is important when medicaments are applied which may irritate, cauterize, or blister adjacent normal skin. Flexible collodion and tincture of benzoin compound are examples of adherent dressings.

IV. SOME SPECIFIC THERAPEUTIC REGIMENS

To conclude this chapter, a few examples of regimens for common disorders of the skin are given to indicate how the foregoing principles can be put into practice.

A. **Psoriasis**

1. Very acute, eruptive forms of the disease are approached with caution to avoid pushing them over into generalized, exfoliative, erythrodermatous processes. Bed rest, sedation, topical corticosteroids, and colloidal baths may be used until the process is sufficiently stabilized to allow more vigorous therapy.

2. Tar and ultraviolet light therapy (modified Goekerman regimen):

5% crude coal tar in Lassar's paste is applied at bedtime. In the morning the excess paste is removed with mineral oil and the patient is exposed to ultraviolet light, with daily increase of dose from minimal erythema dose to one sufficient to maintain good tanning. This exposure is followed by a bath to which has been added a tar preparation such as Polytar or Balnetar bath oil. Packer's tar soap can also be used. The therapy is applicable to widespread eruptions that are resistant to other agents, and usually requires hospitalization.

3. Localized lesions in small numbers with minimal scaling can be treated with topical fluorinated corticosteroids in cream base three times a day and at night with plastic occlusive dressing. Intra-lesional corticosteroids are practical only if lesions are few and small.

4. Larger, more numerous, thick, indolent lesions can be attacked vigorously with twice daily inunction of one of the following:

   a) LCD   1.8 to 6.0
   Sulfur (precipitated)   1.8 to 3.0
   Salicylic acid   0.3 to 1.8
   Aquaphor   qs   60.0

   b) Anthralin 0.1% in vas alba. If this concentration is well toler-ated, the strength can be increased to 0.25%, 0.5%, and 1.0% at intervals of 7 days. It is effective with ultraviolet light and is not to be used in intertriginous areas.

5. Scalp lesions can be treated with corticosteroid solutions and occa-sionally creams massaged in 2–3 times a day. A tar, sulfur, and salicylic acid preparation such as Pragmatar is massaged in at bedtime. It can be washed out in the morning with shampoo (e.g., Sebutone or Zetar).

6. Patients with generalized eruptions and/or arthritis who are resis-tant to the above regimens and who are incapacitated by their disease may be treated with systemic methotrexate. It is a dan-erous drug and should be administered only by those who are experienced in its use. As with sulfur, tar, and ultraviolet light, it is effective through inhibition of epidermal proliferation.

B. Contact dermatitis

1. Avoidance of contactants is obvious and effective.

2. The most important therapeutic procedure is the application of wet compresses. The frequency of application is gradually decreased from 6–8 times a day to once a day as the eruption comes under control.

3. Topical corticosteroids are applied in cream or lotion form after each wet compress.

4. Sedatives, antihistamines, and antipruritics suppress the itching enough to reduce the urge to scratch.

5. It is not unusual for one of these eruptions to be extensive enough to require a short course of oral corticosteroid therapy.

C. Fungus infections of the skin   Laboratory confirmation of the diagnosis should always be in process before therapy is started.

1. **Tinea versicolor** can be treated with twice daily application of 25% sodium thiosulfate (Tinver) or nightly application of selenium sulfide (Selsun) followed in one hour by bath and application of 25% sodium thiosulfate. One or 2 weeks may be required for clearing the lesions. Hypopigmented spots will persist until the skin is exposed to sunlight long enough to retan. Tolnaftate is effective but expensive. Recurrences are frequent after all forms of therapy.

2. **Candidiasis** does not respond to griseofulvin. Nystatin (as in Mycolog) is applied 3–4 times daily with good results. Amphotericin B is also effective in topical preparations. Gentian violet and iodochlorhydroxyquin are less specific but have been used successfully for many years. Wet compresses are very useful in acute stages. Drying and ventilation are necessary for maintenance of remission in intertriginous areas. Remember that sexual partners can reinfect one another.

3. **Dermatophyte infections of small areas of glabrous skin and feet** Whenever there are vesiculating, raw, weeping areas, wet compresses are indicated. 1% salicylic acid in 70% alcohol applied daily is an economical form of therapy. Tolnaftate in a propylene glycol vehicle has been found very effective: it is applied twice a day.

4. **Tinea capitis or dermatophyte infection of the body which is too widespread to treat topically** Griseofulvin (or micronized griseofulvin) is the treatment of choice. Adult dosage is 1–2 gm/day in divided doses for the regular preparation and 0.75 gm/day for the micronized form. Therapy is continued until cultures or Wood's light examinations are negative (approximately 4–6 weeks for tinea capitis; 3 weeks for tinea corporis; and 6–8 months for infection of the fingernails). In patients who may be unreliable about taking medication regularly, tinea capitis (microsporum type only) can be treated with a single 2-gm dose of micronized or 3-gm dose of regular griseofulvin. Cutting the hair short and keeping the fingernails cut as short as possible shortens the duration of therapy. To avoid spreading the infection to others, children with tinea capitis should wear caps until the infection is clear.

   Griseofulvin is remarkably free of serious side effects. The regularly occurring leukopenia reverses itself as therapy is continued. To enhance absorption, the drug should be given with milk or other fatty food. Concomitant administration of phenobarbital reduces the effectiveness of griseofulvin. **Caution:** Griseofulvin interferes with the effectiveness of coumarin anticoagulant therapy and may precipitate acute porphyria.

5. **Dermatophyte infection of toenails** does not clear with griseofulvin therapy unless it is in its very early stages. Painstaking efforts to keep the feet dry and well ventilated are important. Drying powders can be used. Laborious trimming of involved nails will allow topical preparations such as Tolnaftate or 5% thymol in chloroform to soak into the area of involvement.

Proper management of fluid and electrolyte disturbances requires knowledge of their pathogenesis and manifestations and of the principles and dangers of therapy. Each problem should be analyzed in terms of preexisting deficits or excesses, continuing abnormal losses, and basal or maintenance needs. If more than one abnormality is present, priority must be assigned to that which is life-threatening or causing the greatest physiologic disturbance. The integrity of the patient's cardiac and renal function should be assessed in planning therapy. Only then can one prescribe the composition and volume of electrolyte solution and the route and rate of its administration; even then it is wise to reevaluate the efficacy of therapy after partial administration of the initially prescribed dose.

The first section of this chapter presents practical information about salts and solutions. The second section considers maintenance requirements. Subsequent sections (salt and water, potassium, acid-base) are concerned with deficits and excesses. The fluid and electrolyte management of patients with abnormal renal function is discussed in the chapter on renal disease.

I. SALTS AND SOLUTIONS

A. Commonly used conversions

	mEq of anion or cation/gm of salt	mg of salt/mEq
$NaCl$	17*	58
$NaHCO_3$	12	84
Na_3 citrate $\cdot 2H_2O$	10	98
Na lactate	9	112
$Na_2SO_4 \cdot 10H_2O$	6	161
KCl	13	75
K acetate	10	98
K_3 citrate $\cdot 1H_2O$	9	108
K gluconate	4	234
$KHCO_3$	10	100
$CaCl_2 \cdot 2H_2O$	14	73
Ca gluconate$_2 \cdot 1H_2O$	4	224
Ca lactate$_2 \cdot 5H_2O$	6	154
$MgSO_4 \cdot 7H_2O$	8	123
NH_4Cl	19	54

*The sodium content of diets is often expressed in grams of $Na+$ rather than in grams of NaCl; one gram of $Na+$ is 43 mEq, whereas 1 gm of NaCl is 17 mEq.

B. IV solutions

	Glucose (gm/L)	NaCl	Na lactate	KCl	CaCl$_2$	MgCl$_2$	NH$_4$Cl
				(mEq/L)			
5% D/W	50						
10% D/W	100						
20% D/W	200						
5% D/S	50	145					
2.5% dextrose in half-isotonic saline	25	73					
0.85% saline (isotonic saline; N/S)		145					
0.9% saline		154					
3% saline		513					
5% saline		856					
1/6 molar sodium lactate (1.9%)			167				
1/6 molar ammonium chloride (0.9%)							167
2% ammonium chloride							374
Ringer's solution		147		4	5		
Hypotonic Ringer's solution (modified)		103		5	5	3	
Lactate-Ringer's solution		103	27	4	4		

Hypertonic solutions should be administered slowly to prevent circulatory overload.

When 15 drops = 1 ml, the number of drops/minute $\times$ 4 = ml/hr.

Only isotonic fluids should be administered subcutaneously; isotonic saline is ideal for hypodermoclysis. Five percent D/W although isotonic may result in contraction of plasma volume and thus precipitate vascular collapse if the patient is already volume-depleted. When 5% D/W is administered subcutaneously it must be given very slowly.

C. Additives   Listed are the volume and number of mEq of anion and cation present in commonly used commercially available ampules of concentrated solutions.

	Volume (ml) in ampule	mEq in ampule (not concentration)
7.5% sodium bicarbonate	50	45
28.0% sodium lactate	40	100
7.5% potassium chloride	20	20
14.9% potassium chloride	20	40
10.0% calcium chloride	10	14
10.0% calcium gluconate	10	4
25.0% magnesium sulfate	2	4
26.8% ammonium chloride	20	100
		Gm in ampule
25.0% mannitol	50	12.5
50.0% glucose	50	25

II. **MAINTENANCE THERAPY** This section deals with the needs for water, sodium, potassium, and carbohydrate in patients who are unable to take food or fluids orally but who do not have abnormal fluid or electrolyte losses, preexisting deficits or excesses, or inadequate renal function.

  A. **Feeding by stomach tube is preferable** to administration of intravenous fluids when normal alimentation is prohibited for more than a few days (see section on tube feedings in Chapter 1). Nutritional needs can be provided more adequately and the hazards of rapid fluid and electrolyte administration are reduced.

  B. **Parenteral maintenance fluids** are indicated when artificial feeding is required for only a short period of time, or when tube feeding is contraindicated.

  1. **Obligatory water losses** amount to nearly 1500 ml/day: 800–1000 ml sensible and insensible loss, 400 ml urine, and 100 ml fecal water. Since 300 ml of water is gained each day from exogenous or endogenous oxidation, a minimum intake of 1200 ml water is required, assuming maximum urinary concentration, which sick patients may be unable to achieve. One generally administers 2000 ml water daily in order to allow for a reasonable volume above the obligatory minimum.

  2. **Sodium** virtually disappears from the urine after several days of sodium-free intake, but in the interval a mild deficit accrues (in addition, continuing losses may occur in the sweat and feces). It is customary, therefore, to supply about 70 mEq Na+ (4 gm NaCl) daily. **Potassium** excretion cannot be curtailed sufficiently, as a rule, to prevent significant depletion; 20–60 mEq/day should be provided if renal function is adequate. **Carbohydrate** is necessary to minimize protein catabolism and to prevent ketosis; 150–200 gm glucose should be given daily.

  3. **Adequate daily parenteral maintenance** may be provided by administering 1500 ml 10% D/W with 30 mEq KCl, and 500 ml 5% D/S with 10 mEq KCl. These solutions may be given as a slow infusion over 6–12 hours, or preferably as two infusions some hours apart.

  If parenteral therapy must be continued for longer than one week, consideration should be given to replacement of calcium, magnesium, phosphorus, vitamins, and protein.

III. **REPLACEMENT OF OBSERVED ABNORMAL LOSSES** Observed losses of water and electrolyte must be replaced as well as the maintenance requirements met.

  A. **Insensible and sensible losses** Insensible loss of water (evaporation from skin and lungs) increases with hyperventilation, fever (50–75 ml/24 hours/degree Fahrenheit elevation), high room temperature, and low humidity. Insensible losses should be replaced with 5% D/W.

  Sensible perspiration (sweat), because of its role in body temperature regulation, varies greatly in volume (0–2000 ml/hour). It is extremely difficult to estimate the volume of sweat; in circumstances in which sweat losses may be large, accurate replacement is best guided by changes in body weight. Roughly 500 ml/day may be lost if body temperature is above 101°F or room temperature above 85°F, and twice this amount if sweating is continuous or room temperature above 90°F. Losses should be replaced with hypotonic saline (one-third isotonic saline and two-thirds 5% D/W).

  B. **Gastrointestinal losses** Diseases of the GI tract may cause a marked variation in the volume and composition of its secretions. When precise replacement of losses is necessary the electrolyte content of secretions should be measured. It is usually sufficient, however, to calculate replacement on the basis of measured volume and assumed electrolyte composition. Table 2-1 serves as a guide in replacement.

TABLE 2-1. Electrolyte Content of GI Secretions

	Electrolyte concentration, mEq/L					Replace each liter lost with:			
						Isotonic saline	5% D/W	KCl	NaHCO$_3$
	Na+	K+	H+	Cl−	HCO$_3$−	ml	ml	mEq	mEq
Sweat	50	5	—	55	—	300	700	5	—
Gastric secretions	40	10	90*	140	—	250	750	20†	—
Pancreatic fluid	135	5	—	50	90	250	750	5	90‡
Bile	135	5	—	105	35	750	250	5	45‡
Small-intestine fluid	130	10	—	115	25	750	250	10	22‡
Diarrheal fluid	50	35	—	40	45	—	1000	35	45

* Variable; e.g., achlorhydria.
† Administration of more than the observed loss of potassium is advised because of enhanced urinary potassium excretion in alkalosis.
‡ One ampule of 7.5% NaHCO$_3$ contains 45 mEq HCO$_3$−.

C. **Urinary losses** Because the kidney is the final arbiter of fluid and electrolyte balance, no specific electrolyte content may be designated for urine and no single replacement solution advocated. Under normal conditions the amount of sodium and potassium in the urine approximates that in the diet, but under abnormal conditions the amounts may vary widely. Urinary **sodium loss** may be great in patients receiving diuretics, recovering from tubular necrosis or obstructive uropathy, or with adrenal insufficiency or salt-wasting nephritis. Urinary **potassium loss** may be great in patients receiving diuretics or corticosteroids, in the diuretic phase of tubular necrosis, and in renal tubular acidosis. In prolonged polyuric states, therefore, laboratory determination of the urinary sodium and potassium is the only accurate guide to quantitative replacement.

D. **Internal shifts of fluid** Fluid losses need not be external; fluid may be sequestered in locations inaccessible to the body economy. When such shifts of fluid occur rapidly, replacement therapy is often necessary to preserve intravascular volume. Conditions in which such rapid fluid shifts may occur include (1) the development of edema in the lower extremities following thrombophlebitis or caval ligation, (2) occurrence of ascites in peritonitis, pancreatitis, or following portacaval shunt, (3) development of anasarca in extensive burns or fulminant nephrotic syndrome, and (4) intestinal accumulation in ileus or bacterial enteritis.

IV. SALT AND WATER

A. **Physiology** Rational therapy of altered salt and water balance and distribution requires knowledge of the normal distribution of salt and water, the regulation of tonicity and volume, the disturbances which may occur, and the clinical manifestations of the latter. The percentage of water is higher in thin than in obese persons, in infants than in adults, and in males than in females. Total body water constitutes 60% of body weight in the average adult and remains remarkably constant (within 1–2%) for a given individual. Approximately two-thirds of body water (TBW) is intracellular (ICF) and one-third extracellular (ECF). Approximately three-fourths of extracellular fluid is interstitial (IF) and one-fourth intravascular (plasma).

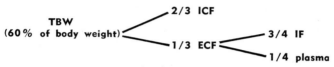

Physiologic disturbances may be discussed as four clinical entities—ECF volume depletion (isotonic loss), ECF volume excess (isotonic gain), hyponatremia (hypotonic gain or hypertonic loss), and hypernatremia (hypertonic gain or hypotonic loss).

B. **Volume depletion** (extracellular volume depletion; saline or sodium depletion)

1. **Pathophysiology** Depletion of extracellular volume results from loss of sodium and water, usually in isotonic proportions; tonicity and therefore intracellular volume are unaffected. Loss of water without salt (as in prolonged severe sweating) is rarely of sufficient magnitude to result in clinically apparent extracellular volume depletion, because water shifts from the ICF to ECF as the extracellular tonicity increases. The change in tonicity is usually more apparent than the change in volume, and this condition is therefore discussed in the section on hypernatremia.

2. **Causes**

   a) Volume depletion is usually caused by loss of gastrointestinal fluid (as in vomiting, diarrhea, gastric or intestinal suction, or surgical drainage). When sodium is lost via the GI tract, urinary excretion of sodium is generally reduced to less than 10 mEq/day.

   b) Less commonly, sodium may be lost in the urine (greater than 20 mEq/day) because of diuretic administration or renal or adrenal disease. Inability to reabsorb sodium maximally is common in renal disease and may result in sodium depletion if dietary salt is restricted. Salt-losing nephritis (urinary sodium loss sufficient to result in sodium depletion despite normal dietary salt intake) is rare but may occur in medullary cystic disease and occasionally in chronic pyelonephritis.

   c) Sequestration of fluid (as in thrombophlebitis, peritonitis, or following caval ligation, paracentesis, or extensive burns) may also cause intravascular or "effective" extracellular volume depletion.

3. **Manifestations** As in all fluid and electrolyte disturbances care-

ful evaluation of historical information and ward observations (intake, output, body weight) will greatly simplify diagnosis and treatment. Symptoms of volume depletion include anorexia, nausea, vomiting, apathy, weakness, and orthostatic syncope.

Signs include poor skin turgor (best tested on the forehead or sternal region), shrunken and furrowed tongue (also occurs in mouth breathers), sunken eyes, postural hypotension, weak pulse, and, when severe, shock and coma.

There is no practical laboratory method of measuring extracellular volume. The serum sodium concentration is *not* a guide to sodium depletion (rather, it reflects the relationship between total body sodium and total body water); in volume depletion it is often normal. The serum creatinine is usually elevated; the urine specific gravity is high and the volume decreased, although the urine sodium concentration is low (except in renal or adrenal salt-wasting). The hematocrit and serum protein concentration rise, and the changes in these values may be useful in approximating the decrease in plasma volume. The plasma volume can routinely be determined by measuring the dilution of ^{125}I-tagged albumin 30 minutes after its IV administration.

4. **Treatment** When very severe volume depletion and shock are present, transfusion of whole blood may be indicated to restore intravascular volume immediately. In other situations infusion of isotonic saline usually suffices and is preferable, since saline, not blood, is deficient. If acidosis is also present, part of the sodium should be given as $NaHCO_3$. Mild degrees of volume depletion may be repleted orally (10 gm NaCl and 2–3 liters of fluid daily).

There is no formula to calculate the amount of saline required to correct volume depletion. If the loss of weight accompanying the sodium depletion is known, an accurate estimate of the amount of saline required to correct the volume depletion can be made; otherwise, the adequacy of repletion must be assessed clinically by reevaluating the patient's physical signs, renal function, and hematocrit or serum protein concentration after the infusion of a given amount of saline.

C. **Volume excess** (extracellular volume excess; saline or sodium excess)

1. **Pathophysiology** Multiple and complex mechanisms result in sodium retention and volume expansion. Although the initiating mechanism is often extrarenal (cardiac or hepatic disease), the common denominator is invariably an abnormality in the renal handling of sodium, usually due to decreased glomerular filtration rate or excessive aldosterone secretion.

2. **Causes** Common causes of volume excess are heart failure, cirrhosis, nephrosis, renal insufficiency, administration of excessive amounts of saline in any of these disorders, and hypoalbuminemia.

3. **Manifestations** The cardinal manifestations of extracellular volume excess is edema. Other manifestations of circulatory overload (dyspnea, tachycardia, venous engorgement, cardiac enlargement, pulmonary congestion) are uncommon in patients without heart disease.

4. **Treatment** Life-threatening volume excess may require treatment by phlebotomy, plasmapheresis, hemodialysis with ultrafiltration, or peritoneal dialysis, especially when heart failure or oliguric

renal disease also exists. Dialysis via the gastrointestinal tract using 50% solution of sorbitol (a nonabsorbable hypertonic solution) given by enema or nasogastric tube may also be effective. More commonly, the administration of diuretics (and digitalis, when indicated) suffices; when heart failure is the primary cause and volume excess is mild, digitalis administration alone may be sufficient. In all situations, however, sodium should be restricted (at least temporarily); water intake should be curtailed when acute circulatory overload is life-threatening.

D. **Hyponatremia (hypo-osmolality)** The tonicity of body fluids is determined largely by electrolytes; nonelectrolytes contribute less than 2% of ECF osmotic activity. Sodium is the principal cation of the ECF; tonicity in milliosmoles/liter, therefore, can be estimated by doubling the serum sodium concentration in mEq/L. In two circumstances, however (hyperglycemia and hyperlipemia), the serum sodium concentration is low without an associated decrease in the osmotic activity of the serum. With those exceptions, hyponatremia always reflects reduced tonicity of body fluid and thus represents insufficient renal excretion of water relative to the excretion of salt. *Hyponatremia per se does not imply a deficit of sodium in the body;* in fact, hyponatremia is frequently associated with an excess of body sodium. Total body sodium is a function of the volume of extracellular fluid as well as the concentration of sodium and cannot be estimated from the latter alone.

1. **Sodium depletion** Hyponatremia may result from sodium depletion. Loss of sodium without water, of course, does not occur as such; the hyponatremia is actually the net result of loss of isotonic (or even hypotonic) fluid which is replaced by administration of water without salt. Water excretion must also be impaired in order for hyponatremia to be sustained.

   Administration of isotonic saline is the treatment of choice, since volume depletion is more serious than hypotonicity, and the ability to have a water diuresis may be restored when volume depletion alone is corrected.

2. **Water intoxication,** though not a distinct syndrome, is deserving of separate mention because of its therapeutic importance; except for severe volume depletion, it represents the only hyponatremic state which may require emergency treatment. Water intoxication is usually iatrogenic, resulting from administration of water to a patient unable to have a water diuresis (e.g., postoperatively, or in the presence of renal insufficiency). When chronic or mild, weakness or apathy may be the only manifestations; when acute or severe, however, confusion, stupor, muscle twitching, or grand mal seizures may occur.

   Hypertonic saline (available as 3% NaCl containing 51 mEq Na+/100 ml or 5% NaCl containing 86 mEq Na+/100 ml) should be administered in most situations in which the patient is symptomatic and the serum sodium concentration is markedly depressed (less than 125 mEq/L), even though total body sodium may be increased. The amount of sodium necessary to correct the hyponatremia may be calculated by multiplying the difference between the desired and observed sodium concentrations in mEq/L by the volume of total body water in liters. Although sodium is restricted to the ECF, calculations must be based on total body water, since

H_2O is withdrawn from cells to equalize tonicity as hypertonic saline is administered. *Other fluids must be restricted when hypertonic saline is given.*

Circulatory overload and pulmonary edema are potential complications of therapy. Hypertonic saline should be administered slowly (at a rate of less than 100 mEq sodium/hour as a rule) and the patient reevaluated frequently (auscultation of the lungs for rales, inspection of the neck for venous distention, or measurement of venous pressure). It may be wise to divide the prescribed amount of fluid into several different infusion bottles so that the entire amount cannot be infused inadvertently at a rapid rate.

3. **Defective urine dilution** Hyponatremia occurring in congestive heart failure, cirrhosis, nephrosis, or adrenal insufficiency is usually due to impaired water diuresis. In these conditions, except for adrenal insufficiency, the hyponatremia is accompanied by edema, i.e., increased total body sodium. The hyponatremia itself is usually asymptomatic and rarely requires therapy, although moderate water restriction may be beneficial in patients with congestive heart failure, cirrhosis, or nephrosis. Administration of hypertonic saline is frequently hazardous and seldom, if ever, of benefit. Isotonic saline is required for the treatment of adrenal insufficiency.

4. **Inappropriate secretion of ADH** (Schwartz-Bartter syndrome) Severe hyponatremia which has been ascribed to the inappropriate secretion of ADH may occur in a variety of disorders (most often pulmonary and cerebral disorders). The hyponatremia is due primarily to water retention but is compounded by urinary loss of sodium. The essential criteria for diagnosis of this syndrome are: (1) hyponatremia, (2) urine that is hypertonic to plasma at all times, even during water administration, (3) inappropriately large amounts of urinary sodium even during water loading, (4) normal glomerular filtration rate, and (5) disappearance of all abnormalities following adequate restriction of water. The ECF volume is normal or expanded.

The serum sodium concentration may fall to dangerous levels if water intake is great, but symptoms rarely appear until the serum sodium concentration falls below 110 mEq/L. The disorder may disappear spontaneously (usually in association with improvement in the underlying disease) and not require therapy. When the serum sodium concentration is significantly lowered, however, water intake should be restricted to less than sensible and insensible losses; when the serum sodium concentration rises to the desired level water may be given in amounts that are equal to losses. If the serum sodium concentration is below 115 mEq/L, hypertonic saline may be administered. In severe cases with impending seizures or coma, peritoneal dialysis is the treatment of choice.

5. **"Sick cell syndrome"** (primary cellular dilution; new steady state) The sick cell syndrome is an asymptomatic dilutional hyponatremia which occurs most frequently in patients with pulmonary or cerebral disease, although it may complicate any chronic debilitating illness. The mechanism of the hyponatremia is not well defined, but the apparent result is a "resetting of the osmostat at a lower level"; a normal response occurs to administration of salt or water, but at a hypotonic level. In contrast to the syndrome of

inappropriate ADH secretion, water restriction results in increased sodium excretion, thus preventing restoration of tonicity. Diagnosis may be confirmed by demonstrating excretion of water and salt (following administration of water on one occasion, salt on another) in such proportion as to maintain the low serum sodium concentration. The hyponatremia is usually modest (serum sodium often greater than 120 mEq/L) and no specific therapy is required.

6. **Artifactual hyponatremia** Hyperglycemia increases extracellular tonicity which, because cell membranes are not freely permeable to glucose, causes water to shift from cells to the ECF. This dilution of extracellular fluid decreases the concentration of extracellular electrolytes: an increase in blood glucose of 180 mg/100 ml causes a fall in serum sodium of 5 mEq/L. When tonicity cannot be restored to normal by excretion of glucose, as in uncontrolled diabetes, hypertonicity may persist or may be decreased by retention of water or excretion of sodium. In each instance tonicity is underestimated by doubling the serum sodium concentration, and it is in this sense that the hyponatremia is "artifactual."

Hyperlipemia decreases the proportion of serum that is water, often by as much as 10%–20%. Since sodium is restricted to the aqueous phase, sodium concentration of whole serum is low even though the sodium concentration of serum water is normal. The hyponatremia associated with hyperlipemia (of practical significance only when serum is lactescent) is artifactual since osmolality is normal.

E. **Hypernatremia** (hyperosmolality; dehydration)

1. **Pathophysiology** Hypernatremia may result from loss of water or gain of sodium; tonicity (osmolality) of both fluids is increased. When hypernatremia is due to loss of water, both ICF and ECF compartments are diminished in volume; when it is due to gain of salt, ECF volume is increased and ICF volume decreased.

2. **Causes** Because thirst normally protects against its development, hypernatremia occurs most commonly in patients unable to obtain water or ask for it. Hypernatremia may result from insufficient water intake (as in coma, vomiting, hypothalamic lesions with loss of thirst sensation), excessive sweating, hyperpnea, diarrhea, and polyuria due to renal (potassium depletion, hypercalcemia, pyelonephritis, Fanconi syndrome) or extrarenal (diabetes insipidus, diabetes mellitus, administration of high-protein tube feedings) causes. Hypernatremia due to gain of salt is uncommon (usually iatrogenic, as in infants inadvertently fed sodium mixtures), although it may occur in hyperaldosteronism and Cushing's syndrome.

3. **Manifestations** Thirst is the major symptom of hypernatremia but may be absent or poorly communicated for the very reason that hypernatremia was allowed to develop (e.g., hypothalamic lesions); water depletion itself may cause confusion and weakness. Urine volume is diminished and specific gravity increased except when hypernatremia is due to polyuria. The hematocrit is usually not increased because of proportionate loss of plasma and red-cell water. The change in ECF volume is small (unless water depletion is very severe) because the extracellular hypertonicity draws fluid from cells; as a result skin turgor, postural changes in blood pres-

sure, and serum protein concentration are minimally affected. Sweating is diminished and fever may result.

4. **Treatment** Solute-free water is required. If the serum sodium concentration is less than 160 mEq/L, water may be given orally (if the patient can take it); if hypertonicity is more marked, 5% D/W should be administered intravenously. In order to guide further therapy and to prevent water intoxication from overtreatment, the serum sodium concentration should be determined after administration of approximately half the calculated water requirement. This is particularly important in comatose patients in whom water intoxication may be inapparent.

The volume of water necessary to restore serum sodium concentration may be estimated by the following calculations:

$$\text{Normal volume body water (L)} = 0.6 \times \text{body weight (kg)}$$

$$\text{Current volume body water} = \frac{\text{normal serum [Na}^+] \times \text{normal volume body water}}{\text{measured serum [Na}^+]}$$

$$\text{Body-water deficit} = \text{normal volume} - \text{current volume}$$

V. POTASSIUM

A. **Balance** The normal diet contains 50–100 mEq potassium per day. Only about 10 mEq are excreted in the stool and sweat; the remainder is excreted in the urine. Thus, the kidney normally determines potassium balance. The kidney can greatly increase excretion to adjust to high potassium intake but is less capable of adjusting to very low potassium intake. In fact, in the absence of potassium, the kidney is unable to maintain potassium balance. Unlike sodium, which is eliminated from the urine after several days of a sodium-free diet, 5–10 mEq potassium daily may continue to appear in the urine even after a week or more of a potassium-free diet.

B. **Serum potassium concentration** The serum K^+ concentration (normally 3.8–5.0 mEq/L) generally reflects total body potassium content even though only 2% of body potassium is extracellular. Thus, when total body potassium is high, the serum concentration tends to be elevated; when body potassium is low, the serum concentration tends to be low. The serum K^+ concentration is also influenced by the pH of the extracellular fluid (serum K^+ concentration higher in acidosis, lower in alkalosis) as depicted diagrammatically in Figure 2-1. Changes in the ECF volume also alter the serum potassium concentration, but only transiently.

The magnitude of potassium depletion cannot be estimated precisely from the value of the serum potassium concentration alone. With moderate potassium deficits, for example, the serum potassium level may be increased if the patient is acidotic, minimally or moderately decreased, or markedly decreased if the patient is alkalotic.

C. **Hypokalemia**

1. **Causes** Hypokalemia results either from loss of potassium from the body or from shift of potassium into cells. Losses may be gastrointestinal (urine potassium less than 20 mEq daily) or urinary (urine potassium greater than 30 mEq daily).

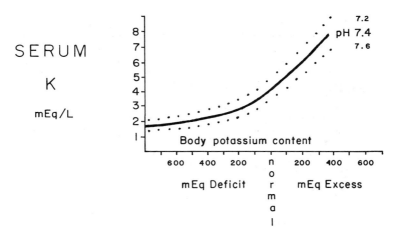

SERUM

K

mEq/L

Fig. 2-1. Schematic illustration of the relationship between serum and tissue potassium. As body potassium rises above normal the serum potassium concentration rises proportionately. As body potassium falls below normal, however, the decrement in serum potassium concentration becomes less and less. Thus, the serum potassium concentration may not be substantially lower after a 600–1000 mEq deficit than after a 300–500 mEq deficit. As noted previously, the serum potassium concentration is higher in acidosis and lower in alkalosis.

a) **Gastrointestinal losses of potassium** occur with diarrhea, intestinal or biliary fistulas, ureteroenterostomy, or vomiting. In the last situation, the potassium deficit may be greater than that which can be explained by loss of potassium by emesis and is usually due to the enhanced urinary excretion of potassium that occurs in alkalosis.

b) **Urinary loss of potassium** occurs in renal tubular disorders (renal tubular acidosis, recovery phase of acute tubular necrosis, occasionally pyelonephritis), in osmotic diuresis (uncontrolled diabetes, mannitol administration), in patients receiving diuretics (particularly thiazides or ethacrynic acid) or corticosteroids, and in Cushing's syndrome and hyperaldosteronism.

c) **Inadequate intake of potassium** is an uncommon cause of hypokalemia except in patients whose only intake is potassium-free parenteral fluids; they may develop a 200 mEq potassium deficit in one week because of continued urinary excretion of potassium.

d) **Hypokalemia due to shift of potassium into cells** may result from alkali administration (particularly to acidotic patients) or parenteral administration of glucose or insulin.

e) **Profuse sweating** may cause a potassium loss of 15–20 mEq/day, but rarely causes hypokalemia per se.

2. **Manifestations** of hypokalemia rarely develop before the serum potassium concentration has fallen below 3.0 mEq/L unless the

rate of fall has been rapid. Signs and symptoms include neuro-muscular disturbances (weakness, hyporeflexia, paresthesias, and rarely flaccid paralysis or tetany) and cardiac abnormalities (arrhythmias, increased sensitivity to digitalis, and ECG changes). The ECG abnormalities occur sequentially and include flat or inverted T waves, prominent U waves, depressed S-T segments, prolonged P-R interval, tall P waves, and widening of the QRS complexes.

Additional manifestations that may be present include nephropathy (impaired urinary concentrating ability and mild depression of the glomerular filtration rate), central nervous system symptoms (irritability, stupor), GI symptoms (nausea, paralytic ileus), metabolic abnormalities (carbohydrate intolerance and negative nitrogen balance), and alkalosis. Polydipsia is a common manifestation.

Metabolic alkalosis and hypokalemia are often associated, primarily because both may have a common origin (e.g., vomiting, diuretic administration) and alkalosis begets hypokalemia (shift of potassium into cells, increased renal excretion).

3. **Prevention** Patients treated with diuretics or corticosteroids are susceptible to potassium depletion and should be advised to take adequate dietary potassium (particularly supplemental fruit or fruit juices). The serum potassium should be measured at intervals if therapy is prolonged, and potassium supplements should be prescribed if indicated. Particular care to prevent potassium depletion is necessary in patients taking digitalis, since severe cardiac arrhythmias may otherwise develop. Patients receiving only parenteral fluids should be given 40 mEq potassium daily unless oliguria or other contraindications exist. Lethal hypokalemia may occur during the treatment of diabetic ketoacidosis; prevention of this complication is discussed in Chapter 15.

4. **Treatment**

   a) **Orally** Hypokalemia is not usually an emergency; therapy always runs the risk of hyperkalemia, since potassium must traverse the tiny extracellular pool (65 mEq) to replenish cellular stores (3000 mEq). Slow oral therapy is desirable, therefore, and generally adequate.

   Dietary supplementation with natural foods may suffice; when this is inadequate, **the drug of choice is potassium chloride.** It is best administered in liquid form (a 10% solution of KCl contains 0.5 gm KCl or 6.5 mEq K+ per teaspoonful), and should be diluted in juice and given immediately after meals in order to minimize gastric irritation. Enteric-coated tablets of KCl should not be given because of undependable absorption and the risk of small-intestinal ulceration (see Chapter 5).

   Potassium Triplex (a solution of potassium acetate, bicarbonate, and citrate containing 15 mEq K+/5 ml), **Kaon** (potassium gluconate, available as Kaon Elixir containing 20 mEq K+/15 ml or tablets containing 5 mEq K+), or **K-Lyte** (effervescent tablets of potassium bicarbonate each containing 25 mEq K+) are more palatable than KCl, however, and are useful when potassium depletion is mild and unaccompanied by alkalosis, and dietary chloride is adequate. When hypokalemic alkalosis occurs, however, KCl should be given because chloride is required both to correct the alkalosis and associated chloride deficit and to allow complete potassium repletion.

b) Intravenously If the patient is unable to take potassium orally or if hypokalemia is severe, parenteral therapy is necessary. The serum potassium level must be known and the adequacy of urine output established before treatment; potassium should rarely be given IV to the oliguric patient.

The potassium deficit should be estimated and the urgency of repletion determined before selecting the dosage and rate of administration of KCl. If the serum potassium level is greater than 2.5 mEq/L and ECG manifestations are absent, potassium should be given at a rate not faster than 10 mEq/hour and in a concentration not greater than 30 mEq/L. Not more than 100–200 mEq/day should be given, even though it may take several days to replace the estimated deficit.

If urgent treatment is evident (i.e., serum potassium level less than 2.0 mEq/L, presence of ECG abnormalities or paralysis), potassium may be given at rates up to 40 mEq/hour and in concentrations up to 60 mEq/L; as much as 400 mEq/day may be given. The ECG should be monitored and the serum potassium level checked after the first 50–100 mEq replacement and frequently thereafter. In critical states potassium should be administered in saline (unless contraindicated) rather than in D/W, since the infusion of glucose-containing fluids may cause the serum potassium level to fall further; cardiac arrhythmias may develop, particularly in patients receiving digitalis. If glucose solutions must be given, use 5% D/W with a potassium concentration of 60 mEq/L.

D. Hyperkalemia

1. **Causes** Hyperkalemia may result from decreased renal excretion of potassium, rapid release of potassium from cells, or administration of potassium.

   Decreased excretion is common in acute renal failure (although uncommon in chronic renal failure unless the patient is terminally oliguric, is acidotic, or has been inadvertently given large amounts of potassium) and adrenal insufficiency. Rapid cellular release of potassium results from severe acidosis or increased tissue breakdown (e.g., following surgery, crush injury, extensive infection, massive hemolysis); these conditions may also be associated with impaired renal excretion of potassium. Exogenous potassium is an uncommon cause of hyperkalemia except in patients with renal insufficiency.

   In patients with significant elevation of the platelet count, or in situations in which the tourniquet has been left in place for a prolonged period of time before venipuncture, the blood sample hemolyzed or refrigerated, or separation of red blood cells from the plasma delayed, the potassium value in the serum sample may be high although the patient's true serum potassium concentration is normal.

2. **Manifestations** may be absent; when they do occur they are enhanced by concomitant hyponatremia, hypocalcemia, or acidosis. Neuromuscular manifestations of hyperkalemia are similar to those of hypokalemia and include paresthesias, areflexia, and muscular or respiratory paralysis. Cardiac manifestations are

frequent when the serum potassium level exceeds 8.0 mEq/L (uncommon at concentrations of less than 7.0 mEq/L) and include bradycardia, hypotension, ventricular fibrillation, and cardiac arrest. The sequential ECG manifestations are tall peaked T waves, depressed S-T segments, decreased amplitude of R waves, prolonged P-R interval, diminished to absent P waves, and widening of the QRS complexes with prolongation of the Q-T interval, resulting in a sine-wave pattern.

3. **Prevention** Hyperkalemia can often be prevented by the prompt recognition of oliguria and elimination of excessive potassium intake in patients with renal insufficiency. Frequently overlooked sources of exogenous potassium are low-salt milk (containing about 60 mEq potassium/L), salt substitutes, bank blood (which may contain as much as 30 mEq potassium/L in the plasma after storage for ten days), and penicillin G (1.7 mEq potassium/million units).

4. **Treatment** Hyperkalemia may be treated by measures that antagonize the effects of potassium, force cellular entry of potassium, or actually remove potassium from the body. Which measures should be used depends upon the degree of hyperkalemia and the severity of the manifestations. Urgency should be assessed on the basis of both the serum potassium concentration and the ECG changes; the situation is urgent if the serum potassium level is greater than 8.0 mEq/L or the ECG reveals absent P waves or a broad QRS complex. However, a very high serum potassium level may result in sudden death despite a normal ECG, or a severe arrhythmia may develop despite only moderate elevations of the serum potassium concentration.

The following tabulation lists the time of onset and duration of effect of the measures commonly employed in the treatment of hyperkalemia.

	Onset of effect	Duration
Calcium gluconate, IV	1–5 minutes	½–2 hours
Sodium bicarbonate, IV	5–10 minutes	2+ hours
Glucose-insulin, IV	½–1 hour	6–24 hours
Resins, orally or rectally	½–2 hours	As long as continued
Dialysis	2+ hours	As long as continued

a) **Calcium** antagonizes the cardiac toxicity of hyperkalemia, particularly if hypocalcemia is also present. (If the patient is receiving digitalis, however, calcium administration is sufficiently hazardous so that calcium should not be given.) Calcium gluconate, 5–10 ml of a 10% solution, may be injected IV over a 2-minute period (preferably with constant ECG monitoring). If ECG abnormalities persist, the injection may be repeated after 5 minutes; if ineffective, further calcium is unlikely to be of benefit. In cardiac arrest or ventricular fibrillation associated with hyperkalemia, similar or slightly smaller doses of calcium may be injected directly into the ventricle.

b) **Sodium bicarbonate** causes potassium to shift into cells; 45 mEq may be injected IV over a 5-minute period and repeated after 10–15 minutes if ECG abnormalities persist. $NaHCO_3$ may also be added to glucose infusions as described in the next paragraph.

c) **Glucose-insulin infusions** reduce the serum potassium level by causing potassium to shift into cells; 300–500 ml 20% glucose containing 20–35 units regular insulin may be administered IV over a 30–60 minute period.

Many observers prefer the rapid infusion of 1000 ml 5% D/S containing 90 mEq $NaHCO_3$; the first one-third of the infusion may be given in 30 minutes and the balance over 2–3 hours. Ten units of regular insulin may be given subcutaneously at the same time. The recommended solution is hypertonic with respect to sodium, however, and may cause rapid volume expansion.

d) **Resins** Cation-exchange resins reduce the serum potassium level more slowly than the previously described measures but have the advantage of actually removing potassium from the body (removing approximately 1 mEq K^+/gm of resin). Sodium-cycle resins, although exchanging 1 mEq Na^+ for each mEq K^+ removed, are preferable to hydrogen-cycle carboxylic resins, which are less palatable and induce acidosis.

   i) **Rectal administration** Fifty grams of polystyrene sulfonate **(Kayexalate)**, a nonabsorbable sodium-cycle cation-exchange resin, and 50 gm sorbitol are added to 200 ml water and given as a retention enema. If sorbitol is unavailable, the Kayexalate may be suspended in 200 ml 10% or 20% D/W. Retention of the enema for the desired 30–60 minutes may be facilitated by the use of an inflatable rectal catheter. Several enemas may be given at hourly intervals and at 6-hourly intervals thereafter if necessary. A single enema may reduce the serum potassium concentration by 0.5–1 mEq/L.

   ii) **Oral administration** is often preferred by alert patients despite the side effect of nausea. Resins are more effective when administered orally and should be given by this route if possible; should vomiting occur, rectal administration will be necessary. Because Kayexalate is constipating, it is desirable to facilitate its passage through the GI tract; therefore, 15 ml 70% sorbitol are given by mouth every 30 minutes until diarrhea is produced. When diarrhea commences 20–50 gm Kayexalate (2 heaping teaspoonfuls = 15 gm) suspended in 15 ml sorbitol are given four times daily.

e) **Dialysis** Hyperkalemia can usually be controlled with the methods described above; dialysis is indicated when conservative methods fail. Hemodialysis has the disadvantage of the time required for preparation of equipment and cannulation of vessels, but once instituted it can remove potassium more rapidly than any other measure. Peritoneal dialysis is indicated for less urgent situations but may be inadequate in the presence of massive tissue necrosis (e.g., crush injuries, overwhelming sepsis).

VI. ACID-BASE DISTURBANCES

A. **General comments** Acids are hydrogen-ion (proton) donors; bases are proton acceptors. These terms are not synonymous with the terms *anion* and *cation*, for the cations $Na+$ and $K+$ are neither bases nor acids, the cation NH_4+ is a weak acid, the anions $Cl-$ and $SO_4=$ are weak bases, and at normal blood pH the anion HCO_3- is a weak base and the anion H_2PO_4- a weak acid.

1. Metabolism both produces and consumes acid. Neutral carbohydrate and fat, when incompletely oxidized, release protons, although this proton release is transient because complete combustion yields CO_2 and H_2O. The CO_2 is a potential acid because, when hydrated, it forms carbonic acid ($CO_2 + H_2O \rightleftharpoons H_2CO_3 \rightleftharpoons H+ + HCO_3-$). These reactions are reversible, however, and the 22,000 mEq CO_2 produced each day by metabolism are excreted by the lungs; if ventilation is not disturbed the production and elimination of volatile acid has no net effect on pH. Metabolism also results in the production of fixed (nonvolatile) acid that requires renal excretion. The average diet yields about 70 mEq/day of fixed acid, derived from such sources as organic sulfur-containing amino acids, some phosphoesters (phosphoprotein), and those carbohydrates and fats that are oxidized to organic acids but not combusted to $CO_2 + H_2O$ because they cannot be metabolized further or because their anions escape into the urine before combustion.

2. The lungs, the kidneys, and buffers provide defense against acid-base disturbances. Chemical buffers (HCO_3-, PO_4-, proteinate, hemoglobin, and bone carbonate) react immediately with acid or alkali to minimize changes in pH, but are thereby consumed, leaving the organism less able to withstand further stress on neutrality. Respiratory adjustments, which also occur promptly, minimize pH changes by increasing or decreasing the excretion of volatile acid (CO_2), but such adjustments in ventilation are also limited. The ultimate correction of acid-base disturbances and restoration of buffer are dependent upon the kidney, even though renal excretion of acid and, to a lesser extent, alkali occurs slowly. The role of the kidney in acid-base regulation is to restore bicarbonate to the blood.

3. Acid secreted by renal tubular cells may be excreted in the urine as hydrogen ions, titratable acidity ($H+$ buffer by HPO_4-), or NH_4+ ($H+$ buffered by NH_3). Although the kidney can achieve an $H+$ concentration in the urine (at pH 4.0, maximum urine acidity) 1000 times that in the blood (at pH 7.4), very little acid can be excreted as free $H+$, and the great majority is excreted as titratable acid and ammonium in approximately equal amounts.

B. **The simple disturbances of acid-base equilibrium** (disturbances caused by single etiologic mechanisms) are metabolic and respiratory acidosis and alkalosis. Each of these four disturbances evokes compensatory responses that tend to minimize the changes in pH, but overcompensation does not occur.

In **metabolic acidosis** the primary mechanism is retention of fixed acid or loss of alkali (i.e., a decrease in HCO_3- or total CO_2); the compensatory response is hyperventilation and a resultant fall in pCO_2. In **respiratory acidosis** the primary mechanism is pulmonary retention of CO_2 (i.e., increase in pCO_2) resulting in a small increase in total CO_2. The quantitatively significant increase in total CO_2 is due to compensatory renal regeneration of HCO_3- (equivalent to renal excretion of acid). In **metabolic alkalosis** the primary mechanism is loss of fixed acid or gain of alkali (i.e., an increase in HCO_3^- or total CO_2); the compensatory response is hypoventilation and a resultant increase in pCO_2. In **respiratory alkalosis** the primary mechanism is hyperventilation and a resultant fall in pCO_2; the compensatory response is a decrease in HCO_3^- or total CO_2 due to increased endogenous acid production and decreased renal acid excretion.

The following chart summarizes the abnormalities that occur in the partially compensated, simple acid-base disturbances. Primary mechanisms are indicated by $\longrightarrow$, the resultant pH by $\longrightarrow$, and the compensatory response by $-\rightarrow$.

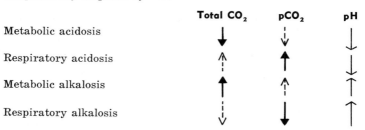

	Total CO_2	pCO_2	pH
Metabolic acidosis	↓	↓	↓
Respiratory acidosis	↑	↑	↓
Metabolic alkalosis	↑	↑	↑
Respiratory alkalosis	↓	↓	↑

C. Laboratory diagnosis

1. Co₂ alone Diagnosis of acid-base disturbances is often made on the basis of a single laboratory determination, the "CO_2," interpreted in light of clinical information. Although a low CO_2 is indicative of either metabolic acidosis or respiratory alkalosis, and a high CO_2 is indicative of either metabolic alkalosis or respiratory acidosis, the clinical setting usually indicates whether the primary etiologic factor is metabolic or respiratory. The CO_2 determination alone, therefore, often but not always suffices to indicate which of the four acid-base disturbances is present.

Several different methods may be used to determine the "CO_2"; it is important to understand how each test is performed and what it measures (see below). Serum contains HCO_3^-, physically dissolved CO_2 (the amount is proportional to the pCO_2), and H_2CO_3 (the amount is proportional to the dissolved CO_2). At normal blood pH the ratio of HCO_3^- to the sum of dissolved CO_2 and H_2CO_3 is 20:1.

a) Total CO₂ or CO₂ content This is the preferred method for measuring CO_2 in difficult acid-base problems. Blood is collected anaerobically, and plasma or serum is separated and analyzed without exposure to air (usually by keeping the sample under mineral oil). The total amount of CO_2 (i.e., HCO_3^-, dissolved CO_2, and H_2CO_3) liberated by acidification of the sample is measured.

Some laboratories measure the CO_2 content of blood allowed exposure to air. Since the pCO_2 of the atmosphere is only 0.3 mm Hg, very little dissolved CO_2 remains in the blood sample, and the total CO_2 that is measured is almost exclusively bicarbonate; the test results are about 1–2 mEq/L lower than the true total CO_2 content or CO_2 combining power if serum is promptly separated from cells.

b) CO₂ combining power or CO₂ capacity rather than the CO_2 content is usually performed by most clinical laboratories when a

"CO_2" is ordered. The blood sample is permitted exposure to air, and dissolved CO_2 thus escapes (less than 2 mEq/L in normal persons, more when the patient's pCO_2 is elevated or when the serum is not separated promptly from the red cells). Before analysis the sample is equilibrated with gas that has a pCO_2 of 40 mm Hg (serum or plasma is equilibrated when the CO_2 combining power is performed, whole blood when the CO_2 capacity is measured). If the patient has a normal pCO_2 and the serum is separated from red blood cells promptly, the CO_2 combining power is virtually the same as the CO_2 content (except for small corrections necessary because of use of serum or plasma rather than whole blood and equilibration at room temperature rather than at body temperature).

The CO_2 combining power has become a popular test because blood can be handled more conveniently, and the assumption has been made that only metabolic (not respiratory) derangements would be detected. This assumption is essentially correct for acute respiratory disturbances (the patient's dissolved CO_2 diffuses into the atmosphere, which has a pCO_2 of 0.3 mm Hg, and is replaced with a "normal" amount of dissolved CO_2 by equilibration with a pCO_2 of 40 mm Hg), but not for respiratory disturbances of duration sufficient for physiologic compensation to occur (since the compensatory change in HCO_3^- concentration is not eliminated by equilibration with a normal pCO_2).

2. **Total CO_2, pH, and pCO_2**   Although the most reliable evaluation of acid-base status is afforded by measurement of pH or pCO_2 in addition to total CO_2 content, the latter value alone usually permits correct diagnosis (since most of the CO_2 is HCO_3^- under abnormal as well as normal conditions) if clinical information is interpreted correctly. In certain circumstances, however (as in the hyperventilating patient with either respiratory alkalosis or metabolic acidosis), correct diagnosis may require the measurement of blood pH and/or pCO_2.

Both pH and pCO_2 may be measured simply with electrodes. Because pH meters are more commonly available than pCO_2 electrodes, the pH and total CO_2 are usually measured and the pCO_2 is then calculated. Acid-base status may also be defined by the Astrup technique by measuring the initial pH of an anaerobic blood sample and the pH of the same sample equilibrated at two different known levels of pCO_2.

a) Arterial blood samples are not necessary for determination of acid-base status. Venous blood is quite adequate if samples are properly collected, if peripheral circulation is not impaired, and if the difference between arterial and venous values is appreciated. Normal values are listed below.

	pH	pCO_2	Total CO_2
Arterial blood	7.38–7.43	35–45 mm Hg	24–29 mEq/L
Venous blood	7.35–7.40	40–50 mm Hg	26–32 mEq/L

The syringe should be coated with heparin (1000 units/ml) to serve as anticoagulant and to seal the barrel against air leaks. Venipuncture should be performed without use of a tourniquet if possible; if not possible, the blood sample should be drawn *before* the tourniquet is released. Air bubbles should be expressed from the syringe and the syringe then capped (or the attached needle inserted into a cork or rubber stopper). If pH and total CO_2 cannot be measured promptly the capped syringe may be stored in ice water for as long as 2–3 hours.

b) From any two of the three variables (total CO_2, pH, pCO_2) the third may be calculated; the pCO_2 may be read from standard nomograms or easily *estimated* by utilizing the derived equation below. One thus avoids use of complicated formulas or logarithm tables in order to solve the Henderson-Hasselbalch equation.

$$pCO_2 = \frac{[H^+] \ [\text{total } CO_2 \text{ content}]}{25}$$

$[H^+]$ is expressed in nanoequivalents/L (nEq/L, millimicroequivalents/L) and can be derived readily from the pH by remembering that a pH value of $7.40 = $ an $[H^+]$ of 40 nEq/L, and that each 0.01-unit increase in pH is roughly equivalent to a 1.0 nEq/L decrease in $[H^+]$ within the pH range of 7.28–7.45. (For example, a change in pH from 7.47 to 7.30 is accompanied by a rise in $[H^+]$ from 33 nEq/L to 50 nEq/L.) The maximum error in pCO_2 calculated by this simplified formula is 7% or less when the pH is between 7.10 and 7.50 (*New Eng. J. Med.* 272:1067, 1965).

D. Metabolic acidosis results from accumulation of fixed (nonvolatile) acid (by ingestion, increased endogenous production, or decreased excretion) or from loss of alkali. It is clinically useful to divide metabolic acidoses into two groups, i.e., those in which protons are retained in association with chloride (metabolic acidosis with hyperchloremia) and those in which protons are retained in association with other anions (metabolic acidosis with increase of unmeasured anions). The concentrations of these unmeasured anions (designated $\triangle$) is arbitrarily defined as the concentration of the serum sodium minus the sum of the concentrations of chloride and total CO_2:

$$\triangle = [Na^+] - \Big([Cl^-] + [CO_2] \Big)$$

Normally, $\triangle = 8 \pm 4$ mEq/L. If *delta* is normal the acidosis is one of the hyperchloremic acidoses; if it is increased one of the "anion-gap" acidoses exists. When there is a *large* increase in unmeasured anions a metabolic acidosis almost always exists; although cellular production of organic acids also occurs in alkalosis, particularly respiratory alkalosis, this compensatory mechanism rarely results in an increase of unmeasured anions greater than 10 mEq/L above the normal value.

1. Causes

a) **Metabolic acidosis with increase of unmeasured anions** may occur in uremia (impaired NH_4^+ excretion and HCO_3^- reabsorption; the retention of $PO_4^=$, $SO_4^=$, and organic-acid anions is coincidental), diabetic ketoacidosis (accumulation of betahydroxybutyric and acetoacetic acids), lactic acidosis, and intoxication with salicylate, methanol, ethylene glycol, or paraldehyde.

b) **Metabolic acidosis with hyperchloremia** may occur in ammonium chloride ingestion, prolonged or severe diarrhea (loss of HCO_3^- in the stool), chronic pyelonephritis prior to development of azotemia (diminished H^+ excretion), renal tubular acidosis (diminished H^+ secretion by renal tubule cells), and ureteroenterostomy (loss of HCO_3^-, which exchanges for urinary chloride across the intestinal mucosa).

2. **Diagnosis** Definitive diagnosis of metabolic acidosis requires demonstration of decrease in pH and pCO_2 in addition to a decrease in total CO_2. Although the total CO_2 is low in both metabolic acidosis and respiratory alkalosis, a value of less than 15 mEq/L is uncommon in respiratory alkalosis. Hyperventilation occurs in both respiratory alkalosis and metabolic acidosis but may not be clinically noticeable in conditions characterized by chronic acidosis.

3. **Treatment** Underlying disorders should receive appropriate therapy. Treatment of lactic acidosis is discussed in paragraph **5**; treatment of diabetic ketoacidosis is discussed in Chapter 15.

a) **Treatment of acidosis per se is urgent when the patient is acutely ill** (e.g., comatose, hypotensive) or the blood pH is less than 7.2. $NaHCO_3$ is the preferred alkali for parenteral administration; sodium lactate has no known advantages and may be ineffective if cellular metabolism is deranged. The alkali requirement cannot be calculated precisely. Although $NaHCO_3$ remains in the ECF, only about one-half the desired rise in plasma concentration is achieved if replacement is calculated on the basis of ECF volume alone (because hydrogen ion is buffered intracellularly as well as extracellularly). In calculating the amount of $NaHCO_3$ required to correct the acidosis, 40% of body weight (twice the ECF volume) should be considered as the apparent volume of distribution of HCO_3^-. The *approximate* number of mEq $NaHCO_3$ required to correct the acidosis equals $0.4 \times kg$ body weight $\times$ (desired CO_2 concentration $-$ measured plasma CO_2 concentration in mEq/L). Generally, one to four ampules of 7.5% $NaHCO_3$ are added to 1000 ml 5% D/W for parenteral administration. One-half to two-thirds of the calculated amount may be infused over a 2-hour period if the patient is severely acidotic and critically ill; subsequent rate of administration should be prescribed only after reevaluation of the clinical situation. In the presence of hypokalemia, aggressive correction of acidosis should not be initiated without first initiating correction of K^+ deficit (see Chapter 15). Partial correction of acidosis associated with hypokalemia may precipitate the fatal manifestations of hypokalemia by further decreasing the extracellular/intracellular ratio of K^+.

b) **Chronic acidosis** is tolerated well by most patients; in renal insufficiency treatment is seldom required until the CO_2 falls below 18–20 mEq/L. With this degree of acidosis, the $CaCO_3$ of bone is probably the principal buffer in maintaining the plasma pH. Although the patient may be asymptomatic, therapy is necessary to prevent osteomalacia, nephrocalcinosis, and nephrolithiasis. For chronic acidosis of moderate degree, therapy may be initiated with $NaHCO_3$ 1 gm (12 mEq Na^+) or 10% sodium citrate 15 ml (15 mEq Na^+) three times daily. Sodium citrate is more efficacious when nephrocalcinosis and nephrolithiasis are present because of the probable inhibition of stone formation in addition to systemic alkalinization. In patients with an additional renal phosphate "leak" and hypocalcemia, calcium carbonate and neutral sodium phosphate may be used to aid the reversal of osteomalacia and maintain the bone buffer. Adjustments in dosage may be made after the effects of initial therapy are evaluated. It is reasonable and generally sufficient to raise the CO_2 to approximately 20 mEq/L; raising the CO_2 to higher levels often requires inordinately large doses of alkali and may result in alkalosis, edema, tetany, or hypertension.

4. **Complications of therapy**   Since sodium salts are generally administered, alkali therapy is complicated frequently by volume overloading and occasionally by hypertension. Rapid parenteral administration of large amounts of sodium may precipitate acute pulmonary edema, but continued oral administration of alkali may also precipitate congestive heart failure, particularly in patients with heart disease or impairment of salt excretion. Oral alkali therapy may often be continued despite volume overloading if dietary salt is rigidly restricted; those patients who can tolerate an increased potassium intake (particularly those with renal tubular acidosis) may be given potassium salts of alkali instead.

Tetany may develop if alkali is administered rapidly or excessively. Although tetany may not be due to a decrease in ionized calcium concentration, as often assumed, calcium administration may be of therapeutic value. Calcium salts must not be given in the same infusion as bicarbonate, for precipitation will occur.

Hypokalemia may also occur, since the potassium originally displaced from cells as acidosis developed reenters cells as alkali is administered.

5. **Lactic acidosis,** although uncommon, deserves special mention because of the frequently fatal outcome and the increasing recognition of the entity in clinical practice. Lactic acidosis may occur in the presence of severe circulatory or respiratory depression (e.g., in shock, cardiac arrest, severe congestive heart failure, or pulmonary disease) in which tissue hypoxia may be expected (**secondary lactic acidosis**). **Idiopathic or spontaneous lactic acidosis,** however, occurs in a variety of disorders (particularly uremia, diabetes, severe bacterial infections, pancreatitis, leukemia) not apparently characterized by tissue hypoxia; patients with idiopathic lactic acidosis do not appear to be suffering from any of the well-recognized causes of disordered lactate-pyruvate metabolism, and the pathogenesis of the syndrome is unknown at present.

a) **Diagnosis** of lactic acidosis should be considered when the clinical picture of a metabolic acidosis develops in a setting in which tissue hypoxia is likely, or when seriously ill patients (particularly those with the diseases mentioned above) develop tachypnea and hyperpnea of abrupt onset followed within several hours by stupor and coma. Laboratory studies reveal a marked decrease in total CO_2, a large increase in unmeasured anions, and marked increase in blood lactate concentration. Definitive diagnosis, however, requires the demonstration of a decrease in pH as well, for increases of lactate and pyruvate may also occur in metabolic alkalosis and respiratory alkalosis with marked hyperventilation.

b) **Treatment** is generally unsatisfactory, and more than 90% of patients die. Supportive measures should be instituted promptly, remediable causes of tissue hypoxia should be corrected, and large doses of $NaHCO_3$ should be given parenterally. Patients with lactic acidosis are usually markedly resistant to therapy and in some instances may require 200–400 mEq or more of bicarbonate during the first few hours of treatment just to prevent further fall in the serum bicarbonate concentration. Frequent evaluation of the patient's acid-base status is necessary to ensure that adequate alkali is being given and to prevent alkalosis (for resistance to therapy occasionally disappears suddenly and a metabolic alkalosis may supervene). Although other modes of therapy (e.g., hemodialysis, administration of methylene blue) have been tried, they are of unproved value.

E. Metabolic alkalosis

1. **Causes** include loss of fixed acid (from vomiting, nasogastric suction, and rarely diarrhea), Cushing's disease, hyperaldosteronism, ingestion of alkali, prolonged administration of corticosteroids or diuretics (particularly thiazides, ethacrynic acid, and mercurials), and potassium and chloride depletion. Although the metabolic alkalosis accompanying potassium depletion has been attributed to shift of $Na+$ and $H+$ into cells as $K+$ is lost from cells, recent data suggest that the alkalosis may be due to altered renal tubular function—i.e., increased HCO_3- reabsorption—that is augmented by the concomitant chloride deficiency often accompanying potassium depletion (decreased availability of chloride limits proximal reabsorption of sodium and enhances distal exchange of $H+$ and $K+$ for $Na+$). The extracellular alkalosis, once developed, is maintained by the kidneys.

2. **Diagnosis** usually may be made by demonstrating an elevation of the serum CO_2 concentration in one of the conditions previously listed; other tests are generally unnecessary unless conditions that predispose to the development of respiratory acidosis are also present. In these circumstances measurement of the pH or pCO_2 in addition will allow differentiation of metabolic alkalosis from respiratory acidosis.

3. **Treatment** is directed at the underlying condition. Volume depletion, if also present, should be corrected by the administration of isotonic saline; potassium deficits should be replaced by administration of potassium chloride. Oral or parenteral administration of acid (e.g., NH_4Cl) is rarely necessary and may be deleterious by causing further loss of potassium and sodium. When extraordinary degrees of alkalosis are present, however, NH_4Cl may be administered cautiously; dosage should be based on an apparent volume distribution of 40% of body weight.

F. Respiratory acidosis is due to inadequate pulmonary excretion of CO_2 with a resultant increase in pCO_2 and hence in H_2CO_3.

1. **Causes** are discussed in the section on respiratory failure in Chapter 8.

2. **Diagnosis** should be strongly suspected when elevation of the serum CO_2 content occurs in the presence of any condition known to predispose to the development of respiratory acidosis. Because the normal ratio of dissolved $CO_2 + H_2CO_3$ to HCO_3- is 1:20, a small

rise in dissolved CO_2 results in a profound fall in pH. Although endogenous buffers rapidly generate bicarbonate to minimize this fall in pH, this small rise in total CO_2 (several mEq/L) may go unnoticed. Hours to days may elapse before renal compensation (via reabsorption of HCO_3-) effects a clearly significant rise in total CO_2. For these reasons diagnosis often requires measurement of pH or pCO_2 in addition to the total CO_2. In simple disturbances the pH is low (differentiating respiratory acidosis from metabolic alkalosis) and the pCO_2 elevated (differentiating respiratory acidosis from metabolic acidosis), usually to levels higher than those occurring as a compensatory response to metabolic alkalosis.

Unfortunately, the clinical situation is more complicated, for patients with acute respiratory acidosis often have complex acid-base disturbances; varying degrees of metabolic acidosis or alkalosis frequently coexist, and interpretation of laboratory data becomes difficult. Recent studies by Schwartz et al. have provided data that may be helpful in deciding whether a given bicarbonate (total CO_2) level represents a compensatory change because of an elevated pCO_2, or reflects instead a second primary acid-base disturbance.

They have studied the uncomplicated response to acute, graded hypercapnia in man and to chronic hypercapnia in the dog. Table 2-2, which lists for varied levels of pCO_2 the limits of pH and total CO_2 that may be anticipated with 95% probability during acute and chronic hypercapnia, is based on their data and clearly shows that in chronic hypercapnia the serum HCO_3- is higher and the fall in pH less than in acute hypercapnia. These data may be helpful in allowing the physician to detect those patients with pulmonary insufficiency who have a metabolic acidosis or alkalosis superimposed on acute respiratory acidosis (see *J. Clin. Invest.* 44:291, 1965; *New Eng. J. Med.* 272:6, 1965).

3. **Treatment** of uncomplicated respiratory acidosis is directed at improving ventilation and is discussed in Chapter 8. The administration of alkali is rarely necessary (unless a severe complicating metabolic acidosis is also present) and may actually be harmful (since the low pH is an important stimulus to ventilation in chronic hypercapnia). Potassium and chloride deficiency, often accompanying the metabolic alkalosis superimposed on chronic respiratory acidosis, should be treated by the administration of KCl.

TABLE 2-2. pCO_2, pH, and Total CO_2 in Hypercapnia

pCO_2 (mm Hg)	pH		Total CO_2 (mEq/L)	
	Acute	Chronic	Acute	Chronic
40	7.45–7.38	7.46–7.36	24–28	23–29
50	7.36–7.31	7.41–7.33	26–29	27–32
60	7.29–7.24	7.38–7.31	27–30	31–36
70	7.23–7.19	7.34–7.28	28–31	34–39
80	7.18–7.14	7.32–7.25	29–31	36–42
90	7.13–7.09	7.30–7.22	29–32	39–45
100	—	7.28–7.20	—	41–48
110	—	7.26–7.17	—	42–51
120	—	7.24–7.14	—	44–54

G. **Respiratory alkalosis** is due to a low pCO_2 (and hence reduced H_2CO_3 concentration) because of hyperventilation.

1. **Causes** include psychogenic hyperventilation (the most common), hypermetabolic states (e.g., fever, thyrotoxicosis, delirium tremens), gram-negative bacteremia, and excessive ventilation by mechanical ventilators. Some degree of respiratory alkalosis may also occur in pregnancy and in patients with cirrhosis or certain cardiac, pulmonary, or central nervous system lesions. Early stages of salicylate intoxication may also result in respiratory alkalosis, but metabolic acidosis may quickly supervene, especially in children.

2. **Diagnosis** should be suspected when symptoms suggestive of respiratory alkalosis (e.g., irritability, light-headedness, paresthesias, tetany, and even syncope) occur in a patient with a disorder that predisposes to the development of respiratory alkalosis. Increased ventilation may not be apparent in patients who have an increased depth of respiration without associated tachypnea.

   Although the pCO_2 and pH are markedly abnormal in acute hyperventilation, the total CO_2 and other commonly measured electrolytes are not usually altered detectably. Only when compensatory changes have occurred does the total CO_2 fall perceptibly; laboratory values may then resemble those seen in mild metabolic acidosis. Definitive diagnosis requires measurement of pH or pCO_2 in addition to total CO_2. Measurement of the urine pH may give misleading information.

3. **Treatment** is generally directed at the underlying disorder; the alkalosis per se requires no therapy as a rule. Tetany or syncope associated with acute hyperventilation may be relieved by rebreathing into a paper bag. If hyperventilation is suddenly terminated (as in the readjustment of a mechanical respirator, for example), an acidosis may develop (increase in pCO_2 in presence of decreased HCO_3^-); although the kidney normally restores buffer composition, alkali administration may occasionally be necessary for more prompt correction.

VII. CALCIUM

A. **General** Approximately 60% of serum calcium is bound to protein, primarily albumin, and is in equilibrium with ionized calcium, which constitutes the remaining 40%. Changes in serum proteins are reflected in proportional changes in the total serum calcium, with approximately 0.8 mg/100 ml Ca associated with each 1.0 gm/100 ml change in serum albumin. Although acidosis and alkalosis may shift the bound-ionized calcium equilibrium, this shift by itself is of little physiologic significance. Observed neuromuscular irritability with alkalosis and its absence with acidosis is a manifestation of other ion shifts in addition to calcium at the level of the cell membrane. Remember that hyperkalemia potentiates the cardiac and neuromuscular irritability of hypocalcemia and vice versa.

B. **Hypocalcemia** Hypocalcemia in the absence of azotemia or hypoalbuminemia is a relatively uncommon clinical problem because of the large calcium reserve provided by the skeleton. With the exception of patients with hypoparathyroidism in whom a paradoxical hypercalciuria is observed, the diagnosis of hypocalcemia can rapidly be excluded with a positive Sulkowitch test of the urine.

1. **Acute management** Acute symptomatic hypocalcemia is a medical emergency requiring the prompt administration of 20–30 ml of 10% calcium gluconate intravenously over 10–15 minutes. Subsequent calcium needs may be titrated with an IV drip of 10% calcium gluconate until these requirements can be met with oral calcium supplements. Intramuscular parathyroid extract, 200–300 units every 4–6 hours, is a beneficial adjunct to the acute management of patients with postoperative hypoparathyroidism. The adequacy of therapy may be evaluated by monitoring the Chvostek sign or the appearance of muscle spasm in the patient's forearm after occlusion of the arterial pulse up to 5 minutes with a blood pressure cuff (Trousseau's sign). Of the two, Chvostek's sign is probably the least specific and reliable.

2. **Chronic hypocalcemia** The long-term management of hypocalcemia is directed toward increasing intestinal absorption of calcium; this can be achieved to a limited extent by increasing dietary calcium.

   a) **Calcium** Dietary calcium supplementation is necessary in order to achieve a total daily calcium intake of 1800–2400 mg. Calcium lactate and calcium gluconate are superior to other forms of supplemental calcium, particularly the calcium phosphates, which are relatively insoluble and poorly absorbed. It is important to note that elemental calcium constitutes only a small fraction of the calcium preparation. For example a 600 mg tablet of calcium lactate contains 79 mg of elemental calcium, so that an average dosage schedule would be 5 tablets QID.

   b) **Vitamin D** Chronic and resistant hypocalcemia requires the use of vitamin D to enhance gut absorption when calcium supplementation alone is inadequate. In vitamin D-resistant and -deficient rickets and renal tubular acidosis the therapeutic aim is restoration of the serum calcium and alkaline phosphatase to normal and, in the child, the maintenance of good growth. When the serum calcium has returned to normal, the 24-hour urinary excretion of calcium may be monitored to avoid the hypercalciuria of vitamin D toxicity and the hypocalciuria of inadequate therapy. Vitamin D requirements are quite variable and depend upon the age of the patient, the severity of the disease, and calcium intake. The usual starting dose is 50,000 units of calciferol (vitamin D_2) per day which may be increased to 800,000 units or more in vitamin D-resistant rickets. Patients with hypoparathyroidism are occasionally resistant to vitamin D_2 or D_3, with persistent elevation of serum phosphorus during vitamin D therapy. These patients should be treated with AT 10 (dihydrotachysterol, Hytakerol). One mg crystalline dihydrotachysterol is equivalent to 3 mg or 120,000 units of vitamin D_2. It is not unusual to control a patient previously requiring 8–12 mg of D_2 with 1 mg AT 10. Commercially available preparations of AT 10 have in general from 1/4 to 1/5 the potency of the crystalline preparation. In women desiring pregnancy the vitamin D should be reduced to 20,000 units or less two to three months prior to conception, to avoid the congenital abnormalities associated with vitamin D toxicity and idiopathic hypercalcemia of infancy. Vitamin D is known to cross the placenta, but unfortunately the level of vitamin D toxic to the fetus is not known.

C. **Hypercalcemia** The patient with hypercalcemia may have anorexia, nausea, vomiting, abdominal pain, constipation, polyuria, polydipsia, dehydration, psychoses, obtundation, and finally coma. The most important therapeutic measure, regardless of etiology, is rehydration of the patient.

1. **Saline** Urinary calcium excretion is enhanced by saline infusion, since there is some evidence that sodium competitively inhibits tubular reabsorption of calcium.

2. **Sodium sulfate** For more rapid calcium diuresis isotonic sodium sulfate may be given intravenously at a rate of 1 L every 3–6 hours, depending upon the severity of the clinical situation and the cardiac and renal status of the patient. The sulfate anion further inhibits tubular reabsorption by chelating the filtered calcium. Because of the invariable and often marked lowering of serum potassium with sodium sulfate infusion, it is advisable, in most patients, to add 20–40 mEq of KCl to the IV fluids. Note that isotonic sodium sulfate is hypertonic with respect to sodium, and hypernatremia is also a potential complication.

3. **Corticosteroids** Large doses of Solu-Cortef intravenously (250–500 mg/L every 8 hours) will also lower the serum calcium. Although poorly understood, the mechanism of corticosteroid action probably involves a combination of decreased bone turnover, decreased gut absorption, and decreased renal tubular absorption. Great caution should be taken regarding hypokalemia and hypernatremia if corticosteroids and sodium sulfate are administered simultaneously.

4. **Phosphate** Intravenous phosphate has been successful in rapidly lowering the serum calcium in those patients with severe impairment of renal function in whom increased excretion of calcium by the above methods would be inadequate. 500 cc of a 0.1M solution of disodium phosphate and monopotassium phosphate (50 mM or 1.5 gm phosphorus) has been given over 6–8 hours without significant complications (*New Eng. J. Med.* 274:1, 1966). In addition to increasing calcium deposition into bone, there is evidence suggesting that phosphate infusions may also result in extraskeletal precipitation of calcium. Larger doses or more rapid infusion rates have resulted in hypocalcemia, renal cortical necrosis, shock, and death.

5. **EDTA** Because of serious renal toxicity EDTA (ethylenediaminetetraacetic acid) infusions should be used only in the acute management of life-threatening cardiac arrhythmias resulting from hypercalcemia.

6. **Long-term management of hypercalcemia** of hyperparathyroidism, sarcoidosis, thyrotoxicosis, myeloma, etc., is directed at the treatment of the underlying disease. In those patients in whom the underlying disease cannot be reversed (malignant tumors) management of the associated hypercalcemia is a therapeutic challenge. It is important to distinguish between two recognized forms of hypercalcemia of malignancy without obvious metastatic involvement of bone. The first is characteristically associated with carcinoma of the breast in which the tumor is probably producing an osteolytic sterol. The serum phosphorus in these patients is normal or elevated. The associated hypercalcemia has been successfully managed with small doses of corticosteroids equivalent to 5–15 mg of prednisone daily. A second form of hypercalcemia of

malignancy is characteristically seen with carcinomas of the lung, ovary, and kidney, and is usually associated with hypophosphatemia and low tubular reabsorption of phosphate. These tumors have been shown to produce a substance similar to parathyroid hormone. Inasmuch as the hypercalcemia of hyperparathyroidism is relatively refractory to corticosteroids, it is reasonable that hypercalcemia associated with such tumors would also be refractory. Oral phosphate therapy as neutral sodium phosphate, however, will effectively lower serum as well as urine calcium in most of these patients and in patients with primary hyperparathyroidism. The mechanism of action of phosphate repletion in these patients is not clearly understood. The amount of phosphate required to achieve therapeutic effects depends upon the severity of hypercalcemia and hyperphosphaturia. One teaspoonful of Fleet Phospho-Soda (600 mg/tsp) TID with meals is well tolerated as a starting dose. Phosphate supplementation should be reduced or discontinued if the serum phosphorus becomes abnormally elevated.

VIII.. MAGNESIUM Hypomagnesemia is an occasional cause of seizures and tetany, clinically mimicking hypocalcemia. Chronic diarrhea, continuous gastric drainage, and postoperative hyperparathyroidism superimposed on malnutrition constitute the usual setting for symptomatic hypomagnesemia. The diagnosis should always be considered when tetany fails to respond to adequate intravenous calcium therapy. Magnesium is administered as magnesium sulfate, 2–4 ml of a 50% solution every 4 hours intramuscularly.

3. Renal Disease

Rational treatment of patients with renal disease requires a thorough understanding of basic pathophysiology. Clinical manifestations of renal insufficiency largely reflect changes in hydration, in electrolyte concentration, and in acid-base, calcium, and phosphorus balance. Most of these abnormalities are at least partially reversible; their correction can contribute to the increased well-being and comfort of the chronically ill patient and may be lifesaving in cases of acute renal failure. For purposes of discussion, renal diseases are grouped into four categories based on current concepts of renal pathophysiology: acute renal failure, chronic renal insufficiency, the nephrotic syndrome, and infections of the urinary tract.

I. **ACUTE RENAL FAILURE** refers to a group of conditions characterized by progressive azotemia usually, but with important exceptions, associated with decreased urine volume. Determination of the creatinine and sodium concentrations in the plasma and urine (in addition to the other studies usually performed) should be made as a part of the differential diagnostic study. Microscopic examination of the sediments of centrifuged and uncentrifuged fresh urine specimens should be performed by the physician.

The conditions that may result in acute renal failure can be classified in terms of the functional abnormality involved.

A. **Conditions reflecting an uncompensated decrease in glomerular filtration rate per nephron**

1. **Volume depletion** (e.g., dehydration or blood loss) is often referred to as "prerenal azotemia." Therapy is directed at correction of the primary extrarenal causes for the abnormality.

Volume depletion must be differentiated from acute tubular necrosis. Table 3-1 lists laboratory studies that may be helpful in differential diagnosis; in most situations, however, such studies are adjunctive in establishing the diagnosis, and the response to administration of synthetic extracellular fluid (synthetic ECF), saline, ethacrynic acid, or mannitol should be determined. Mannitol 12.5 gm or 25 gm may be administered IV over 5–10 minutes, or one liter of synthetic ECF* or saline may be infused IV rapidly (over 30 minutes). Mannitol infusion will cause the excretion of large amounts of sodium and water; because the amount of water excreted is proportionately greater, preexisting mild hypernatremia may be made worse. Mannitol when not excreted remains largely within the intravascular space and carries the risk of

---

*Synthetic ECF is made by mixing 750 ml isotonic saline, 225 ml 5% D/W, and 25 ml NaHCO$_3$ (3.75 gm/50 ml). Each liter provides 137 mEq sodium, 115 mEq chloride, and 22.5 mEq bicarbonate.

precipitating cardiac decompensation in susceptible patients. Judicious administration of synthetic ECF is a more physiologic means of accomplishing ECF volume expansion. Ethacrynic acid when administered intravenously as a single injection of 100 mg will produce at least a threefold increase in urine volume within 5–30 minutes; the possibility of overexpansion of the plasma volume during the diagnostic procedure is avoided.

The diagnosis of volume depletion may be established if the urine volume increases in response to one of the above measures; additional amounts of synthetic ECF should then be administered. If urine flow does not increase, another diagnosis (particularly acute tubular necrosis) should be considered; administration of fluids should be regulated as for the treatment of acute tubular necrosis in order to avoid overhydration.

2. **Hepatorenal syndrome** Certain patients with advanced liver disease, especially those with severe portal hypertension or those who have been treated by vigorous diuresis, may develop an inability to excrete appropriate quantities of sodium and water; they elaborate a small volume of urine which is practically free of sodium. ECF volume increases, edema and ascites frequently develop, and the serum osmolality and sodium concentration fall. Oliguria and increasingly severe azotemia ensue. Diuresis may be achieved by the administration of ethacrynic acid or furosemide. Successive doses should be doubled until urine volume and sodium excretion increase. Concomitant hypokalemia, if present, must be treated. Overall results are generally disappointing, despite effective diuresis, since the underlying hepatic disease is usually severe.

3. **Acute glomerulonephritis**

   a) **Rest** Bed rest should be required during the acute stage as long as hematuria, proteinuria, hypertension, and edema are significant. During the 4–8-week phase of rapid improvement, modified bed rest may be allowed, but if resumption of activity significantly increases the 24-hour protein excretion or microscopic hematuria, complete bed rest should be resumed for several weeks more; ambulation may then be attempted again.

   b) **Diet** Rigid salt restriction (1–2 gm daily) is the most important measure during the acute edema-forming phase. Dietary protein need not be restricted (unless acute renal failure develops) and should average 60–70 gm daily. If anuria or oliguria and uremia develop, the diet should be the same as that for patients with acute tubular necrosis.

   c) **Hypertension and hypertensive encephalopathy** Treatment is described in Chapter 7 (Hypertension). Hydralazine and methyldopa may be particularly beneficial, since they are not regularly associated with decreases in glomerular filtration rate (GFR) and renal blood flow. Reserpine, 2.5 mg intramuscularly, may be given for the treatment of hypertensive crises. Magnesium sulfate is not recommended for the treatment of hypertension associated with acute glomerulonephritis.

   d) **Edema and congestive heart failure**

      i) Salt should be restricted to 1–2 gm daily; bed rest should be enforced. Diuresis occurs spontaneously in most patients, and other measures to reduce the ECF volume are usually unnecessary.

    ii) If pulmonary edema develops, venesection or plasmapheresis may be very effective; dialysis may be necessary in severe cases. Digitalis and nonmercurial diuretics may be given, even in the presence of azotemia, but their efficacy is questionable.

  e) **Antibiotics** A course of eradicative therapy for beta-hemolytic streptococci should be given routinely, as described in Chapter 4, to the patient and close contacts. Prophylactic therapy should be continued during the period of convalescence.

  f) **Corticosteroids** Evidence does not suggest that routine administration of ACTH or steroids favorably influences the course of acute glomerulonephritis except in rapidly progressive acute glomerulonephritis and acute glomerulonephritis secondary to lupus erythematosus or hypersensitivity angiitis. In these situations high-dose corticosteroid administration (60–80 mg/day of prednisone or equivalent) may be lifesaving. Renal biopsy should precede steroid therapy in such cases.

B. **Conditions reflecting diffuse nephron damage (acute tubular necrosis, nonoliguric renal failure, bilateral cortical necrosis)** Acute tubular necrosis (ATN) frequently develops following sudden unexpected trauma, usually in individuals without underlying renal disease. Hypotension of variable duration can be documented in many cases, but its influence on the development of ATN is often difficult to assess. In general, the precipitating events are numerous; the clinical course and chemical abnormalities vary considerably. The recovery rate in relatively uncomplicated cases, properly managed, is greater than 70%.

    Nonoliguric renal failure (NORF) can be defined as ATN that develops without an initial period of oliguria. It must be differentiated from hypercalcemia and hypokalemia in which rapidly progressive renal failure may develop in the presence of normal or high urine volumes.

    Bilateral cortical necrosis (BCN) infrequently follows obstetric accidents and generalized Shwartzman reactions but may occur in other circumstances, particularly when hypotension is severe and prolonged. Although the prognosis of BCN is considerably worse than that of ATN, the disease is not always fatal. Management of these conditions is discussed below. Results of laboratory studies which may be helpful in establishing the diagnosis are listed in Table 3-1; the

TABLE 3-1. Laboratory Studies in Acute Renal Failure

	U/P Creatinine	Urine Sodium Concentration
Decreased GFR/nephron	Usually > 20; often > 50	Usually < 20 mEq/L; often < 10 mEq/L, especially in the hepatorenal syndrome
Diffuse nephron damage	Usually < 20; often < 15	Usually > 30–40 mEq/L
Nonoliguric renal failure	Usually < 20; often < 15	Usually < 20; often < 15
Obstructive uropathy	Variable; often high in short-term obstruction, and low after prolonged obstruction	Variable; may be low in short-term partial obstruction

values given are general ones and may diverge significantly from the ranges listed because of the effects of underlying renal disease, state of hydration, residual urine in the bladder, gross hematuria, etc.

1. **Oliguric phase**   The oliguric phase may last from several days to three weeks (rarely longer), averaging 10–12 days. Urine output is usually, though not always, less than 400 ml/day; often it is less than 50 ml/day for several days. Complete anuria is very rare in ATN but may occur in BCN; when present, other disease processes, such as obstruction, acute glomerulonephritis, etc., should also be considered. The severity and rapidity of development of hyperkalemia, hyperphosphatemia, and acidosis are increased in patients with severe trauma and extensive tissue destruction.

   a) The underlying disease must be treated, with particular attention to debridement of devitalized tissue in cases of trauma.

   b) **Infection**   Antibiotics should not be administered prophylactically, but if infection, especially of the urinary tract, does occur, they should be properly chosen on the basis of sensitivity studies and given in correct (usually reduced) dosage. Instrumentation of the urinary tract and indwelling catheters should be avoided, if possible; if mild urinary retention occurs, Urecholine 5–10 mg TID–QID may be tried. Intravenous catheters should be protected with antibiotic ointment and sterile dressings at the point of entry; they should be changed every 2–3 days. An often overlooked source of large amounts of potassium is crystalline penicillin for intravenous administration (approximately 17 mEq potassium/10 million units); if large doses of penicillin must be given intravenously, the sodium salt may be used.

   c) **Diet and fluids**   If the patient is normally hydrated, fluid intake should be 400 ml/24 hours plus urine and unusual losses. At least 100–150 gm of carbohydrate daily are required; the total daily caloric intake should be 1500–2000 calories. When the patient can take oral feedings, carbohydrate-fat mixtures should be given; butter-sugar mixtures are not unpalatable and are a good source of calories. Commercially available preparations include Ediol (5 cal/ml) and Lipomul (6 cal/ml); 50–60 ml may be given 3–4 times daily, or the mixture frozen and served as sherbet. If parenteral feedings and fluids are required, give 25% glucose by continuous IV infusion through a catheter inserted into the superior vena cava; 15–20 mg heparin should be added to each day's aliquot of fluids. When the patient is not ambulatory, cannot take adequate calories orally, and must therefore rely on the 800–1000 calories provided by IV glucose, he should lose 0.5–1.0 pound daily during the oliguric phase; failure to lose weight suggests that too much fluid is being administered.

   d) **Anabolic steroids,** when used in an attempt to stimulate anabolic activity and decrease endogenous protein breakdown, may be of distinct value in the patient with acute renal failure; their long-term use in patients with chronic renal disease or other debilitating illnesses is of questionable value. Anabolic steroids may produce virilism in women, abnormalities in liver function tests (BSP retention and transaminase elevation), and, rarely, cholestatic jaundice.
      For use in acute renal failure: methandrostenolone (Dianabol)

5–10 mg/day orally for 10–20 days; nandrolone phenpropionate (Durabolin) 25–50 mg IM weekly; norethandrolone (Nilevar) 25 mg/day orally or IM for 10–20 days; stanozolol (Winstrol) 6–10 mg/day orally for 10–20 days; or equivalent amounts of other preparations. In other situations repository preparations may be used: testosterone cypionate (Depo-Testosterone) or testosterone enanthate (Delatestryl) 200–400 mg IM every 3–4 weeks; nandrolone decanoate (Deca-Durabolin) 50–100 mg IM every 3–4 weeks.

e) **Convulsions** Short-acting barbiturates should be given IV or IM; Dilantin should be administered concurrently. If hypocalcemia is symptomatic, inject IV 20–30 ml 10% calcium gluconate. If water intoxication is suspected, restrict water; rarely, when water intoxication is marked, dialysis is required. If acidosis is severe, attempt to correct it partially but observe the patient closely for symptoms of hypocalcemia. Treat hypertension, if severe, as described in Chapter 7.

f) **Nausea, pruritus, and hiccups** may be controlled with a phenothiazine (Thorazine or Compazine, in reduced dosage; e.g., 5–10 mg Thorazine every 4 hours). **Aphthous stomatitis** may be prevented by keeping the pH of the mouth acid with lemon juice or 1% HCl. Symptoms due to severe uremic enterocolitis may occasionally be lessened by the administration of a course of broad-spectrum antibiotics.

g) **Anemia** Patients with acute renal failure tolerate anemia well; the hematocrit should usually be maintained between 22% and 27%. Transfusions are indicated if the hematocrit falls below 22%, if active bleeding occurs, or if the anemia per se is symptomatic or contributes to heart failure or hypotension. Fresh blood should be used; the survival time of fresh red blood cells is longer, and less potassium is released into the plasma acutely. Those patients who tolerate a hematocrit lower than 22% without symptoms need not necessarily be transfused; occasional patients will require elevation of the hematocrit beyond 30% to be kept comfortable.

h) **Congestive heart failure** Usual measures are indicated. Digitalization should be carried out slowly, preferably with digoxin; digitalizing and maintenance doses should be reduced about 50%. Diuretics are of no value in conditions characterized by diffuse nephron damage, and dialysis or plasmapheresis will be required if circulatory overload is marked.

i) **Hyperkalemia and hypokalemia** Treatment is discussed in Chapter 2. Hypokalemia is rare in acute renal failure except in the diuretic phase; the treatment of hyperkalemia is directed at reducing both endogenous and exogenous sources of potassium.

j) **Acidosis and alkalosis** Treatment is discussed in Chapter 2. Acidosis per se does not usually require treatment unless the CO_2 is less than 15 mEq/L and symptoms are present.

k) **Adjustment of drug dosage** Drugs that are excreted by the kidney, especially long-acting barbiturates and certain antibiotics, should be given in decreased dosage, proportional to the degree of renal insufficiency.

i) **Barbiturates** If required, short-acting preparations which are metabolized primarily in the liver should be used.

ii) **Digitalis** If required, a short-acting preparation such as digoxin should be given; digitalizing and maintenance doses should be reduced about 50%. Hyperkalemia and hypocalcemia partially antagonize the effects of digitalis, and correction of these chemical abnormalities should proceed slowly in order to avoid precipitating digitalis intoxication (particularly cardiac arrhythmias). Digoxin is cleared by hemodialysis at rates approximating one-tenth normal renal clearances and in insignificant amounts by peritoneal dialysis. Therefore, no adjustments in maintenance doses usually are required unless hemodialyses are frequent or prolonged.

iii) **Antibiotics Penicillins, cephalothin, erythromycin,** and **lincomycin** may be given in the usual dosage. **Tetracycline** should be given in reduced dosage when renal function is less than 25% of normal. If the glomerular filtration rate is less than 30 ml/min give 0.5–1.0 gm orally initially, then 0.5 gm every 24–48 hours (equivalent dosages may be given parenterally); if the GFR is less than 10 ml/min, 0.5-gm doses should not be given more frequently than every 2–4 days. With **streptomycin** 1–2 gm are given IM initially, then 0.5–1.0 gm every 2–3 days. **Chloramphenicol** should be given in one-half the usual dosage because metabolites that accumulate may increase the incidence of erythropoietic depression. **Kanamycin, colistin,** and **polymyxin** must be given in significantly reduced dosage for the treatment of life-threatening infections with organisms resistant to other antibiotics; their administration to patients with renal failure otherwise is not justified because of the high incidence of toxicity.

l) **Dialysis** should be used as an adjunct to conservative management. A detailed discussion of the indications for extracorporeal or peritoneal dialysis is beyond the scope of this Manual, but one must remember that dialysis is an integral part of the management of patients with acute tubular necrosis and does not represent a last heroic effort to save a dying patient. One should not wait until the patient is in extremis before recommending dialysis.

2. **Diuretic phase** Twenty-five percent of the deaths due to acute renal failure occur during this phase of the disease, often because of infection. Onset of diuresis is usually heralded by stepwise increments in urine volume, but on occasion increases in volume may occur rapidly. The BUN and serum potassium may continue to rise for the first few days after diuresis begins; urinary sodium losses may be in excess of 300 mEq daily, and the urine sodium concentration may drop substantially and suddenly toward the end of the first week of diuresis. The total urine volume and solute excretion are in part determined by the previous state of hydration. Urinary losses of sodium, potassium (if hyperkalemia is not present), and water (if gross overhydration is not present) must be replaced quantitatively. Twice-daily body weights, daily values for serum and urine electrolytes, and daily hematocrits must be obtained. Creatinine clearance values should be checked frequently; if the GFR is increasing and the body weight is remaining steady, it is unlikely that excess fluids are being administered. However,

if the urine volume continues to rise for 5–6 days after the onset of diuresis, fluids may be restricted for about six hours and the urine output carefully measured; a distinct decrease in urine volume strongly suggests that excess fluids are being given.

C. **Nonoliguric renal failure** Treatment of this disorder requires replacement of electrolytes and water as dictated by urinary losses. Therapeutic errors occur when fixed urine volumes are not recognized and overhydration is produced, or when mercurial diuretics or inordinate amounts of potassium are administered.

D. **Obstructive uropathy** has formerly been called "postrenal azotemia." Obstruction, which may occur at any point in the urinary tract, must be considered in all cases of acute renal failure (especially in cases with anuria), for it is a potentially reversible lesion; when not relieved in 4–7 days permanent renal damage will result. It is preferable to avoid instrumentation of the urinary tract in establishing the diagnosis. Intravenous pyelography combined with laminagraphy of the kidneys and excretory tract may be valuable in determining the presence of obstruction; even when the serum creatinine has risen to 5 mg/100 ml, concentration of the dye may be adequate to demonstrate dilatation of the ureters and calyceal system. When there is a strong suspicion that ureteral obstruction may be present, one ureter should be catheterized to ascertain its patency.

Postobstructive diuresis describes the clinical state that can occur after relief of severe urinary tract obstruction. Marked polyuria, associated with the excretion of large amounts of sodium and potassium, may occur. Although self-limited, the diuresis may be of such degree and duration as to cause marked contraction of extracellular fluid volume and peripheral vascular collapse. Effective therapy requires the prompt quantitative replacement of urinary losses of water, sodium, and potassium. If infusions of electrolyte solutions are given rapidly, they should be warmed to body temperature.

II. **CHRONIC RENAL INSUFFICIENCY** Chronic progressive renal diseases are characterized by irreversible loss of a large part of the functional nephron population. In many instances a specific etiologic diagnosis cannot be established; chronic pyelonephritis and chronic glomerulonephritis are the most common causes. Most patients with chronic progressive renal disease (except for those with such conditions as diabetic nephropathy, amyloidosis, multiple myeloma, and the collagen diseases) have small, contracted kidneys; laminagrams of the kidneys may therefore aid in differentiating these patients from those who have acute renal failure. Management is directed toward maintaining the functional capabilities of the residual urine-forming nephrons. Patients with advanced degrees of renal insufficiency may be maintained in relative comfort and continue as productive members of society. Reversible decreases in renal function contribute significantly to the morbidity and mortality of patients with chronic renal disease. When the glomerular filtration rate is less than 30 ml/min, small reductions in GFR result in large increments in urea nitrogen concentration, and apparent deterioration of renal function should not be automatically considered as evidence of a preterminal disease. Sodium and water depletion, obstruction, infection, physiologic stress, congestive heart failure, hypercalcemia, and nephrotoxic agents are the most important causes of reversible decreases in renal function. Accurate estimations of GFR are important in management, and the importance of serial determinations cannot be overstated. At glomerular filtration rates < 20 ml/min the urea clearance underestimates and the creatinine clearance overestimates the true GFR. However, a simple mean of these two values approaches satisfactorily the inulin clearance (true GFR).

A. General measures　Patients should be encouraged to be as active as possible in order to minimize protein catabolism. Therapeutic multivitamins should be given to those patients with anorexia and limited food intake. Adjustments in drug dosage and the management of convulsions, nausea, pruritus, hiccups, anemia, and infection are discussed in the preceding section, I. Acute Renal Failure.

B. Diet

   1. Calories　Caloric intake should exceed 2000 cal/day ideally. When anorexia, nausea, or vomiting is severe, as is often the case in patients with "end-stage" renal disease, butter-sugar mixtures or commercially available carbohydrate-fat supplements, as previously described, may be given.

   2. Protein　Most patients with azotemia are in negative nitrogen balance and should be given 50–60 gm of protein daily unless progressive acidosis, hyperkalemia, or hyperphosphatemia is present. In these situations protein should be limited to 20–30 gm daily and should be of high biologic value (i.e., high in essential amino acids) to minimize negative nitrogen balance.

   A strict Giovannetti-type diet (18–20 gm protein supplemented by essential amino acids) can be expected to alleviate uremic symptoms in patients whose GFR is between 2–5 ml/min if followed for over one month. Glomerular filtration rates greater than 10 ml/min do not require protein restriction (*Proc. Roy. Soc. Med.* 59:665, 1966).

   3. Salt　Uremia per se is not an indication for salt restriction; most patients with chronic renal disease can be given 4–7 gm salt daily (essentially a normal diet without added table salt). However, in certain situations there may be either a sodium-losing tendency or elaboration of urine that is practically salt-free. In instances in which the patient's exact sodium requirement is unknown, give a 1-gm NaCl diet for four days; on the fourth day measure the 24-hour urinary sodium. Then give 8 gm NaCl/day for four days; on the fourth day again measure the 24-hour urinary sodium. (Better balance data will be obtained if the patient is given a 1–2-gm salt diet throughout this 8-day period, and the additional salt supplied in packets of known amount; this can be added to certain foods, and the patient instructed to eat the entire portions of those foods to which the salt has been added.) From these two values, plus daily measurements of plasma sodium and body weight, the optimal salt intake may be estimated. Patients who require more than 8–9 gm salt daily frequently need supplemental salt in the form of NaCl tablets (enteric-coated tablets should be avoided because they are irregularly absorbed) or bouillon (one cube contains about 3.5 gm salt). Some patients requiring $NaHCO_3$ for the treatment of acidosis will tolerate the increased sodium load without fluid retention and weight gain. If these do occur, the intake of NaCl should be decreased by 1.5 gm (25 mEq Na+) for each 2 gm of $NaHCO_3$ (24 mEq Na+) given.

C. Fluids　Relatively fixed urinary osmolalities and an obligatory solute load render most patients with renal failure unable to conserve water and salt; they cannot withstand prolonged periods of fluid deprivation. Dehydration with reduction of extracellular fluid volume further compromises renal function and must be avoided. If appetite is unimpaired no arbitrary value need be set for fluid intake, which should be ad lib with an additional 200–400 ml at bedtime. Supplemental fluids will be required during very hot weather to compensate for sweat losses, and during intercurrent illnesses with fever, nausea, vomiting, or diarrhea. In those cases in which it is necessary to expand the ECF volume, the synthetic ECF mixture previously described will be useful.

D. Congestive heart failure Use of digitalis is described in the preceding section on acute renal failure. Although diuretics have previously been thought to be of limited value (response to mercurials and to thiazides is poor when the GFR is below 20 ml/min, and both drugs reduce the GFR in experimental situations), newer compounds have been found to be useful. Furosemide and ethacrynic acid are usually effective even in the face of severe renal impairment. Large doses of either drug are surprisingly well tolerated and do not result in postdiuresis reduction in creatinine clearance if the plasma volume is not depleted. A more rational approach to diuresis in the uremic patient with edema involves restriction of salt and water intake so that negative balance is induced. A rice diet with less than 500 mg NaCl/day may be given, but the patient must be observed closely because true sodium depletion may develop.

E. Hypertension Mild elevations of diastolic blood pressure do not require treatment, and attempts to reduce these to normal may result in deterioration of renal function; diastolic pressures of 100–110 mm Hg are optimal in many patients. When hypertension is either more severe or symptomatic, treatment is then necessary; methyldopa 250 mg 1–4 times daily is particularly useful in managing hypertension in many patients with chronic renal insufficiency. The blood pressure must be "titrated" against the glomerular filtration rate to arrive at the proper balance (i.e., the best control of blood pressure which can be achieved without deleterious effects on renal function) for each patient. A minority opinion holds that most patients will eventually tolerate diastolic pressures of near normal values (90 mm Hg) if they can be maintained through the period of deterioration which follows reductions of this magnitude. The management of hypertension in general, and of hypertensive encephalopathy, is discussed in Chapter 7.

F. Hyponatremia may be dilutional; or a true sodium deficit may exist associated with signs of ECF volume contraction and deteriorating renal function. In this latter situation urgent correction with synthetic ECF (and $NaHCO_3$ in addition if acidosis is present) is necessary.

Remember: An extremely common cause of clinical deterioration in patients with chronic renal disease is uncontrolled negative salt balance, which may occur without concomitant hyponatremia. This complication tends to develop because of low-salt diets and/or anorexia with limitation of food intake. Many uremic patients seen for the first time have true salt depletion and are markedly benefited by cautious expansion of the ECF volume with synthetic ECF.

G. Hyperkalemia and hypokalemia Minimal to moderate nonprogressive elevation of the serum potassium in severe chronic renal failure generally requires no treatment; occasionally it is necessary to restrict dietary potassium. Marked hyperkalemia does not develop, as a rule, until renal function has deteriorated most severely.

Hypokalemia resulting from anorexia, vomiting, diarrhea, or potassium loss by the kidneys may require administration of potassium supplements.

H. Acidosis per se is not treated unless the CO_2 is less than 15 mEq/L and/or symptoms are present. Reduction of protein catabolism is an important measure, since the majority of metabolic acids are derived from this source; administration of exogenous acids (e.g., methionine, NH_4Cl, etc.) should be discontinued.

I. Hypocalcemia and hyperphosphatemia The major therapeutic goal in controlling abnormalities of calcium-phosphorus metabolism is reduction of the elevated phosphate level, which may be attempted by decreasing protein catabolism, eliminating foods high in protein and phosphate (e.g., milk), and binding phosphate in the gut, thereby decreasing its absorption. The last may be achieved by administering aluminum carbonate gel (Basaljel) 30–50 ml QID; its phosphate-binding capacity is greater than that of aluminum hydroxide gel. Gelusil should not be given because it contains added phosphate. The tendency to hypermagnesemia has been aggravated by magnesium-containing antacids, and their use is not recommended.

Hypocalcemia is frequently asymptomatic, particularly if some degree of acidosis is present; as the elevated phosphate level falls the serum calcium will rise. Generally no other therapy is required. Oral administration of calcium alone is rarely beneficial, but administration of moderate to large doses of vitamin D may partially correct the hypocalcemia in some cases in which absorption of calcium is impaired. When frank tetany occurs 10–30 ml 10% calcium gluconate should be given IV slowly. Calcium carbonate tablets or liquid (2 tablets or 30 ml QID) may be used. Caution must be exercised when vitamin D and $CaCO_3$ are administered, especially when $NaHCO_3$ is given concomitantly. Life-threatening hypercalcemia has resulted in some patients given this combination of drugs.

J. Osteomalacia and osteitis fibrosa Hyperparathyroidism routinely accompanies advanced renal insufficiency. In some patients the accompanying bone disease is a major part of their illness and should be treated with vitamin D and calcium under close supervision. In addition the hyperfunctioning parathyroid glands sometimes become autonomous (so-called tertiary hyperparathyroidism). Subtotal parathyroidectomy may be indicated for some patients with renal osteodystrophy.

K. Hyperuricemia Modest hyperuricemia may develop in renal insufficiency but rarely reaches concentrations > 10–12 mg/100 ml. Frank gouty attacks are rare except in those individuals with associated gout. Present evidence suggests that allopurinol in usual doses decreases serum uric acid levels in these patients without adversely affecting GFR (*Ann. Rheum. Dis.* 25:681, 1966).

L. Dialysis When an intercurrent event such as congestive heart failure, severe infection, or surgical operation contributes to clinical deterioration, dialysis may be very beneficial in ameliorating the uremic symptoms and restoring the patient to his previous state; peritoneal dialysis is usually preferred in these circumstances. (A brief discussion of chronic dialysis and transplantation appears at the end of this chapter.)

III.   NEPHROTIC SYNDROME   The nephrotic syndrome is characterized by increased glomerular permeability to protein, resulting in marked proteinuria (usually greater than 3.5 gm daily in adults without marked depression of the glomerular filtration rate), and the urinary excretion of doubly refractile fat bodies; edema, hypoproteinuria, and hyperlipemia occur to a variable degree. More common underlying diseases include glomerulonephritis, diabetes mellitus, systemic lupus erythematosus, amyloidosis, and renal vein thrombosis; the nephrotic syndrome may also occur in association with constrictive pericarditis or prolonged severe right-sided congestive heart failure, and exposure to certain allergens, drugs, or nephrotoxins. An underlying disease may not be demonstrable.

By correlating clinical and physiologic data and by carefully examining the urinary sediment, a reasonable diagnosis may be reached in some cases; in others, however, histologic examination of renal tissue (preferably with electron microscopy as well as light microscopy) may be required in order to establish a definitive diagnosis. Percutaneous needle biopsy is a relatively safe and effective means of obtaining renal tissue in most patients; open biopsy (through a small flank incision), however, should be performed in those patients who are uncooperative, severely hypertensive, or have a GFR of less than 20 ml/min. In order to minimize postbiopsy complications, markedly uremic patients should be dialyzed prior to open biopsy, and severely edematous patients diuresed, if possible. The protocol for renal biopsy is given at the end of this chapter.

Whether or not corticosteroids are used in the treatment of the nephrotic syndrome will usually depend on the etiology, the level of renal function, and the degree of apparent irreversible structural changes seen in the biopsy sections. Most observers agree that corticosteroids are ineffective in the treatment of nephrosis due to amyloid disease, Kimmelstiel-Wilson disease, or advanced glomerulonephritis; in other situations, however, their administration may favorably influence the natural history of the disease. Treatment of the nephrotic syndrome is discussed below.

A. General measures

1. If edema is severe, a low-sodium diet (500 mg/day) should be prescribed.

2. Protein intake should be 90–120 gm/day unless uremia is present.

3. Total caloric intake should be 25–50 cal/kg body weight/day.

4. All infections should be treated promptly; antibiotics should not be given prophylactically.

5. Diuretics may be used if renal insufficiency is not severe. Combination of spironolactone and a thiazide may be especially beneficial. Careful monitoring of the serum potassium should be employed in patients whose creatinine clearance is < 50 ml/min. When the GFR is < 25 ml/min, the use of spironolactone is not indicated because severe hyperkalemia may ensue. Some observers recommend that mercurials not be given to patients with the ne-

phrotic syndrome because of reports of oliguria and increasing renal insufficiency following their administration.

6. Salt-free albumin is of only transient value in inducing diuresis. In a severe emergency situation 25–50 gm may be given IV over a 30–60-minute period.

B. Corticosteroids Those patients who would appear to benefit from steroid administration, as discussed previously, should be given prednisone 40–60 mg/day (or equivalent dosage of another preparation) ; therapy should be initiated in the hospital. When proteinuria ceases or stabilizes at a lower value, maintenance doses of steroids may be given. If no significant response (as manifested by decreasing values for 24-hour excretion of protein) has occurred by 28 days, continued daily steroid administration is of little value, as a rule, except for promoting diuresis in those patients who are refractory to other diuretic measures.

1. Evidence suggests that side effects of steroids may be reduced by giving them intermittently (see discussion of steroids in Chapter 16) ; prednisone 40–60 mg once every 48 hours may be given for maintenance therapy. The BUN rise often seen following steroid administration does not necessitate discontinuing therapy unless a significant decrease in GFR can be demonstrated.

2. Treatment should be continued for at least one year, perhaps indefinitely. The GFR and 24-hour protein excretion should be measured frequently and the patient carefully reevaluated at yearly intervals in order to decide whether or not to continue therapy; unfortunately, well-defined criteria to assist in making this decision do not exist.

3. Steroid administration may be continued during periods of infections.

4. For severe anasarca that is incapacitating and unresponsive to the usual measures, the following regimen produces diuresis in a high percentage of cases, but it is fraught with dangers, especially sudden expansion of intravascular volume and cardiac decompensation. This program must be used only in hospitalized patients.

a) Give hydrocortisone 400–500 mg daily for 10 days. Diuretics and salt restriction may be continued as needed.

b) Discontinue hydrocortisone on the tenth day.

c) After 24 hours give 400 ml 12% dextran in water mixed with 50 ml 50% glucose IV over a period of six hours. Observe the patient closely for signs of intravascular volume expansion, and measure the central venous pressure frequently. The dextran mixture may be repeated in 48 hours if diuresis does not occur.

d) If no response occurs after the second dextran infusion, repeat the entire regimen, administering the hydrocortisone for 18 days instead of 10 days; on each of the last 7 days of treatment give IV 12.5 gm salt-free albumin in addition.

C. Other measures Recent studies indicate that immunosuppressive agents, particularly antimetabolites such as 6-thioguanine, 6-mercaptopurine, and azathioprine may be of benefit in the treatment of certain patients with the nephrotic syndrome. This includes those individuals responsive to corticosteroids but debilitated by the complications of large dosage (who may respond well to antimetabolites either alone or in combination with reduced dosage of steroids) and certain patients not responsive to corticosteroids (who may obtain significant benefit from antimetabolites alone). The toxicity of these drugs, however, dictates that they be used only in special circumstances and by experienced personnel under carefully controlled conditions.

IV. **URINARY TRACT INFECTIONS** Pyelonephritis is the most common cause of chronic renal insufficiency, accounting for the majority of all deaths (in autopsy series) due to renal failure; the 2–20% incidence of pyelonephritis at autopsy remains essentially unchanged despite the widespread use of antibiotics. In most instances it is virtually impossible to distinguish lower urinary tract infections from actual infection of the renal parenchyma; furthermore, as many as 40% of patients with bacteriuria have or will develop renal involvement. For these reasons, treatment of lower urinary tract infections should be just as vigorous as if the kidney itself were involved.

The goal of therapy in pyelonephritis is preservation of nephrons; to achieve this goal one must delineate any predisposing causes to infection (vascular abnormalities, obstruction, reflux, etc.) and deal with them appropriately. In acute pyelonephritis bacteriuria should be eradicated. In chronic pyelonephritis that is not usually possible, but repeated efforts should be made to suppress bacteriuria in an attempt to decelerate progression of the disease process. There may be an advantage in urging high fluid intake if renal insufficiency is not severe; protoplasts, which may play a role (even though not precisely defined at present) in chronic infections, can be lysed in a hypotonic medium.

A. Diagnosis

1. A properly collected and promptly plated clean-voided midstream urine specimen (CVS) that yields 100,000 or more bacteria/ml on quantitative culture is usually diagnostic of a urinary tract infection. (If immediate plating of the urine is not possible, the specimen should be refrigerated until it can be processed.) The presence of more than 10^5 bacteria/ml carries an 80% likelihood that a second CVS will give a similar count; two positive clean-voided specimens (or one catheterized specimen) give approximately 95% correlation with the presence of a urinary tract infection.

2. If bacteria are seen with methylene blue stain of fresh unspun urinary sediment, at least 10^5 bacteria/ml of urine are usually present.

3. Catheterization should be avoided if possible. The incidence of recognizable bacteriuria after a single catheterization is 1–3%, but bacteria are seeded into the bladder in much higher percentage; these are frequently organisms that are resistant to many antibiotics and therefore difficult to eradicate.

   In a few situations in which an uncontaminated CVS cannot be obtained, a single careful catheterization may be performed by the physician, using sterile technique and lubricating the catheter tip with neomycin ointment. An alternative technique, used routinely in some institutions, is the aspiration of bladder urine by midline suprapubic needle puncture after surgical preparation and local anesthesia of the puncture site. Advantages claimed for this technique are virtual elimination of contamination of the bladder by bacteria and minimal discomfort to the patient. The patient should be well hydrated and instructed not to void so that the bladder is easily palpable at the time of the procedure.

B. Treatment For proper treatment the organism should be identified and antibiotic-sensitivity studies performed. In acute pyelonephritis it is necessary to begin therapy with a broad-spectrum antibiotic before culture results are known; a different antibiotic may be substituted subsequently if the results of sensitivity studies so dictate.

1. Asymptomatic bacteriuria in pregnant women should be treated because a significant percentage of these patients, if untreated, will develop clinical pyelonephritis during the course of their pregnancy.

2. On rare occasions patients present with a picture strongly suggestive of pyelonephritis and with abnormal sediment but negative urine cultures; renal biopsy evidence suggests that carefully obtained urine cultures occasionally may be negative in face of active interstitial pyelonephritis or complete obstruction. In such cases a course of antibiotic therapy is warranted.

3. Bladder neck obstruction, when present, should be relieved surgically.

4. Antibiotic selection is discussed in Chapter 9.

5. Papillary necrosis is a fulminant variety of pyelonephritis. This complication should be considered in patients with infections associated with diabetes mellitus, lower urinary tract obstruction, and instrumentation of the urinary tract, and in those who are phenacetin abusers. The diagnosis is substantiated by identification of sloughed tissue in freshly voided urine filtered through cheesecloth, or occasionally by radiographic contrast procedures. These patients are more resistant to bacteriologic cure, have more symptomatic relapses, and have a higher incidence of hypertension than patients with less severe pyelonephritis.

6. Noneradicable infections, which may be present in up to 80% of patients with chronic pyelonephritis, are often asymptomatic; bacteriostatic therapy and urinary acidification may be of great importance in suppressing bacteriuria. The following agents may be used for long-term bacteriostatic therapy:

   a) **Sulfisoxazole** 1–2 gm/day in divided dosage, or other sulfa preparations as listed in Chapter 9. Remember that patients with renal insufficiency may develop very high blood levels of the drug, and dosage may require reduction accordingly.

   b) **Nitrofurantoin (Furadantin),** though more expensive and associated with a higher incidence of adverse reactions, may be given in a dosage of 50–100 mg 3–4 times daily.

   c) **Methenamine mandelate (Mandelamine)** 1.0 gm QID. Urine pH must be kept at 5.0 or less if bacteriostasis is to be effective; it is for this reason that DL-methionine is often given concurrently.

   d) **DL-methionine** The sulfur group of this amino acid is oxidized to sulfate with the release of hydrogen ions into the blood; a profound decrease in urine pH results. Because marked systemic acidosis may develop after administration of large doses (particularly in patients with renal insufficiency), the drug should not be given to patients with preexisting acidosis. DL-methionine is available as a powder costing 1–2 cents/gm (in capsule form its cost is many times higher) ; the initial dose is 6 gm/day in divided dosage, and the amount given may be increased up to 15 gm/day if necessary to maintain the urine pH at less than 5. The drug may be administered in cranberry juice, which has a high concentration of hippuric acid. The patient should be taught to monitor the pH of his urine once or twice daily and be given instructions in adjustment of the drug dosage to keep the pH below 5.0. Plasma CO_2 concentration and/or blood pH should be determined once or twice during the first several weeks of therapy.

7. When an indwelling catheter is inserted, the routine administration of antibiotics favors the emergence of resistant organisms; antibiotics, therefore, should not be given prophylactically. The indwelling catheter should be inserted under strict aseptic conditions; when the catheter is in place an antibiotic ointment, such as bacitracin or neomycin, should be applied to one or two inches of the catheter extending from the urethral meatus, and this area then wrapped in sterile gauze. All joints in the catheter collecting system should be prepared in the same manner; closed systems with a minimum number of joints are preferable. Continuous irrigation of the bladder with antibiotic solutions instilled through a triple-lumen catheter may more effectively reduce the incidence of infections (see Chapter 9).

V. **DIALYSIS AND TRANSPLANTATION**   The optimal method of dialysis varies with facilities available, training of personnel, and the specific clinical situation. A discussion of specific indications for dialysis in acute renal failure is beyond the scope of the Manual; in general, the trend in most centers is toward early and frequent dialyses in the management of patients with a worsening clinical picture or progressing chemical abnormalities; the procedure no longer represents a last heroic effort for dying patients.

The Renal Division at Washington University Medical Center employs peritoneal dialysis when possible; hemodialysis is performed only when the former is contraindicated or ineffective (as in the removal of certain drugs, such as glutethimide). Multiple hemodialyses have been made feasible by the development of Teflon-Silastic or all-Silastic arteriovenous shunts. Peritoneal dialysis is not associated with the acute fluctuations of blood pressure (in response to rapid changes in blood volume) that may occur with the artificial kidney, and the mechanics of the procedure (except for the insertion of the peritoneal catheter and prescription of the dialysis fluid) may be carried out by a nurse.

A 16–20-exchange peritoneal dialysis (one exchange per hour) is usually as effective as five to six hours of hemodialysis on the twin-coil artificial kidney. Hypertonic peritoneal exchanges (4.25% dextrose) are extremely effective in removing excess sodium and water and may be employed in the treatment of refractory edema of cardiac origin.

The feasibility of repeated dialysis in the management of patients with advanced chronic renal failure has been demonstrated, although the efficacy of long-term therapy cannot be completely evaluated at present; both chronic dialysis and transplantation (except in the case of identical twins in whom transplantation may be regarded as an established means of therapy) are still in the developmental stages. Neither must be undertaken without full consideration of the multiple facets involved. Until these techniques become generally established means for the treatment of patients with end-stage renal disease, one should manage such patients with the conservative measures previously described.

VI. PROTOCOL FOR PERCUTANEOUS RENAL BIOPSY Percutaneous renal biopsies should be performed only by experienced personnel. Open biopsy, rather than percutaneous, should be performed when patients are uncooperative or would not survive the loss of the biopsied kidney.

A. Preoperatively, obtain the following:

1. Consent.

2. Complete blood count (including platelet count), prothrombin time, clotting time, bleeding time, clot retraction, and Rumpel-Leede's test.

3. Intravenous pyelogram or other evidence that the patient has two functioning kidneys.

4. Blood type and cross-match of two units of whole blood to be on call in the blood bank on the day of biopsy.

5. Urine sediment examination within 24 hours before biopsy.

B. Postoperatively, note the following:

1. The patient should remain prone, on a sandbag, in the biopsy position, for one hour after completion of the procedure.

2. Vital signs should be checked very closely for 48 hours (at least every 5 minutes for the first hour, every 15 minutes for the next two hours, then every 30 minutes for the following two hours, etc.).

3. Complete bed rest should be enforced for 24 hours.

4. Fluid intake of at least 3000 ml, if tolerated, should be urged during the first 24 hours after biopsy.

5. Hematocrit or hemoglobin should be measured within 8 hours of biopsy, and then daily for at least 3 days.

6. Intake and output should be measured carefully for at least 3 days. All urine should be saved during this period, and the sediment examined daily. Once hematuria has disappeared, progressive ambulation may be allowed. Because delayed bleeding (up to two weeks after biopsy) may occur on rare occasions, the patient should be instructed to look at each urine specimen for discoloration suggestive of hematuria.

ANGINA PECTORIS

The pathophysiology of angina pectoris remains poorly understood. Although it is generally accepted that anginal pain originates in an area of ischemic cardiac muscle and does not occur in the normal heart, there is little new information to demonstrate the manner in which the pain is produced. The pain is influenced by so many factors, particularly emotional ones, that evaluation of treatment programs is almost impossible. Atypical chest pain may be mistakenly labeled as angina, and evaluation of therapy may be then further impaired. When serious question exists as to the etiology of atypical chest pain after thorough routine evaluation, selective coronary angiography may be indicated; in experienced hands this technique is becoming increasingly valuable in confirming or excluding the diagnosis of coronary artery disease. Even when the diagnosis of angina is clear, the objective evaluation of beneficial effects of antianginal drugs is difficult despite studies of coronary blood flow, selective coronary angiography, etc. The only point of consistent agreement is that nitrites are beneficial in relieving anginal pain (despite failure of abnormal ECG patterns to improve). The treatment of angina pectoris is designed to reduce the frequency and severity of attacks of chest pain; most important is a positive physician-patient relationship in which the physician maintains a supportive, reassuring, optimistic attitude. Measures that may be helpful are discussed below.

I. GENERAL CARE

A. Bed rest Patients should be instructed to avoid activity that produces chest pain. Bed rest is recommended when other efforts fail to reduce the frequency of attacks, when the pattern of chest pain changes and increases in severity, and when ECG changes of myocardial injury or ischemia develop. In these cases 1–2 weeks of bed rest followed by a period of reduced activity may be required. Specific periods of rest during the day, especially 30–60 minutes after meals, are advisable. Patients should be advised to sit in a chair rather than to lie in bed immediately after meals.

B. Exercise and exposure Mild forms of exercise that do not precipitate anginal attacks should be encouraged. Especially recommended is a twice-daily 15–20-minute walk on level ground (walking up an incline of 15% doubles the work of the heart). Patients should be cautioned to reduce activity during very cold or hot humid weather, when angina is often more severe.

C. Work The psychologic value of encouraging continuance of normal occupational duties, if possible, cannot be overestimated. Most persons may continue at their occupation, but when manual labor is involved and attacks of angina are frequent, it may be necessary to restrict activity or recommend a relatively sedentary job.

D. Diet   Important goals are restriction of calories for overweight patients and reduction of fat intake. The obese patient should reduce to normal body weight. The diet should contain 50–60 gm fat; saturated fats should probably be limited to one-third to one-half of the total fat intake. Large meals and heavy bedtime snacks should be discouraged; functional GI disturbances that may precipitate attacks of angina should be managed appropriately. Tea and coffee may be allowed in moderate quantities unless they interfere with sleep or precipitate chest pain or cardiac arrhythmias.

E. Reduction of serum lipids   Atherosclerosis is a disease process associated with disordered lipid metabolism. Abnormalities (usually elevation) may occur in the serum concentration of total lipids, phospholipids, cholesterol, triglycerides, and lipoproteins, but no diagnostic pattern can be defined. Although data from current prospective epidemiologic studies, such as the Framingham study, do suggest that hyperlipemia (as well as other factors such as obesity, hypertension, diabetes, cigarette smoking, etc.) is associated with an increased risk of coronary heart disease, there are no unequivocal data to indicate that lowering of serum lipids will affect the incidence of coronary heart disease or reverse established atherosclerotic changes. Nonetheless, numerous drugs have been used in attempts to reduce serum lipids; most are of limited efficacy, and some are associated with significant side effects. Whether or not to administer such agents remains a matter of personal philosophy at present, but most physicians do recommend dietary restriction of fat as discussed above. Clofibrate (Atromid-S) has been shown to lower plasma lipids significantly in about 75% of patients, especially in those with high plasma levels of both cholesterol and triglycerides. Adverse reactions include weight gain in about 40% of patients, prolongation of prothrombin time in patients receiving prothrombin-depressant medication, and an occasional rise in SGOT and SGPT of doubtful clinical significance. Administration of the drug should be discontinued if there is no reduction in lipid levels after 3 months. The daily adult dose is 2 gm; the drug is not recommended for pregnant women and patients with renal or hepatic impairment.

Nicotinic acid in doses of 1.0–1.5 gm TID with meals may lower serum cholesterol, triglycerides, and to a lesser extent phospholipids, but numerous undesirable side effects may occur: nausea, vomiting, gastric irritation, dryness and brownish pigmentation of the skin, hyperuricemia, decreased glucose tolerance, hepatic dysfunction, and occasionally cholestatic jaundice. Dextrothyroxine also may lower serum cholesterol, but in truly effective dosage calorigenic effects are significant and angina may be aggravated or cardiac arrythmias precipitated. Sitosterol in doses of 3–6 gm immediately before meals and 1–2 gm before snacks may retard intestinal absorption of cholesterol. Other agents recommended with varying enthusiasm include estrogens and cholestyramine.

F. Smoking   Cigarette smoking is associated with an increased risk of coronary heart disease; nicotine per se may induce vasospasm and aggravate preexisting angina. Patients should be encouraged to discontinue smoking if possible, bearing in mind that anxiety symptoms, increased appetite, and weight gain are frequent sequelae to cessation.

G. **Other contributing factors** Tension and anxiety are common precipitating causes of angina, and administration of sedatives or tranquilizers is an important part of the therapy. Diseases of the GI and biliary tracts (particularly duodenal ulcer, hiatus hernia, cholelithiasis) that may precipitate attacks of angina should be treated appropriately.

II. DRUG THERAPY

A. **Nitrites** Their mechanism of action is a subject of controversy. Although nitrites cause general vasodilatation, relief of anginal pain is not believed related to coronary-artery dilatation and increased coronary blood flow, but rather to the effectiveness of nitrites in reducing cardiac workload. The drugs reduce systemic and pulmonary arterial pressure and decrease cardiac output. Myocardial oxygen consumption is not changed. It is important to start therapy with a minimum dose, e.g., 0.3 mg, and increase until an optimum level is reached. Nitrites are generally contraindicated in glaucoma. They should be used cautiously in patients suspected of having an acute myocardial infarction.

1. **Glyceryl trinitrate (nitroglycerin)** is dispensed in tablets of 0.3, 0.4, and 0.6 mg (1/200, 1/150, 1/100 gr); they should be dissolved sublingually or in the buccal pouch. Tablets usually dissolve within 20 seconds and produce lasting relief of pain within 2–3 minutes. Unpleasant side effects include sensations of warmth, flushing, occasional throbbing headaches, and varying degrees of dizziness. The drugs should be used prophylactically during activity that is likely to produce pain. If any episode of chest pain does not subside with rest and 3–6 tablets taken at 3-minute intervals, the patient should be instructed to call his physician. Advantages of nitroglycerin tablets include ease of carrying, relatively long duration of action, and uniformity of effect. Patients should be instructed to purchase a month's supply of tablets rather than larger quantities, for the tablets may become hard, dry, and inert with aging.

2. **Long-acting nitrates** The clinical effectiveness of such preparations remains disputed despite animal experiments reporting drug-induced stimulation of collateral circulation after occlusion of a main coronary artery. Nonetheless, they are widely used in the hope of reducing the frequency of attacks of chest pain; they are valueless in acute attacks when administered orally. Many observers believe that maximum beneficial effects are not achieved because of inadequate dosage and rigid dosage schedules that are not tailored to the patient's pattern of activity. The drugs are usually given orally, although onset of action is more rapid and reduction of pain more consistent after sublingual administration. Several of the available preparations and the usual dosage are listed below; larger doses may be given if they are required and if the side effect of headache does not become too annoying.

    a) **Isosorbide dinitrate (Isordil)** is available in 5-mg sublingual tablets, and 10-mg tablets or 40-mg sustained-action tablets (Isordil Tembids) for oral administration. Usual dose range is

5–10 mg sublingually every 4 hours (preferred), 5–30 mg orally QID, or one 40-mg Tembid BID.

b) **Pentaerythritol tetranitrate (Peritrate)** is available in 10- and 20-mg tablets, and in 80-mg sustained-release tablets (Peritrate-SA); the usual dosage is 10–20 mg QID, but may be raised to 40 mg TID if necessary. The dose of sustained-release tablets is 80 mg BID.

c) **Erythrityl tetranitrate (Cardilate)** is available in tablets of 5, 10, and 15 mg; usual dosage is 5–15 mg QID sublingually (preferred) or orally, but may be raised to 30 mg TID if necessary. The drug can cause a drop in systolic blood pressure.

B. **Dipyridamole (Persantine)** is said to be an effective antianginal agent which increases coronary blood flow and enhances myocardial utilization of oxygen, but careful evaluation of the clinical effectiveness of this drug is lacking. At least one recent double-blind controlled study found no significant difference between the drug and placebo (*J.A.M.A.* 201:865, 1967), but the literature should be watched for further controlled studies. Recommended average dosage is 25 mg TID–QID. Side effects include mild gastrointestinal distress, nausea, weakness, dizziness, and (after large dosage) hypotension and syncope.

C. **Propranolol (Inderal)** is a beta adrenergic blocking agent with fewer and less serious side effects than the original prototype drug, pronethalol. Several studies have now shown this drug, in adequate dosage, to be an effective antianginal agent (*Amer. J. Cardiol.* 18:345, 1966). Although without significant effect in the normal person at rest, propranolol decreases heart rate, cardiac output, mean arterial pressure, left ventricular work, and maximum O_2 uptake; and increases A-V oxygen difference, ventricular size, stroke volume, and systolic ejection time during exercise. Mild coronary vasoconstriction has been found in some cases, blockade of vasoconstriction in others. It is thought to be beneficial in angina by favorably altering the balance between available oxygen and myocardial work. The dose range for significant antianginal activity appears to be between 90 and 400 mg daily, with a mode of 200–400 mg daily. The effect appears to be dose-related. Initially low doses are given, e.g. 10 mg QID. Increasing the dose to obtain a pulse rate of 55–60 beats/min after 2 minutes rest supine is a reasonable guide. Side effects are usually minor: nausea and vomiting, mild diarrhea, visual disturbances, fatigue, dizziness, and rash. Rarely, hypotension occurs. Congestive heart failure may be precipitated or aggravated. Heart block is usually worsened. Asthma and pulmonary insufficiency are other relative contraindications to its use. (Mechanism of action, clinical applications, and toxic effects are summarized in *New Eng. J. Med.* 275:1106, 1175, 1966.)

D. **Xanthines** These drugs, particularly theophylline, dilate coronary arteries and increase coronary blood flow, but they increase cardiac work; their exact mechanism of action in relieving anginal pain is unknown. Intravenous administration is more effective than oral because oral preparations are poorly absorbed. The best oral xanthine is a hydroalcoholic solution of theophylline (Elixophyllin) containing 80 mg theophylline per 15 ml. Recommended dose is 30–45 ml QID.

E. **Digitalis** Several studies have shown that left heart failure as manifested by increased wedge pressure and pulmonary artery pressure occurs during attacks of angina pectoris. Although symptoms of overt congestive heart failure are absent, administration of full doses of digitalis and/or diuretics may benefit patients with "refractory angina."

III. **SURGERY** Selective revascularization of the myocardium by internal mammary artery implantation into a blind tunnel in the myocardium appears to be a promising development in the treatment of intractible angina pectoris (*New Eng. J. Med.* 275:283, 1966; *Amer. J. Cardiol.* 19:344, 1967). In experienced hands the procedure results in long-term patency of the implanted artery in 80% of patients, sustained relief of angina in 60–80% or more after a lapse of 3 to 6 months postoperatively, and objective improvement in myocardial metabolism and vascularization; unfortunately no suitable control group exists for the surgically treated patients.

Another indication for surgery at present is a history of multiple myocardial infarctions in a young patient. Further selection of acceptable patients depends on selective coronary angiography. Currently, significant left coronary disease is prerequisite; more than 50% stenosis (either single or multiple) of the left anterior descending artery or of the left circumflex artery, or both, is an ideal pattern for selection. Associated disease of the right coronary artery is acceptable, provided it does not predominate. These current selection conditions may broaden in the near future if more extensive and more successful revascularization procedures gain acceptance.

Current contraindications to this surgical approach include a myocardial infarction within the last 6 months, severe congestive heart failure, marked left ventricular dilatation, and multiple or massive ventricular aneurysms. Operative mortality at the present time is around 4% for patients with angina only on effort, and around 20% for patients with angina at rest. The pertinent literature should be followed closely in this rapidly advancing area.

IV. **ANTICOAGULATION** The administration of anticoagulants to patients with angina pectoris remains controversial. The problem is discussed briefly in the paragraphs on anticoagulants in the section on myocardial infarction.

V. **RADIOACTIVE IODINE** Radioactive iodine (RAI) therapy is rarely used now at Washington University Medical Center for the treatment of angina pectoris. Its use should be reserved for those few patients with incapacitating angina, constant for more than 6 months, who are refractory to standard therapeutic measures and are unacceptable for surgical therapy. The aim of RAI administration is ablation of thyroid function; a "balanced hypothyroidism" is then maintained with thyroid hormone therapy so as to allow the patient the least amount of angina with the least possible degree of hypometabolism. Contraindications to RAI therapy include preexisting myxedema and recent myocardial infarction. Approximately 70% of patients will note a decrease in the severity of their angina pectoris.

MYOCARDIAL INFARCTION

Myocardial infarction is a medical emergency requiring careful management during the acute phase; once the infarct has healed the prognosis for a long and useful life may be good.

I. **GENERAL MEASURES** Rest is of prime importance. The room should be quiet; visitors should be limited to members of the immediate family and visits should be brief. Rectal examinations should not be performed; oral rather than rectal temperatures should be recorded. The seriously ill patient should not shave or feed himself initially; cigarette smoking should not be allowed. Nurses should be instructed to answer the patient's calls immediately.

Many medical centers have established coronary-care centers in the hope of significantly reducing mortality by providing constant electrical monitoring of cardiac rate and rhythm, constant nursing and house-staff care, and ready availability of electrical equipment for the treatment of cardiac arrhythmias. Patients may remain in such units for the first 5–7 days of their illness, when complications are most common. Data from such centers show a definite decrease in mortality from arrhythmias and asystole following acute myocardial infarction. Evaluation of the effect of the coronary-care unit on overall mortality is more difficult because of variability in admission policies, diagnostic criteria for acute infarction, length of stay, competence of nursing and house staff, population characteristics at the various centers, etc. Nevertheless, it does appear that overall survival is improving, some centers recently reporting as much as 20–30% reduction in overall mortality.

II. **REST**

A. Although the average myocardial infarction requires 6 weeks to heal, hospitalization with enforced rest must be adjusted to the individual case; generally the patient is hospitalized 3–4 weeks.

B. **Bed rest vs. armchair treatment**

1. Many physicians believe that most patients, even "poor risk" patients when not in shock, do better if allowed to sit in a bedside chair for a short period several times daily. Advantages include increased mental and physical comfort, easier ventilation, decreased risk of peripheral venous stasis with thrombosis and embolism, and decreased incidence of hypostatic pneumonia, urinary retention, and severe constipation. The patient must be transported from bed to chair with an absolute minimum of effort on his part, for active exertion nullifies all the advantages of chair rest.

2. Most physicians at the Washington University Medical Center enforce bed rest for 7–10 days, then allow chair rest. Patients kept in bed should be instructed to move their toes and feet actively to prevent venous congestion; the legs of patients with venous insufficiency or edema should be wrapped with elastic bandages or stockings.

C. Gradually increasing ambulatory activity is allowed after 3–4 weeks, depending on clinical and laboratory evidences of healing. Resumption of former activities in the 2–6-month postconvalescent period is also dictated by the clinical course. Some patients may never return to their previous pace.

III. DIET For the first few days the diet should be liquid or soft, low in salt, fat, and carbohydrate, and easily digestible. Very hot or cold liquids and solids should not be given during the first several weeks, for they may cause vagal stimulation and cardiac arrhythmias. As the patient improves and appetite increases, a more liberal diet may be allowed.

IV. BOWEL CARE Constipation is an almost constant problem and should be prevented, if possible, by the routine administration of stool softeners and mild laxatives. Most patients undergo much less physical and emotional stress if allowed the use of a bedside commode rather than a bedpan; they must be helped to and from the commode.

V. CONTROL OF PAIN Pain engenders severe anxiety; it should be treated promptly with adequate doses of effective drugs. Morphine, the drug of choice, in doses of 10–15 mg may be given every 2–4 hours (occasionally more often) as needed. Atropine may be given to block the vagal effects. Demerol, in doses of 75–125 mg, is slightly less effective and may cause significant parasympatholytic effects and tachycardia. Oxygen should be administered routinely as long as significant pain persists. Recurrent or persistent pain may indicate progressive myocardial damage and is a bad prognostic sign; other causes, particularly pulmonary infarction, must be considered.

VI. SEDATION Adequate sedation is most important. Phenobarbital or short-acting barbiturates (amobarbital, butabarbital), chloral hydrate, and chlordiazepoxide (Librium) are effective drugs.

VII. **OXYGEN** administration is indicated in the presence of shock, heart failure, cyanosis, persistent pain, dyspnea, and Cheyne-Stokes respirations, but caution must be exercised in patients with chronic lung disease and pulmonary insufficiency. Oxygen is often administered routinely during the first 24 hours or so to the patient with an uncomplicated myocardial infarction.

VIII. COMPLICATIONS

    A. Congestive heart failure represents a serious complication of myocardial infarction (mortality rate almost doubled) and should be treated promptly as described in the chapter on that subject. Careful auscultation for a ventricular or a new atrial diastolic gallop, chest x-ray examination for hilar congestion, and measurement of central venous pressure are important in its early detection before the more overt signs and symptoms of congestive heart failure supervene. Because patients with recent myocardial infarction may be more sensitive to digitalis (and thus the incidence of digitalis-induced arrhythmias may be increased), digitalization should be undertaken cautiously.

    B. Arrhythmias Cardiac arrhythmias, including VPCs, occur in 80–90% of patients with acute myocardial infarction and in the past have accounted for 40% of deaths. Emphasis is placed on prevention of death-producing arrhythmias or block by early and prompt treatment of the more benign electrical abnormalities which almost always precede them. (See Chapter 6, Cardiac Arrhythmias, for therapy in patients without acute myocardial infarction.) Special considerations in the treatment of these complications in patients with acute myocardial infarction are as follows:

1. Routine use of prophylactic quinidine, procaine amide, or other antiarrhythmic agent for the prevention of arrhythmias during the acute postinfarction phase is not advocated. The literature should be watched carefully for controlled studies on this subject.

2. If atrial premature contractions (APCs) occur frequently (2–3 per minute), in runs, or in a regular pattern, give quinidine 0.3 gm TID–QID. Larger doses may be required.

3. Supraventricular tachycardias unresponsive to the usual measures (see Chapter 6, Cardiac Arrhythmias) or causing rapid deterioration with shock and/or congestive heart failure should be terminated with cardioversion.

4. VPCs occur in 50–70% of patients with acute myocardial infarction and may herald ventricular tachycardia or fibrillation. They should be treated if they occur (a) in the vulnerable period of the cardiac cycle at or near the peak of the T wave, (b) in salvos of two or more, (c) frequently, e.g. more than 3–5 per minute, (d) from multiple foci. Such VPCs should be stopped promptly with a 25-mg, 50-mg, or up to 1–2-mg/kg injection of 2% lidocaine given rapidly IV; or procaine amide 50 mg IV every 1 or 2 minutes, monitoring blood pressure. Once the VPCs are terminated, prophylaxis is maintained for a variable interval with either a continuous IV infusion of 0.2–2.0% lidocaine to deliver 20–50 µg/kg/min (1.4–3.5 mg/min in a 70-kg patient), or procaine amide 500 mg p.o. or IM q8h up to 1000 mg p.o. or IM q6h if necessary (watching carefully for toxicity). Rarely other drugs such as diphenylhydantoin (Dilantin), propranolol (Inderal), or quinidine may have to be tried. Refractory ventricular irritability may respond to a temporary transvenous catheter pacemaker of sufficient rate to keep the ectopic focus suppressed.

5. Ventricular tachycardia unresponsive promptly to the usual IV medications (described in Chapter 6) should be terminated by cardioversion, with light thiopental anesthesia, if anesthesiologist and drug are immediately available, but without anesthesia if necessary in the emergency situation.

6. Sinus bradycardia, when transient, needs no treatment, but, if sustained, can cause a marked decrease in cardiac output with symptoms and signs of shock or can progress to nodal rhythm, ventricular escape beats, and ventricular tachycardia or fibrillation. Atropine 0.3–1.2 mg IV q4h, or an intravenous infusion of 0.1–0.2 mg isoproterenol per 100 ml 5% D/W sufficient to abolish the bradycardia without inducing ectopic beats, is effective. Refractory bradyarrhythmias may require a temporary transvenous catheter pacemaker.

7. Conduction disturbances occur in about 10% of patients, usually in the presence of congestive failure or shock. First-degree AV block may need no treatment per se but may progress to second-degree and complete AV block, the latter complication associated with a 50% mortality in this group of patients. Some centers

advocate the prophylactic insertion of a temporary transvenous catheter pacemaker on a stand-by basis in high-grade first-degree and second-degree AV block; it is then immediately available should complete block and its attendant complications of standstill, shock, congestive heart failure, or ventricular arrhythmias rapidly develop. Second-degree block is initially treated with an IV injection of 0.3–1.2 mg Atropine or, failing prompt abolition of the block, with IV infusion of a 0.1–0.2 mg/100 ml-solution of isoproterenol adjusted to maintain a heart rate of at least 60 beats per minute without evoking ectopic beats. Either inadequate response to these drugs or progressive block requires prompt insertion of a temporary transvenous catheter pacemaker. Complete heart block is treated at once with such a pacemaker.

C. Shock "Cardiogenic shock" occurs in about 10% of patients with an acute MI; the mortality is over 50%. Hypotension alone is not prima facie evidence of shock; the evanescent drops in blood pressure that may occur following acute MI, if unaccompanied by clinical signs of shock, generally do not require treatment with vasopressor drugs. The treatment of shock is discussed in Chapter 17.

D. **Postmyocardial-infarction syndrome** This relatively infrequent syndrome is characterized by pericarditis (usually occurring between the second and eleventh weeks after infarction), pleuritis, pneumonitis, fever, severe precordial pain characteristically worse with inspiration, leukocytosis, and elevated sedimentation rate, all running a lengthy course with remissions and exacerbations. Therapy is symptomatic, with reassurance and salicylates (exert caution in their use if patient is taking anticoagulant drugs), and, if symptoms are severe, steroids (prednisone 40 mg daily, decreasing over a period of six weeks, or equivalent dose of other steroids with less tendency to cause salt retention). Exacerbations are common as steroids are discontinued. Administration of anticoagulants need not be discontinued, although hemorrhagic pericarditis with tamponade is a distinct possibility; the prothrombin concentration should not become lower than 25%.

E. Anterior chest wall syndrome Pain may be confused with that of coronary origin. Symptomatic relief may be obtained with injection of procaine into painful areas; Freon or ethyl chloride spray is occasionally helpful.

IX. ANTICOAGULATION

A. **General information** The use of anticoagulants in the treatment of patients with coronary artery disease remains an area of great controversy. Studies designed to evaluate the efficacy of anticoagulants in the treatment of angina pectoris (by reducing the incidence of subsequent infarction), in acute myocardial infarction (by reducing death rate and thromboembolic complications), and in long-term prophylaxis after an acute myocardial infarction (by reducing reinfarction and mortality rates) have shown conflicting results. Many of these studies have been criticized for their failure to select similar patients for control and treatment populations and to make subsequent treatment programs identical in all respects except for the selected variable. Controversy has also arisen over the adequacy of present laboratory procedures in evaluating the level of hypocoagulability, the optimum therapeutic level for maintenance of effective anticoagulation, the incidence and nature of hemorrhagic complications, and the danger that heparin administered early in an acute myocardial infarction may increase the chances for subintimal hemorrhage; a detailed evaluation of these problems is beyond the scope of this Manual.

B. **Indications** The administration of anticoagulants to the majority of patients with peripheral arterial emboli, deep venous thrombosis (and occasionally superficial thrombophlebitis), and pulmonary embolization is seldom debated. Definitive criteria for selection of patients with coronary heart disease do not exist; however, many observers consider the use of anticoagulants in the groups of patients listed below, provided that the patient is cooperative and amenable to careful follow-up and there are no contraindications to the administration of anticoagulants.

The discussion of heparin and coumarin drugs applies to any situation in which their administration is clinically indicated.

1. **Acute myocardial infarction** Anticoagulants are given to the majority of patients with an acute infarction, especially "poor risk" patients (those with previous infarction, intractable pain, shock, marked cardiac enlargement, heart failure, arrhythmias, a history of previous deep vein thrombosis or pulmonary embolism, and other complicating diseases, such as diabetes or obesity). Anticoagulant therapy in this group can be expected to result in a decreased mortality of around 3% to 4% and perhaps more, primarily by preventing thromboembolic episodes. Although the gain may be relatively small, the population at risk is great and a large number of patients can be salvaged.

2. **Long-term therapy after acute myocardial infarction** The controversy over the effects of long-term anticoagulation on reducing reinfarction and mortality rates is still unresolved despite a voluminous literature. Of the better-designed clinical trials to date, about half have shown small but statistically significant reduction in recurrent infarction and a less significant reduction in mortality, usually only in males less than 55–60 years of age, and usually only during the first 6–12 months of therapy. The rest have shown no significant benefit. Comparisons between such studies are difficult or impossible because of differences in design, patient selection, anticoagulants given, control of anticoagulation, method of allocation into treatment and control groups, etc. Since little statistical evidence of harm has come from the long-term use of anticoagulants in these trials, their administration may be justified in selected patients (especially males less than 60 years of age) for up to 1 year, provided good laboratory control of anticoagulation can be assured. The literature should be carefully followed for further data in this important area.

3. **Angina pectoris and impending myocardial infarction** Anticoagulants are given to a significant number of patients (the lower the ages, the higher the percentage) with angina of less than one year's duration, especially if a recent change in pain pattern (increased frequency and intensity) has occurred. Data from studies of anticoagulant therapy in impending myocardial infarction or acute coronary insufficiency syndrome suggest favorable effect on pre-

venting progression to infarction and on reducing mortality; however, these studies lack true control groups, and the conclusions, therefore, are of questionable validity. The literature should be followed.

C. Contraindications In general anticoagulants should not be administered to patients with a hemorrhagic diathesis, severe hypertension (diastolic pressure greater than 110–115 mm Hg), suspected intracranial bleeding, dissecting aneurysms, active ulceration or overt bleeding from the GI tract, bleeding from the genitourinary or respiratory tract (excluding hemoptysis due to pulmonary embolism or mitral stenosis), or threatened abortion. Other contraindications are less stringent, and the urgency of therapy must be weighed against the risk involved: subacute bacterial endocarditis, severe hepatic or renal disease, the presence of thoracic or abdominal aneurysms, surgical procedures in general (but particularly those for the lung, prostate, eye, and central nervous system) and pericarditis complicating acute myocardial infarction; long-term anticoagulation must also be considered carefully in patients with moderate hypertension, vasculitis, diabetes, emotional disorders, or mental retardation.

D. Heparin

1. **General information** Many observers believe heparin to be the anticoagulant of choice, but its expense and the need for parenteral administration generally preclude its long-term use; it is given primarily to postoperative patients and to those patients with acute thromboembolic complications requiring immediate anticoagulant action. It is also the preferred anticoagulant during pregnancy, since it does not cross the placental barrier.

2. **Action** The most important effect of heparin is its inhibition of thrombin formation. Large doses may inhibit platelet aggregation; there are no significant clinical effects on the fibrinolytic system. Other actions of heparin, which are of unknown clinical significance, include "clearing" of postprandial lipemic serum by activation of the enzyme, lipoprotein lipase, interference with reactions involving complement and antigen-antibody interaction, depression of aldosterone production, and transient depression of the platelet count.

3. **Laboratory control** Lee-White clotting times are followed; technique should include a clean entry into the vein, two-syringe collection of blood, clean glassware, and a rigidly standardized procedure that gives reproducible results. The objective of treatment, i.e., the maximum interference with coagulation with minimal risk of hemorrhage, can be achieved when the clotting time is 2–3 times the normal control.

4. **Preparations** Sublingual tablets are of no value; Depo-heparin, a repository preparation in gelatin-dextrose menstruum for deep IM injection, is not recommended because of irregularity of absorption and frequent hematoma formation at the injection site. Sodium aqueous heparin, the preparation of choice, is available in a variety of concentrations; those most often used are 1000, 5000, 10,000, 20,000 units/ml. Standardized preparations must contain at least 120 USP units of anticoagulant activity per milligram. Because preparations vary in potency and because manufacturers no longer report concentration in milligrams/milliliters,

it is wiser to order dosage in USP units, although many physicians prescribe dosage in milligrams because of convenience.

5. **Administration** Sodium aqueous heparin may be administered IV (continuously or intermittently), IM, or subcutaneously (usually into the abdominal fat pad or lateral thigh). When a single dose is given IV, the anticoagulant action and disappearance rate from the plasma are dose-dependent; effects become evident immediately after injection, reach maximum in less than ½ hour, and are nearly gone in 4 hours; anticoagulant effects may vary significantly from patient to patient. When heparin is administered subcutaneously, effects are more erratic; onset of action is slower, and anticoagulant activity may last 6–8 hours (occasionally up to 12 hours after repeated doses).

Based on control of antithrombotic effect, reliability, and safety, the intravenous administration of heparin on a 4–6-hour schedule is at least as satisfactory as any other regimen. Administration may be facilitated by the use of a pediatric winged-needle (21-gauge) scalp-vein infusion set, the plastic-tubing end of which is sealed by a rubber cap through which heparin is injected with a fine intradermal needle. The method is practical, well tolerated, and avoids the use of indwelling catheters and their associated hazards.

Opinion varies as to the dose of heparin necessary for adequate therapy; some observers give 60,000–70,000 units (approximately 500–600 mg) IV, in divided dosage, on the first day when treating patients with thrombophlebitis and pulmonary embolism, then 40,000 units (approximately 300 mg) daily without control by clotting times. A more satisfactory regimen would be the injection of 5000–10,000 units IV every 4 hours, the dosage being controlled by clotting times. The dosage selected should be calculated to induce, 4 hours after its injection, a clotting time 2–3 times that of the pretreatment value. Some observers give intermittent IV injections every 6 hours, the dosage selected as before to induce a clotting time 2–3 times the pretreatment value at 4 hours after the injection. They feel that a clotting time falling toward normal near the sixth hour further lessens the risk of hemorrhagic complications without interfering with the therapeutic effect of the heparin; however, no definitive data have yet been published. After the dose requirement has been established, the clotting time should be determined once daily—4 hours after the last dose—to exclude possible increase in the anticoagulant effect of the drug and to allow for variations in heparin requirements during the course of treatment. (Patients who are actively clotting not infrequently require more heparin during the first 24–48 hours of treatment than will be required several days after institution of therapy.)

When it is chosen to administer heparin subcutaneously, another satisfactory regimen consists of determination of control clotting time, then injection of 5000–10,000 units IV and 7500 units subcutaneously; clotting-time determinations are repeated every 6–8 hours for 48 hours; each subsequent dose of heparin is dependent on the clotting-time result but is usually in the range of 5000–10,000 units subcutaneously every 6–8 hours. The IV heparin is not repeated. After 48 hours the clotting time is determined once daily, or less often if the response is stable.

6. **Toxicity** Heparin is essentially nontoxic in short-term treatment

except for the hazard of hemorrhage. Hypersensitivity reactions (ranging from sneezing, rhinitis, conjunctivitis, lacrimation, and urticaria to bronchospasm, chest pain, and hypotension) are uncommon; transient alopecia may occur 3–4 months after therapy; thrombocytopenia occurs rarely; osteoporosis and spontaneous fractures may occur in patients who have received the drug in high doses for six months or longer.

7. **Antidotes** An excessive dose of heparin leading to a profoundly prolonged clotting time or minor bleeding can usually be managed by cessation of heparin therapy. In the face of major bleeding, the anticoagulant effect of heparin may be reversed within minutes by the administration of **protamine,** which has a strong electrostatic affinity for heparin and combines with it to form a salt devoid of anticoagulant activity. Dilute 5 ml of a 1% solution to 25 ml with isotonic saline (giving a concentration of 2 mg/ml), and give IV slowly an amount (in milligrams) equivalent to one-half the last dose of heparin (in milligrams), but not in excess of 100 mg (excess protamine itself may induce anticoagulant effects). The drug should be administered over 3–5 minutes so as to diminish the likelihood of reactions such as flushing, dyspnea, bradycardia, and hypotension.

Although blood transfusions are necessary to replace blood lost from hemorrhage, they are not specific antidotes against heparin as they are against coumarin drugs.

E. Coumarin derivatives

1. **General information** Bishydroxycoumarin and warfarin are the safest and most widely used preparations. The coumarin preparations vary primarily in solubility and in onset and length of action. They are usually administered once daily in the late afternoon; individual response is variable, and adjustments in dosage are necessary from time to time. Their action is potentiated by salicylates, phenylbutazone, diphenylhydantoin, broad-spectrum antibiotics (which suppress the normal intestinal flora important for the synthesis of vitamin K), corticosteroids, quinidine, quinine, alcohol, ACTH, clofibrate (Atromid-S), and nonspecific factors such as fever and stress; action is antagonized by vitamin K, gastrointestinal disturbances with diarrhea, chloral hydrate, and barbiturates if taken within 5 hours of ingestion of the anticoagulant tablet.

Patients taking coumarin drugs may be given acetaminophen as an antipyretic, or acetaminophen, propoxyphene, or codeine for relief of mild pain; they may take salicylates occasionally but not in sustained dosage.

2. **Actions** The major effect is inhibition of synthesis of four clotting factors: prothrombin (II), proconvertin (VII), Christmas (IX), and Stuart (X).

3. **Laboratory control** The Quick one-stage prothrombin time determination is the guide most often used to evaluate and control therapy. However, when it is necessary to assess coumarin therapy while a patient is receiving heparin (and it is not convenient to await the disappearance of a prior dose of heparin), one may use the Owren prothrombin and proconvertin (P and P) test, which uses the patient's plasma diluted 1/10 or 1/20, thereby diluting out

the heparin effect (the one-stage prothrombin time uses undiluted plasma).

Therapeutic range should be maintained at 25–30 seconds when the control is 12 seconds (i.e., approximately 2–2½ times the control in seconds). Outside the hospital, prothrombin times should be checked every two weeks after stability of control is established.

4. Preparations   Bishydroxycoumarin (Dicumarol) is supplied in tablets or capsules of 25, 50, and 100 mg. Warfarin is supplied as Coumadin (in tablets of 2.0, 2.5, 5.0, 7.5, 10, and 25 mg) or Panwarfin (in tablets of 2.5, 5.0, or 10 mg).

The peak action of each dose of bishydroxycoumarin is usually reached in 36–48 hours and that of warfarin in 24–36 hours. Some observers feel that the more rapid and complete absorption of warfarin from the gastrointestinal tract allows greater ease of control; furthermore, the drug may be given IV or IM (in essentially the same dosage).

5. Administration

   a) Bishydroxycoumarin   300 mg are usually given on the first day, 200 on the second, 50–100 on the third, and thereafter as dictated by the prothrombin time. Maintenance dose, though variable, is usually in the range of 37.5–75 mg daily.

   b) Warfarin   1 mg/kg body weight, up to 40–50 mg (or 60 mg for very large patients) is usually given the first day; none is given the second day; dosage on the third day and thereafter is dictated by the prothrombin time. The maintenance dose varies from 2–15 mg daily, but is usually in the range of 5–10 mg.

6. Toxicity   Reactions to all the coumarins are rare; Dicumarol is the least toxic. Rash is usually the first manifestation, but other reactions include nausea, vomiting, diarrhea, fever, jaundice, leukopenia, thrombocytopenia, leukemoid reaction, and vasculitis. Coumarin drugs can cross the placenta and can cause lethal fetal or neonatal hemorrhage.

7. Antidotes   Vitamin K_1 (phytonadione) is the drug of choice; AquaMEPHYTON, Mono-Kay, and Konakion are water emulsions of phytonadione (which is fat-soluble) for parenteral use. Mephyton and Mono-Kay may be given orally. When parenteral administration is required, the drugs are usually given IM; in those rare situations in which IV administration is believed necessary, injection should be slow (over 5–10 minutes) in order to avoid such reactions as chills, fever, flushing, sweating, chest tightness, and more serious effects as hypotension, convulsions, cyanosis, and hemoglobinuria; fatal reactions, although exceedingly rare, have been reported.

   a) Excessive prolongation of the prothrombin time unaccompanied by bleeding does not require treatment with vitamin K_1; omission of one or two daily doses of the anticoagulant will usually allow the prothrombin time to return to the therapeutic range.

   b) Mild bleeding associated with excessive prolongation of the prothrombin time can usually be controlled by the oral administration of 5–10 mg vitamin K_1; the prothrombin time returns to a safe range, as a rule, within 12–20 hours. Anticoagulant administration can usually be resumed within 24 hours.

c) **For moderate bleeding** 10–20 mg vitamin K_1 are given IM; if hemorrhage is severe 10–25 mg may be given IV slowly. Effects may begin in 1–2 hours (frequently longer), and a safe prothrombin level is often achieved in 4–8 hours. The patient is often refractory to coumarin anticoagulants for 3–4 days following administration of such large doses of vitamin K_1.

d) **Bleeding without an excessively prolonged prothrombin time**   If bleeding is mild, 5–10 mg of vitamin K_1 may be given orally.

e) **Transfusion** of whole bank blood or plasma most quickly antagonizes the effects of excess coumarin; transfusions should be given when bleeding is persistent or blood replacement necessary.

8. **Bleeding**   Treatment of bleeding is discussed above. **Remember:** Significant bleeding occurs in 3% or more of patients receiving anticoagulants; hemorrhage suggests the possibility of some underlying organic lesion, especially if prothrombin level is greater than 15% of control value at the time of hemorrhage, and should not be attributed to the depressed prothrombin level per se. Appropriate diagnostic measures should be carried out.

9. **Surgical operations**   If tooth extraction or elective minor or major surgery is anticipated, discontinue the drugs until the prothrombin time falls below 1½ times (usually above 30%) the control value; reinstitute therapy after the procedure has been performed. If an operation is required within 2–3 hours, give 25 mg vitamin K_1 IV slowly and administer 1000–1500 ml plasma; if a longer period of time may be allowed, the plasma need not be given, and whole blood may be transfused as needed.

10. **Termination of therapy**   Although previous studies suggested that an increased frequency of thromboembolic phenomena followed abrupt termination of anticoagulant therapy after long-term administration, recent studies have failed to demonstrate this so-called rebound phenomenon. If therapy is to be discontinued, it is probably safe to do so abruptly, although some may wish to continue the regimen of gradually reducing the dosage over a period of several weeks until this question has been definitely resolved.

ACUTE RHEUMATIC FEVER

The diagnosis of acute rheumatic fever may be difficult to establish; minor nonspecific illnesses, rheumatoid arthritis, sickle-cell anemia, and systemic lupus erythematosus may simulate rheumatic fever. Throat cultures may fail to reveal the presence of beta-hemolytic streptococci, and standard serologic tests (antistreptolysin O) may not show elevation of antibody titers. Sequential measurement of several streptococcal antibodies, such as antistreptokinase, antihyaluronidase, and antideoxyribonuclease B, however, will almost always show that a group A streptococcal infection is associated with every case of acute rheumatic fever.

The modified Jones criteria (*Mod. Conc. Cardiov. Dis.* 24:291, 1955) should be fulfilled in order to make the diagnosis as precise as possible. These criteria are satisfied by at least two of the major, or one of the major and two of the minor, manifestations listed below:

Major manifestations: Carditis, polyarthritis, chorea, subcutaneous nodules, and erythema marginatum.

Minor manifestations: Fever, arthralgia (in the absence of arthritis), prolonged P-R interval in the ECG, elevated erythrocyte sedimentation rate, presence of C-reactive protein or leukocytosis, evidence of preceding beta-hemolytic streptococcal infection, and history of previous rheumatic fever or the presence of inactive rheumatic heart disease.

Feinstein has further modified these criteria; he accepts chorea alone as evidence of rheumatic fever (as do most physicians); he accepts monoarticular arthritis as a major manifestation; and he eliminates the history of previous rheumatic fever or the presence of inactive rheumatic heart disease as a minor manifestation.

As many as 40% of streptococcal infections may be asymptomatic. Patients with the first attack of rheumatic fever most often seek medical help for fever and arthritis, but any of a variety of manifestations may occur. Rheumatic or choreic symptoms may be absent. Chorea may occur as the sole manifestation months after the initial streptococcal infection; other evidences of recent streptococcal infection may not be present at this time. There is not necessarily a correlation between the severity of the arthritis and carditis; recurrent attacks of carditis may be unrecognized unless the patient is examined regularly. Recent evidence suggests that patients with cardiac damage (from previous attacks of rheumatic fever) tend to have more severe cardiac involvement and less arthritis during recurrences; in patients with no or questionable carditis during previous attacks, rheumatic recurrences may be less likely to result in permanent valvular damage. Some of the above comments have been taken from the long-term study performed at Irvington House (*Ann. Intern. Med.* 60:Suppl. 5, 1964). Treatment is discussed below.

I. **REST** Bed rest is necessary when the patient is acutely ill or exhibits signs of significant cardiac involvement. As he feels better and signs of carditis subside, he may be allowed to sit in a chair at the bedside and use an adjacent bathroom rather than a bedpan. When the patient becomes asymptomatic and evidence of carditis is no longer present, gradually increasing ambulatory activity should be encouraged. Most patients can return to normal activity 8–12 weeks after treatment has been started, although it may be desirable to control strenuous exercise for a somewhat longer period.

II. **SALICYLATES** often relieve fever, tachycardia, and polyarthritis rapidly (often within 24–48 hours). In general they should be given in the maximum dose tolerated to all patients with acute rheumatic fever. There is no convincing evidence that salicylate administration affects the natural history of the disease or the subsequent occurrence or incidence of rheumatic heart disease.

   A. **Preparations and dosage** Salicylates should be given orally, if possible; acetylsalicylic acid (aspirin) is the preparation of choice. Other dosage forms are described in Chapter 1. Therapy should be initiated with 1 gm every 1–2 hours and continued until mild toxicity occurs (seldom more than 8–10 gm during the first 24 hours for most adults). The dosage is then reduced to that amount which does not produce toxic symptoms. For most adults this will be 5–8 gm/day, administered in divided doses of 1 gm each. A blood salicylate level of 25–35 mg/100 ml is necessary for maximum anti-inflammatory effects, but polyarthritis and fever will often respond well at lower serum levels.

   B. **Toxic effects** are described in the section on salicylates in Chapter 1.

C. **Results**   Almost complete relief of joint symptoms should occur within 48–72 hours in the majority of cases. The diagnosis of acute rheumatic fever should be questioned if the symptoms (not carditis) do not abate within this period.

D. **Duration of therapy**   Salicylates should be continued for 4–8 weeks after signs of active inflammation subside. If symptoms recur therapy should be restarted.

III.   **CORTICOSTEROIDS** may be lifesaving in acutely ill, toxic patients with severe pericarditis and myocarditis. Some patients in whom salicylates fail to control the disease respond quickly to corticosteroids. Their non-specific anti-inflammatory effects may be invaluable in reducing the burden upon a failing heart. There is no convincing evidence that administration of corticosteroids modifies the duration of the acute disease or reduces the incidence of residual heart damage. Generally, corticosteroids should be given to acutely ill patients with significant carditis; they are not required in mild cases with minimal or no carditis. In other situations the decision to administer corticosteroids remains a matter of personal conviction.

A. **Dosage**   Prednisone 40–60 mg/day (or equivalent dosage of another preparation) should be given for 2–3 weeks, then slowly reduced to maintenance levels of 15–30 mg daily. (The correct maintenance dose is that which suppresses all evidence of inflammatory activity.)

B. **Side effects** are discussed in the section on corticosteroids in Chapter 16.

C. **Duration of treatment**   Therapy should be continued for 6–8 weeks. If relapse occurs, treatment should be restarted. Relapses are commoner in patients treated with corticosteroids than in those given salicylates.

IV.   **ERADICATION OF STREPTOCOCCI**   Each patient should be treated for acute streptococcal pharyngitis regardless of results of throat cultures and serologic tests.

A. Adults should be given procaine penicillin 600,000 units once or twice daily IM for 10 days, procaine penicillin with aluminum monostearate in oil 600,000 units IM every third day for 3 doses, phenoxymethyl penicillin 250 mg TID orally for at least 10 days, or a single injection of benzathine penicillin 1,200,000 units. The last is the least desirable.

B. Patients allergic to penicillin should be given erythromycin 250 mg QID orally for at least 10 days.

V.   **PROPHYLAXIS**

A. All patients who have had a well-documented history of rheumatic fever, or who have rheumatic heart disease, should have prophylaxis against streptococcal infections and recurrences of rheumatic fever. The Council on Rheumatic Fever of the American Heart Association recommends that prophylactic therapy be continued indefinitely (as a rule) even though streptococcal infection rates decrease with increasing age. If therapy for life is not feasible, prophylaxis should be continued for that period of life when exposure to streptococcal infections is the greatest hazard. Factors which influence the decision to continue prophylaxis are the patient's general health, presence of valvular heart disease, school attendance, armed forces service, contact with small children in the home environment, and occupation (e.g., teacher, medical personnel, etc.). The following prophylaxis regimens may be used:

> Benzathine penicillin 1,200,000 units IM every 4 weeks
> Buffered potassium penicillin G 200,000 units twice daily
> Sulfadiazine 1 gm/day in a single dose

Parenterally administered benzathine penicillin is more effective in the prevention of streptococcal infections and recurrences of rheumatic fever than either of the oral agents. Penicillin 200,000 units twice daily and sulfadiazine are almost equally effective in preventing streptococcal infections; each is significantly less effective than benzathine penicillin.

Although benzathine penicillin is statistically the agent of choice for prophylaxis, there are circumstances in which oral prophylaxis is desirable; furthermore, local or systemic reactions (which occur in about 10% of patients) may preclude administration of benzathine penicillin. The effectiveness of oral medicines in prophylaxis depends in great part on the patient's cooperation; most failures occur in those patients who fail to take the drug regularly.

B. If pharyngitis occurs, nasopharyngeal cultures should be carefully obtained to determine the presence of beta-hemolytic streptococci. If they are present, a course of therapy, as previously outlined, should be given. Because cultures may be falsely negative, however, many physicians treat each episode of pharyngitis occurring in a patient with a history of rheumatic fever as if streptococci were present.

C. Because the dosage regimens employed for long-term prophylaxis against streptococcal infections are inadequate for preventing bacterial endocarditis, patients with rheumatic heart disease (or congenital heart disease) should be given penicillin at the time of minor surgical procedures (e.g., dental extractions, tonsillectomy); women should receive penicillin at the time of delivery. Dosages are listed in the section on subacute bacterial endocarditis in Chapter 9.

5. Congestive Heart Failure

I. **GENERAL MEASURES** Congestive heart failure may occur in any type of heart disease. The therapeutic measures described do not alter the basic disease process but are directed toward improving circulatory dynamics.

A. **Rest and activity** Since diuresis is favored by the recumbent position, and since many patients have a significant diuresis with bed rest alone, slight to moderate restriction of activities during periods of increasing congestive failure, and modified bed rest (for 2–3 days) during periods of active diuresis are important measures.

B. **Prophylactic anticoagulation** Fifty percent or more of patients with congestive heart failure and longstanding edema of the lower extremities have pulmonary embolization, frequently without associated infarction. Recurrent showers of pulmonary emboli may be asymptomatic but result ultimately in a picture of pulmonary hypertension, progressive ventilatory insufficiency, or "intractable heart failure." Administration of anticoagulants, therefore, should be considered for those patients highly suspected of recurrent pulmonary embolization; some physicians recommend anticoagulants for all patients with persistent edema of the lower extremities secondary to heart failure.

C. **Supportive measures** Venous congestion may be lessened by wrapping the legs in elastic stockings or bandages. Legs should be kept elevated. Edematous skin which is especially vulnerable to injury should be kept clean and soft. Routine measures for sedation and bowel care are described in Chapter 1; sleeping with the head of the bed elevated may improve rest; diuretics should not be given late in the day, as a rule, in order to avoid disturbance of sleep by diuresis; heavy bedtime snacks should be avoided.

D. **Diet** Restriction of salt intake is one of the most important measures. Most patients can be managed on a 2.0-gm salt diet; diets with more severe salt restriction offer little therapeutic advantage (as a rule), are highly restrictive and unpalatable, and generally impractical outside the hospital. Diets should be ordered according to the classification of the American Heart Association:

250 mg sodium (0.6 gm salt)	750 mg sodium (1.9 gm salt)
500 mg sodium (1.3 gm salt)	1000 mg sodium (2.5 gm salt)

Fluid intake up to 2500–3000 ml daily may be allowed, but larger quantities in face of sodium restriction and diuretic therapy may result in hyponatremia.

1. The average diet without salt restriction contains 6–15 gm salt daily; this value is reduced to 4–7 gm by restricting addition of salt at the table, and to 3–4 gm by restricting addition of salt during cooking. One level teaspoonful contains almost 6 gm salt.

2. A palatable low-salt diet (1000 mg sodium) can be built around salt-free bread and milk, unsalted butter and cottage cheese, meat, freshwater fish, and various vegetables except spinach, celery, beet greens, and frozen peas, lima beans, or mixed vegetables. One gram of salt by shaker may be added (surface salt is more palatable than that added during cooking). Diet manuals contain specific instructions, but it is important to point out that the following must be avoided: mineral water, club soda, bicarbonate, certain sodium-containing medications as sodium salicylate, canned soups and juices and most vegetables, salad dressings, most condiments, canned fish, cheese, cured and smoked ham, sausages, pickles, nuts, crackers, breads prepared with baking soda, most candies, proprietary antacids (unless sodium-free), excessive milk ingestion (800 ml contain 1.0 gm salt), and most prepared cereals except cracked wheat, oatmeal, puffed wheat and rice, Instant Ralston, and shredded wheat.

3. Salt substitutes are available, and several may be tried until a palatable preparation is found; Diasal contains KCl with a trace of glutamic acid; Neocurtasal contains KCl, KI, potassium glutamate, glutamic acid, calcium silicate, and tricalcium phosphate; and Co-Salt contains KCl, NH_4Cl, choline, and tricalcium phosphate.

II. DIGITALIS

A. **Mechanism of action** The main pharmacologic effects of digitalis are due to its inotropic action, i.e., the ability to increase the force of myocardial contraction; the manner in which digitalis influences cellular biochemical events to produce these effects is not established. Numerous studies, although yielding inconsistent results, show that digitalis influences the movement of sodium and potassium ions across heart-muscle membrane, resulting in a loss of cell potassium; affects the contractile proteins; and, possibly, induces shifts in intracellular calcium concentration; but the specific relationship of these actions to increase in contractile force of the myocardium is not known. Electron microscopy studies have shown the drug to be localized in the sarcoplasmic reticulum between the myofibrils.

B. **Effects of digitalis administration in low-output failure**

1. **On heart muscle** Increase in the force of systolic contraction results in more complete emptying and decrease in diastolic size of the heart; the mechanical efficiency of the heart muscle is increased (less oxygen consumption per unit of work). The myocardial action of digitalis is its most important action.

2. **On heart rate** Slowing of the ventricular rate is primarily a result of circulatory improvement resulting from the beneficial effects on the myocardium. Direct effects on the A-V node increase the refractory period and slow the rate of conduction.

3. **On cardiac output** Increase in cardiac output is seen only in the failing heart and is secondary to improvement in cardiac contraction and emptying.

4. **On venous pressure** The reduction in venous pressure is due to

improved circulatory dynamics. It seems unlikely that the peripheral effects of arteriolar and venous constriction, with resultant decrease in venous return, are of clinical importance.

5. **On the kidney** There is some evidence that digitalis has a direct effect on the kidney, inhibiting renal reabsorption of salt and water directly without changes in renal blood flow or glomerular filtration rate; these effects are of doubtful clinical significance.

C. Signs of digitalis effect

1. **Improvement of congestive heart failure** Subsidence of dyspnea and orthopnea, disappearance of rales, slowing of the heart rate, especially in atrial fibrillation; disappearance of gallop rhythm; decrease in heart size; diuresis; weight loss.

2. **ECG changes** Classic changes consist of depression or scooping of the ST segment, followed by flattening or inversion of the T waves. The Q-T interval is shortened and the P-R interval prolonged. These changes, however, are nonspecific and may be seen with myocardial disease. They cannot be used to predict digitalis intoxication; their absence does not preclude recent digitalis administration.

D. Toxic manifestations Gastrointestinal symptoms and cardiac irregularities are the commonest findings. There is no good evidence that the incidence or type of toxic manifestations is affected by the type of digitalis preparation used. Manifestations of digitalis toxicity are listed below; treatment is discussed in paragraph **K**.

1. **Cardiac alterations occur in irritability** with tachycardias or premature systoles from any focus (commonest are ventricular premature contractions) ; **in conductivity** with any degree of heart block (in the presence of atrial fibrillation toxicity may be manifest as A-V dissociation with a regular nodal rhythm or nodal tachycardia) ; **in contractility** with increasing heart failure. This latter manifestation is not uncommon and is all too often overlooked, being mistaken for underdigitalization with resultant increasing cardiac failure. The commonest cause of death from digitalis overdosage is ventricular tachycardia and fibrillation.

2. **Gastrointestinal** Anorexia, nausea, vomiting (both local and central mechanisms), diarrhea, and abdominal pain.

3. **Cerebral and neurologic** Headache, drowsiness, disorientation, confusion, delirium; less frequently, convulsions, dizziness, syncope, paresthesias, and neuralgias.

4. **Visual (uncommon)** Blurred vision, yellow vision, white halos around dark objects, diplopia, scotomata, optic neuritis.

5. **Others (uncommon)** Skin rashes, gynecomastia, eosinophilia, thrombocytopenia, and true idiosyncratic reactions.

E. Indications for digitalis Digitalis is indicated for the treatment of certain arrhythmias (see Chapter 6, Cardiac Arrhythmias) and congestive heart failure of any etiology. Digitalis is of greatest value in low-output cardiac failure, but it should be given to patients with normal cardiac output and failure, or those with high-output congestive failure, even though beneficial effects in the latter may be

negligible; therapy in these situations is directed primarily at the underlying disease. The administration of digitalis routinely before major surgery in patients with compensated heart disease is controversial, and the matter remains one of individual preference. Some experts state that digitalis should not be administered routinely to such patients, since they obtain no significant hemodynamic effects, and the treatment of arrhythmias which might develop postoperatively becomes complicated. Other observers argue, however, that preoperative digitalization is not detrimental, and that the drug should be considered for short-term treatment of patients with cardiac disease and enlarged hearts (despite absence of signs and symptoms of cardiac decompensation) to reduce the chances for development of arrhythmias (particularly atrial fibrillation) postoperatively.

F. Digitalis preparations are derivatives of the foxglove plants, *Digitalis purpurea* and *Digitalis lanata*. They may be whole leaf or purified glycosides. The glycosides are said to offer certain advantages: They are given by weight, not biologic units; absorption from the GI tract is relatively complete and constant; and injectable forms are available.

Chemically, the digitalis nucleus is a phenanthrene ring. When an unsaturated lactone ring is added to the 17 position, the resulting compound is called an aglycone, which has weak cardiotonic actions. When a sugar is added to the 3 position of the aglycone, the resulting compound is the cardiac glycoside.

Table 5-1 lists the more commonly used preparations, trade names, and dosage forms available.

G. Principles of administration of digitalis preparations Response to digitalis varies widely and is influenced by many factors. Because no tests are available to assist in the adjustment of digitalis dosage, because the physician must rely solely on the clinical status of the patient in the treatment of congestive heart failure, and because any plan of therapy requires a guess at the amount of the drug required to produce a desired effect, the physician should always answer the following questions before administering digitalis.

1. Are there contraindications to the administration of digitalis to this patient?   There are no absolute contraindications except for idiosyncrasy and digitalis intoxication. Recent studies repudiate the concept that digitalis should not be given to patients with acute myocardial infarction for fear of inducing rhythm disturbances; the drug should be given, when indicated, although digitalization should proceed more slowly because of the myocardial hyperirritability. Digitalis may be given, when indicated, to patients with first-degree A-V heart block and congestive heart failure, but its use in patients with higher degrees of A-V block is controversial.

2. Do I have a control ECG?   An ECG must be obtained before administration of digitalis because the drug may induce changes (often marked), as previously described, identical to those seen with myocardial damage.

3. Have I planned the correct route of administration?   Digitalis preparations must be given IV or IM for acute pulmonary edema or life-endangering arrhythmias, but in other situations oral administration, if possible, is preferred. Note that the IV dose of digitoxin is the same as the oral, but for other preparations it is less. For

TABLE 5-1. Digitalis Preparations

Preparation	Trade Name	How Supplied: Oral (Tablets, Unless Specified)	Color of Tablets	Parenteral	Comments
Digitalis, powdered U.S.P.	Digitalis	0.05 and 0.1 gm; Tincture: 0.1 gm/ml	Brownish-green	Available, but rarely used	If the tincture is used, measurement should be made with calibrated droppers; increases in potency with standing
Powdered leaf	Digifortis	0.1 gm (capsule)	Gray with green band	For IM or IV 0.1 gm/ml	Main disadvantage is the long period of dissipation
Digitoxin	Purodigin Crystodigin Digitaline Nativelle	0.05, 0.1, 0.15, and 0.2 mg 0.05, 0.1, 0.15, and 0.2 mg 0.1, 0.15, and 0.2 mg	0.05 — Orange 0.10 — Pink 0.15 — Blue or Yellow 0.20 — White	For IM or IV 0.2 mg/ml in 40–50% alcohol	
Digoxin	Lanoxin	0.25 and 0.5 mg	0.25 — White 0.50 — Green	For IM or IV 0.5 mg/2 ml in 40% propylene glycol and 10% alcohol	Rapid action and excretion make this the favored drug for parenteral maintenance, especially if renal insufficiency is present; IM injections are painful
Gitalin	Gitaligin	0.5 mg	Pale green	—	
Lanatoside C (tablets)	Cedilanid	0.5 mg	Coral pink	—	
Deslanoside (parenteral)	Cedilanid-D	—	—	0.2 mg/ml in 2 and 4 ml ampules; for IV use	A widely used preparation for rapid digitalization; it is not often used for maintenance because of rapid dissipation

parenteral therapy the IV route is preferred, since absorption after IM injection may be variable in the presence of congestive heart failure.

4. Has the patient had digitalis in the preceding three weeks?   Neglect in establishing this point is a major cause of digitalis intoxication. In an emergency situation requiring digitalis, but where doubt exists about the level of previous digitalization, give small doses of a rapidly acting preparation (e.g., 0.2 mg Cedilanid or 0.125 mg digoxin) IV; observe the patient closely, monitor the ECG continuously, and repeat in 1–2 hours as the situation warrants.

5. Will this patient be less tolerant to digitalis and require smaller doses? Such is the case in elderly, debilitated, or small patients; in those with myxedema, myocarditis, acute myocardial infarction, renal insufficiency, electrolyte disturbances (hypokalemia, hypercalcemia), and advanced pulmonary disease associated with hypercapnia and/or hypoxia; and in those receiving drugs such as ephedrine, epinephrine, reserpine, procaine amide, or quinidine, which, when given concurrently with digitalis, may predispose to the development of cardiac arrhythmias.

6. Does the patient have digitalis intoxication or increasing congestive heart failure?   It is frequently impossible to be certain whether the patient has digitalis intoxication or has increasingly severe myocardial decompensation and congestive heart failure, which will be benefited by more digitalis. The signs and symptoms (particularly anorexia, nausea, and extrasystoles) of both may be similar, and the problem may be further compounded by the patient who develops worsening congestive failure as a manifestation of digitalis toxicity. Although the mechanism responsible for the latter is not known, this may be the only cardiac manifestation of digitalis toxicity. One may stop digitalis administration, give potassium, and observe the patient over 48 hours. If the severity of the situation dictates immediate action, Cedilanid may be given as described above (paragraph **4**); however, it probably is safer and more effective to withhold digitalis, and institute or increase diuretic therapy while maintaining the serum potassium level.

7. Do I know the intricacies of the particular preparation I am using? Difficulties often arise from use of unfamiliar preparations; learn to use two or three with different properties and know them well!

H. Methods of digitalization   Table 5-2 lists dosages for various commonly used digitalis preparations. Table 5-3 outlines some practical regimens for initial digitalization. The amount of drug required to attain full digitalization depends upon the rate of digitalization; if rapid, the dose approximates those given in the table; if carried out over 48 hours or longer, the total dose will exceed those given in the table because of excretion (e.g., digitoxin, 10% per day; digoxin, approximately 30% per day). Recently doubt has been cast upon the necessity for giving digitalizing doses in nonacute situations (*Circulation* 34:865, 1966); if rapid digitalization is not necessary, one may merely begin the chosen maintenance dosage.

Rapid digitalization should be avoided when slower methods suffice; oral administration is safer than parenteral. As noted previously, a major problem is that of determining a digitalizing dose for any given patient. Some physicians give the drug in moderate dosage until toxic symptoms develop, then omit it for several days before starting maintenance therapy; others administer somewhat less than the amount suggested in statistically derived dosage tables, and then "titrate" the patient to what is considered a maximum clinical response. Although the latter seems vague, it is definitely the preferable approach; toxicity should be avoided, for the initial manifestation may be a severe or fatal cardiac arrhythmia. It is crucial to remember that the digitalizing doses listed in Table 5-2 are the average doses; it is wise to individualize and go slowly rather than push to a predetermined amount.

I. Maintenance of digitalization Table 5-2 lists average maintenance doses, but the amounts required differ significantly from patient to patient and must be determined by the clinical response. Furthermore, the state of digitalization does not remain constant in all patients, and dosage schedules should be evaluated periodically even though most patients may not require adjustment in dosage. Difficulties are most frequently encountered with digoxin (patients become under-digitalized) and digitoxin (digitalis intoxication). Patients with advanced renal or hepatic disease must be followed closely for dosage adjustments.

J. Changing digitalis preparations Following oral digitalization the patient may be maintained with any of the preparations. Following initial rapid digitalization with IV preparations such as Cedilanid or digoxin, partial redigitalization appears to be unnecessary and potentially dangerous.

K. Management of digitalis intoxication Digitalis toxicity is estimated to occur in more than 5% of patients taking the drug. The most serious manifestations are cardiac arrhythmias; the more common ones are paroxysmal atrial tachycardia with block, nonparoxysmal nodal tachycardia, multifocal VPCs, ventricular tachycardia, and complete or incomplete atrioventricular dissociation. Prolonged tachycardias may precipitate pulmonary edema and cerebral or coronary insufficiency; a high degree of A-V block may cause Adams-Stokes attacks. Unfortunately, the development of digitalis intoxication is difficult to anticipate. The ECG may give little evidence of digitalis effect, GI symptoms may be minimal or absent, and transient cardiac irregularities may be the first evidence of digitalis excess. Because of the latter, digitalis administration should be stopped at the first suspicion of toxicity; the serum potassium level should be measured to exclude hypokalemia. Methods of treatment are listed below.

1. Mild symptoms (as previously described) or occasional ectopic beats require no specific therapy; withdrawal of digitalis for several days is usually sufficient. If ectopic beats are very frequent, however, 5.0–8.0 gm KCl may be given orally (in divided dosage) each day for several days; Dilantin, procaine amide, or propranolol may be given as described in Chapter 6.

2. Cardiac toxicity in most instances is treated by the administration of potassium, but when high degrees of A-V block are caused by digitalis intoxication, potassium salts should not be given; in this situation (except for PAT with block) potassium may potentiate the effects of digitalis on the conduction system, thereby further depressing A-V conduction and ventricular responsiveness, and induce more dangerous arrhythmias.

The treatment of PAT with block is discussed in the chapter on

TABLE 5-2. Dosages for Digitalization
(Doses are in gm for digitalis leaf; in mg for all other preparations)

Preparation	Oral						IV or IM			Dissipation	
	Digitalization		Absorption	Max. Effect (hrs)	Maintenance		Digitalization		Max. Effect (hrs)	Action Regressing	Action Gone
	Avg.	Range			Avg.	Range	Avg.	Range			
Digitalis leaf	1.2	1.0–2.0	20%	8–10	0.15	0.05–0.3	—	—	—	2–3 days	2–3 wks
Digitoxin	1.2	1.2–2.0	100%	8–10	0.15	0.05–0.3	1.2	1.0–2.0	4–12	2–3 days	2–3 wks
Digoxin	2.5	1.0–4.0	90%	3–6	0.5	0.25–1.0	1.5	1.0–2.0	1–3	8–10 hrs	2–6 days
Gitalin	5.0	4.0–8.0	50–100%	—	0.5	0.25–1.0	—	—	—	—	
Cedilanid	6.0	5.0–10.0	10%	3–5	1.0	0.25–1.0	1.6	1.2–2.0	1–3	16–36 hrs	3–6 days
Ouabain	—	—	—	—	—	—	0.8	0.5–1.0	0.5–2	8–12 hrs	2–3 days

TABLE 5-3. Regimens for Initial Digitalization

Preparation	Very Rapid Digitalization (12 Hrs. or Less)	Digitalization over 12–24 Hours	Digitalization in 2 Days	Slow Digitalization (3–7 Days)
Intravenous				
Cedilanid (mg)	0.8 mg followed by 0.4 mg q2h as needed	—	—	—
Digoxin (mg)	0.5 initially, then 0.25 every 2–4 hrs as needed	—	—	—
Oral				
Digitalis (gm)	—	0.5 initially, then 0.2 every 6 hrs till digitalized	0.2 TID × 2 days	0.1 TID till digitalized*
Digitoxin (mg)	—	0.5 initially, then 0.2 every 6–8 hrs till digitalized	0.2 TID × 2 days	0.3 daily till digitalized*
Digoxin (mg)	—	1.0 initially, then 0.5 every 6 hrs till digitalized	0.5 TID × 2 days	0.75 daily till digitalized*
Gitalin (mg)	—	2.0 initially, then 0.75 every 6 hrs till digitalized	0.75 TID × 2 days	1.0–1.5 daily till digitalized*

* Or begin with maintenance therapy.

cardiac arrhythmias. First-degree heart block, common with digitalis administration, does not require specific therapy unless the P-R interval is markedly prolonged; digitalis administration may then be discontinued for several days. Complete A-V block, when digitalis-induced, may be treated temporarily by infusions of disodium versenate (as described below); isoproterenol should be given cautiously for fear of precipitating further arrhythmias (particularly ventricular tachycardia).

3. **For life-endangering ventricular irritability** the following may be used (additional comments about specific arrhythmias may be found in Chapter 6).

   a) **Potassium** Give 20 mEq KCl in 500 ml 5% D/W IV over 1–2 hours; monitor the ECG frequently. Intravenous administration of potassium is probably preferable to oral because the exact amount given to the patient can be controlled and the administration stopped immediately if untoward effects occur. However, 5 gm KCl may be given orally in one dose, followed by 2 gm every 3–4 hours as needed. **Remember:** The serum potassium level should be determined; if marked hypokalemia is present, significantly larger amounts of potassium should be given.

   b) **Lidocaine (Xylocaine)** is especially valuable for ventricular irritability (frequent VPCs, bigeminy, ventricular tachycardia). It is given initially by rapid injection of 25–50 mg IV followed by a constant infusion of 1–4 mg/min to suppress the irritable focus. The injection may be repeated. See Chapter 6 for more details on Xylocaine and the drugs mentioned below.

   c) **Procaine amide (Pronestyl)** may be used if lidocaine is not effective as the initial therapy. IV: 100 mg every 1–2 minutes until the arrhythmia converts, but total dose not to exceed 1.5–2.0 gm. IM: 0.5 gm every 2–4 hours. Orally: 1 gm immediately and again 2 hours later, then 0.5 gm every 4–6 hours.

   d) **Diphenylhydantoin (Dilantin)** is effective in suppressing ventricular irritability that is digitalis-induced. When it is given too rapidly, however, hypotension and death may ensue. The optimal IV dose has not yet been determined, but 250 mg or 5 mg/kg **given over a period of no less than 5 minutes** has been safe and often effective. The usual maintenance dose is 300–600 mg per day orally or IM (see Chapter 6).

   e) **Propranolol (Inderal)** appears to be effective in digitalis-induced arrhythmias, especially VPCs and ventricular tachycardia. Give 1 mg IV every 5 minutes (up to 5–10 mg total) until an effect is achieved. The oral maintenance dose is 5–10 mg every 4–6 hours (this is usually 10 times the IV maintenance dose). (See chapter 6.)

   f) **Calcium binding** Chelation of calcium with disodium EDTA (disodium versenate) has been of value in many cases, but the results are erratic, the beneficial effects are of short duration, and renal damage is a possible complication of large dosage. Dissolve 600 mg EDTA in 250 ml 5% D/W and give IV over 30–60 minutes while monitoring the ECG frequently. (Some observers have given as much as 3.0 gm EDTA over 20–30 minutes without observing toxic manifestations; the smaller dose is safer.)

g) DC countershock may restore sinus rhythm in patients with digitalis-induced arrhythmias, but fatal results have been more frequent after attempts at cardioversion in these patients. Despite the increased risk, DC shock is indicated for ventricular fibrillation and for ventricular tachycardia that does not respond to drugs or is accompanied by circulatory collapse.

4. Do not give diuretics (they cause kaliuresis) or large infusions of carbohydrate (they cause intracellular shift of potassium) to a patient with severe digitalis intoxication, for the resultant lowering of the serum potassium concentration may aggravate the cardiac manifestations.

III. DIURETICS are useful in the treatment of a variety of diseases associated with abnormal retention of salt and water. In congestive heart failure they are adjunctive in control of edema and are not to be used in lieu of digitalis, salt restriction, and (when indicated) reduced physical activity.

Diuretics must be used judiciously and their mechanism of action clearly understood, for numerous electrolyte abnormalities may follow their administration. The most serious is hypokalemia, since patients concomitantly receiving digitalis may develop severe cardiac arrhythmias as a manifestation of digitalis toxicity precipitated by the reduction in serum potassium concentration. Furthermore, the development of drug-induced electrolyte abnormalities is the commonest cause of failure to respond to a good diuretic program, even though other factors, as inadequate salt restriction or multiple pulmonary emboli, may also play a role.

Although the effectiveness of diuretics may be enhanced by bed rest, the drugs are usually administered early in the day rather than at bedtime so as to avoid disturbing sleep by diuresis.

A. Mercurial diuretics (parenteral)

1. Mechanism of action Organic mercurial diuretics appear to act all along the nephron, mainly by inhibiting sulfhydryl enzymes and thus the reabsorption of sodium and chloride, which are then excreted with osmotically equivalent amounts of water. Their action is blocked by dimercaprol (BAL). More than 85% is excreted by the kidneys in patients with normal renal function.

2. Preparations most commonly used are the two discussed below. Each contains about 40 mg mercury/ml.

a) Meralluride (Mercuhydrin) may be given IM or IV (this latter route is rarely necessary). It contains 5% theophylline, which facilitates absorption, reduces local irritation, and may add to the diuretic effect.

b) Mercaptomerin (Thiomerin) is a sulfhydryl compound complexed with thioglycolate. It is less stable in solution than meralluride (aqueous solutions must be kept refrigerated) but less irritating; it may be given subcutaneously.

3. Administration A dose of 0.5 ml should be used initially to test for response and hypersensitivity; 1–2 ml are then given at intervals to produce and maintain adequate diuresis. Daily injections lead to excessive electrolyte loss and are not justified; after the initial diuresis, mercurials should not be given more often than every 3–5 days. Their action is enhanced by a prior course of ammonium chloride (see below) or subsequent administration of aminophylline, 500 mg IV 1–2 hours after injection of the mercurial. Injections should be in nonedematous areas; local reactions may be reduced by adding 1 ml 1% procaine. An increase in urine flow is usually evident within 1–2 hours, reaching maximum in 6–9 hours. The response depends on numerous factors (particularly the ECF volume, the glomerular filtration rate, and the serum chloride concentration).

4. **Contraindications** are anuria and drug hypersensitivity. Patients with acute glomerulonephritis may develop increased hematuria, proteinuria, and, rarely, anuria after mercurial administration. Mercurials may be given cautiously, if indicated, to patients with mild to moderate renal insufficiency.

5. **Toxic and undesirable effects**

   a) **Mercurialism** Very rare; due to accumulation of mercury over a period of time in patients with renal insufficiency; manifested by stomatitis, marginal gingivitis, metallic taste in the mouth, diarrhea, proteinuria.

   b) **Hypersensitivity** Pruritus, various skin rashes, asthma, fever, flushing, nausea, vomiting. A change to another preparation may occasionally eliminate further reactions. Severe reactions, when they occur, almost always follow IV injections; fatal reactions are due to anaphylaxis or ventricular fibrillation.

   c) **Bone marrow depression** or agranulocytosis is rare. **Thromboembolic phenomena** may occur after massive diuresis; acute urinary retention may develop in patients with bladder neck obstruction.

   d) **Electrolyte disturbances** are common after excessive use of mercurial compounds; hypokalemia, hyponatremia, and/or hypochloremic alkalosis may develop (the latter may be corrected by administration of ammonium chloride). Symptoms include cramps, tetany, profound weakness, and psychoses.

B. **Ammonium chloride** potentiates the action of mercurial diuretics; it is of little value when used alone. It is given for 2–3 days prior to the administration of the mercurial in order to produce a hyperchloremic acidosis; the dose is 1–3 gm QID with meals (in order to reduce gastric irritation). It should not be given in the presence of severe renal or liver disease or marked respiratory acidosis.

C. **L-Lysine (or arginine) monohydrochloride** may be used as acidifying agents instead of NH_4Cl. Although these amino acids are not more effective than NH_4Cl, they may be advantageous in certain situations because they supply chloride ions without ammonium. The amino acid is deaminated and enters the citric acid cycle. Each gram of the monohydrochloride yields 5 mEq chloride. **Side effects** after oral administration are minimal and include abdominal cramps and diarrhea; severe metabolic acidosis may result from prolonged administration. The recommended **oral dose** is 10–40 gm (usually 40 gm) L-lysine daily in divided dosage (in fruit juice or low-sodium milk) for 3–4 days prior to administration of the mercurial. L-arginine monohydrochloride may be administered intravenously over 2–4 hours in a dosage of 40 gm (dissolved in 500 ml 5% D/W).

D. Acetazolamide (Diamox) inhibits the enzyme carbonic anhydrase, with resultant increased urinary excretion of sodium, potassium, and bicarbonate ions, decreased excretion of titratable acid and ammonia, and little or no increase in excretion of chloride. Its action is on the proximal and distal tubules. Diuresis begins in about one hour, reaches maximum in 2 hours, and is complete in 5–8 hours. With continued administration its natriuretic action is lost and potassium excretion becomes excessive. The **dose** is 250–750 mg once daily for 3–4 consecutive days of each week. **Side effects,** which are minimal, include drowsiness, lassitude, paresthesias, and other symptoms associated with electrolyte abnormalities. The drug is not frequently used as a diuretic since the development of more effective compounds, but it is often given by ophthalmologists to lower intraocular pressure in patients with glaucoma. In long-term use there appears to be a tendency toward renal calculus formation.

E. Xanthines probably act by increasing cardiac output and glomerular filtration rate. They are ineffective when used alone, but may potentiate the effect of a mercurial (see paragraph **A**). Aminophylline 500 mg may be given IV or by rectal suppository.

F. Benzothiadiazides (thiazides), used correctly, are the oral diuretics of choice because of their natriuretic potency, repetitive effectiveness, and relative lack of side effects and toxicity. These drugs are effective antihypertensive agents as well.

    1. Mechanism of action Thiazides exhibit properties of both carbonic anhydrase inhibitors and mercurials, primarily the latter. Excretion of sodium, bicarbonate, chloride, and potassium ions is enhanced, ammonia excretion is depressed, concentration of ammonia in renal-vein blood is increased, and the urine becomes alkaline.

    2. Preparations and dosage Listed in Table 5-4 are the commonly used preparations with trade names, dosage range for maintenance therapy, and duration of action.

        A large number of thiazide compounds are available; their basic mechanisms of action are similar, and the differences reside in dosage, degree of natriuresis, and duration of action.

        Chlorthalidone (Hygroton) is a phthalimidine compound; quinethazone (Hydromox) is a quinazoline compound; the pharmacologic actions of both, and their clinical and side effects, except perhaps hypersensitivity, are essentially the same as those of the thiazides.

    3. Administration of supplemental potassium

        a) Whether or not to give potassium supplements when thiazides are administered for long-term therapy remains controversial. Some authors state that potassium supplements are not required unless the diet contains less than 1 gm salt daily and is inadequate in meat and fruit; others give potassium supplements routinely, since the majority of patients appear to require them. The matter is one of individual preference and experience for the most part, except that potassium supplements should be given routinely to those patients who are capricious in their food intake, and probably to the majority of those taking digitalis concomitantly, unless renal insufficiency is present. The chances for the development of hypokalemia may be lessened by administering other diuretics (particularly

TABLE 5-4. Some Thiazide Preparations

Generic Name	Trade Name	Size of Tablets (mg)	Daily Maintenance Dosage (mg)	Duration of Action (hrs)	Comments on Administration
Chlorothiazide	Diuril	250 and 500	500–1000	6–10	Therapy is often initiated with doses larger than those listed. The maintenance dose suggested is only an average value to provide guidelines; the dosage must be adjusted to suit each patient's particular needs
Hydrochlorothiazide	HydroDiuril Esidrix Oretic	25 and 50	50–100	8–12	
Benzthiazide	Exna	50	50–100	12–18	
Bendroflumethiazide	Naturetin Benuron	2.5 and 5.0 5.0	2.5–5.0	18–24	Thiazides may be given concurrently with other diuretics. Combinations of a thiazide and either triamterene or spironolactone may be particularly useful
Cyclothiazide	Anhydron	2.0	1.0–2.0	18–24	
Hydroflumethiazide	Saluron	50	50–100	18–24	
Methyclothiazide	Enduron	2.5 and 5.0	2.5–5.0	24+	For edematous states the thiazides are usually given once daily in the morning, or intermittently
Trichlormethiazide	Naqua Metahydrin	2.0 and 4.0	2.0–4.0	24–36	
Polythiazide	Renese	1.0, 2.0 and 4.0	1.0–4.0	24–36	
Quinethazone	Hydromox	50	50–100	18–24	
Chlorthalidone	Hygroton	100	50–100	48–72	

triamterene or spironolactone) concurrently with thiazides, or by using intermittent therapy (e.g., two days on, two days off).

b) Those patients given potassium supplements should be given about 45–75 mEq daily (those with hypokalemia require larger amounts initially). **Several preparations are available:**

Potassium Triplex, a solution of potassium acetate, bicarbonate, and citrate, contains 15 mEq potassium/5 ml.

Kaon Elixir is potassium gluconate and contains 20 mEq potassium/15 ml; Kaon tablets each contain 5 mEq.

K-Lyte is a citrus-flavored effervescent tablet of potassium bicarbonate; each tablet, which should be dissolved in 3–4 ounces water, yields 25 mEq potassium.

Kato liquid is potassium chloride in low-sodium tomato juice and contains 20 mEq potassium/45 ml.

A 10% solution of potassium chloride for oral use can be prepared by most pharmacies and contains 20 mEq potassium per 15 ml. Potassium chloride is the most physiologic preparation, and it must be used for adequate treatment of hypokalemic alkalosis (see Chapter 2).

c) **Nonspecific small-bowel ulcers,** generally uncommon, have been noted with increasing frequency in patients receiving thiazide diuretics and potassium supplements. Because these ulcerating lesions have been associated with a marked degree of stenosis, the presenting clinical picture is often that of small-bowel obstruction, but perforation and/or hemorrhage may rarely occur. Retrospective clinical surveys and studies in animals have shown so far that potassium (particularly potassium chloride), either alone or combined with a thiazide in a single tablet, appears to be the major causative factor.

Although studies are limited and other possible predisposing factors not defined (the majority of patients reported have been over 50 years of age and have had cardiovascular disease), currently available data implicate high local concentrations of potassium (such as those obtained by release from enteric-coated potassium chloride tablets) as the mucosal irritating agent which initiates changes resulting in the circumferential stenosing ulcer.

The incidence of this lesion, though unknown, appears extremely low, and no correlation can be made in man between the dosage of potassium and the incidence of the lesion. It would seem prudent, however, to ensure that potassium supplements are administered with meals, and to discontinue such preparations in the event of any unusual gastrointestinal symptoms.

4. Toxic and undesirable side effects

a) Skin rashes (papular, photosensitive, exfoliative dermatitis), gastric irritation, nausea, acute pancreatitis (rare), cholestatic jaundice, and, rarely, thrombocytopenia, agranulocytosis, or leukopenia. Weakness, fatigue, anorexia, and muscle cramps are uncommon.

b) Electrolyte abnormalities (especially hypokalemia or hypochloremic alkalosis) have been described previously. Patients with severe liver disease may develop hepatic coma due to electrolyte abnormalities and, perhaps, the increase in blood ammonia levels following thiazide administration.

c) Hyperuricemia is not uncommon; occasionally, acute gouty arthritis or renal colic (due to uric acid stones) may develop. A previous history of gout or the occurrence of hyperuricemia is not a contraindication to thiazide administration; serum uric acid levels may be reduced by the concurrent administration of allopurinol (see Chapter 16).

d) Hyperglycemia may develop in patients not previously known to have abnormal carbohydrate tolerance; known diabetics may require increased dosage of insulin or oral hypoglycemic agents for control. The mechanism appears to be twofold—decreased insulin secretion or release (partially related to hypokalemia) and peripheral insulin antagonism.

G. Spironolactones, aldosterone antagonists, are effective in the treatment of edematous states, such as congestive heart failure, the nephrotic syndrome, and cirrhosis with ascites and edema, even when elevated aldosterone levels cannot be demonstrated. Although satisfactory diuresis may occur when the drugs are employed alone, excellent results may be achieved by the concurrent administration of another diuretic, particularly a thiazide, ethacrynic acid, or furosemide. Actions are also potentiated by corticosteroids (especially when hyponatremia is present) and occasionally potassium, but the latter salts must be given cautiously, for hyperkalemia may occur. Because diuretic actions may be delayed as long as 7–10 days, the drug is not effective in the treatment of edematous states requiring immediate diuresis. It is usually ineffective in patients with renal insufficiency.

1. Mechanism of action Spironolactones are steroidal compounds similar in structure to aldosterone. They exert their effects by competitively inhibiting the action of aldosterone at the renal tubular level. They increase urinary excretion of sodium and chloride and decrease excretion of ammonia, titratable acid, and phosphorus. Glomerular filtration rate is either unchanged or falls slightly.

2. Preparation and dosage Spironolactone (Aldactone-A) is supplied as 25-mg tablets. The usual dosage range is 25–50 mg QID.

3. Side effects, which are rare, include drowsiness, mental confusion, maculopapular or erythematous skin rashes, and occasionally gynecomastia.

H. Triamterene is a pteridine compound unrelated chemically to any of the previously available diuretic agents.

1. Mechanism of action Triamterene acts on the distal renal tubule to depress the exchange of sodium for hydrogen ions and potassium apparently by noncompetitive inhibition of aldosterone. Its actions are additive to those of thiazides, spironolactone, and combinations of the two. It induces increased excretion of sodium (although the natriuresis is much less than that produced by thiazides), water, chloride, bicarbonate, and uric acid; urinary titratable acid and ammonium are decreased, and the urine pH rises. The urinary excretion of potassium is either decreased or not affected; hyperkalemia may result.

The drug is rapidly absorbed from the GI tract; diuretic action starts within 30 minutes and reaches a peak in 2–6 hours. Almost all of the drug is eliminated in the urine within 24 hours. Triamterene is a weak agent by itself; **ameloride,** an acyl-guanidine compound with similar effects, appears to be much more potent. A recommended dosage has not, however, been established, and the literature must be followed closely.

2. **Clinical application**   Triamterene is not a very effective diuretic when used alone; it should be administered concomitantly with other agents. It is most logically used as an adjunct to a thiazide preparation; not only are the effects of the two additive, but triamterene effectively protects against thiazide-induced hypokalemia. The drug should *not* be given to patients with renal insufficiency or hyperkalemia, nor administered concurrently with potassium supplements, for marked hyperkalemia may result. Serum potassium levels should be checked frequently after initiation of therapy, for even patients with apparently normal renal function may occasionally develop hyperkalemia.

3. **Preparations and dosage**   **Triamterene (Dyrenium)** is supplied as 100-mg capsules. Dyazide is a thiazide-triamterene combination, each capsule containing 25 mg hydrochlorothiazide and 50 mg triamterene. The usual dosage of triamterene is 100 mg once or twice daily with meals; occasionally 100 mg every other day will be sufficient, if given in addition to other diuretics. The maximum beneficial dose is 200 mg daily.

4. **Side effects** are not frequent. Nausea, vomiting, other GI disturbances, weakness, headache, dry mouth, skin rashes, hyperkalemia, and BUN elevation may occur. Leukopenia has been reported very rarely.

I. **Ethacrynic acid and furosemide,** structurally different but pharmacologically similar compounds, are the most potent diuretics now available. Ethacrynic acid is an unsaturated ketone derivative of phenoxyacetic acid and is structurally unique. Furosemide is a sulfonamide compound like the thiazides but has an anthrone ring as well. Research to date has shown the two drugs to be similar in their major mechanism of action, potency, clinical application, and side effects, so that the following comments refer to both agents unless otherwise stated.

1. **Mechanism of action; pharmacologic effects**

   a) Both drugs exert their major effect by blocking the reabsorption of sodium along the entire ascending limb of the loop of Henle. Additional effects probably occur in the proximal and distal convoluted tubules, but may not be similar.

   b) Diuresis is associated with increased urinary excretion of sodium, chloride, potassium, and ammonium ions, in a pattern similar to that seen with the thiazides. With ethacrynic acid there is little or no change in bicarbonate excretion and urine pH decreases, along with an increase in titratable acidity. The effect of furosemide on hydrogen ion and bicarbonate excretion is not firmly established. In contrast to the thiazides, neither agent when used for short-term therapy appears to depress glomerular filtration or renal plasma flow. The administration of doses over 100 mg to hypertensive patients results initially in decreased peripheral resistance and blood pressure; long-term antihypertensive effects are still being evaluated.

c) Both ethacrynic acid and furosemide are rapidly absorbed from the GI tract; diuresis begins quickly after oral administration, reaches maximum in 2–3 hours, and is usually complete in 6 hours. After intravenous administration profound diuresis occurs within 30 minutes, reaching maximum in 60–90 minutes.

2. **Clinical application** Ethacrynic acid and furosemide have been markedly effective in patients with edema (particularly those with anasarca due to CHF, cirrhosis, or nephrosis) refractory to other diuretics. Unlike other agents they remain effective in patients with low filtration rates or severe electrolyte abnormalities (e.g., hyponatremia, hypokalemia, hypochloremic alkalosis). The prompt and massive diuresis occurring after IV administration makes the drugs exceedingly useful in the treatment of acute pulmonary edema.

Furosemide and ethacrynic acid must be used judiciously because they may produce profound and prompt diuresis associated with all the complications of a rapid contraction of the ECF volume. There seems to be little advantage to supplanting other diuretics in those patients who respond well, without adverse side effects, to whatever preparation they have been taking.

Whatever the circumstances, however, those patients given the drugs should be given the minimum dose that will produce the desired effects, should be followed closely, and should have frequent determinations of the serum electrolytes.

3. **Preparation and dosage** **Ethacrynic acid (Edecrin)** is supplied in tablets of 25 and 50 mg for oral administration and in vials containing 50 mg powder for dilution and intravenous administration. **Furosemide (Lasix)** is available as tablets of 40 mg and in 2-cc ampules containing 20 mg furosemide for IV or IM injection.

a) **Oral therapy** should be initiated with 25 or 50 mg of ethacrynic acid or 40 mg of furosemide. If there is no marked diuresis, the dose should be doubled until a single dose of 200 mg of ethacrynic acid or 240 mg furosemide is reached. It is best to give the drugs after meals to lessen chances of gastric irritation. In patients with marked renal failure the increase in sodium excretion is not as great because basal sodium excretion per nephron is already markedly increased. Much higher doses (e.g., 800 mg ethacrynic acid) may be necessary to induce diuresis, but use of these doses is still experimental. The usual daily maintenance doses are 50 to 200 mg of ethacrynic acid and 80 to 240 mg of furosemide, preferably in two divided doses because of the short duration of action. Intermittent therapy (e.g., two days on, two off) is probably the most desirable, as this will minimize the incidence of serious electrolyte disturbances. In conditions associated with massive fluid retention, especially cirrhosis with ascites, the profound diuresis is often hazardous, but may be minimized by intermittent therapy, supplemental chloride and potassium, and concomitant use of an aldosterone antagonist. A relatively safe plan for diuresis has been described (*Gastroenterology* 49:531, 1965) and should be carried out in a hospital.

b) **The usual intravenous dose** is 25–100 mg of ethacrynic acid; the comparable dose of furosemide would be 40–120 mg.

4. **Side effects** most commonly reported are related to the GI tract and

include anorexia, nausea, vomiting, abdominal pain, and diarrhea (which may be watery and profuse). These may be minimized by administering the drug with food. Hematologic abnormalities so far reported are rare; those few that have occurred include thrombocytopenia, neutropenia, and questionably agranulocytosis.

Since both ethacrynic acid and furosemide decrease uric acid excretion, hyperuricemia and clinical gout may result from chronic administration. Furosemide shares the hyperglycemic effect of the thiazides, but the effects of ethacrynic acid on carbohydrate metabolism have not been clearly defined. Acute vertigo with deafness or tinnitus may rarely occur, probably due to inner-ear perilymph imbalance. The magnitude of the diuresis has resulted in acute urinary retention in patients with bladder neck obstruction.

The major adverse reactions are related to the pharmacologic actions of the drugs per se. Marked electrolyte abnormalities may occur and hypokalemia may be precipitated. The degree of kaliuresis usually varies directly with the urinary volume and may require prompt replacement. Prevention of hypokalemia is most crucial in patients receiving digitalis, in whom fatal arrhythmias have been induced. Rapid and profuse diuresis with reduction in ECF may result in hypotension, thromboembolic complications, increasing azotemia in patients with renal insufficiency, or hepatic encephalopathy (particularly if hypokalemia occurs concomitantly) in patients with severe liver disease. The reduction in ECF may induce a "contraction alkalosis," requiring chloride and potassium replacement for correction (*Ann. Intern. Med.* 63:979, 1965).

J. Corticosteroids, when given concomitantly with many of the above diuretics, may be beneficial in promoting diuresis, especially when marked hyponatremia is present. They may act by increasing free-water clearance and glomerular filtration rate. The usual dose of prednisone is 5–10 mg TID or QID for 5 days (watch for increase in congestive heart failure).

IV. PULMONARY EDEMA may occur in circulatory overload (e.g., congestive heart failure, acute glomerulonephritis), in association with severe infections, asthma, central nervous system injuries, etc., and following smoke or gas inhalation. The therapeutic goal is reduction of transudation of fluid into the alveoli, in heart failure by reducing pulmonary hypertension, and in chemical or irritative pulmonary edema by decreasing the inflammatory reaction and capillary permeability.

The treatment of pulmonary edema due to congestive heart failure is outlined below; a similar program is used in irritative pulmonary edema, except that digitalis and diuretics are seldom administered, and large doses of corticosteroids are usually given.

A. General The patient should be made comfortable, and his head elevated. If severe hypertension is present, the blood pressure should be reduced (as described in Chapter 7). If hypotension is present, therapy must be modified (see cardiogenic shock, Chapter 17).

B. Digitalis Digitalization should be accomplished with a rapidly acting preparation administered intravenously. If the patient has already been digitalized, additional small doses of deslanoside or digoxin may be given cautiously.

C. Aminophylline decreases bronchospasm and increases cardiac output; 500 mg are given IV initially and every 3–4 hours if required.

D. Morphine is one of the most important drugs during the acute stage; anxiety is allayed and tachypnea is decreased. The dose is 10–15 mg every 2–4 hours. It must be given cautiously to patients with chronic lung disease. The mechanism of action appears to be related to decrease in peripheral and pulmonary vascular resistance with pooling of blood in veins.

E. Oxygen (100%) should be given, preferably through positive-pressure breathing apparatus (except when shock is present). Some authors recommend that the oxygen be bubbled through antifoaming agents such as 50% ethyl alcohol, propylene glycol, or 2-ethylhexanol in order to decrease the respiratory obstruction resulting from the mechanical interference of edema fluid. The use of such agents is controversial.

F. Diuretics Ethacrynic acid, furosemide, or a mercurial drug should be administered parenterally.

G. An attempt should be made to rapidly decrease the intravascular volume when pulmonary edema is severe.

   1. Tourniquets or blood pressure cuffs (inflated to less than systolic pressure) should be applied to three of the extremities and rotated every 15 minutes. If marked edema and/or venous distention is present, however, this measure may be of little value, and phlebotomy may be necessary.

   2. Phlebotomy may be performed by rapidly removing 100–500 ml of blood (by 100-ml increments every 5–10 minutes), using a vacuum bottle or large syringes. This measure may be lifesaving, especially if pulmonary edema has resulted from excessive fluid administration. If the blood is collected under sterile conditions, the packed red cells may be returned to the patient (plasmapheresis). Phlebotomy is contraindicated in the presence of shock.

V.   CARDIAC TAMPONADE is that form of cardiac failure due to increased intrapericardial pressure. It may occur with large or small pericardial effusions or with constrictive pericarditis (dry tamponade). Treatment is specific—removal of the pericardial fluid and/or the pericardium. The relative merits of open versus closed pericardiocentesis are still being debated (*Amer. J. Cardiol.* 16:722, 1965; *Progr. Cardiovasc. Dis.* 10:64, 1967). Practical considerations make closed pericardiocentesis necessary in cases where the patient is deteriorating rapidly and time is critical. In these cases it is advisable to initiate arrangements for an open procedure, so that no further delay need ensue if the closed approach is unsuccessful.

A. Closed pericardiocentesis

   1. Obtain the following equipment:

      a) 5- and 50-ml syringes

      b) 14-, 18-, and 20-gauge needles, 3 inches in length, with short bevels

      c) 3-way stopcock

      d) Rubber connecting tubing

      e) Sterile Intracath set (optional)

      f) 2 alligator clamps

g) Connecting wire

h) ECG machine

i) Defibrillation equipment

Items **a–d** are usually included in a pericardiocentesis or thoracentesis tray.

2. **Position the patient** on an adjustable table at 60-degree elevation. Alternatively the patient may be sitting in a chair or bed with the back supported.

3. **Premedicate** with a barbiturate, meperidine, or morphine if the patient is apprehensive and his condition allows. Atropine 0.5 mg IM will help protect against a vasovagal reaction and should be given.

4. **Cleanse the skin** and use aseptic technique. **Administer local anesthesia** to the skin and subcutaneous tissue of the selected area. Connect a # 20 needle to the three-way stopcock and 50-ml syringe. Apply the limb leads of the electrocardiograph to the patient. Connect the shank of the needle to the V lead of the ECG machine via the alligator clamps and connecting wire. **Turn on the defibrillator and ECG machine, and monitor continuously.**

5. Numerous **potential sites** have been used, but the following are the safest and most rewarding.

   a) Subxiphoid   The needle is inserted directly inward at the left xiphocostal angle to the level of the inner rib cage. Then the hub is depressed and the needle is directed toward the left shoulder, keeping it close to the inner rib margin.

   b) Apical   The needle is inserted in the fifth intercostal space, 2 cm lateral to the apex beat (if present), or just inside the left border of dullness. With this route there is less chance of injuring a coronary artery.

   c) Triangle of safety   The needle is inserted in the fifth or sixth left intercostal space at the sternal border and is directed medially to avoid the internal mammary artery.

   d) Right-sided approach   If the effusion appears to be mainly on the right, one can enter the fourth intercostal space just inside the right border of dullness, directing the needle slightly medially.

6. Advance the needle slowly, without sudden movement, and with intermittent gentle suction. Fluid is usually encountered at a depth of 3–4 cm with these approaches, and a sensation of "give" is often felt as the pericardium is entered. Epicardial contact is marked by premature beats or ST or P-R segment elevation, and the needle must be drawn back. After the presence and depth of fluid have been ascertained, a larger needle may be substituted and a polyethylene catheter can be advanced. If the fluid is thick a larger needle may be necessary. With large effusions tamponade is usually relieved by removal of even a small amount of fluid.

7. If no fluid is obtained at one site, others should be tried. Possible causes of failure are thick fluid, loculation, tissue in the aspirating needle, and thickened pericardium.

8. Open surgical approach is indicated if the closed procedure fails to relieve tamponade.

9. Dangers of closed pericardiocentesis

a) **Entry into a cardiac chamber** If bloody fluid is aspirated, a rapid hematocrit determination should determine the source of the fluid. Also, sodium dehydrocholate (Decholin) may be injected; if a response occurs, the needle is not in the pericardium and should be withdrawn. In the catheterization laboratory one can determine the location of the needle by simply attaching it to a pressure transducer.

b) Coronary artery damage.

c) **Arrhythmias** Withdraw the needle. If the arrhythmia persists, treat as usual (see Chapter 6).

d) Pneumothorax.

e) Puncture of lung, stomach, or liver.

f) Subepicardial hematoma.

g) Pleuropericardial infection from contamination.
The nature of the above list makes it desirable to have a thoracic surgeon readily available.

B. General measures Maintenance of adequate venous filling pressure is crucial. Although the venous pressure is usually very high in tamponade, this pressure is necessary to maintain adequate cardiac filling. Phlebotomy, tourniquets, and diuretics are, therefore, contraindicated.

1. If blood pressure is falling, a trial of volume expansion is warranted.

2. Oxygen should be given, but positive-pressure delivery is contraindicated, as it will elevate intrapericardial pressure.

3. The use of digitalis and sympathomimetic agents is controversial, probably because they do not constitute definitive treatment.

The cardiac arrhythmias present many challenging problems in diagnosis and treatment. Certain of them are life-threatening (when the ventricular rate is greater than 180/minute, for example, approximately 50% of patients will develop vascular collapse or pulmonary congestion) and require prompt and precise treatment. The mechanism of action, cardiotoxicity, and indications for use of the various antiarrhythmic drugs must be fully understood.

Appropriate therapy requires correct diagnosis. The ECG should be carefully measured and, when indicated, repeated during carotid sinus pressure; it is especially important to look for P waves. Frequent tracings should be obtained during therapy. Every effort should be made to determine whether or not the patient has been taking any type of cardiac drug, particularly digitalis; the heart and lungs should be carefully examined and the jugular pulse observed for A waves; the apical pulse and blood pressure should be monitored frequently.

Which drug to use and by which route it should be administered depend not only on the type of arrhythmia but also on such factors as the severity of the clinical situation (i.e., presence of coronary insufficiency, pulmonary edema, cerebrovascular insufficiency), ventricular rate, age of the patient, electrolyte values, previous administration of digitalis or other cardiac drugs, etc.

Agents available for the treatment of arrhythmias are discussed below; sections dealing with specific arrhythmias follow.

I. **GENERAL MEASURES** The correction of hypotension, hypoxia, and/or electrolyte imbalance may occasionally terminate a cardiac arrhythmia without further specific therapy. Congestive heart failure should be treated by the usual measures unless it is due to a digitalis-induced arrhythmia. Sedation is administered if indicated. Continuous ECG monitoring with the institution of therapy and thereafter is desirable.

II. **ANTIARRHYTHMIC DRUGS**

   A. Digitalis is discussed in detail in Chapter 5.

   B. Quinidine

   1. **Pharmacologic effects** Quinidine exerts beneficial antiarrhythmic effects by depressing myocardial excitability (and thus ectopic impulse formation), slowing conduction velocity (ECG shows widening of QRS complex), and prolonging the refractory period (ECG shows prolongation of Q-T interval). Therapeutic levels also depress myocardial contractility, produce vagolytic effects, and cause varying degrees of peripheral adrenergic blockade with resultant peripheral vasodilatation and hypotension.

   2. **Absorption and excretion** Absorption from the GI tract begins within 15 minutes after a single oral dose. Peak plasma concen-

tration occurs in 2–4 hours; 40% disappears from the blood in 6 hours, 75% in 12 hours, and 90% in 24 hours. If repeated doses are given in a single day, however, the decrement in blood level is slower. When quinidine is administered every 2 hours, for example, there are progressively smaller increases in blood levels after each successive dose through the fourth; no increases occur after the fifth or sixth dose because of balance between absorption and metabolic breakdown. When given every 4 hours, the maximum serum concentration occurs in 48–96 hours, then remains stable. Essentially all of the drug is excreted in the urine.

3. **Serum levels** Although there are often discrepancies between the serum concentration of quinidine and therapeutic or toxic effects (primarily because of the presence in the serum of metabolic products that are inactive but are measured by the ordinary photo-fluorometric quinidine assay), it would be ideal to determine serum levels, since clinical effects and toxicity are better correlated with this value than with dosage per se.

No antiarrhythmic effects are noted at serum concentrations of less than 2 mg/L; ideal therapeutic effects occur at levels of 5–8 mg/L. Myocardial toxicity is uncommon in this range but increases significantly at levels above 8 mg/L (e.g., 30% at 8–10 mg/L; 65% at 14 mg/L). Despite the variability of dose-concentration relationships, the therapeutic range of serum concentration is usually achieved by the administration of 0.6–2.0 gm/day orally, or 300–500 mg IV over a period of 30–60 minutes.

4. **Toxic effects** The most common side effects are diarrhea, nausea, and vomiting. Other symptoms of cinchonism (salivation, tinnitus, vertigo, headache, visual disturbances, confusion) may occur; quinidine administration may be continued if the symptoms are mild. Idiosyncratic reactions such as fever, thrombocytopenic purpura, and exfoliative dermatitis are uncommon. Respiratory paralysis and sudden death are rare but recognized complications of quinidine administration. Proteinuria may be observed.

Hypotension most commonly follows parenteral administration, but, rarely, vascular collapse may occur after administration of small doses orally. Myocardial toxicity may be manifested by VPCs, A-V block, 50% or greater increase in QRS duration, ventricular tachycardia, or ventricular fibrillation. Syncope may be an unrecognized manifestation of ventricular arrhythmia due to quinidine toxicity. Any of the above requires cessation of therapy. Unfortunately, these toxic reactions may occur without preceding symptoms of cinchonism or widening of the QRS complex on the ECG. Quinidine may decrease the refractory period and conduction time of the A-V node by its vagolytic effects; this action may cause undesirable increase in ventricular rate in atrial fibrillation or atrial flutter, particularly if quinidine is administered alone without prior digitalization.

5. **Clinical application** Quinidine has proved most useful in the treatment of APCs and the conversion and prophylactic management of atrial fibrillation. It is contraindicated in patients with known quinine sensitivity and in the presence of incomplete or complete A-V block. With the exception of the postoperative period there are probably no circumstances that justify the parenteral use of quinidine, especially since the advent of cardioversion equipment.

It has been used with some degree of success in the management and prophylaxis of the Wolff-Parkinson-White (WPW) syndrome.

6. Preparations Dosage is listed in the sections dealing with treatment of specific arrhythmias. Oral preparations include **quinidine sulfate** in tablets or capsules of 0.2 gm, **quinidine polygalacturonate (Cardioquin)** in tablets containing the equivalent of 0.2 gm quinidine sulfate, and **sustained-release quinidine gluconate (Quinaglute)** in tablets of 0.3 gm. Cardioquin is reported to cause a lesser incidence of local gastric irritation than quinidine sulfate, though a number of observers have failed to note any significant difference; its pattern of absorption and the dosage are essentially the same. Quinaglute is reported to permit a uniform release of the drug and thus maintenance of significant blood levels of quinidine for longer periods of time than quinidine sulfate. The peak serum concentration (4.3 mg/L) is reached in 4–8 hours after administration of a single dose and drops about 1.0 mg/L during the next 4 hours. It is stated that arrhythmias recur less commonly because quinidine blood levels are maintained, but careful clinical studies to document this claim are lacking. The usual dosage of Quinaglute is 0.3–0.6 gm every 8–12 hours.

For parenteral administration quinidine gluconate is the preparation of choice. It is supplied in 10-ml vials containing 80 mg quinidine/ml.

C. Procaine amide (Pronestyl)

1. Pharmacologic effects The cardiac actions of procaine amide are essentially identical to those of quinidine.

2. Absorption and excretion Absorption from the GI tract is rapid; maximal plasma concentration occurs within 60 minutes after administration of a single oral dose. Effects occur immediately after IV administration, and almost as rapidly (5–10 minutes, maximum in 30–60 minutes) after IM injection. Plasma levels decline about 10–15% per hour. About 60% of the drug is excreted in the urine.

3. Toxic effects Severe hypotension, which may occur after IV administration, is much less common after IM injection, and rare after oral administration. Other side effects include nausea, vomiting, anorexia, fever, drug rash, agranulocytosis (rare), mental confusion (not uncommon), a lupus-like syndrome with positive lupus erythematosus preparations, and ventricular fibrillation or cardiac standstill. ECG changes include prolongation of the P-R, QRS, and Q-T intervals. Although the cardiotoxic effects of quinidine and procaine amide are similar, the QRS widening due to quinidine may be accompanied by depression of the atrial pacemaker and A-V dissociation, whereas procaine amide more often induces premature beats and/or paroxysmal tachycardias. Severe cardiotoxic manifestations due to quinidine or procaine amide may be treated by the administration of molar sodium lactate or EDTA.

4. Clinical application Procaine amide is most commonly used for the treatment of VPCs or other ventricular arrhythmias, especially those which are due to digitalis excess. Procaine amide may be given to patients requiring quinidine but sensitive to that drug. More specific comments appear in following sections. Procaine amide must be used cautiously, if at all, in patients with complete A-V block.

5. Preparations   Procaine amide is supplied in capsules of 250 mg for oral administration, and in 10-ml vials (procaine amide hydrochloride) containing 100 mg/ml for parenteral use.

D. Lidocaine (Xylocaine) has a mechanism of action similar to that of procaine amide, but in contrast to procaine amide equivalent doses of lidocaine cause no fall in blood pressure or decrease in myocardial contractility. Its onset of action after IV administration is rapid (within 45–90 seconds) and duration of action brief (effects are dissipated within 20 minutes). The drug has been used most frequently for the treatment of ventricular arrhythmias developing during anesthesia, but more recently has been used for the treatment of unresponsive ventricular tachycardia (or, occasionally, supraventricular tachycardia) in unanesthetized patients. It is probably the drug of choice for digitalis-induced ventricular premature contractions or ventricular tachycardia (a situation in which electrical cardioversion is contraindicated) and also for the treatment of ventricular tachycardia due to other causes if cardioversion equipment is not available. The usual dose is 1 mg/kg body weight IV every 20 minutes, if necessary. Continuous IV infusion in the same dose as above, as well as smaller (50 mg) single IV doses, have not been extensively tried clinically but may prove beneficial in the refractory case. The usual maximum dose is 750 mg IV, but doses exceeding this have been reported. The drug is contraindicated in patients with Adams-Stokes attacks with A-V dissociation and a slow nodal or idioventricular pacemaker. Side effects in unanesthetized patients include analgesia, drowsiness, discomfort in breathing or swallowing, blurred or double vision, numbness, sweating, cerebral irritation, and medullary depression. Coma has been observed. High doses may precipitate convulsions or respiratory arrest. The drug in its available form contains 0.1 mEq $Na+$/ml.

E. Diphenylhydantoin (Dilantin) may be very effective in the treatment of certain cardiac arrhythmias, particularly those due to digitalis intoxication. Its onset of action is very rapid, and toxic effects appear to be few. (A comprehensive review of this drug and its use in treating cardiac arrhythmias appears in *Ann. Intern. Med.* 67:1084, 1967.) The precise mechanism of action awaits further clarification but is probably related to the drug's effect on ion movement across cell membranes.

Reports indicate that a number of arrhythmias may be controlled or terminated. It has proved to be quite ineffective in atrial flutter and chronic atrial fibrillation, but may prove effective in the prevention of paroxysmal atrial tachycardia or fibrillation. A limited number of favorable reports recommends its usefulness in supraventricular tachycardias, including those secondary to digitalis intoxication; its mechanism of action in these arrhythmias is uncertain. Transient ventricular arrhythmias—namely VPCs, bigeminy, ventricular tachycardia, whether secondary to anesthesia, cardioversion, cardiac catheterization and surgery, arteriosclerotic heart disease, myocardial infarction, or digitalis intoxication—may respond satisfactorily to IV administration with oral therapy instituted thereafter for prophylaxis. There is evidence that Dilantin can oppose the automatism induced by digitalis without affecting its inotropic effect.

The drug may be administered orally in a dosage of 100–200 mg TID or QID for maintenance therapy. For treatment of acute arrhythmias a single dose of 125 mg (diluted to 25 mg/ml) may be injected IV over a 3–5-minute period, with a maximum of 250 mg within 15 minutes, 500 mg within 1 hour, and 1 gm within 1 day. Continuous monitoring is advisable. Maintenance therapy is begun with reversion of the arrhythmia.

The toxicity of long-term Dilantin therapy is reviewed in standard sources. Adverse reactions following IV administration include tremors, ataxia, nystagmus, drowsiness, and confusion, but these are relatively infrequent. Sinus bradycardia and A-V conduction disturbances may occur, but are rare, usually transient, and possibly dose-related; preexistence of these conditions probably contraindicates the use of this drug. Hypotension is infrequent. Ventricular fibrillation and asystole have been reported in elderly debilitated patients given rapid IV therapy. It is advisable not to administer the drug to those with hypoxia or acidosis, since its effect in these circumstances may be unpredictable.

F. Vasopressors Rapid cardiac arrhythmias (especially atrial, nodal, and ventricular tachycardias) are often associated with varying degrees of hypotension. Restoration of systemic blood pressure with vasopressor agents may terminate such arrhythmias in a significant percentage of patients, and administration of such drugs is often the first therapeutic measure employed by many physicians. The antiarrhythmic effects of pressor drugs are most likely related to improved coronary perfusion, effects on the carotid sinus and arch, and perhaps a direct myocardial action. Preparations and dosage are listed in Chapter 17; Aramine is one of the most frequently used. Blood pressure must be carefully monitored, for elevation to excessive levels may be complicated by the development of serious ventricular arrhythmias.

G. Propranolol This agent is now available for clinical use, but experience is still relatively limited. The literature should be followed for reports of further clinical results, including adverse reactions and complications.

Propranolol is a competitive beta-adrenergic blocking agent with a therapeutic ratio 10 times that of its isomer, pronethalol. Electron-microscopic studies conducted on experimental animals have revealed myolytic lesions of a focal or confluent variety, dependent on dose.

By inhibiting myocardial response to catecholamines, propranolol decreases the automaticity of the S-A node and prolongs conduction through it, increases the refractory period of the A-V node, and decreases the automaticity of ectopic pacemakers. Because of these actions it is contraindicated in the presence of bradycardia, congestive heart failure, and A-V dissociation or block. It should not be used in patients with asthma or pulmonary hypertension. It will effectively reduce the ventricular rate in atrial flutter and fibrillation and may prove useful in the preparation of patients for cardioversion and in the treatment of rapid ventricular rate not well controlled by digitalis. It has been found to be of benefit in the treatment of PAT, PAT with block due to digitalis, and VPCs secondary to coronary insufficiency, infarction, cardiac surgery, or digitalis. Preliminary reports indicate that it is also useful in paroxysmal atrial flutter and fibrillation, paroxysmal ventricular tachycardia, and obstructive cardiomyopathy.

Side effects include bradycardia, hypotension, headaches, dizziness, nausea, epigastric discomfort, and pulmonary edema. One case of thrombocytopenia has been reported. Long-term toxic effects have not been enumerated. Some recommend the concomitant use of atropine to modify the unopposed vagal action. In case of overdosage, Isuprel may be used.

Initial therapy is 5–10 mg orally TID–QID, with doses ranging up to 160 mg/day. An escape phenomenon has been observed but is not understood or well documented. Use in the treatment of angina is discussed in Chapter 4.

III. CARDIOVERSION The development by Lown of the capacitor-discharge defibrillator which delivers an external electrical impulse that is underdamped, has a duration of 2.5 msec, is released from a 16 microfarad (µf) capacitor through a 100 millihenry inductance, and synchronized to avoid the vulnerable periods (the 30 msec up to and including the apex of the T wave on the surface ECG) has circumvented the hazards of AC discharge (myocardial damage, ventricular arrhythmias, and standstill). The technique has grown beyond its initial application which was limited to patients with atrial fibrillation considered to be drug failures and to those whose critical condition required rapid reversion of an arrhythmia. Fortunately, cardioversion equipment is becoming widely available, its indications are better defined, and its incidence of side effects has proved to be low. Lown has reported successful conversion to sinus rhythm in 93% of the episodes of atrial fibrillation, 97% of atrial flutter, 98% of ventricular tachycardia, and 74% of supraventricular tachycardia. This form of therapy will not obviate the necessity of administering antiarrhythmic drugs in a variety of clinical circumstances. The following guidelines may be used for the discriminate use of this form of therapy.

A. Contraindications Generally speaking, electrical cardioversion is contraindicated in the following circumstances:

1. Sinus tachycardia.

2. Supraventricular tachycardia unless resistant to vagal maneuvers, digitalis, or antiarrhythmic drugs. If there is a rapid ventricular rate with cardiovascular collapse that is not remedied quickly with drugs, cardioversion should be employed.

3. Digitalis-induced arrhythmias. Most of the complications of cardioversion have arisen in the digitalis-toxic patient. This problem and its associated arrhythmias, if present, are best treated by withdrawal of the drug, the administration of KCl, and the use of antiarrhythmic medication.

4. Repetitive tachycardias or recurrent, diverse atrial arrhythmias prior to onset of chronic atrial fibrillation.

5. Atrial fibrillation associated with rheumatic heart disease in the immediate preoperative and postoperative periods. Intractable heart failure may be an exception. Cardioversion may be done during a convenient period (2 weeks–3 months) postoperatively.

   Patients with intolerance to quinidine and other maintenance antiarrhythmic drugs and patients who previously were converted with quinidine and despite adequate maintenance doses revert to atrial fibrillation should not be cardioverted.

   Patients with atrial fibrillation and hyperthyroidism should become euthyroid before cardioversion is attempted.

6. Elderly asymptomatic patients with coronary artery disease and atrial fibrillation with a slow ventricular rate without digitalis.

7. Complete A-V block.

B. Electrical cardioversion may be useful in the following conditions:

1. Chronic atrial fibrillation, especially if of less than 1 year's duration. If peripheral or pulmonary emboli are thought to originate in the atria, the patient should be anticoagulated and cardioversion attempted.

2. Atrial flutter, one of the easiest arrhythmias to cardiovert.

3. Supraventricular tachycardia, associated with WPW syndrome, which is compromising the cardiovascular system. If the situation is not critical, medical therapy with digitalis and/or quinidine may be tried initially. There is some evidence that propranolol may be useful in such disorders.

4. The seriously ill patient with ventricular tachycardia, especially if accompanied by hypotension or pulmonary edema, or if the arrhythmia is sustained or occurs in the wake of an acute infarction. In such a situation drugs (lidocaine preferred to procaine) administered as outlined (this chapter, sec. II, paragraph **D**) may be tried initially, but electrical cardioversion should be quickly employed if rapid, sustained conversion does not occur, if hypotension occurs or persists, or if there is widening of the QRS complex after a brief trial of these drugs.

5. Ventricular fibrillation of any cause.

C. The technique of electrical cardioversion is described in reports by Lown (*New Eng. J. Med.* 269:325, 1963; *Brit. Heart J.* 29:469, 1967). In general the following measures are observed: The procedure is explained to the patient in order to decrease anxiety and thereby decrease the release of catecholamines. Digitalis and diuretics are withheld for 1–2 days and anticoagulants are administered for 2–3 weeks prior to conversion attempt to those with mitral stenosis or a previous history of peripheral or pulmonary emboli. Quinidine 0.3 gm orally QID is begun 24–48 hours before the procedure. Premedication with a sedative such as Nembutal 1–2 hours beforehand is desirable. The synchronizer is adjusted to a setting of 0 msec (intrinsic instrument delay of about 20 msec generally allows discharge to fall during the downstroke of R wave or within the S wave), and the accuracy of the discharge with the cardiac cycle is checked by discharging the paddles against each other. Amnesia is induced with 25–75 mg of methohexital IV. The paddles are coated with electrode paste, and the patient is positioned so that he is lying with the left infrascapular area on the posterior paddle. The anterior paddle is held with pressure over the upper sternum at the level of the third intercostal space. A stable baseline on the oscilloscope is awaited and the discharge is fired. Low-energy settings—25–50 watt-seconds (w-s)—are recommended as initial discharges. (In ventricular tachycardia and fibrillation initial energy settings of 100 w-s with increments of 100 should be used.) Increments of 50–100 w-s to 400 w-s may then be successfully employed until sinus rhythm ensues. If arrhythmias develop prior to successful conversion, one may abandon the procedure or administer drugs, e.g., 50-mg IV doses of lidocaine to suppress VPCs. Procaine amide and Dilantin may also be used.

D. Adverse effects are few. Muscle soreness and erythema or irritation of the skin at the electrode sites are not uncommon; burns may be kept at a minimum by applying adequate amounts of electrode paste. Enzyme rises (in lactic dehydrogenase and SGOT) occur rarely, and are considered to derive from local muscle trauma. Atrial, nodal, or ventricular ectopic beats and other minor arrhythmias may occur transiently after restoration of sinus rhythm. Reports of serious arrhythmias, such as ventricular tachycardia, are few; fatalities due to ventricular fibrillation or cardiac standstill are very rare and almost always have occurred in patients with digitalis excess. Pulmonary edema occurs rarely. Systemic and pulmonary emboli are rare complications occurring in less than 2% of patients, with no fatalities reported.

IV. ECTOPIC BEATS

A. Atrial premature contractions APCs are usually benign, but if frequent and multifocal they may presage a more serious atrial arrhythmia. Quinidine sulfate 200–400 mg every 4–6 hours may abolish the ectopic focus. Digitalis, diphenylhydantoin 100 mg QID, or procaine amide 250–500 mg QID may also be tried.

B. Ventricular premature contractions VPCs may occur in the absence of organic disease, as a manifestation of increased myocardial irritability (especially after a myocardial infarction), or as a result of digitalis intoxication (multifocal, multidirectional, bigeminy). When not a reflection of serious heart disease they may be treated successfully with mild sedation and abstinence from excessive coffee, tobacco, and alcohol. When VPCs are a manifestation of underlying heart disease, procaine amide 250–500 mg every 6 hours, quinidine sulfate 200–400 mg TID–QID, or diphenylhydantoin 100 mg QID (though experience with the latter agent is limited) may abolish the irritable focus. Lidocaine is useful for short-term therapy. Refer to discussion of lidocaine and its use in acute myocardial infarction in Chapter 4. Propranolol may also be useful. When VPCs occur in the setting of cardiac failure, they may respond to digitalis.

V. SINUS TACHYCARDIA
In adults the rate usually varies between 100 and 160, but in children (and in adults with severe hypermetabolic states) the rate may be higher. Clinically the rhythm is basically regular, but minimal cyclic variations may be present. The ECG will show slight but significant changes in rate if monitored over a 5–10-minute period. Response to carotid sinus pressure is variable: There is often slight and gradual slowing, but the arrhythmia is not terminated. Marked sinus tachycardia is rarely a manifestation of congestive heart failure alone and will not respond to digitalis administration; indeed, digitalis given to the anoxic, hypovolemic, or septic patient with sinus tachycardia may produce severe ventricular arrhythmias. Therapy is directed at the underlying cause.

VI. PAROXYSMAL SUPRAVENTRICULAR TACHYCARDIA
may represent paroxysmal atrial tachycardia (PAT), paroxysmal nodal tachycardia, or a group of arrhythmias in which the source of the ectopic focus cannot be determined. The rate varies from 150–250, but most of these arrhythmias are in the 160–200 range; the atrial and ventricular rates are the same. Clinically the rhythm is characterized by a uniform regularity, often of

sudden onset and cessation; a 10–15-minute period of ECG monitoring will show variation of less than 3 beats per minute. Carotid sinus pressure either abolishes the arrhythmia or produces no effects. The ECG shows a more or less normal QRS complex, but confusion may arise when there is marked aberration or bundle-branch block occurring with more rapid rates; this is particularly common in patients with diseased hearts or the Wolff-Parkinson-White syndrome. Supraventricular tachycardias frequently occur in patients with otherwise normal hearts. As a rule they do not constitute severe medical emergencies unless they have precipitated cardiac failure, vascular collapse, or pain of coronary insufficiency. In these latter situations the urgency for immediate restoration of sinus rhythm would weigh strongly for cardioversion as the therapy of choice if carotid sinus massage and administration of vasopressors do not abolish the arrhythmia promptly. In less seriously ill patients the other measures listed below may be tried. Young healthy patients with supraventricular tachycardias often respond to one or more of the first four measures described, but patients with heart disease frequently require digitalis for restoration of sinus rhythm.

A. **Sedation and reassurance** often will restore normal sinus rhythm.

B. **Vagal stimulation** Many attacks can be terminated by increasing vagal tone. Carotid sinus pressure should be tried first. The patient must be recumbent; the ECG should be monitored constantly. The right carotid sinus should be massaged first, for 10–30 seconds, and if this is ineffective then the left. Both carotid sinuses should not be massaged simultaneously (asystole or cerebrovascular thrombosis may result). Valsalva maneuvers or eyeball pressure may be useful if carotid massage fails, but the latter procedure must be done with great care, if at all, because of the danger of retinal detachment. Induction of vomiting by administration of apomorphine or ipecac is decidedly unpleasant and rarely warranted.

C. **Vasopressors** should be used whenever hypotension exists, but in addition they are frequently effective in normotensive patients, probably by stimulating the carotid sinus and aortic receptors, and perhaps by increasing coronary blood flow. They should not be given to hypertensive patients. **Neo-Synephrine** 0.5–1.0 mg, *or* **metaraminol (Aramine)** 0.5–2.0 mg, may be injected intravenously over 2–3 minutes. Ectopic beats and significant rises in blood pressure may occur. Dosage of other preparations is listed in Table 17-1.

D. **Parasympathomimetic drugs**

1. **Neostigmine is the drug of choice.** Give 0.5–2.0 mg subcutaneously; if the arrhythmia does not revert in 30–60 minutes repeat carotid sinus massage.
2. **Mecholyl,** although effective, should not be used because of its tendency to produce marked hypotension.

E. **Rapid digitalization** is the most consistently effective therapy and should be tried if simple measures do not terminate the attack promptly. Digoxin may be given orally to those patients in no great distress, but intravenous administration of drugs is indicated for those whose arrhythmia requires rapid termination. Give **Cedilanid** 0.4–0.8 mg IV over 2–3 minutes, followed by another 0.4 mg 60–90 minutes later. Equivalent doses of **digoxin** are as effective: 0.75–1.0 mg initially followed by another 0.25–0.5 mg in 60–90 minutes. After each dose of digitalis carotid sinus massage should be tried. In many hands the most rapid response occurs to **ouabain**, but the dosage range is variable, and almost continuous ECG monitoring is required. Although ouabain is an exceedingly effective drug, such rapid abolition of the arrhythmia is seldom required. The dosage is 0.25–0.5 mg initially followed by 0.1–0.15 mg every 30–45 minutes thereafter.

F. **Quinidine, procaine amide, or diphenylhydantoin** (though clinical data concerning this last agent are limited) may be useful in certain situations. See discussion of cardioversion.

G. **Prevention of recurrent attacks** Sedation, avoidance of coffee, tea, tobacco, and overfatigue, and, if necessary, maintenance digitalis and/or quinidine. Refer to earlier discussions in this chapter on diphenylhydantoin and propranolol.

VII. **PAT WITH BLOCK** This rhythm, the "great masquerader," may appear clinically as normal sinus rhythm, atrial flutter, or supraventricular tachycardia. More than 75% of cases result from digitalis excess. Cardinal ECG findings include a rapid atrial rate, usually between 150 and 210, rarely faster. (With flutter the atrial rate is usually greater than 240.) In contrast to flutter the ST segments are isoelectric, the P waves are upright in leads 2 and 3, and the atrial rate may vary considerably, demonstrating a "ventriculophasic" effect (the P-P interval surrounding a ventricular complex is shorter than the P-P interval not enclosing a QRS). The P waves are often small, bizarre, and spiked in shape; they may be recognizable in only one lead, often V_1 or other right-sided precordial lead. The ventricular rate varies, depending on the degree of A-V block, and may be almost regular to grossly irregular. Response to carotid sinus pressure varies, but most often there are variations in A-V conduction, while changes in atrial rate are rare. In 40% of cases, VPCs are associated. It is imperative to differentiate PAT with block from atrial flutter; the former is frequently a manifestation of digitalis excess, whereas the latter is rarely so. **Treatment:**

A. Stop digitalis administration if the drug is being given.

B. Give potassium if digitalis toxicity is suspected. In urgent situations give IV 40 mEq KCl in 500 ml 5% D/W over 1–3 hours. In less serious situations KCl may be given orally: 4–5 gm initially, followed by 2 gm every 3–4 hours as needed. Procaine amide, in usual dosage, may be used alone or in addition to potassium salts.

C. When PAT with block is *not* a reflection of digitalis intoxication, digitalis is the drug of choice.

VIII. **ATRIAL FIBRILLATION** is characterized by a rapid rate and irregularly irregular rhythm. In undigitalized patients the ventricular rate is generally over 100 and may even exceed 200. Clinically no jugular A waves are seen; the first heart sound is variable in intensity; a pulse deficit is usually present. Carotid sinus pressure produces gradual and transient slowing of the ventricular rate but no reversion. The ECG shows gross irregularity associated with a QRS complex which is usually normal in configuration, but occasionally widened and bizarre due to ventricular aberration or bundle-branch block. No matter how bizarre the QRS, however, a very rapid, grossly irregular rhythm is usually atrial fibrillation or atrial flutter with varying block; these should not be confused with ventricular tachycardia.

Chronic atrial fibrillation is most often associated with rheumatic heart disease (particularly mitral valve disease), ischemic or hypertensive heart disease, and diffuse myocardial disease; occasionally it may occur in patients with pericarditis, thyrotoxicosis, or the WPW syndrome. In some patients no heart disease is demonstrable. **Paroxysmal atrial fibrillation** may be produced by digitalis intoxication or pulmonary embolism; it may occur in healthy young adults under increased emotional tension, and in other clinical conditions described in standard sources.

The major disadvantages of atrial fibrillation are decrease in cardiac reserve (restoration of sinus rhythm increases the resting cardiac output by 20–25% in those patients who have heart failure associated with the arrhythmia), pulmonary or peripheral embolism (which is especially common in patients with mitral stenosis), and the subjective distress produced by palpitations. Treatment is described below.

A. **Initial treatment Digitalis** is the drug of choice for controlling the ventricular rate. It may be given orally to patients not in distress; more rapid digitalization with IV preparations is indicated for those patients who have very rapid ventricular rates and appear acutely ill. Digitalization should proceed until the ventricular rate is controlled in the range of 60–80 beats per minute at rest or 90–110 beats per minute after slight exercise unless toxic manifestations preclude administration of the required dosage; maintenance doses may then be given.

Refer to section on propranolol in regard to its use in controlling ventricular rate in fibrillation.

Special problems may be presented by the patient who first presents with atrial fibrillation and slow ventricular response rate (e.g., 40–60 beats per minute); these patients are often in the older age groups and have vascular disease or disease of the A-V node. If such patients do not develop excessive ventricular rates after exercise or exhibit evidence of congestive heart failure, there is no immediate indication for digitalis administration; indeed, these patients have a high incidence of further rhythm disturbances (e.g., sinoatrial standstill, sinoatrial block, slow A-V nodal rhythm, etc.) associated with reversion of atrial fibrillation.

During or after digitalization conversion to normal sinus rhythm may occur; if it does not, then the controversial problem arises as to whether further measures should be attempted to restore sinus rhythm.

B. **Methods for conversion** of atrial fibrillation to sinus rhythm may be pharmacologic (by the administration of quinidine or, rarely, procaine amide) or electrical (cardioversion). The use of the cardioverter and the pharmacology of quinidine and procaine amide are discussed in previous sections of this chapter. Electrical (DC) cardioversion is now the treatment of choice. If the specialized apparatus is not available, pharmacologic conversion may be attempted as outlined below. The indications and contraindications are essentially the same for either method of conversion and are outlined in the electrical-cardioversion section.

C. **Regimen for conversion with quinidine sulfate**

1. **The patient should be hospitalized and fully digitalized** This is important because quinidine is vagolytic and enhances A-V conduc-

tion; at the same time it slows and regularizes atrial action, thus allowing more impulses to pass through the A-V node. The result is a more rapid ventricular rate. Without adequate digitalization the patient may develop atrial flutter with 1:1 conduction and resultant vascular collapse or increased congestive heart failure. On the other hand, digitalis dosage should not be raised for those moderate increases in rate which are concomitants of quinidine administration; since digitalis and quinidine have opposing effects on the atrium, increasing digitalis levels may theoretically decrease chances for reversion.

2. **Give a test dose** of 0.2 gm quinidine sulfate to determine whether hypersensitivity or idiosyncrasy exists; if the patient tolerates this, attempts at reversion may be begun.

3. **Dosage schedules** are determined by the rate of absorption of quinidine, the time of peak plasma concentration, and the rate of disappearance. Two popular dosage schedules have been described by Sokolow and Levine; the Sokolow method is the more frequently used. The pharmacology of quinidine, discussed in the introductory sections of this chapter, should be reviewed before proceeding with treatment.

   Both dosage schedules have recommended that as much as 3–4 gm/day of quinidine be given; in view of the safety and effectiveness of cardioversion, however, it would seem wise to use the cardioverter rather than to administer potentially cardiotoxic doses of quinidine, i.e., more than 2.0 gm daily.

   a) **Sokolow method** Give quinidine 5 times a day at 2-hour intervals. Start with 0.2-gm or 0.3-gm doses. Increase each individual dose by 0.1 gm daily until toxicity or reversion occurs. It is wise to limit the maximum total daily dosage to 3.0 gm, but if reversion is felt imperative, if no evidence of toxicity has occurred, if very frequent ECGs can be obtained, and if cardioversion apparatus is not available, a total daily dose of 4.0 gm may be administered.

   b) **Levine method** Give 3 doses daily at 4-hour intervals, starting with 0.2 gm quinidine sulfate and increasing each subsequent dose by 0.2 gm until conversion occurs or a maximum daily dose of 3.0 gm is being administered.

4. **ECGs should be obtained frequently** and before each dosage of the drug at higher levels. Quinidine should be stopped if severe vomiting occurs, if the QRS duration has increased by 50% of the control value (25% if incomplete or complete bundle-branch block was present initially), or if frequent VPCs appear.

5. **Anticoagulation** The incidence of embolization at time of reversion to sinus rhythm is estimated to be about 1%. Although the value of anticoagulation in preventing embolization is unknown, most observers recommend for patients with previous peripheral or pulmonary emboli and those with mitral stenosis the administration of anticoagulants for 2–3 weeks prior to attempting reversion; in other situations the matter is one of individual preference.

6. **Maintenance quinidine dosage** after successful reversion is usually 0.2–0.3 gm QID; as much as 2.0 gm/day may be required by some patients, but these higher doses are frequently associated with significant gastrointestinal symptoms.

7. Results Successful conversion occurs in 50–90% of patients, with the best results in patients with atrial fibrillation of short duration and without severe congestive heart failure.

IX. **ATRIAL FLUTTER** This arrhythmia is very similar to atrial fibrillation. The atrial rate generally varies between 240 and 350, but in certain patients, especially if they are receiving quinidine, it may be 200 or less. With giant atria an impure flutter with an atrial rate of 400 sometimes occurs. The ventricular rate varies with the degree of A-V block, which is usually 2:1 in untreated cases. A 1:1 block is rare, but any regular rhythm with a ventricular rate greater than 270 is almost invariably flutter with 1:1 conduction and constitutes one of the real cardiac emergencies. Response to carotid sinus pressure, if one occurs, is manifested by a sudden jerky mathematical reduction in rate as the degree of A-V block is increased. The diagnosis can often be made clinically by observing rapid A waves in the neck veins. ECG diagnosis may be difficult or easy. With constant 2:1 block the second F wave may not be obvious, but carotid pressure will often make the genesis of the arrhythmia clear. An important point to look for is a characteristic undulating or sawtooth baseline, usually best seen in leads II, III, and aVF. F waves may be clearly seen in right precordial leads, or in any lead where the QRS complex is small. The etiology of flutter is essentially the same as that of fibrillation, but in almost all cases digitalis intoxication can be excluded as the cause.

The most important diagnostic differential is from PAT with block (as discussed previously), especially since the latter arrhythmia is secondary to digitalis excess in more than 75% of cases.

Control of flutter may require 2–3 times the usual digitalizing dose, even when patients are receiving maintenance digitalis, and the drug should be given parenterally when the ventricular rate is rapid. Cedilanid, digoxin, or ouabain may be used intravenously. Following administration of digitalis the degree of A-V block is increased, and the ventricular rate slows. The rhythm may revert to sinus or to atrial fibrillation. If the latter occurs, quinidine may be given in an attempt to convert to sinus rhythm, but occasionally careful withdrawal of digitalis will be followed by resumption of a sinus mechanism. See section on propranolol for its use in controlling ventricular rate.

The *treatment of choice* is electrical cardioversion if available, since atrial flutter is especially amenable to this form of therapy, success being achieved in 95% of cases. Flutter may be followed immediately or later by atrial fibrillation, which may be more easily controlled with digitalis alone. At this point one should follow the guidelines outlined in the section on atrial fibrillation.

X. **VENTRICULAR TACHYCARDIA** is usually a manifestation of severe organic heart disease (arteriosclerotic most often, but occasionally rheumatic or hypertensive) or of digitalis or quinidine intoxication. The rate may vary greatly, but generally is between 150 and 250. The rhythm is often very slightly (but never grossly) irregular. The first sound varies in intensity due to A-V dissociation and varying P-R interval. The second sound is diminished and sometimes inaudible. A prominent protodiastolic gallop may be heard. The ECG shows a regular (or at most slightly irregular) rhythm with rapid rate, a bizarre wide QRS complex greater than 0.12 seconds, A-V dissociation, and occasionally ventricular fusion beats or sinus captures of the ventricle. The last mentioned, when present, are diagnostic of ventricular tachycardia and distinguish this arrhythmia from supraventricular tachycardia with rate-conditioned aberration.

Supportive measures are important. The agitated patient should be sedated, oxygen should be administered, and vasopressors should be given if hypotension is present. Cardioversion is the initial therapy of choice unless the arrhythmia is secondary to digitalis intoxication. Pharmacologic conversion may be attempted (lidocaine 50–75 mg IV, procaine amide 100 mg IV) but if sinus rhythm does not occur quickly, then cardioversion should be undertaken directly.

A. Lidocaine   Refer to section on this form of therapy. It is the drug treatment of choice.

B. Procaine amide is most effective when given parenterally. Many observers prefer intravenous administration (despite the risk of severe hypotension) because ventricular tachycardia usually requires rapid therapy and because intramuscularly administered medications may be poorly absorbed due to impaired peripheral circulation. Other observers argue, however, that with **IM** medication effects appear almost as rapidly (in 5–10 minutes, maximum in 30–60 minutes) and severe drops in blood pressure are less frequent.

　1. IM   0.5–1.0 gm every 2–3 hours.

　2. IV   Start a slow infusion of 5% D/W, preferably using an indwelling catheter for the tubing in case it becomes necessary to administer pressor agents. Inject 100 mg procaine amide every 2–4 minutes into the tubing until the desired effect is achieved, until toxicity precludes further administration, or until a total dose of 1.0 gm has been given. The use of larger and potentially cardiotoxic doses (up to 2.0 gm) is unwarranted if cardioversion equipment is available. If hypotension occurs, give vasopressors as necessary to maintain the blood pressure; hypotension is not a contraindication to continuing therapy unless it is unresponsive to pressor agents. Therapy must be stopped, however, if there is more than 50% widening of the QRS complex.

　3. Oral   For maintenance therapy, dosage is usually 0.25–0.5 gm every 4–6 hours. Procaine amide is seldom given orally for the treatment of attacks of acute ventricular tachycardia.

C. Quinidine gluconate   Because of its high incidence of toxicity, parenteral administration of this drug is warranted only in the preoperative or postoperative setting. The drug should be given **IM** as an 8% solution (0.8 gm in 10 ml). Effects appear in 15 minutes and are maximum in 1–2 hours. The dose is 0.4 gm (5 ml) initially and every 2 hours until reversion or toxicity occurs. Hypotension may be severe.

XI.   CARDIAC ARREST may be secondary to ventricular fibrillation or asystole. External cardiac resuscitation should be applied until the mechanism for the arrest is defined. If ventricular fibrillation is present, external defibrillation should be carried out. The technique for external cardiac resuscitation, basically as described by Kouwenhoven and associates, is listed below.

A.   The patient must be adequate for resuscitation.

B.   Rapid diagnosis of arrest (apnea, no pulse, dilated pupils, cyanosis) must be made. **Time is critical.** Oxygenation must be reestablished in less than 4 minutes. Observe time.

C. As soon as possible obtain ECG to determine type of cardiac arrest (asystole or ventricular fibrillation).

D. Summon help but start resuscitation at once. Alert anesthesiologists; perform tracheal intubation and institute bag breathing.

E. Give 3 or 4 rapid mouth-to-mouth artificial respirations. Continue at 12/minute if possible.

F. Place patient on a solid surface (floor, bedboard) and apply external cardiac compression at 60–80 times/minute (the heel of the hand should be placed on the lower end of the sternum just above the xiphoid).

G. Determine effectiveness of compression (femoral pulsations, constriction of pupils, spontaneous respirations), but not at the cost of interrupting resuscitation.

H. Observe for return of spontaneous cardiac action.

I. Inject Isuprel 1–2 ml into the heart if no spontaneous activity after several minutes.

J. Apply external defibrillator if indicated by presence of ventricular fibrillation.

K. If unable to defibrillate, increase the height of the fibrillatory complexes by intracardiac or intravenous administration of epinephrine 0.5 ml 1:1000 aqueous, or Isuprel 1–2 ml.

L. Inject 10% calcium chloride 5–10 ml or Isuprel 1–2 ml into the heart or intravenously if weak cardiac action occurs.

M. Reverse acidosis with 3.75 gm (44.6 mEq) sodium bicarbonate (one 50-ml ampule) intravenously if arrest persists longer than 5 minutes, and repeat at 5–10-minute intervals until cardiac activity is restored.

N. Give Xylocaine (lidocaine) 50–100 mg into the heart or intravenously, if necessary, to decrease myocardial irritability or to maintain defibrillation. Procaine may be used instead.

O. Perform venous cutdown, if necessary, for infusion of fluids.

P. Continue external cardiac compression and artificial respiration until spontaneous cardiac activity and ventilation adequate to maintain the patient occur.

Q. Give continuous vasopressors to sustain blood pressure, if necessary.

R. Apply postresuscitation hypothermia if neurologic changes have occurred or arrest has persisted for a protracted period. Lower temperature to 33°C, but not below (to prevent increased myocardial irritability and further arrhythmias).

S. Diagnose and treat inciting cause of cardiac arrest, if possible.

T. With "return to life" the resuscitation procedures may stop at any step.

U. Most of the above steps in external cardiac resuscitation require a hospital environment. Have patient transported to hospital as soon as possible if arrest has occurred elsewhere; continue respiration and cardiac compression during transfer.

XII.   WOLFF-PARKINSON-WHITE SYNDROME is usually seen in young otherwise healthy persons, especially females. The essential diagnostic feature is an ECG that shows a short P-R interval (0.10 second or less) and widening of the QRS complex (due to slurring at the onset of the upstroke of the R wave—the so-called delta wave). These patients are subject to recurrent attacks of PAT or atrial flutter (or occasionally atrial fibrillation) which may erroneously be considered ventricular tachycardia because of an aberrant, bizarre QRS pattern. The condition is usually benign, but sudden death may occur during an attack of paroxysmal tachycardia. Recurrent attacks of tachycardia (which may be exceedingly difficult to manage) may be reduced in frequency by administration of sedatives, but if this measure is not effective, quinidine and procaine amide are the drugs of choice. Digitalis should not be given, as a rule, since it preferentially blocks the normal spread of impulse through the A-V node and increases abnormal excitation, with a resultant increase in ventricular rate. On rare occasions, however, arrhythmias not responsive to other antiarrhythmic drugs may respond to digitalis. Electrical cardioversion has been successfully used to terminate the supraventricular arrhythmias associated with this disorder and should certainly be tried if the arrhythmia is refractory to the prescribed medications.

XIII.   ADAMS-STOKES ATTACKS are attacks of acute cerebral ischemia, with or without unconsciousness and convulsions, following sudden changes in cardiac rhythm that markedly decrease cardiac output. Such attacks may occur during bursts of ventricular tachycardia or fibrillation and during prolonged asystole occurring with transition from sinus rhythm to complete heart block (or during shifts between complete and incomplete heart block). Symptoms of impaired consciousness begin 3–10 seconds after transient circulatory arrest, and complete loss of consciousness occurs after 10–20 seconds. In the majority of cases no precipitating factors are demonstrable. The attacks begin suddenly, seldom exceed 1–2 minutes in duration, and are not followed, as a rule, by neurologic sequelae or postictal confusion. During the attack pallor is often marked, and (if asystole or ventricular fibrillation is the mechanism) pulse and heart sounds are absent. Adams-Stokes attacks may present a difficult diagnostic problem in the elderly, and a careful history is mandatory. Acute myocardial infarct or cerebral vascular disorders may be the cause or result of such an attack. Asymptomatic complete heart block probably requires no therapy, but the patient should be followed closely for signs of deterioration.

A.   Treatment during repeated acute attacks

  1.   Direct vigorous thumping on the precordium may initiate cardiac activity.

  2.   Isoproterenol (Isuprel) and epinephrine   Both drugs may be effective in acute attacks, but Isuprel is preferred because its inotropic effect is more marked, its activity is largely restricted to the higher cardiac pacemakers (sinus and A-V nodes), it is five times as potent as epinephrine in increasing rhythmicity of the ventricular pacemakers, it has much less tendency to produce ventricular fibrillation in the presence of previous cardiac damage, and it has essentially no vasoconstrictor action. Epinephrine may cause striking elevation of the blood pressure and may precipitate ventricular tachycardia or fibrillation; it probably should not be used unless it is certain that asystole is present. Both drugs may be given by intracardiac injection for the treatment of cardiac arrest. The drugs are much less effective if acidosis is present, and are contraindicated if the Adams-Stokes attacks are thought to be due to transient ventricular tachycardia or fibrillation.

a) **Isuprel IV infusion:** 1–2 mg are diluted in 200 ml 5% D/W and administered at a rate of 0.5–10 ml/minute. **Subcutaneously:** 0.2 mg every 3 hours. **Sublingually:** 10–20 mg every 2–4 hours.

b) **Epinephrine IV infusion:** 3.0 ml of 1:1000 aqueous epinephrine are diluted in 300 ml of 5% D/W; rate of administration is dictated by adequacy of heart rate. **Subcutaneously:** 0.2–0.3 ml of 1:1000 aqueous epinephrine every 1–2 hours. **IM:** 0.5–1.0 ml of 1:500 epinephrine in oil every 6–12 hours.

3. **Artificial pacemakers,** which monitor ventricular contraction and apply external electric stimulation each time asystole exceeds a certain predetermined length of time, have proved cumbersome and do not always initiate ventricular contraction. For temporary purposes a bipolar electrode catheter may be placed in the right ventricle with fluoroscopic control and sterile techniques and attached to one of a variety of external power supplies which have adjustable controls for rate and milliamperage. Temporary pacing may then be discontinued if indicated by the resumption of normal A-V conduction, or replaced by a permanent type of cardiac pacemaker. The choice between transvenous and epicardial-abdominal permanent pacemakers remains controversial. Excellent evidence exists that artificial pacing by either method definitely prolongs life by a significant margin in symptomatic complete heart block. One must weigh the slight risk in thoracotomy against the relative risk in transvenous pacing with its potential associated complications. **Temporary cardiac pacing** is indicated in the following conditions:

a) Symptomatic complete or incomplete heart block unresponsive to medical therapy.

b) Acute myocardial infarction complicated by significant conduction defect and/or tachyarrhythmia which causes cardiovascular collapse and is unresponsive to medical therapy.

Permanent cardiac pacing is indicated in the following conditions:

a) Adams-Stokes attacks uncontrolled by medical therapy.

b) Congestive heart failure and mental confusion uncontrolled by medical therapy.

c) Complete heart block following cardiac surgery.

After installation of a permanent pacemaker the patient should be instructed to take his own pulse twice daily for a full minute and report any variation greater than 3–5 beats/minute. Electrocardiograms should be repeated if symptoms recur and at reasonable periods of time to determine rate, pacing spike amplitude, presence of competition, or ectopic arrhythmias.

The most common cause of failure of either type of pacemaker is battery exhaustion. Wire breakage is less frequently observed. Infection may occur with either, and if septicemia or bacterial endocarditis supervenes, removal of the transvenous type is usually necessary. Aside from increased cardiac threshold, which may occur with both types of pacemakers, other causes of pacing failure peculiar to the transvenous type are electrode displacement or perforation of the myocardium.

B. Other measures for less urgent situations

1. Sympathomimetic drugs for maintenance

a) Isuprel, sublingually, 10–20 mg every 3–4 hours.

b) Ephedrine 10–20 mg every 3–4 hours.

c) Amphetamine 5–10 mg QID. Severe anorexia usually results.

2. Atropine 0.5–1.0 mg subcutaneously TID–QID is a useful adjunct to improve A-V conduction.

3. Corticosteroids may be beneficial in heart block associated with acute myocardial infarction, according to some observers. They postulate that steroids decrease inflammation and edema in the area of the conducting system, thereby accelerating A-V conduction. Large doses (e.g., prednisone 40–60 mg daily) should be given for several days.

Hypertensive cardiovascular disease is characterized by an abnormality in the small branches of the arterial tree. The most easily measured manifestation of the disease is an elevation in systolic *and* diastolic blood pressure. Systolic hypertension without concomitant elevation in diastolic blood pressure is usually related to loss of elasticity in the great vessels (i.e., atherosclerosis) or increased cardiac output (i.e., hypermetabolic conditions). The term *hypertension* in this chapter means an abnormal elevation in diastolic pressure.

In the general population normal and elevated blood pressures form a continuum with no obvious line of demarcation between them, but it is customary to consider a diastolic pressure of 90 mm Hg as the upper limit of normal. Blood pressure probably tends to rise with age. The young patient tolerates hypertension poorly; a teenage boy with a diastolic pressure of 110 mm Hg is in greater danger from hypertension than is a 65-year-old woman with a diastolic pressure of 125 mm Hg. Nevertheless, we have arbitrarily considered mild, moderate, and severe hypertension as characterized by basal diastolic blood pressures of 90–110, 110–130, and more than 130 mm Hg, respectively. These limits are not absolute and are given only for practical guidance.

I. DIAGNOSIS

A. To confirm the diagnosis Basal blood pressure must be determined. The lowest meaningful supine blood pressure, after several days of hospitalization without treatment, best approximates it. Basal sitting and standing blood pressures are also helpful for the subsequent evaluation of the effectiveness of treatment. Isolated elevated blood pressure readings obtained outside the hospital are often unreliable and misleading, even if recorded after a rest period of several hours.

B. To evaluate the patient's condition The diagnostic work-up has two purposes. The first seeks to discover any underlying surgically correctable cause for the hypertension (e.g., adrenal tumors, coarctation of the aorta, renal vascular and parenchymal diseases). Discussion of the specific diagnostic tests used to differentiate these conditions is beyond the scope of this Manual.

The second and equally important goal is an assessment of the damage, if any, the hypertension has caused to various target organs, particularly the kidneys, and to a lesser extent the heart and blood vessels.

II. THERAPEUTIC RATIONALE

A. The approach to therapy

In **severe or moderate hypertension** complicated by secondary renal or cardiovascular dysfunction, life may be immediately endangered. The more severe the hypertension, the worse the untreated prognosis and the more it can be improved with therapy. Antihypertensive treatment must lower the diastolic pressure acutely and then maintain it at or near the normal level chronically. Acute control of the blood pressure can almost always be achieved in the hospital; maintenance of normotension at home is more difficult, but it is equally important and almost always possible. It is usually inadequate to assess the response of severely hypertensive patients to potent therapy on the basis of occasional measurements of blood pressure in the office. To achieve optimal control the patient should be taught to use a sphygmomanometer and record his blood pressure every day at regular hours, both at home and at work. Only a few patients cannot take these readings satisfactorily.

In **severe or moderate hypertension without complications,** prevention of complications is the main goal of therapy; the evidence is good that treatment does indeed lessen complications.

Patients with **mild hypertension** are liable to die of atherosclerosis but not of the complications of hypertension. Effective treatment would have to prevent cerebral and coronary thrombosis; unfortunately the value of therapy in preventing atherosclerotic disease is not presently proved.

B. **Objective of therapeutic management**   The prognosis in patients with treated hypertension is related to the level at which blood pressure is maintained and not to a particular drug or regimen. The supine diastolic pressure should be kept below 100 mm Hg, if that can be achieved without severe distress to the patient. With ganglioplegic agents and drugs that produce most of their effect when the patient is standing, control is satisfactory if the diastolic pressure of the sitting patient averages less than 100 mm Hg. Therapeutic measures that achieve this control are, in the following sections, called **effective treatment.**

III.   INDICATIONS FOR EFFECTIVE ANTIHYPERTENSIVE TREATMENT

A. **Absolute and urgent:**   Complicated severe—including malignant or accelerated—hypertension. A diastolic pressure exceeding 150 mm Hg is an indication for urgent antihypertensive treatment in any patient. If the diastolic pressure exceeds 130 mm Hg with hospital rest and one of the following conditions is present, treatment should be instituted immediately and any search for an underlying cause of hypertension should be deferred.

1. **Hypertensive encephalopathy or cerebrovascular accident**   The term *hypertensive encephalopathy* has been used to designate at least three distinct pathologic entities: (a) spasm of intracranial arteries; (b) cerebral edema; (c) widespread focal cerebral infarction. The first is often rapidly responsive to antihypertensive therapy, the second is more slowly corrected, and the last is irreversible.

2. **Retinal hemorrhages** and/or soft, cotton-wool exudates with or without papilledema.

3. **Congestive heart failure**   The higher the pressure, the greater the symptomatic response to blood pressure reduction. In patients with diastolic pressure over 110 mm Hg, lowering of the blood pressure will help the heart failure. In patients with acute pul-

monary edema, including those with recent myocardial infarct, hypertension should be treated when the diastolic pressure is above 140 mm Hg.

4. **Acute nephritis or preeclampsia** with rapid rise in diastolic pressure.

5. **Renal azotemia** when the BUN ranges from 20–100 mg/100 ml. (With BUNs of more than 100 mg/100 ml renal reserve is so limited that treatment is of little value, while with BUNs below 20 mg/100 ml there is enough reserve to permit some procrastination.)

B. **Absolute but not urgent:** Uncomplicated severe, and complicated or uncomplicated moderate hypertension.

   1. A diastolic pressure above 130 mm Hg in patients with uncomplicated hypertension.

   2. Patients with diastolic pressures over 110 mm Hg with or without cardiovascular (cardiac enlargement, angina, old myocardial infarction, old CVA, aortic aneurysm) or renal (proteinuria or decreasing glomerular filtration rate of no obvious etiology) manifestations.

C. **Relative and not urgent:** Complicated mild hypertension. Patients with diastolic pressures between 100 and 110 mm Hg and with headaches or with any of the manifestations mentioned above in **B-2**. For such patients effective therapy should be initiated but maintained only if control of the blood pressure improves the patient's condition. If continued effective therapy cannot be justified, the patient should be continued on minimal therapy unless there is some clear contraindication.

IV. **INDICATIONS FOR MINIMAL AND NOT NECESSARILY EFFECTIVE TREATMENT** Diuretic or other minimal therapy is indicated for asymptomatic patients without cardiovascular or renal complications with basal diastolic pressures between 100 and 110 mm Hg or with labile hypertension. Therapy should be pushed for high-risk patients, i.e., young patients, Negro patients, men, and patients with a hypertensive family history.

It is no longer enough merely to reassure hypertensive patients that they have no complications at the moment. Hypertension is a progressive disease that accelerates the rate of progression of atherosclerosis and can lead to progressive renal dysfunction and ultimately death. There is no rationale for withholding treatment until complications develop. Whatever objections there are to treating mild hypertension are related to the side effects and toxicity of the drugs presently available.

V. **PRACTICAL CONSIDERATIONS**

A. **Hospitalization** is advisable for hypertensive patients requiring urgent therapy or initiation of treatment with potent antihypertensive drugs, especially ganglioplegic agents. Hospitalization for 2–3 weeks is usual when therapy is started, and periods of 6 weeks or more may be needed for patients with malignant hypertension. Such patients should not be discharged unless the blood pressure is well controlled. Effective control is arbitrarily defined as an average diastolic pressure below 100 mm Hg with the patient in the sitting position. This level has been chosen because with this degree of control there appears to be a gradual lessening of the severity of the hypertensive process, while with less stringent control no such improvement with time is evident.

B. Side effects at the beginning of treatment are usual; they can be both uncomfortable and incapacitating. Eventually they will regress; however, depending on their severity they may take from days to months to disappear. The physician must recognize that effective control of blood pressure by the presently available drugs is associated with a high probability of significant side effects, including asthenia, anorexia, orthostatic hypotension, and nasal congestion; when ganglioplegic agents are used, all the effects of parasympatholysis should be anticipated. The physician must educate his patient as completely as possible about his disease, describing clearly both the benefit and the side effects of therapy. Side effects may be sufficiently severe to force the physician to accept something less than completely adequate control of the blood pressure.

The physician must also be alert to detect toxic effects in contradistinction to side effects. The most common of these are discussed under the individual drugs. The significance of most of these toxic manifestations is poorly understood; some may necessitate discontinuing the drug.

C. Readjustment of the dosage of antihypertensive medications depends on numerous factors. In conditions in which the circulating volume is reduced (hemorrhage, diarrhea, dehydration) and in circumstances that produce vasodilatation (alcohol ingestion, postprandial periods, hot weather, hot bath, febrile illness) hypotensive episodes may be precipitated, particularly in patients with sympathetic blockade. Conversely, the appearance of edema is often accompanied by reduced responsiveness to guanethidine and ganglioplegic agents.

Drug tolerance, which has been described with most antihypertensive agents when they are used singly, may develop, and increasing dosage may be required to maintain adequate control of the blood pressure. In our experience, however, when hydralazine is used in combination with ganglioplegic agents, tolerance does not develop. In fact, the reverse occurs, and in well-controlled patients less and less antihypertensive agent is needed to maintain control. It is important that dosage be individualized for each hypertensive patient, since it is impossible to predict how a particular patient will respond to a particular drug. A physician should use the smallest possible dose of the fewest possible drugs to maintain adequate control of the blood pressure.

VI. PRINCIPLES OF TREATMENT   By combining drugs that lower blood pressure by different mechanisms, additive effects can be obtained. Judicious combination of drugs often makes it possible to decrease the total incidence of side reactions by reducing the necessary dosage of the individual drugs. Moreover, in some instances the side effects of one drug can be used to counteract those of another. For instance, the tachycardia associated with hydralazine can be reduced by concomitant use of guanethidine, which produces bradycardia, and the diarrhea induced by guanethidine can be countered by the constipation induced by ganglioplegic agents.

Good control is rarely achieved with a single drug. Thiazides, unless contraindicated primarily by diabetes or a strong family history of diabetes, probably should be part of the antihypertensive regimen because of their usually unimportant side effects. Their antihypertensive effects are additive to those of all other antihypertensive drugs, and the required dosage of other antihypertensives can be lowered.

Important adjunctive measures in the treatment of hypertensive patients include adequate rest, with sedation if necessary, loss of excess weight, and moderate restriction of dietary salt.

A. **Mild hypertension** Therapy may be instituted on an outpatient basis and should be started with thiazides. If after two weeks the blood pressure is not well controlled, small doses of hydralazine or methyldopa should be added. Reserpine may also be used instead, but it is a far less effective antihypertensive agent, and the danger of insidious depression, particularly in old people, is very real.

B. **Uncomplicated moderate hypertension** Treatment may be instituted on an outpatient basis and should be initiated with thiazides together with methyldopa or hydralazine. If blood pressure control is not achieved after two weeks, small amounts of guanethidine may be added.

C. **Severe or complicated moderate hypertension** If parenteral therapy is not required and control of the blood pressure in a matter of days is sufficient, initial oral therapy should include thiazides and guanethidine or a ganglioplegic agent. Within 48–96 hours either hydralazine or methyldopa should be added to the regimen. In our hands long-term therapy of such hypertension is more successful when the patient uses a sphygmomanometer and records his blood pressures at home. The therapeutic regimen most commonly used for such patients by the Hypertension Division at Washington University includes a thiazide derivative and hydralazine, usually administered in combination with a ganglioplegic agent.

D. **Coronary artery disease** In patients with severe hypertension coronary artery disease is not a contraindication to antihypertensive therapy. Control of markedly elevated blood pressure usually reduces the severity of angina pectoris. The early prognosis is better in hypertensive patients who have adequate blood pressure control at the time myocardial infarction occurs. Therapy of mild or moderate hypertension should not be started during the first two weeks following myocardial infarction but should be restricted to the recovery period if the hypertension persists. Because it increases cardiac output, hydralazine alone should not be given to patients with angina pectoris, although it may be administered concurrently with other drugs which lower cardiac output.

E. **Cerebrovascular accidents** Hypertensive encephalopathy and cerebral hemorrhage are both indications for treatment. They may be indistinguishable, and a diagnosis of hypertensive encephalopathy can often be confirmed only in retrospect by a remarkable improvement in response to pressure reduction. Cerebral thrombosis, again in the presence of markedly elevated blood pressure, is an indication for treatment. In patients with moderate hypertension adequate control of blood pressure can reduce the incidence of strokes; there is no evidence that blood pressure reduction, unless excessive, causes cerebral thrombosis.

F. **Renal insufficiency** Therapy is usually of little help in patients with renal, as opposed to prerenal, azotemia with blood urea levels over

100 mg/100 ml. In patients with less advanced renal damage, blood pressure reduction may slow down renal destruction. Therefore, patients with blood urea levels of less than 100 mg/100 ml should always be treated. Careful attention should be paid to renal function. The institution of therapy in an azotemic patient may result in a temporary rise of BUN. After several weeks of effective control, however, the BUN will usually return to its pretreatment level, where it can often be maintained for long periods. More than doubling of the initial BUN, on the other hand, is an alarming sign.

Patients with coronary or cerebrovascular disease or with significant azotemia are almost certainly in danger from episodes of hypotension; their blood pressures should be reduced gradually and wide fluctuations in pressure avoided as much as possible. They also may not tolerate a normal blood pressure; in these patients one must sometimes be content with a lesser reduction in pressure.

G. Surgical procedures When an elective surgical operation is scheduled, administration of long-acting antihypertensive drugs should be discontinued, especially those which produce sympathetic blockade and inhibit cardiovascular reflexes. The therapeutic problem should be discussed with the anesthesiologist. Reserpine and guanethidine should be stopped two weeks before operation and the blood pressure controlled with hydralazine, methyldopa, or parenteral ganglioplegic agents. Circulating blood volume should be measured, and care should be taken that it is adequate. Whenever possible some control of blood pressure should be obtained in severely hypertensive patients before a surgical operation.

H. Pregnancy The absolute indications for treating hypertension are unaltered by pregnancy. Furthermore, the available data suggest that the higher the pressures, the greater the probability of fetal loss and of maternal complications. Any diastolic pressure above 90 mm Hg should be treated. Both preexisting hypertension and toxemia are treated with the same drugs used for nonpregnant women, with the exception of ganglioplegic agents. Guanethidine may be used since it does not have parasympatholytic effects. A disadvantage of reserpine in the treatment of toxemia of pregnancy is increased susceptibility to convulsions and, with parenteral administration, the danger of hypotension.

Intravenous diazoxide consistently and effectively lowers the blood pressure in toxemia. Its tendency to cause salt and water retention apparently is not a problem in emergency use; if treatment is continued for several days diazoxide can be antagonized by a thiazide diuretic if necessary. Its disadvantage in prolonged parenteral and oral use is hyperglycemia.

I. Pheochromocytoma Although the only recommended therapy is surgical removal, pheochromocytoma deserves special comment because of the antihypertensive agents used in the control of blood pressure before and during operation. Alpha-adrenergic blocking agents, which act specifically on the peripheral vascular system, are used for control of the hypertension in the preoperative period, in the prolonged treatment of cases not amenable to operation, and for the prevention or treatment of paroxysmal hypertension during operative manipulation of the tumor. Phenoxybenzamine (Dibenzyline, 10-mg capsules) is the drug of choice in long-term management because of its longer duration of action (12–24 hours), while phentolamine

(Regitine, 5-mg ampules) is preferred during surgery because of its short duration of action (5–10 minutes). The tachycardia induced by the alpha-adrenergic blocking agents may be controlled with beta-adrenergic blocking agents.

Most important in the adequate preparation of patients with pheochromocytoma for surgical exploration is correction of their diminished circulating blood volume. This preparation can be achieved either by determining the blood volume and correcting the deficit or by blocking peripheral vasoconstriction with alpha-adrenergic blocking agents for several days before operation to allow the circulating blood volume to correct itself. The use of alpha- and beta-adrenergic blocking agents in the preoperative management of patients with pheochromocytoma has been reported in detail (*Brit. Med. J.* 1:196, 1967).

The use of antihypertensive drugs that may release catecholamines or produce sympatholysis and thereby potentiate the effect of endogenous catecholamines is contraindicated; one should not use reserpine, methyldopa, guanethidine, or ganglioplegic agents.

VII. ANTIHYPERTENSIVE DRUGS The antihypertensive drugs available for oral use in this country are listed in Table 7-1. Relative potency and hemodynamic effects are presented in Table 7-2. Parenteral treatment of hypertension is discussed separately.

A. Rauwolfia alkaloids appear to act by inhibiting transport and binding of norepinephrine and epinephrine at an intraneuronal level. The resultant depletion of catecholamine in the peripheral sympathetic system and in the brain leads to failure of impulse transmission at the sympathetic neuroeffector junctions. Blood vessels therefore do not constrict in response to sympathetic stimulation nor to infusions of tyramine; their response can be restored to normal after infusion of norepinephrine. The alkaloids are readily absorbed from the gastrointestinal tract, and their metabolic products are excreted in the urine.

1. Preparations include the crude root, the alseroxylon fraction, the pure alkaloids (reserpine, rescinnamine, deserpidine), and the synthetic alkaloid syrosingopine. Reserpine is the most potent of the alkaloids, which all have essentially similar clinical effects. Equivalent doses are 0.25 mg reserpine (Serpasil), 200 mg crude root (Raudixin), 4 mg alseroxylon fraction (Rauwiloid), 0.5 mg deserpidine (Harmonyl), 0.35 mg rescinnamine (Moderyl), and 1 mg syrosingopine (Singoserp).

Many combinations of rauwolfia alkaloids with other antihypertensive agents are marketed, but they cannot be recommended. In addition to the disadvantages of a fixed ratio of drugs, therapy with such mixtures is complicated by the fact that the rauwolfia component has a much greater cumulative effect than the other constituents.

2. Clinical effects The antihypertensive effect of oral rauwolfia alkaloids is mild and gradual in onset, appearing within 3–6 days and requiring 3–6 weeks to reach a maximum effect. Oral doses of 0.75–1.5 mg reserpine daily are effective and will lower diastolic blood pressure; such doses, however, are no longer used for prolonged treatment because of excessive sedation and other side effects. On the other hand, the usual prescribed doses of less than

TABLE 7-1. Oral Antihypertensive Preparations

Generic Name	Sizes of Available Tablets (Mg)	Starting Dose (Mg)	Duration of Action (Hrs)	Doses Per Day	Increment Per Dose (Mg)	Interval Between Increment (Days)	Usual Range of Total Daily Effective Dose (Mg)
Pentolinium	20, 40, 100	20	4	4–6	20	1	60–1500
Mecamylamine	2.5, 10	2.5	6	3–4	2.5	1–2	10–120
Guanethidine	10, 25	25	10 days	1	10–12.5	4–5	20–200
Hydralazine	10, 25, 50, 100	10	6	4	25	2–3	100–500
Methyldopa	250	250	8	3	250	3	750–4000
Hydrochlorothiazide	25, 50	25–50	8–12	2	—	—	50–100
Reserpine	0.1, 0.25	0.25	2–6 wks	1	0.25	7	0.5–1.0

Starting dose, interval between increments, and usual range of total daily effective dose are for hospitalized patients with adequate renal function, given one drug alone. With the exception of hydralazine, for patients with azotemia, for outpatients, and for patients in whom treatment is started with a combination of drugs, therapy should be initiated at a lower level and increased more gradually (about half the above indicated starting and increment doses should be used).

TABLE 7-2. Hemodynamic Effects of Oral Antihypertensive Drugs

Type of Drug	Potency	Venous Pooling	Renal Blood Flow	Cardiac Output	Pulse Rate	Peripheral Vascular Resistance
Ganglion blocker	+++	++	Decreased	Decreased	Increased	Unchanged or increased
Guanethidine	+++	++	Decreased	Decreased	Decreased	Unchanged or increased
Hydralazine	++	No effect	Increased, later normal	Increased, later normal	Increased, later normal	Decreased
Methyldopa	++	+	Essentially unchanged	Unchanged or decreased	Decreased	Decreased
Thiazide	+	No effect	Decreased, later normal	Decreased, later normal	Unchanged	Increased, later decreased
Reserpine	+	+	Unchanged	Unchanged	Decreased	Decreased

0.5 mg daily have a negligible effect on blood pressure. Parenterally administered reserpine is considerably more effective and reduces the blood pressure by producing effective sympathetic blockade with secondary pooling of blood in the venous system, decrease in cardiac output, and orthostatic hypotension.

The bradycardiac effect of reserpine may be used to reduce or counteract the tachycardiac effect of hydralazine.

3. **Side effects** are many, the most important being depression, peptic ulceration, and weight gain. Depression may be insidious in onset and may include suicidal tendencies; it occurs particularly in elderly patients. Other side effects are nasal stuffiness, fluid retention, lassitude, decreased libido, nightmares, lactation, diarrhea, dizziness, drowsiness, and extrasystoles in patients taking digitalis.

B. Diuretics

1. **Benzothiadiazides** have now become commonplace in the treatment of hypertension. Their precise mode of action is poorly understood. The antihypertensive effects during the first few weeks of treatment have been related to decreased circulating blood volume and decreased cardiac output; however, diazoxide, a nondiuretic thiazide analog, causes salt and water retention yet lowers the blood pressure. If treatment continues, blood volume and cardiac output return to pretreatment levels, but the fall in blood pressure persists and systemic peripheral resistance decreases. The different preparations, their equivalent dosages, and side effects are described in Chapter 5.

   a) **Clinical effects**   The antihypertensive actions of all benzothiadiazides are comparable. The other sulfonamide diuretics, chlorthalidone, quinethazone, furosemide, and the diuretic ethacrynic acid are also effective in lowering blood pressure but offer no advantages over the thiazide diuretics in the treatment of hypertension. A fall in diastolic blood pressure of about 10–20 mm Hg will result from the chronic oral administration of 50–100 mg/day hydrochlorothiazide (or equivalent dose of an analog), 100–200 mg/day furosemide, or 100–200 mg/day ethacrynic acid. Neither thiazides nor their analogs by themselves often effectively control diastolic pressures greater than 110 mm Hg, but they are often combined with other antihypertensive drugs to permit smaller doses of the latter. The dose of ganglioplegic agents or of guanethidine should be reduced when administration of diuretics is started, in order to avoid profound falls in blood pressure.

   b) **The incidence and severity of adverse effects,** particularly of potassium depletion, are related to the dosage of the drug. Various claims for greater efficacy and less danger from a particular benzothiadiazide are not supported by any clinical evidence. Diuretics must be used cautiously in patients with impaired renal function.

2. **Aldosterone antagonists**   These diuretics differ from benzothiadiazides in that they decrease potassium excretion slightly and cause some potassium retention, whereas thiazides increase potassium excretion and cause potassium depletion. They have been used in patients in whom thiazides produce severe hypokalemia. The pteri-

dine derivative, triamterene (Dyrenium), is supplied in tablets of 100 mg; it often corrects the potassium deficit induced by thiazide but has little or no antihypertensive effect itself. Circulating potassium must be carefully followed when triamterene is combined with thiazides, for this combination may result in fatal hyperkalemia. The antihypertensive effects of 100 mg spironolactone (Aldactone) given in divided doses are mild and comparable to those of thiazides, but more gradual in onset. Spironolactone, as opposed to all other diuretics mentioned above, does not produce hyperuricemia or hyperglycemia. Side effects of spironolactone include epigastric distress, drug rash, drowsiness, breast tenderness, and gynecomastia. Aldactone should not be given to patients with renal insufficiency because of the danger of hyperkalemic acidosis.

C. **Methyldopa (Aldomet)** inhibits the decarboxylation of a number of amino acids but has no significant inhibitory action on the synthesis of endogenous norepinephrine. It is metabolized into alpha-methyl norepinephrine, a far less potent pressor agent than norepinephrine. It probably acts via this metabolite, which displaces stored norepinephrine at nerve endings.

1. **Clinical effects** Some observations in man suggest a degree of sympathetic inhibition; the drug causes postural hypotension, bradycardia, nasal stuffiness, and failure of ejaculation. These reactions resemble those of reserpine and guanethidine. It furthermore resembles reserpine in causing sedation and, following a large dose, in depleting catecholamines in the brain. The fall in blood pressure when the patient is supine appears largely due to decreased peripheral resistance. The blood pressure is, however, reduced to a larger extent with the patient erect, but postural hypotension is less marked than with guanethidine or ganglioplegic agents. Like other drugs which produce sympathetic denervation, methyldopa increases sensitivity to injected norepinephrine. Its effect appears 3–5 hours after a single large dose. When given orally, about half the administered dose is excreted in the first 12 hours. Although the rate of excretion is much slower in patients with uremia, methyldopa may be particularly useful in patients with impaired renal function because it does not affect renal blood flow. It should be emphasized that doses even as high as 4 gm/day are ineffective for a number of patients; hence the drug has limited use in complicated severe hypertension.

2. **Side effects** are uncommon and rarely severe. Most frequent are dry mouth, mild gastrointestinal symptoms (either diarrhea or constipation), postural hypotension, and drowsiness. The latter is most common and is seen in over 50% of patients during the first several weeks of therapy and then regresses to varying degrees. Less common side effects include fever, skin rash, depression, lactation, fluid retention, impairment of liver function (including elevation of the transaminases, with jaundice, cellular necrosis, and eosinophilic infiltration), decreased libido, and hemolytic anemia. The finding of positive antinuclear factor and positive direct Coombs tests has been reported recently in 10–25% of nonanemic patients ingesting methyldopa; the incidence is dosage-related. Fortunately hemolytic anemia occurs only rarely in this drug-induced Coombs-positive state.

D. Hydralazine (Apresoline) acts directly on the vascular smooth muscle to decrease peripheral resistance. The relaxant effect of hydralazine on the arterioles is more marked than that on the veins. Hydralazine possibly produces its antihypertensive effect by blocking alpha-adrenergic receptors, and it increases cardiac output, pulse rate, and renal blood flow by stimulating beta-adrenergic receptors. Some of the latter effects usually disappear when the drug is given for prolonged periods. The increase in cardiac output may be prevented by administration of ganglioplegic agents, but the renal vasodilatation is unaffected. Hydralazine is well absorbed after both oral and parenteral administration. Blood levels are maximal 3–5 hours after oral administration. Very little is known about the metabolism of hydralazine. Less than 5% of an oral dose is excreted unchanged in the urine.

1. **Clinical effects** Hydralazine has a more pronounced effect on the diastolic than on the systolic blood pressure. The fall in blood pressure is rarely postural and occurs in the supine and the upright positions. Hydralazine is the drug of choice in the treatment of patients with hypertension complicated by renal insufficiency, since it does not adversely affect renal function and does not depend upon renal function for its inactivation. When the initial dosage of hydralazine given alone is higher than 50 mg daily, headache, palpitation, flushing, and dyspnea on exertion usually occur. Doses larger than 500 mg daily should be reserved for severe and unremitting hypertension, since the incidence of adverse effects is related to dose.

2. **Side effects** When properly used, hydralazine is generally well tolerated. The high incidence of side effects reported in early therapeutic trials was apparently related to the prolonged use of large doses (500–1000 mg/day). The most common side effect is headache, which appears soon after therapy is initiated and usually disappears in 7–10 days if the drug is continued. Headaches can usually be prevented by small doses of ganglioplegic agents (10–20 mg pentolinium QID). To counteract the tachycardia and palpitation caused by hydralazine at the beginning of treatment, reserpine, guanethidine, or ganglioplegic agents may be concurrently administered. Anorexia, nausea, vomiting, and diarrhea may occur. Nasal congestion, conjunctivitis, and febrile reactions occur less frequently. Because the drug may aggravate angina pectoris or precipitate attacks of chest pain, hydralazine administered alone is usually contraindicated in patients with coronary artery disease. A collagen–vascular disease occurs in a small percentage of patients treated with hydralazine for longer than 6 months and seldom appears in patients who have taken less than 400 mg/day. The disease begins with transient arthralgia and progresses to an arthritis which may be undistinguishable from rheumatoid arthritis. Arthralgia, myalgia, and skin rash are usually considered indications for discontinuing the drug. If treatment is continued, fever, anemia, splenomegaly, impaired liver function, skin rash, hematuria, and leukopenia may appear. The resultant disease resembles disseminated lupus erythematosus, and LE cells have been observed in the peripheral blood. The clinical syndrome is completely reversible when the drug is discontinued, but antinuclear factor may persist in the serum for years.

E. Guanethidine (Ismelin) produces selective adrenergic postganglionic blockade by preventing the release of norepinephrine at the sympathetic myoneural junction, but it does not produce parasympatholysis. Guanethidine also partially depletes peripheral stores of norepinephrine; it has no effect on the brain, as it does not cross the blood-brain barrier. When given intravenously, guanethidine may release sufficient norepinephrine to produce a transient hypertension lasting about 15 minutes. Guanethidine also produces bradycardia and decreases cardiac output and renal blood flow with little change in peripheral vascular resistance. The marked orthostatic hypotension frequently associated with guanethidine results from pooling in the peripheral venous system, decreased central venous pressure, and fall in cardiac output. Urinary excretion of guanethidine is slow, and the action of the drug, maximal after 72 hours, lasts for more than a week. Maximum dosage need be limited only by the development of side effects. There are no criteria to predict the sensitivity of the individual patient; the drug must therefore be titrated in each case. Decrease in circulating volumes, as may occur with diarrhea, vomiting, febrile illness, bleeding, salt depletion, trapping of blood in the legs, or standing still, will potentiate the effect of guanethidine. Tolerance to the drug has not been reported.

1. **Clinical effects** Guanethidine should be reserved for patients with moderate or severe hypertension who cannot be controlled satisfactorily with other antihypertensive agents. In nonazotemic patients guanethidine has largely replaced the ganglioplegic agents because of its prolonged therapeutic response and the absence of side effects associated with parasympatholysis. In azotemic patients the drug is often poorly tolerated. Orthostatic and exercise hypotension are the great disadvantages of the drug and may be particularly dangerous in patients with ischemic disease of the heart or brain. When symptomatic hypotension appears, the dose of guanethidine should be reduced by 20–30%. In some patients it may be impossible to lower blood pressure when the patient is lying down without causing profound hypotension on standing or on exercise; for these individuals guanethidine is relatively contraindicated, and control of hypertension may be more adequate with a shorter-acting ganglioplegic agent. In order to avoid severe postural hypotension, patients must be instructed not to stand up rapidly, and to sit or lie down if dizziness occurs.

2. **Side effects** Morning hypotension and fall in blood pressure with exercise are frequent problems. They can be lessened by decreasing the dose of guanethidine and adding other drugs that do not produce such effects. Guanethidine nearly always produces some looseness of the stools and may cause diarrhea. The diarrhea may be explosive and lead to fecal incontinence; since the diarrhea represents unopposed parasympathetic activity, it can be controlled with atropine or another parasympatholytic drug (Pro-Banthine 15 mg QID) ; the addition of small doses of a ganglioplegic agent may occasionally be useful. Other side effects include dry mouth, muscle tremor, and failure of ejaculation.

F. **Ganglioplegic agents** are very potent antihypertensive drugs. They block the transmission of impulses through the ganglia of the autonomic nervous system by interfering with the action of acetylcholine on the ganglion cells. In contrast to guanethidine the ganglioplegic agents produce parasympathetic as well as sympathetic blockade. The former is responsible for virtually all the unpleasant side effects and the latter for the blood pressure reduction. The hypotensive action is primarily due to reduced venomotor tone, increased capacity of the venous bed, decreased venous return, and lowered cardiac output.

The commonly used preparations in the United States include the quaternary ammonium derivative **pentolinium (Ansolysen)** and the secondary amine **mecamylamine (Inversine)**. The quaternary ammonium compounds are poorly and variably absorbed from the gastrointestinal tract (10–50% of an oral dose) ; they are not metabolized and are excreted by the kidney in the same way as inulin. Mecamylamine is better absorbed; it also is not metabolized and is entirely excreted by the kidney, but it may be reabsorbed by the tubules, depending on the pH of the urine. Alkalinization of the urine reduces, and acidification promotes, renal excretion of the drug. Even if the urine is acid, the excretion of mecamylamine is slower than that of pentolinium. Because of its toxic effects on the nervous system, mecamylamine is contraindicated in azotemic patients. Therapy with ganglioplegic agents should be initiated in the hospital and should not be continued for outpatients who are not recording their own blood pressure at home, since an effective control of the blood pressure usually requires that each dose be adjusted according to the blood pressure.

1. Clinical effects   Ganglioplegic agents are indicated only for patients with severe hypertension. Because of their rapid onset of action they have considerable advantages over guanethidine in the treatment of patients with hypertensive encephalopathy or malignant hypertension. Their action also is considerably shorter, and cumulative effects therefore are not a problem. They provide the possibility of a better control of the blood pressure, but their administration requires more careful attention. The remarks of the previous paragraph about guanethidine in regard to orthostatic hypotension and sensitivity of individual patients to the drug are entirely applicable to the ganglioplegic agents. Although administration of the drug to patients with renal disease or ischemic conditions of the heart or brain is associated with some hazard, it is less than that associated with guanethidine.

Patients must be instructed not to cease therapy on their own, because withdrawal of a ganglioplegic agent is often followed by a rapid return of severe hypertension that may be refractory to these drugs when they are readministered. Hydralazine, with its different mechanism of action, decreases the wide swings in blood pressure that characterize the use of ganglioplegic agents alone. A decrease in severity of the hypertension may occur following prolonged effective control of blood pressure by the combination of hydralazine and ganglioplegic agents.

2. Side effects   If severe postural faintness on awakening is a problem, the nighttime dose of the medication must be reduced. With overdosage the blood pressure may fall to such low levels that anuria results and excretion of the drug ceases. Treatment involves tilting the patient's head down, and if necessary raising the blood pressure with pressor agents sufficiently to maintain adequate flow of urine. If norepinephrine is given, one must remember that patients with sympathetic blockade will be very sensitive. All other side effects are referable to paralysis of the parasympathetic ganglia and may be mitigated by parasympathomimetic drugs. Severe constipation is common, and paralytic ileus may occur. The latter is not always accompanied by a very low blood pressure. If constipation has been mild, the patient may prevent its continuing by taking the first dose of the day after a bowel movement. Severe constipation may be prevented by administering orally with each dose of the ganglioplegic agent 5–10 mg neostigmine (Prostigmin) or 5–10 mg bethanechol (Urecholine), or by taking at bedtime milk of magnesia, cascara, or magnesium citrate. Daily bowel movements must be ensured to prevent accumulation of the drug in the gut.

Mecamylamine should not be given to patients with azotemia, since effective doses usually induce a neurologic syndrome (characterized by severe tremor and incoordination) that necessitates discontinuing the drug.

G. Monoamine-oxidase (MAO) inhibitors These drugs are relatively impotent antihypertensive agents, and they may produce serious side effects (see Chapter 1). The potential hazards of monoamine-oxidase inhibitors outweigh the limited advantages they may have.

VIII. PARENTERAL TREATMENT OF HYPERTENSION Parenteral antihypertensive preparations are used in hypertensive emergencies. A hypertensive emergency exists when the diastolic blood pressure is elevated above 150 mm Hg (whether or not symptoms are present) or when pulmonary edema, cerebral hemorrhage, or encephalopathy is associated with a diastolic pressure greater than 120–130 mm Hg. In any of these situations the blood pressure must be reduced immediately. When properly used, shorter-acting agents are more effective and less dangerous than long-acting antihypertensive drugs, but they require more effort and cautious attention of the medical staff. Patients must be monitored constantly. Initially the blood pressure must be recorded frequently (every 5 minutes with trimethaphan and pentolinium), changes in cerebral status often evaluated, and urine output carefully measured. Vasopressors should be immediately available in case severe hypotension develops. Parenteral preparations must never be used in nonhospitalized patients.

A reasonable goal in the treatment of hypertensive emergencies is reduction of the diastolic blood pressure to 110 mm Hg, even though disturbing (usually temporary) manifestations may be associated with the rapid reduction in blood pressure. Renal insufficiency may be worsened, and mental confusion may increase in severity or appear de novo; cerebral or coronary thrombosis, however, is rarely a complication unless hypotension occurs. As soon as the blood pressure has been reduced to a satisfactory level, oral therapy should be initiated.

A. Trimethaphan camsylate (Arfonad) is supplied in 10-ml multidose vials containing 50 mg/ml. One vial should be diluted to 500 ml with 5% D/W (giving a concentration of 1 mg Arfonad/ml); the dilute solution should be administered IV at an initial rate of 50–60 drops/min (3–4 mg/min); adjustment in the rate of administration should be determined by response of the blood pressure. Onset of action is immediate, and the antihypertensive effect of the drug quickly disappears when its infusion is discontinued. When the desired level has been obtained, oral therapy with other agents should be initiated as previously described.

B. Pentolinium (Ansolysen) when given IM acts within 3 minutes and produces maximal effects within 15 minutes. The drug is supplied in a multidose vial containing 10 mg/ml; 1.0 mg (0.1 ml) is drawn into a tuberculin syringe and diluted to 1.0 ml with isotonic saline. Therapy is initiated with 0.1 mg injected IM into the deltoid muscle so that a tourniquet may be placed above the injection site if severe hypotension results. The patient should be kept in a sitting position in bed; if this is not possible, his head should be elevated. The dose of pentolinium is doubled every 10 minutes until the first decrease of at least 5 mm Hg in systolic blood pressure occurs. Therapy should then be stopped until the maximum fall in systolic pressure has occurred; when this reading is stable for 15 minutes, therapy may be resumed with the same regimen if the diastolic pressure is still above the desired level. When the desired diastolic pressure is reached, the largest dose required to achieve this level is then administered every 2–4 hours as needed. If the dose of pentolinium has reached 50 mg and no response has occurred, hydralazine should be given in addition.

C. Hydralazine (Apresoline) is very useful for the treatment of hypertensive emergencies arising in patients with acute glomerulonephritis or toxemia of pregnancy. A dose of 10–25 mg may be given IM (or injected IV over a 5-minute period) and repeated every 30 minutes until 100 mg have been given or the desired diastolic pressure has been achieved. The effective dose of hydralazine is then repeated every 2–4 hours. Onset of action is within 10–20 minutes, maximum response is usually in one hour, and effects may persist as long as 12 hours.

D. Methyldopa (Aldomet) is supplied in 5-ml vials containing 50 mg/ml. Like that of reserpine the antihypertensive action of intravenous methyldopa is delayed for 3–5 hours. Methyldopa may be given as an IV drip—250–500 mg over 30–60 minutes and repeated if necessary every 6 hours. The maximum recommended dose is 1 gm. Parenteral methyldopa has produced liver damage in about 5% of patients in some series.

E. Reserpine should be given in a dosage of 2.5–5.0 mg IM initially and repeated every 4–12 hours as needed. Larger doses are of no additional benefit. When the blood pressure is well controlled, oral therapy may be initiated. Reserpine is usually effective but has the two disadvantages of slow onset of action (1–3 hours) and long and variable duration of action. The fact that at any particular instant the level of blood pressure is the result of the drug given several hours to several days earlier makes precise control impossible. Parenteral reserpine may therefore produce serious and prolonged hypotension.

F. Diazoxide (Hyperstat) is not commercially available. The drug has mild antihypertensive effects when given orally but is strongly antihypertensive when given intravenously. It has been used especially in the treatment of toxemia of pregnancy. It does not cause orthostatic hypotension and appears to lower the blood pressure by directly dilating the arterioles, with an increase in cardiac output and renal blood flow. The full dose of diazoxide, 5 mg/kg, injected rapidly undiluted has an immediate and striking hypotensive effect that lasts from 3–24 hours. A slow injection or an infusion of the drug is without effect on the blood pressure. Restriction of dietary salt is indicated in order to prevent salt and water retention by the drug. A thiazide diuretic may have to be given in combination with diazoxide to eliminate this problem. Diazoxide produces greater hyperglyecmia than the benzothiadiazide diuretics.

8. Pulmonary Disease

During recent years, knowledge in the field of pulmonary diseases has increased as rapidly as in any area of medicine. Logical therapy of pulmonary disease must be based on an understanding of the physiologic mechanisms involved in the disease process, the interrelation between lung function and other systems, and current principles of treatment.

PHYSIOLOGIC CONSIDERATIONS

I. **VENTILATION** The delivery of air into the alveoli is a complex, well-coordinated process, dependent upon the central and peripheral nervous systems, various chemoreceptors, the thoracic musculoskeletal system, and the diaphragm.

Alveolar ventilation is the only useful ventilation available. It is that volume of fresh air which ventilates alveoli perfused with capillary blood. Other ventilation, which does not participate in gas exchange, essentially is wasted and is called dead-space ventilation (the physiologic dead space includes anatomic dead space). Dead-space ventilation is increased when the ventilation to alveoli greatly exceeds the blood flow.

1. **Normal alveolar ventilation** is sufficient to meet the metabolic demands of the body, i.e., to fulfill the O_2 requirements and excrete the CO_2 generated in tissue metabolism. In the normal resting male, at pH 7.40 the arterial blood PO_2 should be greater than 90 mm Hg and the P_aCO_2 should be 40 mm Hg $\pm$ 2 mm; females have a slightly lower P_aCO_2. Since the major buffering system of blood is the CO_2-HCO_3^- system, the pH is influenced by the P_aCO_2 as stated by the Henderson-Hasselbalch equation.

2. **Measurement of alveolar ventilation** The assessment of alveolar ventilation clinically is done by measuring the arterial blood P_aCO_2. The CO_2 content of arterial blood is dependent upon the rate of CO_2 production and the magnitude of alveolar ventilation. The P_aCO_2 of arterial blood has an inverse, linear relationship to the level of alveolar ventilation over physiologic ranges; i.e., as alveolar ventilation increases, the P_aCO_2 in arterial blood falls. **Alveolar hypoventilation** is defined as an increase in the P_aCO_2 of arterial blood (> 45 mm Hg at sea level) and **alveolar hyperventilation** as decreased arterial P_aCO_2 (< 35 mm Hg).

II. **BLOOD FLOW** The even distribution of blood flow throughout the lungs is dependent upon normal cardiac function and an intact pulmonary vascular bed, with low vascular resistance.

III. **GAS EXCHANGE** occurs at the alveolar capillary interface. Parameters for adequate function at this site include: the overall surface area, the distance between alveolar gas and capillary blood, the even distribution of gas and blood flow at each gas-exchanging site. Abnormalities of the various components, either pulmonary or extrapulmonary, may lead to abnormal gas exchange.

Mechanisms of abnormal gas exchange Arterial blood gas measurements frequently show a reduction of P_aO_2 as the initial sign of impaired gas exchange. Impaired oxygenation of blood occurs by:

1. **Impairment of diffusion**—abnormal transfer factor. The diffusion of O_2 molecules across the alveolar-capillary region is impaired by a pathologic process which alters and lengthens the diffusion pathways. As a result there is insufficient time for the oxygenation of hemoglobin as it traverses the capillary bed. Exercise aggravates this abnormality, causing a greater fall in P_aO_2. The P_aCO_2 usually is low secondary to alveolar hyperventilation. Diffusion defects are most notably seen with diffuse interstitial pulmonary disease or with reduction in the alveolar-capillary surface area.

2. **Abnormal ventilation–blood flow relationship** is the most frequent abnormality of gas exchange. It occurs with nonuniform distribution of air, nonuniform distribution of blood, or combinations that disturb the balance between ventilation and blood flow. Normally the overall ratio of alveolar ventilation ($\dot{V}_A$) to alveolar capillary perfusion ($\dot{Q}_c$) is about 1.0:1.2. The value is slightly higher in upper lung zones than in the lower lung zones because of gravitational effects in the upright position. Disease may greatly alter the ventilation-perfusion ratio in regions of the lung and lead to a reduced P_aO_2 in arterial blood, but the P_aCO_2 may be normal, slightly increased, or decreased. Segments of the lung with abnormally high $\dot{V}/\dot{Q}$ ratios compensate for underventilating regions. This mechanism probably is operative to some extent in all forms of intrinsic pulmonary disease.

3. **Venous to arterial shunting** Systemic venous blood may bypass ventilated alveoli in either intrapulmonary or intracardiac channels. Breathing 100% O_2 for 20 minutes raises intra-alveolar P_aO_2 to levels around 650 mm Hg by displacing nitrogen. This maneuver normally results in an arterial P_aO_2 of > 600 mm Hg, but shunt flow is not considered grossly abnormal unless arterial P_aO_2 is < 500 mm Hg. The P_aCO_2 may be normal, low, or slightly increased.

4. **Alveolar hypoventilation** Major reductions in alveolar ventilation result in the accumulation of CO_2 and arterial hypoxemia. The hypoventilation can arise from both intrapulmonary and extrapulmonary causes.

5. **Hemoglobin defects** Abnormal hemoglobin may preclude adequate gas transfer, as in carbon monoxide poisoning or with methemoglobinuria or sulfhemoglobinemia.

IV. **MECHANICAL ABNORMALITIES OF THE PULMONARY SYSTEM**

A. **Reduction of compliance** Reduced pulmonary compliance requires increased energy to expand the lungs and is characteristic of those disorders generally called restrictive pulmonary disease. The vital capacity is decreased. Restrictive disease can result from altered elastic properties of the thoracic wall (kyphoscoliosis) or changes within the lung parenchyma (interstitial disease of any etiology), or may be found with increased surface tension in alveoli with widespread atelectasis. Restrictive disease can be demonstrated simply by finding a reduced vital capacity on spirometry.

B. Increased airway resistance is the major mechanical abnormality in obstructive pulmonary disease. Increased airway resistance may result from mechanical obstruction of airways by secretions, edema of respiratory mucosa, or bronchial smooth-muscle contraction, or it may occur from defective elastic performance of the lung, as in emphysema. Spirometry reveals reduction in the timed vital capacity (during a forced expiration 83% of the vital capacity is normally expired in 1 second, and 97% in 3 seconds), reduced maximal midexpiratory flow rate, and maximum breathing capacity.

V. CONTROL OF RESPIRATION

A. The major stimuli to respiration are the P_aCO_2 and the $H+$ concentration, acting primarily on the medullary respiratory centers. However these stimuli are indirectly influenced by (a) peripheral chemoreceptors in the carotid bodies and aortic arch, (b) pulmonary stretch receptors, (c) baroreceptors in the carotid bodies and aortic arch, (d) stretch and tension receptors in muscle and joints, (e) thermoreceptors mediated via the hypothalamus, and (f) higher centers in the pons and cortex.

B. The hypoxic drive   This mechanism, normally unimportant, assumes major importance in respiratory failure when the medullary respiratory centers become insensitive to P_aCO_2 by acclimatization to chronic CO_2 retention. The stimulus to respiration then originates from the carotid bodies and aortic arch chemoreceptors, which are sensitive to low P_aO_2. Their influence on ventilation normally is minimal until the P_aO_2 falls below 60 mm Hg, at which time hypoxia becomes a progressively more powerful stimulus to respiration as the P_aO_2 continues to fall. With medullary respiratory center depression, the administration of O_2 may further depress respiration by suppressing the hypoxic stimulus.

C. Respiratory depression   A number of pharmacologic agents, such as barbiturates, morphine, anesthetic agents, and various tranquilizers, depress respiration by directly depressing the medullary centers. Tranquilizers with no direct influence on the medullary centers may have nonspecific depressive effects on the higher centers. Thus, in patients with respiratory disease these agents should be used with caution. In patients with CO_2 retention they are contraindicated.

MANAGEMENT OF OBSTRUCTIVE PULMONARY DISEASE

Obstructive pulmonary disease encompasses a group of disorders (asthma, chronic bronchitis, emphysema, bronchiolitis, etc.) characterized by increased airway resistance. This group is the most common mechanical abnormality encountered clinically, and represents a major cause of death and disability.

I.   MECHANISMS OF INCREASED AIRWAY RESISTANCE   In general, resistance to air flow is caused by extensive narrowing of the air passages.

For therapy to be effective, it must counteract the mechanisms responsible, listed below:

A. Potentially reversible mechanisms

1. **Excessive secretions** which obstruct and narrow the smaller airways can result from (a) excessive overproduction secondary to infection or irritation (gases, cigarette smoke, etc.); (b) decreased efficiency of the normal cleansing mechanisms, resulting in secretions not being mobilized and cleared from the air passages (decreased bronchial ciliary activity—a known effect of cigarette smoke—or an ineffective cough mechanism); and (c) increased viscosity of secretions, resulting in difficulty in mobilization from airways; hyperviscosity may result from infection or the use of antihistaminics or may be part of a metabolic disorder of exocrine glands, e.g., cystic fibrosis.

2. **Bronchospasm**

   a) **Immune mechanism,** characteristic of asthma, in which following an antigen-antibody reaction chemical substances are released which constrict the airways.

   b) **Neurogenic mechanisms** may arise from higher centers in the CNS, as exemplified by the association of acute asthma with emotional factors or reflex arcs initiated by irritation of the nasal passages, larynx, or bronchi.

   c) **Irritants** of a wide variety may invoke bronchospasm, probably most often via neurogenic means (dust, fumes, cold air, etc.).

   d) **Chemical mechanisms**   There are a number of substances which can constrict airways, such as acetylcholine and other cholinergic agents, serotonin, histamine, etc.

3. **Mucosal swelling**   Thickening of the bronchial mucosa by edema, inflammation, or luminal compression by bronchial-wall or peribronchial edema can narrow the air passages.

B. Irreversible mechanisms

1. **Bronchial and peribronchial fibrosis**   A previous severe inflammatory process in the peripheral airways (bronchiolitis) may leave residual damage. Some of the bronchi and bronchioles are surrounded or replaced by fibrous tissue, resulting in narrowing, kinking, and obliteration of air passages.

2. **Check-valve mechanism in peripheral airways**   The small airways are normally kept patent by the tractional forces of the surrounding lung parenchyma. With parenchyma destruction and loss of supporting tissue, these airways prematurely collapse during expiration, resulting in air trapping and alveolar distention. This form of obstruction is most prevalent in obstructive emphysema.

3. **Defective support of trachea and bronchi**   Rarely, there may be congenital abnormalities of the cartilaginous rings of the trachea and major bronchi resulting in collapse during expiration. Recently, there have been a few reports of collapse of major airways with obstructive emphysema; the importance of such a defect in the pathogenesis of emphysema is not clear at present.

II. GENERAL PRINCIPLES, TECHNIQUES, AND PHARMACOLOGIC AGENTS IN OBSTRUCTIVE DISEASE

- **A. Attitude** Each patient requires an individualized, comprehensive therapeutic program. The chronicity of the illness must not invoke an attitude of hopelessness or abandonment in the physician. Psychologic support of these patients is a major part of therapy.

- **B. Removal of bronchial irritants** is of major significance in order to reduce those stimuli which increase airway resistance. Cigarette smoke is the leading irritant, and every effort must be made to remove it. Avoidance of such environmental factors as allergens by asthmatics, dusts, fumes, jobs with high risks of respiratory complications (coal mining, etc.), and exposure to extremely cold air, is an important therapeutic step. Treatment of upper respiratory tract disease (postnasal discharge, chronic sinusitis) must be undertaken to prevent their complications in the lower respiratory tract.

- **C. Control of secretions** The initial step is removal of bronchial irritants.

    - **1.** Cough is the major mechanism for tracheobronchial clearance of secretions. Most aspects of therapy aid and support this mechanism. The major harmful effect of sedation in obstructive pulmonary disease may be interference with cough. **Do not suppress cough!**

    - **2. Reduce viscosity** The thinning of secretions markedly aids their mobilization from distal segments of the lung, often via the normal cleansing mechanisms.

        - **a) Hydration** The state of hydration is important in the management of secretions. Fluids are encouraged and dehydration is corrected by appropriate means. However, restoring total body water to normal only stimulates the flow of thinner secretions to a limited extent. **Water must be delivered to the mucus-covered surface to hydrate it effectively.**

            - **i) Administration** The simplest way to deliver aerosolized water is by a steam vaporizer or various nebulizers. The particle size of the aerosol is extremely important, and the most effective machines for delivering a specific particle-sized mist are the ultrasonic aerosol generators. To achieve deposit on the smaller bronchi and bronchioles, a particle size of less than 10 μ is required. If therapy is aimed at the larynx or trachea, a particle size of greater than 10 μ is required. The steam vaporizer has the advantage of delivering relative sterile moisture particles.

            - **ii) Aerosolized water** is best given for 10–15 minutes just prior to IPPB and bronchodilator therapy. (It can be on a QID basis or more frequent, depending upon the situation.)
              A longer period of mist inhalation (20–25 minutes) may be desirable when the patient arises in the morning, since the greatest accumulation of secretions occurs during sleep. The purpose is to facilitate sputum production, and inhalation can be continued as needed to accomplish this end.

            - **iii) Dry gases should never be inhaled for prolonged periods,** since they dry secretions and are irritating to the airways. The flow of gas should be through moisturizers or nebulizers filled with water or saline.

b) **Mucolytic agents** can be administered by aerosol to alter the structure of mucus, pus, or fibrin.

i) **n-Acetyl-L-cysteine (Mucomyst)** probably is the most effective of the currently available agents. It lowers viscosity presumably by breaking disulfide bonds. The dose is usually 3 to 5 ml of 20% solution given by aerosol every 4 to 6 hours. It should be accompanied by a bronchodilator during administration (e.g., both agents aerosolized and given via IPPB), since acetylcysteine may cause bronchospasm that can be severe in hypersensitive patients. Direct instillation into the trachea should not be done routinely, since severe bronchospasm and respiratory distress can occur. The immediate liquefication of mucus may result in a copious volume of material, and ability to clear the secretions is essential (especially during the first 24 hours of therapy). Other uncommon effects include stomatitis, rhinorrhea, nausea, and vomiting. Prolonged administration of acetylcysteine is not advisable.

ii) **Pancreatic deoxyribonuclease (dornase) (Dornovac)** has little effect against mucus per se; however, it may be of use if the secretions are purulent. In those cases in which Mucomyst appears ineffective (usually marked purulence), Dornovac may be effective. Dose is 50,000 to 100,000 units in 2 ml of diluent, given by aerosol 1 to 4 times a day. An occasional anaphylactoid reaction has been noted after prolonged use. Pharyngeal irritation may occur.

iii) **Other mucolytic agents** include the proteolytic enzymes (trypsin, chymotrypsin) which are felt to be of no real benefit for they have irritative effects and a tendency to induce hypersensitivity reactions; and the surface-active agents (Alevaire, Tergemist, Tween 80), which behave as emulsifiers and are of doubtful value. They have no effect on mucus or pus and theoretically may do harm by altering the surface tension of the alveoli, leading to their collapse.

c) **Expectorants** allegedly promote watery bronchial secretions. There are numerous such preparations, but the most widely used are SSKI (saturated solution of potassium iodide) and glyceryl guaiacolate. The effectiveness of these agents is disputed. Clinical experience over the years suggests some patients may benefit from SSKI or glyceryl guaiacolate. SSKI is given 5 to 10 drops in water TID or QID. Side effects of iodides are discussed in Chapter 14. Other agents (terpin hydrate, ammonium chloride, eucalyptol) are probably of no value.

3. Removing secretions (see also Respiratory Failure)

a) **Postural drainage** utilizes gravity to drain the bronchial tree and aid the cough mechanism in secretion clearance. In localized secretions (e.g., bronchiectasis of a single lobe), the patient assumes a comfortable position, with the bronchial orifice and trachea below the segment being drained. With secretions generally distributed (most of which are usually in the lung bases) the best position is with the thorax lower than the hips, so that the bases are drained. Positions can be changed periodically (lying flat, on right side, then left side) to promote drainage from the various bronchial segments. Some patients do not tolerate their heads lower than the hips; in them, lying flat with periodic rotation of positions will suffice. The positions assumed should not be so uncomfortable as to cause the patient distress. Postural drainage is gradually increased to 5–10 minutes until it is tolerated without difficulty. During and following drainage, coughing is encouraged. Just prior to postural drainage, inhalation of heated aerosolized water mists (10 minutes), followed by bronchodilators and IPPB (10 minutes), is given to obtain maximum benefit. Physiotherapy is advocated by some to expedite postural drainage, and the thorax is thumped with cupped hands. Postural drainage should be continued, if it aids the removal of secretions.

b) **IPPB** (intermittent positive-pressure breathing) serves a number of purposes, which are discussed in appropriate sections. It is effective in the mobilization of secretions in those with or without respiratory failure. In conscious, cooperative patients, ventilation to high-resistance areas is improved enough to augment expulsive forces to mobilize secretions. Besides being an effective means of delivering bronchodilators, IPPB alone dilates bronchi during inflation of the lung. The secretions can be effectively managed by giving IPPB for 10 minutes QID or more, with bronchodilator.

D. **Bronchodilation** The aim of bronchodilator therapy is to reduce abnormally high airway resistance. Bronchodilator drugs are of limited value, if the other factors contributing to obstruction are neglected (secretions, infections, smoking). These drugs are not a regimen in themselves, but are an important *part* of the therapeutic regimen. Bronchodilator therapy must be individualized, since response varies greatly. It is useful to document by spirometry the patient's response to bronchodilator drugs. Since this therapy is entirely symptomatic, dosage and route of administration frequently require adjustment. Intensive therapy is indicated during periods of severe or acute obstruction, and maintenance therapy may be necessary on a long-term basis. Pharmacologic agents include:

1. **Adrenergic drugs** (isoproterenol, phenylephrine, racemic epinephrine, epinephrine, ephedrine) are potent bronchodilators and can be given by a variety of routes. Generally, the most effective form of therapy is via aerosols. Combination aerosol and oral administration can be effective, especially in outpatient care. Subcutaneous epinephrine has been used primarily in acute asthma. Side effects include tremor, palpitations, tachycardia, and cardiac arrhythmias. Great caution must be taken in patients with hypertension, coronary, cerebral, and peripheral vascular disease.

a) **Aerosols** The most effective are isoproterenol, racemic epinephrine, and phenylephrine, administered by hand bulb nebulizers, powered nebulizers, inert-gas-propelled cartridges, or IPPB.

i) **Correct technique of inhalation** is important in hand bulb and cartridged nebulizers in order to get the best possible distribution of aerosol in the lungs. After maximal exhalation, the aerosol is inhaled slowly to full inspiration, and the breath is then held for several seconds. After a pause of 1 minute the cycle may be repeated. Powered nebulizers appear to be more effective when used with an IPPB device rather than alone.

    ii) **Dosage** In the hand bulb nebulizer 2.25% racemic epinephrine or 1:200–1:400 isoproterenol. For cartridges, each "puff" has a fixed amount of medication. Powered nebulizers or IPPB: 0.5–1.0 ml 1:200 isoproterenol, or 2.25% racemic epinephrine are diluted with enough saline or water to assure aerosol therapy for at least 10 minutes (e.g., 0.5 ml of 1:200 isoproterenol with 2.5–3.5 ml saline).

    iii) **Administration** In uncomplicated situations (not in respiratory distress, nor acute or severe failure), aerosol therapy 3–4 times per day often suffices. With hand bulb or cartridges, 2–4 inhalations (see Technique) per treatment are usual; with powered aerosols or IPPB, 10–15 minutes per treatment. The first treatment of the day should be promptly upon arising in the morning, since secretions tend to accumulate during sleep. Therapy can be given PRN for symptoms. In acute situations, medications can be given every 30–60 minutes. However, frequent administration may result in systemic reactions or rarely a paradoxical episode of bronchospasm due to bronchial irritation.

  b) Oral route The best oral agent is ephedrine. Sublingual isoproterenol has been used, but its systemic effects and transient action limit its usefulness. Ephedrine is more useful in the long-term management of mild to moderate symptoms than in the severe symptoms of acute respiratory infection. The usual dose of ephedrine is 25 mg TID or QID. It is best used in combination with an aerosol bronchodilator, staggering their administration (i.e., oral ephedrine given 1–2 hours after the aerosol bronchodilator). Many preparations combine ephedrine with other agents, but ephedrine is essentially the only effective agent in the combination. Tolerance may occur after several weeks, but effectiveness usually is restored if the drug is discontinued for 4–7 days. Gastric irritation or urinary retention may occur.

  c) Parenteral route Epinephrine is the only adrenergic agent given subcutaneously. Short-acting preparations are used frequently in the initial treatment of acute asthmatic attacks because the response is rapid and the dose can be repeated. Epinephrine hydrochloride (1:1000 solution) 0.2–0.5 ml is given subcutaneously as often as every 30 minutes (for several doses) if necessary. Resistance to epinephrine may develop in prolonged attacks secondary to respiratory acidosis. Some claim the effect may be restored by intravenously administered sodium bicarbonate; however, sodium bicarbonate should not be injected without knowledge of the arterial blood gases (pH, P_aCO_2, P_aO_2). Great caution with alkali therapy is warranted, since the precipitation of metabolic alkalosis can be catastrophic. (See page 166.) Great caution must be taken not to inject directly into the systemic circulation.

2. Xanthines Aminophylline and theophylline are excellent bronchodilators with minimal toxicity. Side effects include nausea, vomiting, and flushing. Rapid IV infusion can lead to hypotension, cardiac arrhythmias, and death.

a) **Parenteral route** IV aminophylline is excellent in any condition of respiratory distress with bronchospasm (acute asthma, chronic lung disease with acute decompensation). Frequently, patients with cardiogenic pulmonary edema (left ventricular failure, mitral stenosis) present in respiratory distress with bronchospasm that may be effectively relieved by aminophylline. Pulmonary disease may be mistaken for cardiogenic pulmonary edema, and morphine administration is contraindicated in obstructive pulmonary disease. **When doubt exists as to the etiology of respiratory distress, aminophylline is the drug of choice.**

In acute situations, 250–500 mg aminophylline given IV over 5–10 minutes often gives relief. Similarly, 250–500 mg in 100–200 ml 5% D/W given over a period of 30 minutes to 2 hours is effective with less risk. In hospitalized patients with resistant bronchospasm, 500–1000 mg aminophylline in 500 ml 5% D/W every 6 hours IV for several days is effective, unless side effects (nausea, vomiting, headache, hypotension, arrhythmias) occur.

b) **Rectal administration** Enemas of aminophylline or theophylline, 250–500 mg in 20–30 ml of water are quite effective. Packaged rectal units of theophylline are available which can be administered every 6–8 hours and control moderately severe symptoms or nocturnal attacks. Use at bedtime is effective to reduce nocturnal increases in airway resistance secondary to the accumulation of secretions.

The suppositories (250–500 mg), although more frequently used, are less effective because of variable absorption.

c) **Oral administration** A number of preparations contain aminophylline or theophylline alone or in combination with other agents. The usual dose is 120–200 mg QID. The oral route is not the preferred route. The amount present in most preparations is usually insufficient, and when the amount is adequate, gastric irritation is common.

E. **Control of infection** Infection is a frequent cause of acute decompensation in obstructive pulmonary disease and may play a significant role in the progression of the disease. In many acute asthmatic attacks infection is the inciting factor. Thus, prompt attention to all infections, including those which may appear trivial, is mandatory. When the sputum suddenly becomes purulent, or the volume of sputum suddenly changes, infection should be assumed. Examination of sputum with Gram stain is very helpful. Most studies indicate that pneumococcus and *H. influenzae* are the most frequent organisms, but cultures often show no pathogens. **The antibiotics of choice are penicillin, tetracycline, and ampicillin,** unless culture indicates otherwise.

1. **Acute respiratory infection** Antibiotic therapy should be initiated at the first definite signs of upper respiratory tract infection. Although most of these infections are viral in origin, bacterial complications are so common as to indicate therapy. In moderately severe chronic bronchitis, chronic asthma, or emphysema, antibiotics should be continued for 10–14 days, even if the cultures are negative.

2. **Prophylactic therapy** with antibiotics for chronic bronchitis and emphysema is controversial, with strong arguments for and against antibiotic prophylaxis. In general, most tend to treat each infection vigorously as it arises. In moderately severe cases it is

recommended the patient have several days' supply of tetracycline available to initiate therapy at the first signs of infection. Antibiotic coverage, continuously or for 3 to 5 days out of the week, may be justified during the winter months in those patients with repeated respiratory infections or those who chronically produce large volumes of purulent sputum.

3. **Influenza vaccine** Influenza in patients with chronic lung disease can be disastrous. Polyvalent influenza virus A and B vaccine should be given yearly. In the primary course of immunization, two 1-ml subcutaneous injections are given two months apart. A booster injection of 1 ml subcutaneously is given yearly, preferably in the fall.

III. **OBSTRUCTIVE DISEASE SPECIFICS** The previous discussion described features and principles of therapy which are applicable to all forms of obstructive disease. This section will deal with more specific problems.

A. **Bronchial asthma** may present in two forms:

1. Classical **extrinsic asthma** is extremely common and is characterized by hereditary predisposition; a history of atopy; has its onset predominantly in the young and is episodic (i.e., intermittent airway obstruction, which is reversible). It appears to be a genetically determined immunologic disorder involving antigen and a reagenic antibody, recently classified as a gamma E immunoglobulin.

2. One also encounters an adult-onset, nonatopic type of obstructive disease that is more or less continuous, and seems to warrant a separate term, **intrinsic asthma**. The mode of hypersensitization is not clearly understood, but the final pathway is felt to be mediated via immune mechanisms. Features common to asthma and chronic bronchitis may be present. One must refrain from calling all that wheezes "asthma." The diagnosis must be established, since wheezing may be seen in a variety of illnesses (mitral stenosis, left ventricular failure, inhalation of noxious agents, partial obstruction of the trachea, carcinoid, various vasculitides, pulmonary embolism).

a) **Control of etiologic factors** The avoidance of allergens, irritants, extreme cold, and infections, which may precipitate attacks, is obvious. Other aspects of management are:

i) **Emotional** factors play a significant role in precipitating acute asthma. Supportive psychotherapy is warranted. Tranquilizers may be useful in episodic asthma, where emotional factors are the inciting event. However, they must be used with caution. In severe attacks with a tendency to CO_2 retention, they should not be used. The use of sedatives or narcotics is contraindicated in acute attacks.

ii) **Environment** In those with a strong allergic history, who are susceptible to airborne allergens and irritants, certain precautions can be taken. The rooms (especially bedrooms or hospital rooms) should have adequate humidity and be as allergen-free as possible (e.g., dustproof covers, window filters, foam rubber pillows, avoidance of pets).

iii) **Desensitization** has been of value in treating extrinsic asthma in atopic children and allergic young adults. It is for this reason that anyone with asthma should undergo careful skin testing for hypersensitivity. Even though the best results have been obtained in young asthmatics, if specific hypersensitivity is present in one who has been significantly troubled by asthma, a course of desensitization is warranted. In adult late-onset intrinsic asthma, where no history of allergy exists, desensitization with various bacteria antigens has been of less value.

iv) **Drugs precipitating asthmatic attacks**   Some asthmatics are extremely sensitive to aspirin. Indomethacin has been implicated also in recent reports. Penicillin may be a potential hazard in asthmatics. Other drugs may have a similar effect and the awareness of such potential hazards is warranted.

b) **Corticosteroid therapy in asthma**   These agents can be effective in severe acute asthma, status asthmaticus, and debilitating chronic asthma, which fail to respond to the more usual measures. Their use in ordinary episodic attacks is not warranted. Corticosteroids are supplemental to the usual measures.

i) **In acute severe asthma** not responding to usual measures, large doses of corticosteroids are used (e.g., 300 mg hydrocortisone IV, or 40–60 mg prednisone orally per 24-hour period). Following relief of the acute episode, improvement is maintained for 2–3 days, and the steroid dosage is rapidly reduced and stopped. If symptoms soon recur, the course may be repeated and the lowest dose effective to maintain remission is determined. Attempts to stop steroids are then withheld until some later time.

ii) **In chronic asthma,** corticosteroid therapy should be confined to those unresponsive patients with severe or persistent symptoms. Again, it is emphasized that steroids are supplemental and not alternative to the usual measures. The smallest dose to maintain remission is used, usually 20 mg prednisone on alternate days. Aerosol preparations of steroids mixed with bronchodilators are available. Aerosolized steroids may have significant systemic absorption, and dosage becomes uncertain with their use.

c) **Management of acute asthmatic attacks**   Therapy is individualized depending upon the severity of the attack. Vigorous initial efforts usually provide prompt symptomatic relief and should be followed by a program adequate to maintain long-term remission.

i) **Mild episodic attacks** that occur infrequently often respond to IV aminophylline or subcutaneous epinephrine. In elderly patients aminophylline is preferred. Follow-up therapy with aerosol bronchodilators (2–3 inhalations, QID, PRN) or the addition of oral and/or rectal agents should be kept up for at least one week, if required. An inciting etiologic factor should be sought and treated.

ii) **Severe asthmatic attacks** include those which do not respond to initial therapy. Frequently bronchospasm is reduced, but dyspnea and "tightness in the chest" persists, usually due to secretions in the peripheral airways. The following plan may be instituted:

(a) Repeat aminophylline or epinephrine if initial administration does not relieve symptoms. The aminophylline is best given IV, 500 mg in 500 ml 5% D/W over 2–3 hours.

(b) Loosen secretions and reduce airway resistance with aerosol bronchodilators. Hydrate secretions with water mists or nebulized water aerosols, followed by bronchodilator given via IPPB. Treatments can be given hourly or more frequently, until a satisfactory response is achieved. (Aerosolized bronchodilator is not necessary in the IPPB during all treatments, since vigorous use of bronchodilators may occasionally result in increased bronchospasm.)

(c) Obtain sputum smears and cultures, since infection is a common inciting agent. If secretions are purulent, antibiotic therapy is advisable.

(d) If no response or little improvement occurs in several hours, corticosteroid administration should be considered (see above).

(e) Blood gas analyses are useful to determine the level of alveolar ventilation and whether respiratory acidosis is present. Severe acidosis in resistant cases may inhibit the effects of bronchodilators. The results are within normal limits in a majority of instances, but it is best to improve the arterial pH by increasing the alveolar ventilation.

(f) Serial measurements of the vital capacity with a portable spirometer can be of value in following the response to therapy.

(g) Narcotics and sedatives should not be given at any time.

(h) The patient should be hospitalized if the attack does not subside within 6 hours with therapy, since delay only makes subsequent therapy more difficult. Hypoxia should be promptly corrected, if present.

iii) **Status asthmaticus** refers to a severe refractory attack which can be fatal. Typically, the tracheobronchial tree is filled with tenacious mucus plugs, which may cause respiratory failure with alarming rapidity. Management is outlined above, plus management for respiratory failure if it occurs. The most critical aspect of therapy is to remove viscid secretions and maintain a patent airway. It may be necessary to assist ventilation initially by endotracheal intubation. Intubation is preferred to tracheotomy for the removal of secretions and for short-term assisted ventilation.

iv) **Interim management between acute attacks** Effective care during the interim periods following acute attacks may prolong remissions. In patients with mild infrequent attacks, no interim therapy may be required. However, airway resistance has been shown to be significantly increased in many completely asymptomatic asthmatics. Minimum effective therapy should be maintained (e.g., cartridged aerosol bronchodilator, 2–3 inhalations TID or QID) in these patients along with follow-up evaluation. In more severe cases, individualized programs, following the general principles in obstructive disease, should be maintained.

B. Chronic bronchitis and emphysema These disorders are discussed together, since they frequently coexist, and many principles of management are similar. Chronic bronchitis is characterized by a productive cough due to a generalized bronchial hypersecretion (not due to a specific disease process, e.g., lung abscess, primary cardiac disease, bronchogenic carcinoma, etc.) and may be subdivided into the following: simple chronic bronchitis, chronic or recurrent mucopurulent bronchitis, and chronic obstructive bronchitis. Emphysema is characterized by enlargement of the air spaces distal to the terminal nonrespiratory bronchiole, accompanied by destruction of the alveolar walls. The pathogenesis of these disorders is not completely understood, but several things appear clear. Severe chronic obstructive disease is primarily a disease of cigarette-smoking men over the age of 50 who commonly live in cities and who frequently have had chronic bronchitis for many years.

Emphysema is not always associated with bronchitis. Its occurrence occasionally in young persons suggests possible intrinsic parenchymal defects associated with heredity, deficiency of serum $alpha_1$-antitrypsin, and Marfan's syndrome.

In chronic bronchitis, depending upon severity, there may be a fair degree of reversibility. In moderate disease, if smoking is discontinued and therapy is vigorous, respiratory function may improve dramatically. In emphysema, improvement may occur, especially relief of symptoms, following a good therapeutic regimen aimed at the reversible components. Although tissue destruction is fixed in emphysema, the decreased activity of the patient reduces the need for ventilation. Even though cure may not be possible, the aim of therapy is to bring symptomatic relief and to prevent respiratory and circulatory failure.

1. Management of chronic bronchitis and emphysema has been discussed.

2. Special considerations in management

a) Corticosteroid in chronic bronchitis and emphysema If a mixed picture of both asthma and chronic bronchitis is present, the use of corticosteroids may be of benefit. A brief course of high doses of corticosteroids (40–60 mg of prednisone), along with the usual measures, has benefited acute respiratory insufficiency in chronic bronchitics. Although short courses of high-dosage corticosteroids may benefit some patients, long-term corticosteroid therapy in chronic bronchitis and emphysema has been shown to be of no benefit.

b) IPPB at home is indicated when the patient is unable to take a deep breath and effectively use a nebulizer, when persistent P_aCO_2 elevation (greater than 60 mm Hg) is present, and when the patient requires repeated hospitalizations for respiratory failure.

c) Central nervous system stimulants in ambulatory patients are of no established value.

d) Physical therapy

i) **Breathing training** can be of use, especially under the guidance of a skilled therapist. The patient is taught to inhale through the nose, and then to exhale slowly, evenly, and deeply against pursed lips while contracting the abdominal muscles. The techniques are learned first supine, then in a sitting position, and finally while walking.

ii) **Graded exercises** Some have advocated a program of gradually increasing exercises to recondition muscles that have become inactive from the limited physical activity of advanced obstructive disease. The aim is to improve the ability to perform more activity before dyspnea develops. In severely handicapped patients, the program can be instituted while the patient breathes O_2 at low flow rates (2–4 L/min). The services of a therapist are desirable.

RESPIRATORY FAILURE

Respiratory failure can result from a variety of causes both intrinsic and extrinsic to the lung. When associated with intrinsic lung disease, all the abnormalities of gas exchange may be operative. When it is due to extrinsic causes, the primary mechanism is alveolar hypoventilation (see Physiologic Considerations at beginning of chapter).

I. **RESPIRATORY FAILURE AS HYPOXIA ALONE** is primarily seen in widespread involvement of the pulmonary parenchyma. The most notable pathology is diffuse interstitial infiltrative or inflammatory disease, with a number of etiologies (e.g., sarcoidosis, berylliosis, histiocytosis X, alveolar cell carcinoma, lymphangitic carcinomatosis, Hamman-Rich syndrome, etc.). Reduction of the pulmonary vascular bed may have similar results (pulmonary embolism). Even though hypercapnia is usually not present, it may occur late in the course of the disease or if obstructive disease is superimposed.

Therapy primarily is directed at the underlying disease. Respiratory care is supportive including treatment of hypoxia and prevention or treatment of superimposed airway disorders. (See also IV. Special Considerations, later in this section.)

A. **Mild hypoxemia** If the arterial PO_2 is greater than 60 mm Hg, oxygen therapy usually is not required, for this degree of reduction in the P_aO_2 can usually be tolerated by most patients.

B. **Severe hypoxemia** A P_aO_2 of less than 50 mm Hg without elevation of the P_aCO_2 usually indicates extensive parenchymal disease. Therapy is aimed primarily at the relief of hypoxia with oxygen. It usually is unnecessary to use inspired O_2 concentrations of greater than 40%. (At sea level, 40% oxygen gives an inspired PO_2 of approximately 280 mm Hg.) The induction of hypercapnia by oxygen therapy is usually of no concern, since alveolar hyperventilation commonly is present and the respiratory centers remain sensitive to CO_2.

Cor pulmonale with acute right ventricular failure is common. In the hospital, bed rest and O_2 therapy can reduce the work of the right ventricle, as well as relieve some symptoms. IPPB and bronchodilator therapy usually are not indicated unless a superimposed obstructive problem arises.

II. **RESPIRATORY FAILURE WITH HYPOXIA AND HYPERCAPNIA (ALVEOLAR HYPOVENTILATION)** refers to sudden deterioration in the clinical status of the patient and determines the need for vigorous therapy. Usually, when the arterial blood pH is less than 7.25, the P_aCO_2 greater than 60 mm Hg, and the P_aO_2 less than 50 mm Hg, the situation is critical, and the need for therapy is urgent. Etiologies include:

A. **Intrinsic lung disease**   A number of diseases involving the pulmonary parenchyma can result in respiratory failure with hypercapnia. The most frequent cause is obstructive pulmonary disease. The degree of airway obstruction usually is increased by secretions and bronchospasm, with infection frequently the precipitating factor. Superimposition of a major complication (pulmonary embolism, pneumothorax, atelectasis, extensive pneumonia, etc.) on obstructive or extensive parenchymal disease may precipitate acute failure.

B. **Extrinsic causes**   Respiratory failure as a result of alveolar hypoventilation can arise from extrapulmonary causes, even when the lungs are normal. Although intrinsic lung disease may be present, an extrinsic disorder must be excluded in each episode of acute failure. In this situation, the addition of an extrinsic component leads to further compromise of function. A few examples are cited below:

   1. **Depression of respiration** can be caused by drugs (morphine, barbiturates, glutethimide, certain tranquilizers, anesthesia), cerebral trauma, increased intracranial pressure, prolonged anoxia, cerebral ischemia, electrocution, and high P_aCO_2.

   2. **Abnormalities of the spinal cord, peripheral nerves, or myoneural junctions,** including injured spinal cord, poliomyelitis, Guillain-Barré syndrome, peripheral neuritis, myasthenia gravis, nerve gases, pseudocholine-esterase deficiency, neuromuscular blocking agents (curare, succinylcholine), and nicotine poisoning.

   3. **Abnormalities of the chest wall** including traumatic flail chest, myopathies involving the respiratory muscles, marked elevation of the diaphragms, marked obesity (pickwickian syndrome), kyphoscoliosis.

   4. **Compression of lungs** by pleural effusions, hemothorax, fibrothorax, and pneumothorax.

III. **THERAPY OF ACUTE RESPIRATORY FAILURE** is aimed at the rapid correction of hypoxia and the improvement and maintenance of alveolar ventilation (as reflected by the arterial P_aCO_2).

A. **Diagnosis in respiratory distress**   Clear definition of the disease process must be pursued vigorously. In respiratory failure caused or complicated by extrinsic factors, therapy aimed specifically at each responsible factor is instituted while effective ventilation is supported. In respiratory distress the differentiation between the rhonchi of pulmonary edema due to cardiac failure and the "wheezing" of airway obstruction may be difficult when the patient is seen initially. When in doubt, the drug of choice is aminophylline to treat the acute episode. Morphine used mistakenly can lead to fatal respiratory depression.

B. **Blood gases**   Frequent measurements of arterial pH, P_aCO_2 and P_aO_2 are essential in management. Alveolar ventilation does not usually correlate well with ventilatory rate in respiratory failure. Tachypnea is present frequently in the face of hypercapnia, unless respiratory depression has occurred. The P_aCO_2 is the most accurate way to follow alveolar ventilation.

C. General measures and methods

1. **Apnea and the open airway** When treating an apneic patient, one aims to secure a patent airway, remove secretions, oxygenate the patient, and assist ventilation.

   Mouth-to-mouth insufflation is instituted until some mechanical device can be obtained. However, if the upper respiratory tract is obstructed all methods of resuscitation fail. In the unconscious apneic patient, the upper respiratory tract can be obstructed by the soft tissues of the pharynx or by the tongue falling back. This obstruction is apt to occur when the patient is prone or supine with the chin down toward the chest. Mucus, vomitus, or foreign bodies in the oropharynx may have the same effect. The approach is: (a) clear the oropharynx quickly with the fingers (suction, when available); (b) with the patient supine, soft-tissue obstruction frequently is relieved by extending the head (chin up), with forward displacement of the mandible, and inserting a plastic pharyngeal airway. If there is complete obstruction of the larynx or trachea, tracheotomy must be done.

2. **Reduce airway obstruction in lower respiratory tract**

   a) **Removal of secretions** is a major step toward improving alveolar ventilation. Approach includes promoting cough and passing a transtracheal catheter for irrigation with saline and suction (discussed later).

   b) **Bronchodilators** IV aminophylline and/or aerosol bronchodilators.

   c) Increase alveolar ventilation via **mechanical respirator** (IPPB or by assisted or controlled ventilation).

   d) **Humidification** of inhaled gases by nebulization of water at body temperature.

3. **Treat infection** It is reasonable to assume infection is present, especially in chronic obstructive disease. After cultures and smears are obtained, initiate therapy with ampicillin or tetracycline until culture results are available.

4. **Hypoxia must be corrected** Correction is achieved by increasing alveolar ventilation (including mechanical respirators) and increasing the concentration of O_2 in inspired gases to increase P_aO_2 above 50 mm Hg.

5. **Correction of hypercapnia and respiratory acidosis** is accomplished by lowering the P_aCO_2 by increasing alveolar ventilation with the procedures outlined and the use of mechanical respirators.

   a) **Complications of rapid lowering of P_aCO_2** Even though a P_aCO_2 of greater than 70 mm Hg can lead to respiratory depression, coma, and circulatory collapse, care must be taken in the rate of reduction of the P_aCO_2. In acute CO_2 retention there is no significant increase in $HCO_3{}^-$, and rapid lowering of the P_aCO_2 usually leads to no complication. With chronic CO_2 retention, high $HCO_3{}^-$ levels are present in the tissues and the rapid reduction of the P_aCO_2 can result in severe tissue alkalosis (usually a complication of mechanical respirators used for assisted or controlled ventilation). Most often these patients have low chlorides and frequently hypokalemia. The resultant alkalosis has been associated with tremors, focal and grand mal seizures, and death.

Ideal therapy is (a) careful reduction of P_aCO_2 with frequent blood gas measurements and (b) correction of the $K+$ and $Cl-$ deficit with KCl. Correction of the hypochloremia promotes renal excretion of excess HCO_3-.

b) Mild to moderate hypercapnia (P_aCO_2 of less than 50 mm Hg)   In most situations, the aim of initial therapy is to prevent further increases in the P_aCO_2, especially during O_2 administration. Where hypoxia is present, the Ventimask is an ideal way to give O_2. Vigorous therapy, as previously noted, is undertaken to improve alveolar ventilation. If the P_aCO_2 increases or the alveolar ventilation appears limited, then assisted ventilation with a mechanical respirator appears indicated (see Artificial Respiration).

6. Right ventricular failure is discussed in the section on cor pulmonale. The emphasis during respiratory failure is on correction of the hypoxia and hypercapnia, which frequently will lead to recovery of the right ventricle. Digitalis and diuretics are warranted. However, these agents should not be primary therapeutic agents during the initial phases. The many cardiac arrhythmias that have occurred during digitalis administration in respiratory failure can be ascribed to hypoxia, acidosis, rapid shifts of $K+$, and $K+$ depletion, all of which render the myocardium sensitive to digitalis. The correction of the hypoxia and acidosis will lower the pulmonary vascular resistance and reduce right ventricular work.

7. Correct dehydration by oral and parenteral routes. This common problem frequently is overlooked.

8. Electrolyte and metabolic acid-base disturbances frequently are a part of respiratory failure. They easily can be overlooked unless frequent determinations of electrolytes and pH are made. Hypokalemia and hypochloremia often are present and contribute to potential alkalosis and cardiac arrhythmias (see above). These electrolyte abnormalities are corrected by KCl. With chloride depletion, the $K+$ deficit cannot be corrected with other $K+$ preparations. Abnormalities other than those related to respiratory failure or the effects of prior medications, may alter electrolytes and pH. Their recognition and correction should be prompt.

IV.   SPECIAL CONSIDERATIONS IN RESPIRATORY FAILURE

A. Oxygen therapy   The most serious threat to the patient is O_2 deprivation. *Hypoxia must be corrected promptly.*

1. O_2 therapy when P_aCO_2 is normal or low   The threat of respiratory depression from O_2 administration in this circumstance is minimal. Concentrations of O_2 up to 40% can be given safely. In extensive pulmonary involvement (interstitial fibrosis, widespread pneumonia, pulmonary edema, A-V shunting) the inspired O_2 concentration may have to be adjusted to achieve a minimum P_aO_2 of 50 to 60 mm Hg. Appropriate adjustments of the inspired O_2 concentration should be correlated with direct measurements of arterial P_aO_2. In a majority of instances, 30–40% O_2 is more than sufficient.

2. **O_2 therapy when elevated P_aCO_2 or tendency to elevations of P_aCO_2** The concern of depressing respiration by removing the "hypoxic drive" with O_2 administration is justified; however, the omission of O_2 in a hypoxic patient is unjustified for persistent severe hypoxia may greatly jeopardize recovery. Patients on supplemental O_2 must be watched closely for respiratory depression by frequent measurements of the arterial P_aCO_2, and observing the level of consciousness and respiratory rate. *If O_2 administration leads to a significant rise in the P_aCO_2, then O_2 therapy must be combined with assisted or controlled ventilation* (see Artificial Respiration). Depending upon the delivery system used, the concentrations of O_2 vary from 24% to 40%.

   a) **Low O_2 concentrations** (24–30%) are used to relieve hypoxia, hopefully without depressing the "hypoxic drive." An arterial P_aO_2 of 60 mm is sufficient to relieve the dangers of hypoxia, without completely depressing the hypoxic stimulus of respiration. Recent studies show that the Ventimask is excellent for the administration of low O_2 concentrations. It utilizes the Venturi principle to deliver O_2 concentrations of 24% or 28%. The 24% Ventimask is recommended, since the risks of respiratory depression are less. There is no need to go beyond the 28% Ventimask to reach the minimum arterial P_aO_2. If higher O_2 concentrations are needed, the risks of elevating the P_aCO_2 are such that assisted ventilation should be considered for O_2 administration.

   b) **Low-flow O_2** (1–2 L/min) through nasal cannulas or catheters delivers O_2 concentrations in the 25–30% range. Although low-flow O_2 is equally effective, the Ventimask is preferred, since it requires less attention to assure the proper O_2 concentrations.

   c) Oxygen therapy utilizing assisted or controlled ventilation in delivery is usually given in 40% concentration.

3. **Intermittent use of O_2 in respiratory failure** The practice of administering O_2 intermittently in respiratory failure as a means of avoiding respiratory depression is not condoned, for it can be hazardous (*Lancet* 2:10, 1960). When O_2 is stopped, the ensuing hypoxemia may be more severe than that which was present during air breathing. The continuous administration of O_2 in low concentrations is preferred.

4. **Long-term O_2 therapy** for chronic hypoxia in obstructive disease is beneficial. Even though there is no reversal of pulmonary mechanical abnormalities, clinical status improves (exercise tolerance increases, secondary erythrocythemia reverses, and pulmonary vascular resistance falls). Continuous low-flow O_2 (24 hours/day) via nasal prongs allows the patient to talk, eat, and sleep without interruption. These patients show improvement after one month, and a few have continued as outpatients. These studies indicate that in hospitalized patients continuous O_2 administration for chronically hypoxic patients is safe and may facilitate recovery.

5. **Methods of oxygen administration** The O_2 stream should be moistened by passage through a saline or water-containing heated moisturizer, to prevent the drying effect on the mucous membranes

of the respiratory tree. Contamination of nebulizers by gram-negative organisms occasionally occurs, resulting in pulmonary infections. Prevention of this complication can be achieved by daily cleansing of the apparatus followed by nebulizing a solution of 0.25% acetic acid through the system for five minutes. Administration of 100% oxygen for prolonged periods may be hazardous, for injurious effects have been described in the alveolar-capillary region.

a) **Nasal cannulas** (prongs) are commonly used because of simplicity and comfort. There is no rebreathing of expired air. O_2 flow rates of 2–8 L/min can provide approximate O_2 concentrations between 25% and 40%. They are effective even in mouth breathers.

b) **Nasal catheters** offer no advantage over nasal cannulas and are uncomfortable. If used, the catheter tip should have multiple holes and be well lubricated before insertion; it should not extend beyond the uvula (to prevent gastric inflation). The catheter should be alternated between nostrils every 6 to 12 hours. O_2 flow rates are essentially the same as for cannulas.

c) **Face masks** include the Ventimask* which is a light, comfortable, loosely fitting mask; it employs the Venturi principle to mix 100% O_2 with air to give accurate inspiratory concentrations of O_2. Masks are available which provide 24% or 28% inspired O_2. Numerous other masks are available that deliver high concentrations of O_2. Tight-fitting masks (over nose and mouth) are uncomfortable and not well tolerated for over 60 minutes and must have an exhalation valve to prevent rebreathing of expired CO_2. All masks create problems in eating, speaking, and expectorating.

d) **Oxygen tents** offer a cool, moist, and comfortable environment. However, they often interfere with patient care and are an inefficient means of administering O_2. (Sufficient leakage must be present at the tent edges to prevent CO_2 accumulation). O_2 flow rates of at least 10 L/min are required to reach tent concentrations of 35–40% O_2.

e) **IPPB respirators** are engaged to sources of 100% O_2 and adjusted to deliver maximal air mix, providing inspired O_2 concentrations of 40%.

B. **Maintenance of patent airways**   When secretions cannot be mobilized effectively by the cough mechanism after nebulized water mists, bronchodilators, augmented lung inflation with IPPB, and postural drainage, the following measures may be required.

1. **Tracheal suction**   Nasal tracheal suction is done using sterilized gloves and catheters. The catheters should be resterilized after one use. However, if they must be reused without sterilization they should be rinsed with 70% ethyl alcohol, then with saline, and stored in the folds of a sterile towel. The preferred catheter is a 16-inch, No. 18 to 24F, soft-rubber curved tip, with a single side hole. **Technique:** The catheter is lubricated with viscous tetracaine and is inserted through a nostril and guided into the trachea while the patient is panting or coughing. Preferably, the patient is sitting

*Available from the Bethlehem Co., Bethlehem, Pa.

upright and leaning slightly forward, with the jaw extended during passage. The catheter is applied to a Y tube attached to suction of 40 cm H_2O. Suction is not applied during insertion. The catheter is advanced until obstruction to passage is reached in the trachea. Suction is applied during withdrawal, as the catheter is rotated between thumb and forefinger to sweep the tracheal walls. To get into the right bronchus, the patient's head is rotated to the left, with the curved catheter tip pointing to the right. The reverse is done for insertion into the left bronchus. Suction is applied for no longer than 30 seconds (to avoid asphyxia). For endotracheal tube and tracheotomy, the techniques of tracheal suctioning are similar. For direct catheter passage into the trachea (not through nose) there are certain differences in technique: (a) the catheter is moistened with sterile saline; (b) the cuff of the endotracheal tube or tracheotomy tube is deflated; (c) a 16–18F curved-tip catheter is preferred; (d) the catheter is completely removed from the trachea, and the patient is ventilated between insertions for suctioning; (e) occasionally, 1–5 ml of saline may be flushed into the trachea to dilute the secretions and then suctioned out.

2. **Bronchoscopy** occasionally is necessary in respiratory failure to rule out an obstructing lesion in the airway, especially when there is any question of aspiration.

3. **Endotracheal intubation** is quite useful if maintenance of a patent airway is only a temporary measure (as in depression of respiration due to drugs, aspiration of secretions) and assisted ventilation is required. This procedure averts tracheotomy and secretions can be suctioned through the endotracheal tube. It is preferred initially over tracheotomy in severe asthmatic attacks that lead to respiratory failure. In some asthmatics, failure is a recurrent problem and would necessitate multiple tracheotomies. In chronic obstructive disease with acute respiratory failure it frequently is better to intubate initially rather than to perform a tracheotomy. The reasons are:

   a) The endotracheal tube is removed after 36–48 hours to avoid tracheal injury.

   b) During the 36–48 hours the airway is maintained during the initial phases of therapy, and the situation can be appraised further without the duress of an emergency.

   c) In the acute situation, endotracheal intubation is safer than tracheotomy in individuals who are obese or have short necks.

   d) During the time allowed by endotracheal intubation, the decision to perform tracheotomy can be considered carefully. Dramatic improvement during this period may avert tracheotomy; recovery by more conservative methods can occur. However, if tracheotomy is required, the airway is already secure, and hasty tracheotomy and its complications have been avoided (bleeding into airway; see below).

   After extubation, the patient must be followed closely for laryngeal edema, which occurs occasionally and requires reinsertion of the tube or tracheotomy.

4. **Tracheotomy** If the previously outlined management of respiratory failure is followed, the indication for tracheotomy becomes

apparent. In comatose uncooperative patients, it should be done early. In others, alternative measures can be tried first (including endotracheal intubation). **Advantages:** Tracheotomy affords continuous effective suctioning of secretions from the airways, and the cuffed tracheotomy tube is an excellent connection for continuous artificial respiration with respirators. Other advantages include less interference with swallowing and less trauma to the larynx, and trials of extubation are made easier by simply plugging the tracheotomy opening.

a) Complications

    i) Bleeding is a common postoperative complication. Slow bleeding can usually be controlled by packing the wound. If bleeding is brisk the tracheotomy cannula is removed and an endotracheal tube inserted before investigating the source.

    ii) Subcutaneous and mediastinal emphysema frequently results from suturing the wound too tightly. Skin sutures should be removed and the wound packed.

    iii) Pneumothorax usually occurs because of injury to the apical pleura or dissection of air from mediastinal pleura.

    iv) Bronchorrhea requires frequent adequate suctioning.

    v) Infection Overall tracheal care and sterile techniques in suctioning of secretions must be adhered to rigidly. Cultures should be obtained at the first signs of infection.

    vi) Tracheal trauma usually arises in difficult cases (short necks, obesity) or when tracheotomy is performed under less than ideal conditions. Except on rare occasions tracheotomy should be done in the operating room with an endotracheal tube in place.

b) Tracheotomy care and function The tracheotomy is malfunctioning if the patient can phonate, if a soft-rubber catheter cannot be passed to the carina, or if there is no expiratory gas stream at the tracheotomy orifice. The tracheal cannula should have the largest internal diameter possible to reduce flow resistance to a minimum (9.5 mm or greater). With the IPPB respirator, the outer cannula must have an inflatable cuff; otherwise, leaks around the cannula will prevent delivery of the desired pressures and volumes to the lower respiratory tract. With large leaks the respirator may not cycle, since the cycling mechanisms are dependent upon reaching a critical pressure. The cuff should be deflated periodically to prevent pressure necrosis of the tracheal mucosa.

    i) Sterile techniques during tracheal suctioning must be followed rigidly. Extra care is required, since the normal filtering of organisms by the nasopharynx is bypassed.

    ii) Care in suctioning techniques must be followed to reduce trauma to the trachea and mainstem bronchi.

    iii) The outer cannula should be changed within 48 hours after tracheotomy and every few days thereafter. When possible, the inner cannula should be removed and cleaned several times daily.

iv) All inspired gases must be adequately humidified to keep secretions thin and to avoid crusting, irritation, and erosion of airway mucosa.

v) Oxygen is administered by either yokes or masks specially designed to fit across the tracheotomy opening or by suitable attachment to a respirator during assisted or controlled ventilation. Oxygen should not be given via the direct insertion of a catheter through the tracheotomy opening, since the catheter can produce expiratory obstruction.

vi) Agents that suppress respiration or the cough reflex, or dry out secretions, should be avoided (narcotics, atropine, antitussive agents).

vii) When the tracheal cannula is finally removed the tracheotomy wound is left to close spontaneously.

C. **Artificial respiration; assisted and controlled ventilation**   The object of mechanical respirators is to improve alveolar ventilation by either assisted ventilation (patient-cycled) or controlled ventilation (machine-cycled). Besides ventilation, respirators provide an effective means of delivering aerosolized water and medications to the respiratory tract. (Aspects of IPPB in therapy have been previously outlined.)

1. **Types of ventilation**

a) **Assisted ventilation** can be either intermittent or continuous, depending upon the clinical situation. (Frequent IPPB therapy every hour for 15 minutes may be considered intermittent assisted ventilation.) Continuous ventilation is best done via an endotracheal tube or tracheotomy. The factors that determine the conversion from intermittent to continuous ventilation are failure to lower the P_aCO_2, a rising P_aCO_2, accumulation of secretions, and progressive deterioration of the patient due to exhaustion or weakness.

b) **Controlled ventilation** may be instituted for the reasons noted above. Other factors that influence a decision for controlled ventilation include poor synchronization between the patient and respirator (especially in agitated patients), coma, patient exhaustion with inability to cycle the respirator, respiratory depression due to O_2 even though the patient is on continuous assisted ventilation, or complete depression of the respiratory centers (drugs, cerebral disease). These points serve only as guides to the type of ventilation required; the clinical status is the primary determinant. Blood gas measurements must be made frequently to assess the adequacy of mechanical ventilation, and ventilation must be adjusted accordingly.

On occasion, in order to achieve completely controlled respiration, it is necessary to depress the respiratory centers with morphine or with muscle relaxants such as succinylcholine, etc. These latter maneuvers should not be done unless a well-trained respiratory team is available in an intensive-care setting where continuous care and careful observations can be made.

2. Types of respirators

a) Pressure-cycled respirators (intermittent positive pressure) can be patient- or machine-cycled and can be used for assisted or controlled ventilation.

    i) Assistance to ventilation is given only during inspiration by positive pressure, with the expiratory phase being passive. In assisted ventilation the patient's inspiratory effort initiates flow from the respirator which automatically shuts off flow when a preset pressure is reached. A sensitivity control regulates the inspiratory effort needed to initiate flow.

    ii) Peak positive pressure can be adjusted by suitable control. Peak pressures between 12 to 20 cm H_2O are the most suitable. However, if reduced compliance is present ("stiff lungs" or obese chest wall) or there is marked increase in airway resistance, pressures greater than 20 cm H_2O may be required to deliver an adequate tidal volume.

    iii) Inspiratory flow rates can be independently regulated in some models. In others, rates are automatically determined by the design of the machine. Flow rates of 40–60 L/min are reasonable in lungs with relatively normal airways. With markedly increased airway resistance, lower flow rates (6–30 L/min) are needed to reduce turbulence. (High turbulence may cause rapid pressure build-up in the system, resulting in premature cessation of the inspiratory phase.)

    iv) Respiratory rate in assisted ventilation is determined by the patient's efforts. A frequency control is present for controlled ventilation. High respiratory rates can be deleterious; the lower rates (10–14/min) with large tidal volumes are more desirable.

    v) The connection between the patient's airway and the respirator must be airtight. This is difficult to accomplish with a face mask for prolonged periods because of patient discomfort. For continuous ventilation a cuffed endotracheal or tracheotomy tube is necessary.

    vi) One limitation of pressure-cycled respirators is that in some patients, even at maximal pressure, they may be unable to deliver adequate volumes to maintain effective ventilation. At this point a volume-cycled respirator should be used.

    The most desirable regimen is a slow breathing frequency (10–14/min), low flow rates, large tidal volumes, and an expiratory phase longer than the inspiratory phase.

b) Volume-cycled respirators are machine-cycled and can be used only for controlled ventilation. They basically consist of a motor-driven piston which delivers a predetermined volume to the lungs (Moerch, Emerson, Engström). Spontaneous respiration can be overridden by volume-cycled respirators to gain complete control of ventilation. The major advantage of this type of respirator is the assurance that the desired volumes are delivered (even in the face of high resistances to inflation in the lungs). This feature, on occasion, has resulted in ruptured alveoli because of high airway pressures generated in lungs with high resistance. The frequency, as well as the tidal volume, can be predetermined. Oxygen mixtures, aerosolized medications, and humidification can be delivered by these respirators.

3. Bedside evaluation

a) When the respirator is ventilating the patient, all lung segments should be auscultated frequently to note segmental ventilation.

b) Blood gases (pH, P_aCO_2, P_aO_2) measured in arterial blood are obtained 20 minutes and 60 minutes after the onset of assisted or controlled ventilation, and then hourly until all adjustments between the patient and respirator are adequate.

c) Measurements of respiratory rate, tidal volume, and minute ventilation are made repeatedly and correlated with the blood gases. With rapid respiratory rates, the P_aCO_2 may actually increase (increase in dead-space ventilation). The frequency should be reduced and the tidal volume increased in this case, while still the minute ventilation is maintained (or even increased, if necessary).

If, during assisted ventilation, progress is poor, consider controlled ventilation (see Controlled Ventilation, above).

4. Complications of respirators

a) Rapid lowering of the P_aCO_2 can lead to alkalosis with severe CNS complications (see previous discussion of rapid lowering of the arterial P_aCO_2). Reduction of the arterial P_aCO_2 should not exceed 10 mm per hour, with the arterial pH used as the primary guide for the rate of CO_2 excretion.

b) If the same tidal volume is maintained for a prolonged period, the pulmonary compliance may fall (development of "stiff lungs" due to collapse of small respiratory units). This complication can be averted (at least lessened) by inflating the lungs to full capacity several times each hour ("sighing" the patient).

c) High pressures generated by respirators may reduce the venous return to the heart resulting in a fall in cardiac output and blood pressure.

d) Positive-pressure respirators should not be used in myocardial infarction, pericardial tamponade, mediastinal emphysema, tension pneumothorax, active tuberculosis, massive hemoptysis, or severe coronary insufficiency. If the use of respirators in these cases becomes absolutely necessary, extreme caution must be followed.

D. Respiratory stimulants can increase ventilation by either direct or indirect stimulation of the respiratory centers (doxapram, ethamivan, aminophylline, dichlorphenamide, nikethamide, salicylates, caffeine). They are useful in a limited number of situations. Doxapram and ethamivan used intravenously appear to be the agents of choice. The use of dichlorphenamide, a carbonic anhydrase inhibitor, is controversial. The best indication for these agents is respiratory depression aggravated by or precipitated by drugs (morphine, barbiturates), or

O_2 administration during sleep in patients in whom the lungs are essentially normal or have mild to moderate disease. Analeptic agents are contraindicated in patients with convulsive disorders.

COR PULMONALE

Cor pulmonale is defined as right ventricular enlargement due to a primary disorder within the lungs. Pulmonary hypertension invariably underlies its development. The **reversible components** of pulmonary hypertension are hypoxia, hypercapnia, and acidosis as a result of impaired gas exchange, which cause pulmonary vasoconstriction. Hypoxia has the greatest vasoconstrictor effect, with acidosis potentiating the vasoconstriction of hypoxia. The following pathologic conditions within the lung diminish the pulmonary vascular bed and are usually **irreversible**:

1. Occlusion of vessels (pulmonary emboli, thrombi, fat emboli).
2. Primary vascular disease (endarteritis, sclerosis, polyarteritis).
3. Obliteration or destruction of the vascular bed (emphysema, diffuse interstitial pulmonary disease).
4. Compression of vessels by masses or infiltrative processes.

Therapy should be directed toward pulmonary abnormalities and right ventricular failure.

I. **PULMONARY ABNORMALITIES**

    A. **Hypoxia** is corrected by the administration of O_2; measures must be taken to improve gas exchange to correct the hypercapnia and acidosis. In acute situations a significant portion of the pulmonary vascular resistance may be due to these factors.

    B. **With the nonreversible components, therapeutic aims are** to arrest the disease process, prevent complications that may intensify the pulmonary hypertension, and support the cardiac function.

II. **RIGHT VENTRICULAR FAILURE,** the result of persistent pulmonary hypertension, may arise insidiously or acutely (pulmonary embolism or severe respiratory failure). Measurement of the central venous pressure is useful. The following therapeutic measures should be taken:

    A. **Correction of hypoxia, hypercapnia, and respiratory acidosis** probably is the most important aspect of therapy. Correction of the hypoxia and acidosis may reduce the pulmonary vascular resistance enough so that the right ventricle may recover without additional measures.

    B. **Electrolyte and acid-base abnormalities** often contribute to cardiac arrhythmias complicating right ventricular failure during acute respiratory failure. If the acidosis is rapidly converted to alkalosis (blowing off CO_2 too rapidly or excessive infusion of $HCO_3{}^-$), the acute serum K^+ changes may result in ventricular arrhythmias. Another cause of arrhythmias is the administration of digitalis during periods of serum hypokalemia. The latter frequently is present along with chloride depletion. This deficit can be corrected only by the administration of KCl. In acute right ventricular failure, especially during respiratory failure, the electrolytes and arterial pH must be assessed before the administration of drugs which directly affect the heart.

C. Digitalis can benefit the failing right ventricle of cor pulmonale. However, its efficacy may be limited by the degree of irreversible pulmonary hypertension, persistent hypoxia, and the added burden of a labile acid-base state and abnormal electrolytes. The benefit of digitalis may be difficult to discern clinically, since tachycardia from chronic hypoxia and dyspnea from a primary lung disorder may persist. If right ventricular failure is present, digitalis should be used; however, every effort must be made to correct the hypoxia, pH, and electrolyte disturbances prior to its use, since they predispose to the undesirable side effects of digitalis, especially during periods of acute decompensation; for this reason digitalization during the initial phases must be done with extreme caution. The better alternative is to digitalize slowly after correction of the above abnormalities is well under way. Only short-acting preparations (Digoxin) should be used. Digitalis is an important part of the therapy when used properly (see Chapter 5).

D. Rest, especially during the initial phases of treatment for acute decompensation, will reduce cardiac work and is important. The patient should remain in bed initially, and then be allowed to sit in a comfortable chair, reclining if possible. As improvement occurs, graded exercise is encouraged to tolerance.

E. Diuretics and salt restriction are indicated for fluid retention. Acute diuresis at the onset of therapy probably is unnecessary and may even be dangerous, since improvement of cardiac and pulmonary function seldom is dramatic in cor pulmonale with diuresis alone (as compared to pulmonary edema due to left ventricular failure). Correction of hypoxia alone occasionally will initiate diuresis by the increase of cardiac output resulting in increased renal perfusion. Electrolyte depletion must be avoided and patients on diuretics should be on K^+ replacement (KCl), unless otherwise contraindicated (see Chapter 5).

F. Phlebotomy Increased red-cell mass and blood viscosity may add to the work of the right ventricle. If the hemoglobin is over 18 gm/100 ml, 200–400 ml of blood may be removed every few days until the hemoglobin is under 16 gm. Phlebotomy should not be considered an emergency procedure in cor pulmonale.

PNEUMOTHORAX

A pneumothorax may be open (hole in chest wall, bronchopleural fistula) or closed (not in direct communication with atmosphere). Spontaneous pneumothorax is usually of the closed type and most frequently is due to a ruptured subpleural bleb or alveolar cyst.

Treatment depends on the degree of collapse, the amount of patient discomfort, and the pressures in the intrapleural space. Complete reexpansion of the lung should be attained as soon as possible, since further delay only makes expansion more difficult. In spontaneous pneumothorax of less than 25%, spontaneous reexpansion frequently occurs within 1–3 weeks. Patients should be observed in the hospital, since further collapse of more serious proportions can occur. In a small pneumothorax, simple aspiration through a needle may be sufficient to reexpand the lung. If aspiration fails to control the pleural pressures and air leak continues, catheter drainage with water seal is indicated. Open pneumothorax due to a chest-wall wound requires immediate closure by any means possible (e.g., compression of wound) followed by aspiration of the air. Persistent bronchopleural fistula usually requires surgical intervention.

I. **INTERCOSTAL DRAINAGE WITH SUCTION** Reexpansion is most effectively attained by chest catheter and water-seal drainage. Indications include tension pneumothorax, recurrent pneumothorax, hemopneumothorax, bilateral pneumothorax, underlying diffuse pulmonary disease, pneumothorax with significant extension, and impairment of ventilation and gas exchange.

Under local anesthesia a sterile catheter (18–28F soft-rubber catheter preferably or a 18–26 Foley) is introduced, usually into the second anterior intercostal space, and immediately attached to a water-seal bottle with 10–14 cm H_2O negative pressure (Thoracic Gomco or Emerson). The catheter often can be removed in 48 to 72 hours. Thoracotomy is required if catheter drainage fails.

II. **COMPLICATIONS OF PNEUMOTHORAX**

A. **Tension pneumothorax** is an acute emergency, and air must be removed rapidly by thoracentesis. Chest catheter drainage is then instituted as soon as possible.

B. **Pleural effusion** with spontaneous pneumothorax, though not infrequent, usually is insignificant. For significant effusions, thoracentesis is indicated to rule out empyema and hemothorax.

C. **Hemothorax** usually arises from the chest wall, but can also come from the pulmonary parenchyma. Reexpansion usually controls the bleeding; if not, thoracotomy is indicated.

D. **Pulmonary edema** can complicate catheter drainage with suction, if large pressures are used. This complication occurs when small-gauge catheters (e.g., IV Intracath set) are used. The small-caliber catheters, to maintain significant flow, require large negative pressures which result in pulmonary edema.

E. **Recurrence rate in spontaneous pneumothorax** is between 10–30%. Resection of the involved segment or pleural poudrage may be required.

F. **Other considerations** Approximately 15% of cases of spontaneous pneumothorax are not due to subpleural blebs or bullae. Frequent other causes include rupture of a tuberculous or pyogenic subpleural abscess, erosion of the esophageal wall by a malignant process, or tear of the esophagus during esophagoscopy.

EMPYEMA

Prior to the development of antibiotics, empyema was a frequent complication of pneumococcal pneumonia and was the commonest indication for nontuberculous thoracic surgery. Even though it is less frequent today, empyema still poses a serious problem that requires prompt attention.

The commonest cause of empyema is bronchopulmonary infection; pneumonia accounts for 60% of the cases. Other causes include lung abscess, bronchiectasis, tuberculosis, carcinoma, chest trauma, intra-abdominal abscess, spontaneous pneumothorax, and postoperative complications. Of the latter, esophageal surgery has a relatively high incidence of empyema. The most common organism is the staphylococcus, with an increasing number caused by gram-negative organisms.

Proper management requires complete drainage and obliteration of the empyema space to prevent the development of fibrothorax. Empyema is characterized by three phases; therapy is discussed accordingly.

I. **THE EXUDATIVE PHASE** is the immediate pleural response to infection, resulting in the outpouring of nonviscous fluid with a low cellular content. The primary aim of therapy is antimicrobial, with drainage being supportive. After the appropriate cultures are obtained, vigorous antibiotic therapy is initiated. The effusion is drained as completely as possible with thoracentesis. Further management is dependent upon the rate of fluid reaccumulation, character of the fluid, and the clinical status of the patient. Repeat thoracentesis is performed as indicated. However, if fluid reaccumulation is rapid, or if the fluid is becoming purulent or the patient toxic, an intercostal catheter should be inserted into the pleural space and kept on continuous chest-tube drainage. Open drainage is contraindicated at this stage, since it may result in collapse of the lung.

II. **THE FIBRINOPURULENT PHASE** is characterized by large quantities of pus; the fluid is thick and viscous. Fibrin is deposited on the pleural surfaces. Frequently the fluid is loculated within the pleural space. The lung is compressed, and as the fluid becomes thicker, the lung becomes "fixed." During this phase, drainage is the primary aim of therapy with antimicrobial therapy now being supportive. Thoracentesis is usually inadequate, and the treatment of choice is intercostal chest-tube drainage with continuous suction. Enzymatic debridement with Varidase is of use during this phase, in conjunction with chest-tube drainage (see below). If these measures fail, open drainage is indicated. Antibiotics are given parenterally; the efficacy of intrapleural antibiotics has never been established clearly.

III. **THE ORGANIZING PHASE** is characterized by fibroblastic activity with encapsulation and entrapment of the lung. If left untreated, bronchopleural or pleurocutaneous fistulas may develop. Treatment usually is open drainage with decortication. Thoracoplasty rarely is indicated.

IV. **ENZYMATIC DEBRIDEMENT; VARIDASE (STREPTOKINASE–STREPTODOR-NASE)** The purpose of enzymatic debridement is to liquefy and drain viscid, loculated, and semifixed purulent fluid from the pleural space. Varidase is composed of two enzymes—streptokinase, which initiates the natural fibrinolytic systems by activating plasminogen to lyse fibrin, and streptodornase, which liquefies pus by depolymerizing deoxyribonucleoproteins which are present in high concentration. They are indicated in the fibropurulent stage and occasionally in the early organizing stage of empyema. When these agents are used, provision for adequate drainage must be available, since large volumes of fluid can be generated. Varidase is used in conjunction with closed intercostal tube drainage.

Varidase (an amount which contains 200,000 units of streptokinase and 50,000 units of streptodornase) is mixed with 15–20 ml of saline and injected through the intercostal chest tube into the pleural space. The tube is closed, and the patient is positioned to ensure adequate contact between the enzymes and the empyema. Close observations must be made for the rapid accumulation of fluid in a relatively closed space. After 6 hours the chest tube should be reopened to allow drainage (sooner if fluid rapidly accumulates, or later if no discomfort is apparent). Some have employed two chest tubes, injecting Varidase through a tube inserted "high" in the empyema, and draining from another placed lower. In general, one tube suffices. Daily injections can be carried out for 4 or 5 days, then every several days as necessary (dose can also be reduced if desired response is obtained). **Side effects** include high fever, malaise, generation of large fluid volumes, and rarely hypersensitivity reactions. Varidase should not be used if a bronchopleural fistula is present.

9. Antibiotics and Infectious Diseases

ANTIMICROBIALS

Antibiotics may be divided into bactericidal and bacteriostatic categories on the basis of their activity against microorganisms and further classified by their mechanism of action. The currently available **bactericidal antibiotics** interfere with the synthesis of bacterial cell walls (the penicillins, cephalothin, vancomycin, and bacitracin), disturb the function of the bacterial cell wall and cell membranes (the cyclic polypeptides, such as polymyxin, colistin, tyrocidine, and gramicidin), or cause miscoding for amino acids (the aminoglycosides, such as streptomycin, neomycin, kanamycin, paromomycin, gentamycin, and viomycin). The **bacteriostatic antibiotics,** chloramphenicol, tetracyclines, oleandomycin, erythromycin, and lincomycin, interfere primarily with protein synthesis. Novobiocin, also bacteriostatic, has a complex mode of action, affecting synthesis of protein and altering permeability of cell membranes. The polyene antifungal agents, amphotericin, nystatin, and hamycin, interfere with the function of sterol-containing cell membranes by altering their permeability.

Optimal therapy of some infections requires use of more than one antimicrobial agent. Although certain studies have indicated that, in general, combinations of bactericidal agents tend to be synergistic, combinations of a bactericidal and a bacteriostatic drug tend to diminish the potency of the former, and the combination of two bacteriostatic drugs has only an additive effect; these relationships do not always hold true. Activity of an antibiotic combination against a particular organism can be estimated either by in vitro testing of the combination or by in vitro testing of the patient's serum after therapy is begun. Successful treatment with bacteriostatic antibiotics is dependent upon natural host defenses for eradication of infection; infections in patients with decreased resistance should be treated with bactericidal drugs.

The importance of performing sensitivity tests on infecting organisms cannot be overemphasized despite the occasional difficulty in correlating the results of in vitro testing with clinical results. It is rare for an infecting organism to respond to an antibiotic when it can grow in high concentration of the drug in vitro, but good clinical responses are occasionally obtained with antibiotics that appear of little value on the basis of in vitro studies. Tests should always be performed on those species with a significant percentage of resistant strains; species with a generally predictable sensitivity pattern need not be tested in ordinary circumstances. Serial dilution methods are preferable to disk methods and are always indicated for determining minimum inhibitory concentrations. Guides for correlating disk sensitivities with those obtained by tube dilution are presented in a review of in vitro testing of bacterial sensitivity to drugs (*Amer. J. Med.* 39:766, 1965).

Table 9-1 gives the approximate serum concentration that may be expected following the administration of the usual IM, IV, or oral dosage of the more frequently used antibiotics. Table 9-2 is a guide to initial antimicrobial therapy of infections caused by some of the more common pathogens.

I.   PENICILLINS The penicillin (PCN) nucleus, 6-aminopenicillanic acid, has been modified by the addition of a variety of side chains to produce a number of semisynthetic penicillins with specific properties (e.g., gastric acid resistance, penicillinase resistance, antibacterial activity against gram-negative bacteria). The dosage, type of preparation, and route of administration depend upon the causative organism, the severity of the infection, and the sensitivity of the organism to the specific penicillin congener. Most penicillins are rapidly excreted by the kidney, but penicillinase-resistant penicillins are also excreted in large part in the bile. When high serum levels are required, the penicillin dosage may be raised or urinary excretion may be retarded by the concurrent administration of probenecid 0.5 gm every 6 hours. Tables 9-1, 9-2, and 9-3 summarize much of the information that appears below.

A. Preparations

1. **Benzyl PCN (PCN G)** is susceptible to penicillinase and inactivated by gastric acid. GI absorption of oral preparations is variable.

    a) **Crystalline PCN G,** for administration intramuscularly, intravenously, or intrathecally, is usually supplied as the potassium salt (containing 1.7 mEq K+/million units), but sodium salts are available. Intravenous infusions give sustained blood levels.

    b) **Procaine PCN G,** for IM injection only, gives detectable blood levels for 12–24 hours.

    c) **Procaine PCN G in aluminum monostearate,** for IM injection only, gives blood levels for 48–72 hours.

    d) **Benzathine PCN G (Bicillin)** is for IM injection only; 1.2 million units give detectable blood levels for 4 weeks.

    e) **Oral PCN G** must be taken on an empty stomach at least 30 minutes before meals and in a dosage 3–5 times that of parenteral aqueous PCN because of unpredictable absorption and variable blood levels.

2. **Phenoxymethyl PCN (PCN V) and phenoxyethyl PCN (phenethicillin)** are similar to PCN G in antibacterial activity but are acid-stable, well absorbed, and preferable to PCN G for oral administration. Each 125 mg of the drug equals 200,000 units. The potassium salts of the phenoxymethyl PCN preparations are better absorbed than the free acid, and an equivalent oral dose of the potassium salt yields blood levels of PCN 2–5 times greater than those provided by PCN G. Phenethicillin may produce slightly higher blood levels than phenoxymethyl PCN. Because the absorption of both of these preparations may be enhanced by the presence of food in the stomach, they should be administered immediately before or after meals.

3. **Methicillin** is penicillinase-resistant, inactivated by gastric acid, and much less active than PCN G against pneumococci, streptococci, and nonpenicillinase-producing staphylococci. Its major use is in the treatment of infections caused by penicillinase-producing strains of *S. aureus* not amenable to therapy with PCN G. Methicillin (and other penicillinase-resistant PCNs) should be restricted

to use in the treatment of infections caused by PCN G-resistant staphylococci because the drug is a powerful inducer of penicillinase production; staphylococci may develop resistance, although the number of reports at present is few in this country.

Minimum dosage is 1 gm IM every 4 hours or 1 gm diluted in 50 ml sterile saline and injected IV over 5 minutes every 4 hours. Larger doses may be required for the treatment of severe infections. Solutions of methicillin and kanamycin should not be mixed, since they will inactivate each other. Allergic reactions occur with a frequency similar to that due to PCN G; cross-sensitivity to PCN G occurs frequently but not invariably. Side effects are similar to those of PCN G, but in addition a few cases of bone marrow depression have been reported. Superinfections may occur but are less common than with broad-spectrum antibiotics or PCN G. Methicillin is an irritant, and pain is usually experienced even when the drug is injected deep intramuscularly.

4. **Oxacillin** is stable in gastric acid and resistant to penicillinase. Oral absorption, which is somewhat erratic, may be improved if the drug is taken on an empty stomach (about 60% absorption). Even though 80% of oxacillin is bound to protein in the serum (versus 20% for methicillin), the minimum inhibitory concentration of oxacillin for penicillinase-producing staphylococci is lower than that of methicillin; a given parenteral dose of oxacillin, therefore, may be equivalent in activity to a dose of methicillin that is two to four times larger. Oxacillin is more effective than methicillin in inducing staphylococci to produce penicillinase; organisms may develop resistance to oxacillin in vitro in a stepwise fashion not related to penicillinase production.

The advantages of oxacillin over methicillin, except for the availability of an oral preparation, are not clear-cut; indeed, the oral preparation, if used too freely, may be a liability in terms of inducing resistant staphylococci. Usual dosage is listed in Table 9-1. Side effects are similar to those of other PCN preparations; in addition, transient elevations in transaminase and mild GI disturbances have been reported. Cholestatic jaundice has been reported in association with the administration of oxacillin.

5. **Cloxacillin,** the chlorophenyl analog of oxacillin, is similar to oxacillin in most respects, but it is well absorbed after oral administration and slightly more active than oxacillin against penicillinase-producing staphylococci.

6. **Dicloxacillin** is acid-stable and penicillinase-resistant. Certain strains of methicillin-resistant staphylococci that may also be resistant to oxacillin and cloxacillin are inhibited by dicloxacillin. Usual dosage is listed in Table 9-1.

7. **Nafcillin** is acid-stable and penicillinase-resistant. Oral absorption is less predictable than that of cloxacillin. Its antibacterial activity against penicillinase-producing staphylococci is comparable to that of oxacillin, but nafcillin is more effective than either oxacillin or cloxacillin against streptococci and pneumococci.

Usual dosage is listed in Table 9-1. Side effects are similar to those of other preparations; cross-sensitivity reactions may occur with the other penicillins. Thrombophlebitis and pain at injection sites may follow parenteral administration. Occasional increases in transaminase and BSP retention may occur.

TABLE 9-1. Relation of Antibiotic Dosage to Serum Concentration*

Antibiotic	Route of Administration and Dose			Serum Concentration†
	Intravenous	Intramuscular	Oral	
Crystalline PCN G	1–5 M (million) units every 4–6 hrs	—	—	4
Procaine PCN G	—	0.3–1.2 M units every 6–12 hrs	—	2–3
Phenoxymethyl PCN, phenethicillin	—	—	0.25–1 gm every 6 hrs	0.1–2.0
Benzathine PCN	—	1.2 M units every 2–4 wks	—	0.01–0.1
Methicillin	1–2 gm every 4–6 hrs	1–2 gm every 4–6 hrs	—	6–10
Oxacillin	0.5–1 gm every 4–6 hrs	0.5–1 gm every 4–6 hrs	0.25–1 gm every 4–6 hrs	4–13
Cloxacillin	0.5–1 gm every 4–6 hrs	0.25–0.5 gm every 6 hrs	0.25–1 gm every 4–6 hrs	6–10
Dicloxacillin	0.5–1 gm every 4–6 hrs	0.25–0.5 gm every 4–6 hrs	0.25–0.5 gm every 4–6 hrs	10
Nafcillin	1–2 gm every 4–6 hrs	0.5 gm every 4–6 hrs	0.25–1 gm every 4–6 hrs	5–8
Ampicillin	0.5–1 gm every 6 hrs	0.5–1 gm every 6 hrs	0.25–1 gm every 6 hrs	2–8
Cephalothin	1–2 gm every 4–6 hrs	1 gm every 4–6 hrs	—	20
Cephaloridine	0.25–1.0 gm every 6 hrs	0.25–1.0 gm every 6 hrs	—	10–35
Lincomycin	0.6 gm every 8–12 hrs	0.6 gm every 12 hrs	0.5 gm every 6–8 hrs	2–20
Erythromycin	0.5–1 gm every 6 hrs	0.2 gm every 4–6 hrs	0.25–1 gm every 6 hrs	0.5–10
Oleandomycin	0.2–0.4 gm every 6 hrs	0.2–0.4 gm every 6 hrs	0.25–0.5 gm every 6 hrs‡	1–10
Novobiocin	0.25–0.5 gm every 6 hrs	0.25–0.5 gm every 6 hrs	0.25–0.5 gm every 6 hrs	10–30
Vancomycin	0.5 gm every 6 hrs	—	—	6–25
Streptomycin	1–2 gm daily	0.5–1 gm every 12 hrs	—	20–30

Tetracyclines	0.25 gm every 6 hrs (not over 1 gm/day)	—	0.25–0.5 gm every 6 hrs (0.15 gm every 6 hrs for demethylchlortetracycline)	3–5
Chloramphenicol	0.5–1 gm every 6 hrs	0.5–1 gm every 6 hrs	0.25–1 gm every 6 hrs	10–20
Kanamycin	15 mg/kg/day in 2 doses (not over 1.5 gm/day)	15 mg/kg/day in 2 doses (not over 1.5 gm/day)	—	2–30
Polymyxin B	2.5 mg/kg/day in 4 doses	1.5–2.5 mg/kg/day in 4 doses	—	1–8
Colistin	—	2.5–5 mg/kg/day in 2–4 doses	—	3–5

* See text for more detailed comments.
† Serum concentrations are approximations of those achieved with the lower dosage schedules and are expressed in units/ml for crystalline, procaine, and benzathine PCN, and in µg/ml for all other drugs.
‡ Triacetyl derivative.

TABLE 9-2. Guide to Therapy of Infections Caused by Some Common Microorganisms

Antibiotic	Gram-Positive Organisms						Gram-Negative Organisms											
	Staph. aureus (PCNase negative)	Staph. aureus (PCNase positive)	Str. pyogenes	Viridans strep.	Str. faecalis	Pneumococcus	H. influenzae	Meningococcus	Gonococcus	Klebs. pneumoniae	E. coli	Salmonella	Shigella	Proteus mirabilis (indole-negative)	Proteus (indole-positive)	Pseud. aeruginosa	Aero. aerogenes	M. pneumoniae
Penicillin PCNase-sensitive	⊕	0	⊕	⊕	±	⊕	±	⊕	⊕	0	±	0	0	±	0	0	0	0
Penicillin PCNase-resistant	+	⊕	⊕	±	0	+	±	0	0	0	0	0	0	0	0	0	0	0
Ampicillin	+	0	+	+	+	+	+	+	+	±	⊕	⊕	⊕	⊕	0	0	±	0
Cephalothin	+	⊕	+	+	0,±	+	±	+	+	⊕	⊕	0	+	+	0	0	0	0
Lincomycin	+	⊕	+	+	0	+	0	0	0	0	0	0	0	0	0	0	0	±
Erythromycin	+	*	+	+	0,±	+	+	+	⊕	0	0	0	0	0	0	0	0	⊕
Novobiocin	+	+	+	±	0	+	+	+	+	0	0	0	0	±	±	0	0	?
Vancomycin	+	⊕	+	+	+	+	0	0	0	0	0	0	0	0	0	0	0	0
Streptomycin	±	*	0	±	±	0	+	+	0	+	+	0	0	±	±	0,±	±	+
Tetracyclines	+	*	±	0	0	+	⊕	+	⊕	+	⊕	0	±	0,±	±	0	⊕	⊕
Chloramphenicol	+	*	0,±	0	0	+	+	+	+	⊕	+	⊕	+	+	±	0	±	+

Kanamycin	+	+	0	0	0	0	+	+	+	±	+	+	±	0	+	0	±
Polymyxin B, colistin	0	0	0	0	+	●	0	+	0	+	+	+	0	0	●	±	0
Cephaloridine	+	●	+	+	0,±	+	±	●	+	●	+	+	+	0	0	0	0
Sulfonamides	0	0	+	0	0	±	+	±	±	±	±	±	±	0	0	±	0
Nitrofurantoin†	0	0	+	0	0	±	0	±	±	0	+	0	±	±	±	±	±
Nalidixic acid†	0	0	0	±	±	±	+	+	+	+	+	+	+	0	+	+	?

A plus (+) indicates that the organism is usually sensitive to the antibiotic; ± indicates variable sensitivity; and 0 indicates unlikely sensitivity (or resistance). Gray circle indicates the preferred antimicrobials for each species of infecting organism.

This table is intended only as a guide to the activities of certain antibiotics; selection of the appropriate antimicrobial depends on the clinical circumstances and the antibiotic sensitivity tests. For therapeutic effectiveness, the minimal inhibitory concentration (MIC) of the antibiotic for any specific organism (as determined in a tube-dilution sensitivity test) should be at least 4–8 times less than an achievable serum concentration (see Table 9-1). Dilutions of the patient's serum may be tested directly against the organism as a check on the serum antimicrobial activity.

* Penicillinase is not active against these drugs, but organisms that have been induced to produce penicillinase often have been exposed to these antibiotics and have developed resistance.

† Serum levels are very low; useful only in urinary tract infections. Resistance may develop rapidly to nalidixic acid.

8. **Ampicillin** is acid-stable but not penicillinase-resistant; it is well absorbed after oral administration. Ampicillin is an important PCN congener because of its extended antimicrobial activity against gram-negative bacteria. It is highly effective against *H. influenzae,* alpha-hemolytic streptococci, *Proteus mirabilis,* and moderately active against *Escherichia coli,* enterococci, and certain strains of aerobacter, shigella, and salmonella. It is less active than PCN G against the common nonpenicillinase-producing gram-positive cocci, and ineffective against penicillinase-producing staphylococci.

Usual dosage is listed in Table 9-1. The drug is excreted primarily in the urine; probenecid, which significantly reduces the urine concentration, should not be given when ampicillin is being administered for the treatment of urinary tract infections. Adverse reactions are similar to those produced by other preparations; GI disturbances, superinfections, and cross-sensitivity reactions to PCN G may occur.

B. **Penicillin allergy,** manifested by skin eruptions, angioneurotic edema, serum sickness-like syndromes, etc., is the most common adverse reaction to penicillin. Coombs-positive hemolytic anemias, CNS irritability, and bone marrow suppression are not common. In general, patients with a history of penicillin allergy should not be treated with penicillin; however, in some patients with a history of penicillin hypersensitivity who have life-threatening infections (bacterial endocarditis) the benefits of giving penicillin may be greater than the risk of a penicillin reaction. Ideally, a clinical immunologist should be consulted and after a careful history and skin tests, hyposensitization should be started beginning with very small doses of oral penicillin. In all such patients intravenous fluids should be started and epinephrine readily available.

II. **CEPHALOTHIN (KEFLIN)**   The cephalosporins represent a family of antibiotics produced by the fungus Cephalosporium. With the isolation of the active nucleus of cephalosporin C it became possible to produce semisynthetic compounds with antibacterial activity greater than that of the parent compound. Cephalothin is such a semisynthetic derivative. Because of the structural similarity of the PCN and the cephalothin nucleus, cross-allergenicity between these antibiotics may occur. Cephalothin cannot be considered a uniformly safe substitute for PCN in patients with a history of PCN allergy.

Certain organisms, particularly certain strains of aerobacter, *P. morganii,* and pseudomonas, may produce cephalosporinases that destroy the antibacterial activity of the drug. Cephalosporinases may also break the β-lactam ring of the PCN nucleus, thus acting as penicillinases. Although staphylococcal production of a penicillinase that is also active as a cephalosporinase has been induced in the laboratory, the penicillinase thus far produced by freshly isolated staphylococci has been reported to have negligible cephalosporinase activity. Cephalothin is active against most all the gram-positive cocci except some enterococci, and many gram-negative bacilli except pseudomonas, indole-positive proteus species, and several strains of aerobacter and *E. coli.* Encapsulated klebsiella organisms are usually sensitive. Sixty percent of the drug is bound to serum proteins; 70–80% is excreted unchanged in the urine.

A. **Dosage and administration**   Cephalothin is not absorbed after oral

TABLE 9-3. Some Penicillin Preparations

Generic Name	Brand Name	Route of Administration	Penicillinase-Resistant	Stable in Gastric Acid	Oral Absorption
Phenoxymethyl PCN (Penicillin V)	Compocillin-V, Pen • Vee, V-Cillin	Oral	No	Yes	Good; K+ salts are better absorbed
Phenethicillin	Chemipen, Darcil, Maxipen, Syncillin, and others	Oral	No	Yes	Good
Ampicillin	Omnipen Penbritin Polycillin	Oral, IM, IV	No	Yes	Good
Methicillin	Dimocillin-RT Staphcillin	IM, IV	Yes	No	Poor
Oxacillin	Prostaphlin Resistopen	Oral, IM, IV	Yes	Yes	Variable; should be taken on an empty stomach
Cloxacillin	Tegopen	Oral	Yes	Yes	More regularly absorbed than oxacillin
Nafcillin	Unipen	Oral, IM, IV	Yes	Yes	Irregular
Dicloxacillin	Dynapen, Veracillin	Oral, IM, IV	Yes	Yes	Good

administration and must be given either **IM** or **IV**; usual dose is 4–12 gm/day in divided dosage every 4–6 hours. IM injections must be given deep into the gluteus muscle or lateral thigh. For IV injection the prescribed dosage of the drug is diluted in 10 ml isotonic saline or distilled water and injected IV over 3–5 minutes; the drug may be given by continuous IV infusion but should not be mixed with barbiturates, chlortetracycline, oxytetracycline, or calcium salts.

B. Side effects   Pain and sterile abscesses at the site of IM injections may occur. Thrombophlebitis is common with prolonged IV administration. Hypersensitivity phenomena (eosinophilia, fever, urticaria, skin rashes, serum sickness, and anaphylaxis) may occur in 3–4% of patients. Neutropenia has developed in a few patients. Superinfections, particularly with pseudomonas and aerobacter, may occur.

III.   **CEPHALORIDINE (LORIDINE)** is similar to cephalothin in its antibacterial spectrum. Cephaloridine causes less pain at the site of injection, less binding to protein in the serum, and higher blood levels. Preliminary in vitro studies suggest that cephaloridine may be potentially less satisfactory than cephalothin in the management of serious staphylococcal disease because of its susceptibility to staphylococcal betalactamases. Superinfections with resistant gram-negative bacilli and nephrotoxicity are the major adverse effects of the drug. Cross-sensitization with penicillin may occur. Dosage is listed in Table 9-1.

IV.   **LINCOMYCIN (LINCOCIN),** derived from the actinomycete *Streptomyces lincolnensis*, is chemically distinct from all other available antibiotics. The drug is active against most gram-positive organisms except enterococci; it is not active against most strains of neisseria and hemophilus or other gram-negative organisms. Over 90% of freshly isolated staphylococci were sensitive to lincomycin in a concentration of 5 µg/ml or less in one study. Staphylococci occasionally have been observed to develop resistance to the drug during therapy. Lincomycin is bacteriostatic primarily but occasionally acts as a bactericidal antibiotic. The exact role of lincomycin in antibacterial therapy has not been established, but the drug appears to be an acceptable alternative to penicillin in the treatment of many gram-positive infections in PCN-allergic individuals. For severe infections, however, vancomycin probably should be tried first.

A. Dosage and administration   The drug is rapidly absorbed from the GI tract; 20–35% of an oral dose reaches the bloodstream, peak plasma concentrations occur in 2 hours, and detectable antibacterial activity may persist for 12 hours. Oral preparations may be administered every 6–8 hours and IM injections every 12 hours, or the drug may be administered by continuous IV infusion. The drug is supplied in 250- and 500-mg capsules and in sterile solution containing 300 mg/ml. Dosage is listed in Table 9-1. The drug has significant biliary excretion and limited urinary excretion, but the dosage in patients with significant renal insufficiency should be reduced by 50–75%.

B. Side effects   The most common side effect is diarrhea, occasionally bloody, after oral administration. Other adverse reactions include urticaria, rash, pruritus, rectal irritation, and vaginitis. Neutropenia, leukopenia, transaminase elevation, and jaundice, all disappearing after cessation of therapy, have been reported. Superinfections with nonsusceptible organisms may occur.

V. **MACROLIDE ANTIBIOTICS: ERYTHROMYCIN AND OLEANDOMYCIN** The macrolide antibiotics are derived from two different strains of streptomyces. The drugs are bacteriostatic (occasionally bactericidal) primarily for gram-positive cocci, but also for neisseria, *H. influenzae, Corynebacterium diptheria,* listeria, brucella, rickettsia, and treponema. Bacteria may develop resistance to the drugs during a course of therapy; oleandomycin-insensitive strains are usually erythromycin-insensitive, but bacteria that have developed resistance to erythromycin may still be sensitive to oleandomycin. Erythromycin is a more effective antimicrobial than oleandomycin on a weight-for-weight basis. Erythromycin is well absorbed from the GI tract; oleandomycin is not well absorbed.

Usual dosages are listed in Table 9-1. A number of erythromycin preparations for oral, IM, or IV administration are available. Oleandomycin phosphate for parenteral administration is available without and with lidocaine; the latter must be given IM only. Triacetyloleandomycin (TAO, Cyclamycin) is available for oral administration. IV administration of either drug may lead to thrombophlebitis; IM injections are painful.

Side effects include nausea, vomiting, esophagitis, hypersensitivity reactions (fever, eosinophilia, skin rashes), and diarrhea, but major alterations in intestinal flora are less common than with the tetracyclines. Erythromycin estolate (Ilosone) may cause cholestatic jaundice; it subsides when the drug is discontinued. Triacetyloleandomycin may cause both cholestatic jaundice and hepatocellular damage.

VI. **NOVOBIOCIN** has significant activity against staphylococci, certain strains of proteus, and most gram-positive bacteria. The significant incidence of side effects has limited its use to the treatment of infections with resistant organisms, chiefly proteus and staphylococci, in patients allergic to penicillin. It is rapidly absorbed from the GI tract and slowly excreted; the usual oral dose is 250–500 mg every six hours; the parenteral dose is essentially the same. Side effects include frequent skin eruptions, blood dyscrasias (leukopenia, hemolytic anemia, thrombocytopenia), diarrhea, fever, and, rarely, serious liver damage. A yellowish tint of the skin, sclerae, and plasma may occur. The drug has been shown to be a potent inhibitor of glucuronyl transferase.

VII. **VANCOMYCIN** is bactericidal for gram-positive cocci and is most useful for the treatment of severe staphylococcal and enterococcal infections not responsive to other agents. The usual dose for patients with normal renal function is 2.0 gm daily given in divided dosage IV every 6–12 hours; a continuous IV infusion may be given. Toxic effects include skin rashes, thrombophlebitis, and deafness due to auditory-nerve damage, especially in patients with impaired renal function and excessively high serum levels of the drug. Chills and fever attributed to the drug have been reported in up to 25% of cases.

VIII. **STREPTOMYCIN,** a bactericidal antibiotic effective against gram-positive and gram-negative organisms, is notable for inducing sensitive bacteria to become resistant. Its greatest usefulness is in the treatment of tuberculosis (in combination with INH and PAS), *Klebsiella pneumoniae* infections (in combination with chloramphenicol, tetracycline, or cephalothin), subacute bacterial endocarditis or peritonitis from a ruptured viscus (in combination with penicillin), tularemia, brucellosis, and plague.

The drug must be given parenterally (usually IM, rarely IV) for the treatment of systemic infections. The major part (50–70%) of parenterally administered streptomycin is excreted unchanged in the urine within 24 hours when renal function is normal; a small amount is excreted in the bile.

A. **Dosage and administration** Dosage is listed in Table 9-1. Streptomycin may be given IV by diluting 1–2 gm streptomycin sulfate in 1 liter isotonic saline and administering the solution at a rate of 25 drops/min. Streptomycin in a dosage of 2 gm/day should not be continued for longer than 2 weeks because of the danger of vestibular damage; when required, 1 gm/day may be given for 30 days without danger, as a rule.

B. **Adverse effects** are related to total daily dose and duration of therapy. Auditory-nerve damage is manifested chiefly by vestibular disturbances, but rarely some impairment of auditory function may occur. Intraperitoneal administration, especially when skeletal-muscle relaxants are given concurrently, may cause respiratory arrest due to blockade at the neuromuscular junction. Other uncommon side effects include scotomata due to optic-nerve damage; paresthesias of the hands or perioral areas; renal damage, manifested by proteinuria, cylindruria, and oliguria; and hypersensitivity reactions (skin rashes, exfoliative dermatitis, eosinophilia, fever, blood dyscrasias, stomatitis, angioneurotic edema, and anaphylactic shock).

IX. **TETRACYCLINES** are bacteriostatic antibiotics useful in the treatment of infections caused by rickettsia, the psittacosis-lymphogranuloma venereum group of organisms, mycoplasma, brucella, pasteurella, *Entamoeba histolytica*, shigella, leptospira, clostridia, chancroid, granuloma inguinale, and in the treatment of syphilis and gonorrhea in patients allergic to PCN. Although tetracyclines may be used in the treatment of infections due to *H. influenzae*, *S. aureus*, *Streptococcus pyogenes*, and *Diplococcus pneumoniae*, resistant strains may be found; furthermore, even apparently sensitive organisms may not be eradicated during a course of therapy. Because of these dangers, streptococcal infections and severe infections due to any of the preceding organisms should be treated with antibiotics other than a tetracycline. The frequency of tetracycline resistance among the gram-negative urinary tract pathogens requires that antibiotic sensitivities be performed on the infecting organism.

Tetracyclines are rapidly absorbed from the GI tract. Although absorption is increased when the stomach is empty, gastric distress may be minimized by giving the drug with meals. Aluminum or magnesium hydroxide antacids, which chelate tetracyclines and reduce their absorption, should not be given concurrently. Chlortetracycline is excreted primarily in the bile and the other tetracyclines primarily in the urine.

A. **Preparations and dosage** Available preparations include chlortetracycline, oxytetracycline, tetracycline, demethylchlortetracycline, and rolitetracycline (Syntetrin). The first three preparations may be given orally or IV; the usual dosage is listed in Table 9-1. Demethylchlortetracycline, available for oral administration only, is given in smaller dosage (150 mg every 6 hours); rolitetracycline, for IM or IV use only, is said to be advantageous when IM administration is required, because its high solubility allows more efficient absorption from IM injection sites; the usual IM or IV dose is 150–350 mg every 8–12 hours.

B. Adverse effects

1. **GI symptoms** of nausea, vomiting, diarrhea, and pruritus ani are the most common. Cheilitis and glossitis may occur and usually respond to the administration of vitamins.

2. **Superinfections,** particularly with staphylococci and gram-negative organisms such as proteus and pseudomonas, represent the most serious hazard to patients receiving high-dosage long-term therapy. Staphylococcal enterocolitis may occur. Monilia infections of the mouth, GI tract, and vagina may produce annoying symptoms, but are not usually serious.

3. **Photosensitivity,** manifested by appearance of skin eruptions after exposure to sunlight, may occur after treatment with any of the preparations, but is more common with demethylchlortetracycline. Other skin rashes are rare.

4. Yellowish or brownish **discoloration of deciduous teeth** may occur in children, or in infants of mothers given significant dosages of tetracycline for long periods of time during pregnancy.

5. **Azotemia** may occur, presumably due to the antianabolic effects of tetracycline. Patients with normal renal function may develop elevated BUN values and increased nitrogen and sodium excretion; changes in GFR usually do not occur. Patients with impaired renal function develop effects that are proportional to the degree of renal insufficiency, the dose of the drug, and the duration of treatment. These include azotemia, hyperphosphatemia, acidosis, and rarely hypovolemia. These changes may not be temporally related to the administration of the antibiotic, occasionally appearing as long as 2–6 days after a course of therapy.

6. **Acquired Fanconi syndrome,** with polydipsia, polyuria, glycosuria, aminoaciduria, hypercalciuria, hyperphosphaturia, acidosis, and reduced serum concentrations of potassium, phosphate, and uric acid, may occur following use of outdated preparations; these changes in tubular function are reversible when the drug is discontinued.

7. Extensive, fine-droplet, **fatty infiltration of the liver** progressive to fatal hepatic insufficiency may occur after IV administration of large doses (more than 1.5–2.0 gm/day) of tetracycline (see Chapter 10). Other rare side effects are drug fever, thrombocytopenia, agranulocytosis, and aplastic anemia.

X. **CHLORAMPHENICOL** Originally obtained from *Streptomyces venezuelae,* the drug is now synthesized. It is bacteriostatic, but in high dosage it may be bactericidal against some organisms. It is effective against rickettsiae, a variety of gram-positive and gram-negative bacteria, and useful in the treatment of salmonella infections and in the management of *H. influenzae* meningitis. Rapid absorption occurs from the stomach, and peak serum levels appear 2 hours after an oral dose. The drug is excreted in the urine (70–90% in 24 hours); a small percentage appears as active chloramphenicol, but most appears as inactive aromatic compounds and conjugates, especially glucuronide. *Because aplastic anemia may result from the administration of chloramphenicol, the drug should never be used indiscriminately or for infections which will respond equally well to other antibiotics. Although the incidence of this complication is low, it is fatal in most cases.*

A. Dosage The usual oral dose is 2–3 gm/day given in divided dosage every 6 hours. Chloramphenicol sodium succinate may be given IM or IV in the same dosage.

B. Toxicity

    1. Hematopoietic changes Erythropoietic depression, which may occur in any patient given chloramphenicol, appears to be more common in patients with hepatic or renal disease. Changes include reticulocytopenia, significant rise in serum iron, marked increase in saturation of iron-binding globulin, appearance of vacuolated red-cell precursors in the bone marrow, and a mild anemia. These changes, secondary to a pharmacologic action of chloramphenicol, are related to dosage and duration of therapy and are correlated with the level of free chloramphenicol in the serum. These abnormalities are completely reversible after discontinuance of the drug and do not appear to be of any value in predicting the onset of aplastic anemia; the mechanism of this latter complication is unknown. Patients receiving chloramphenicol should have frequent complete blood counts; the appearance of agranulocytosis, leukopenia, or thrombocytopenia necessitates immediate discontinuance of therapy, but these rare changes do not necessarily foreshadow the development of aplastic anemia, which may appear as long as 5 months after a course of therapy.

    2. Other complications include nausea, diarrhea, occasional superinfections, and rarely allergic manifestations such as skin rashes, fever, and angioneurotic edema. Peripheral and optic neuritis have been reported.

XI. **POLYPEPTIDE ANTIBIOTICS: POLYMYXIN B AND COLISTIN** are bactericidal drugs that are effective only against gram-negative bacteria but possess a high degree of antimicrobial activity against these organisms. These drugs are often effective against pseudomonas, even when the organisms are resistant to all other antibiotics. Certain strains of *E. coli* and aerobacter may also be sensitive; most strains of proteus are resistant. The toxic-to-therapeutic ratios of the two drugs are similar, but colistin appears to be associated with a lower incidence of untoward reactions. The drugs are not absorbed after oral administration; after parenteral administration they diffuse into tissues poorly, and infections of parenchymatous organs may not respond well. They do not cross the blood-brain barrier well, even in the presence of meningeal inflammation, and they must be given intrathecally when required for the treatment of meningitis. Complete cross-resistance exists between polymyxin B and colistin.

A. Preparations and dosage Polymyxin B sulfate may be given IM, IV by infusion, or intrathecally. The IM and IV doses are 1.5–2.5 mg/kg body weight/day (maximum of 200 mg/day) in patients with normal renal function. For IV administration the calculated dose is dissolved in 200–500 ml 5% D/W and infused over 60–90 minutes; two infusions 12 hours apart each containing half the calculated dose may be given instead. For IM administration the daily dosage should be administered in 4 equally divided doses every 6 hours; the calculated dosage should be dissolved in 0.5 ml 1% procaine hydrochloride and given deep in the gluteus muscle or lateral thigh.

Colistin is supplied as the sodium salt of the methane sulfonate derivative of colistin (colistimethate) with dibucaine hydrochloride (for IM injection only). A special preparation without added dibucaine must be used for IV or intrathecal administration. The usual daily dosage should not exceed 5 mg/kg body weight given in 2–4 divided doses; frequently, 150 mg are given IM every 12 hours.

B. Adverse effects of both drugs include circumoral and "stocking" and "glove" paresthesias, ataxia, visual and speech disturbances, dizziness, nystagmus, dermatoses, and, possibly, leukopenia and granulocytopenia. Renal toxicity is more common with polymyxin B, but appearance of formed elements in the urinary sediment, proteinuria, and rise in BUN may occur after administration of either drug. Nephrotoxicity occurs most often in patients with compromised renal function. These side effects tend to increase in severity when therapy is continued but are usually reversible when treatment is discontinued. Apnea due to neuromuscular blockage occurs rarely.

XII. NEOMYCIN is bactericidal against a wide variety of gram-positive cocci and gram-negative bacilli. It may be particularly useful in the treatment of gram-negative infections, especially proteus, but the significant incidence of ototoxicity and nephrotoxicity associated with parenteral administration restricts its use to desperate situations. The IM dose is 1–2 gm/day in divided dosage. The drug is poorly absorbed from the GI tract; oral administration may be useful, however, in sterilizing the gut prior to surgery and in hepatic coma.

Diarrhea and malabsorption associated with histopathologic changes in the small bowel may occur in patients given oral preparations for long periods of time. Respiratory arrest due to a curare-like effect occurs rarely.

XIII. KANAMYCIN is bactericidal for mycobacteria and a broad range of gram-positive cocci and gram-negative bacilli; it is ineffective against some pneumococci, most streptococci, pseudomonas, and anaerobic bacteria. The drug is of greatest usefulness in the treatment of systemic infections due to gram-negative bacilli (except *Salmonella typhosa* and pseudomonas). However, because of ototoxicity and nephrotoxicity, it should not be used for the treatment of infections due to organisms known to be sensitive to less toxic drugs. Cross-resistance is shared with paromomycin, neomycin, and rarely streptomycin. For systemic infections it must be given parenterally, the usual dose in patients with normal renal function being 0.5 gm IM every 8–12 hours (with a maximum of 15 mg/kg body weight/day); it may be given IV.

Pain at the injection site and eosinophilia are common; serious toxic reactions include ototoxicity with vestibular damage and permanent deafness, especially in patients with impaired renal function or those receiving a total dose of more than 20 gm. Glomerular and tubular renal damage (increasing BUN, proteinuria, cylindruria) are usually reversible, and permanent functional impairment is rare. Apnea occurs rarely.

XIV. **BACITRACIN** is a polypeptide antibiotic that is bactericidal primarily against gram-positive organisms. It is widely used topically because of its low incidence of sensitization but rarely given systemically because of serious renal toxicity. Other less toxic antimicrobials now supplant this drug for treatment of systemic infections.

XV. **SULFONAMIDES** are bacteriostatic drugs active against a number of gram-negative bacilli and gram-positive cocci, but they are used primarily in the treatment of nocardiosis and certain urinary tract infections (particularly those due to *E. coli*). Sulfonamides may be used for chemoprophylaxis against shigella, group A beta-hemolytic streptococci, and meningococci, although resistant forms of these organisms have been reported and may limit the use of the drug for prophylaxis in certain situations. Sulfonamides are usually administered orally in the doses listed below in order to provide serum concentrations of 10–20 mg/100 ml. Renal excretion provides urinary levels 10–25 times those achieved in the serum. Chemical and bioassay methods for determining sulfonamide concentration in the serum often give divergent results, and there may be little correlation between the blood sulfonamide level and antibacterial activity; the only certain indication of efficacy is clinical improvement.

A. Preparation and dosage

1. **Sulfadiazine** is slowly and incompletely absorbed from the GI tract; 50% is excreted in the urine in 24 hours; 15–40% is acetylated and thus inactivated. The dose is 4–6 gm/day in 4 divided doses after an initial dose of 4 gm.

2. **Sulfisoxazole (Gantrisin)** is the most soluble preparation and is rapidly absorbed from the GI tract; 95% is excreted in the urine in 24 hours. The dose is 4–6 gm/day in 4–6 divided doses after an initial dose of 4 gm.

3. **Sulfamethoxazole (Gantanol)** is well absorbed after oral administration; excretion is largely in the acetylated form. The dose is 2–3 gm/day in 2 or 3 divided doses after an initial dose of 2 gm.

4. **Sulfamethoxypyridazine (Kynex, Midicel) and sulfadimethoxine (Madribon)** are rapidly absorbed from the GI tract but slowly excreted in the urine. Because of the slow excretion these drugs may readily accumulate in the body; care must be taken to avoid overdosage. The usual dose of sulfamethoxypyridazine is 0.5 gm once daily after an initial dose of 1 gm; the dose of sulfadimethoxine is 2 gm initially, followed by 1 gm once daily.

5. **Succinylsulfathiazole (Sulfasuxidine) and phthalylsulfathiazole (Sulfathalidine)** are poorly absorbed from the GI tract and are used primarily to suppress bacterial growth in the intestine prior to surgery. The usual dosage is 6–12 gm/day.

B. Toxicity The overall incidence of toxic reactions is 5–10%; the reactions are more common with the long-acting preparations, which may result in high blood concentrations, especially in patients with renal insufficiency.

1. **Renal** Crystallization in the kidney may cause tubular obstruction. The risk can be minimized by assuring fluid intake adequate to maintain a urine volume of at least 1200–1500 ml/day. Sulfonamides are more soluble at an alkaline pH, and when large doses

are given the urine should be alkalinized by the administration of $NaHCO_3$, providing there is no contraindication to large doses of sodium. Triple sulfas may offer less danger of crystallization. Toxic tubular necrosis and hypersensitivity angiitis occur rarely.

2. **Hematopoietic** Acute hemolytic anemia (including patients with glucose-6-phosphate dehydrogenase deficiency [G6PD]), agranulocytosis, aplastic anemia, and thrombocytopenia may occur.

3. **Other reactions** include a variety of skin and mucuous-membrane lesions, a serum sickness-like syndrome, and rarely toxic hepatitis. A number of reports have described the Stevens-Johnson syndrome in patients taking the long-acting sulfonamides (Kynex, Midicel, Madribon); some fatalities have occurred. Because of the seriousness of this adverse reaction, the short-acting preparations, which are effective for the same conditions, are preferred.

XVI. **NALIDIXIC ACID (NegGram)** is a naphthyridine derivative excreted in the urine and useful only in the treatment of urinary tract infections. Blood concentrations are not sufficient for the treatment of systemic infections. The drug is clinically effective against certain gram-negative bacilli, particularly *E. coli* and certain proteus species. Best results are obtained in acute infections; occasionally, chronic infections may respond. Since 25% of patients treated with nalidixic acid develop resistant organisms, the usefulness of this drug is sharply limited. The usual dosage is 4 gm/day in 4 divided doses for 7–14 days, then 2 gm/day thereafter if prolonged therapy is required.

Side effects include nausea, vomiting, pruritus, skin rashes, eosinophilia, headache, malaise, drowsiness, dizziness, visual disturbances, and myalgias. A few reports of leukopenia and transaminase elevation have appeared. Skin photosensitivity with bullous eruption has been reported.

XVII. **FURAN DERIVATIVES** include **nitrofurazone (Furacin), furazolidone (Furoxone),** and **nitrofurantoin (Furadantin);** the drugs are bacteriostatic agents active against both gram-positive and gram-negative bacilli. None is useful in the treatment of systemic infections. Nitrofurazone is used as a topical antibacterial agent; furazolidone is most often used for treatment of intestinal infections with shigella or salmonella and, in suppository form, for trichomonas vaginitis.

Nitrofurantoin is useful only in the treatment of certain urinary tract infections, particularly those due to *E. coli*; it is not effective in infections due to pseudomonas and most proteus strains. The usual oral dose is 50–100 mg QID; significant antibacterial levels do not occur in serum or tissues.

Side effects include nausea, vomiting, headache, and skin eruptions. Rarely anaphylaxis, jaundice, polyneuropathy (particularly in patients with renal insufficiency), and pulmonary infiltrations occur. Anemia (megaloblastic, hemolytic, aplastic) has been reported following the administration of this drug.

TREATMENT OF INFECTIOUS DISEASES

I. **GENERAL COMMENTS ABOUT THERAPY**

A. **Supportive care**

1. Adequate supportive treatment of infectious diseases requires the establishment and maintenance of fluid, electrolyte, and nutritional

balance. Other general measures of importance, depending on the clinical situation, are evacuation of pus, removal of foreign bodies, relief of obstruction, and rest.

2. Fever does not require treatment unless it is sufficiently high to produce central nervous system damage or to compromise the cardiovascular system; significant discomfort is a valid indication for lowering elevated temperature, but care must be exercised not to obscure fever indicative of inadequate therapy or emerging complications. *Routine administration of antipyretics is discouraged.*

3. Isolation techniques (contact, respiratory, intestinal, general) should be specified and rigidly enforced.

4. An acute-phase serum is often of value in subsequent diagnosis and probably should be collected and stored until the patient is discharged from the hospital.

B. Antimicrobials

1. Viral infection, unless complicated by bacterial infection, should not be treated with antimicrobial agents. Fever alone is not an indication for antimicrobial therapy, but there may be justification for a therapeutic trial of antibiotics after appropriate diagnostic procedures have failed to reveal the cause of a prolonged temperature elevation.

2. An etiologic diagnosis based on the clinical and laboratory findings should often make possible the rational selection of an antimicrobial for treatment of an acute infection before the culture results are available. When the results of cultures and antibiotic sensitivities have been obtained, adjustment in the drug and dosage may be made.

3. The use of multiple antimicrobial agents is justified in the critically ill patient when the identity of the infecting organism is not apparent, when the suspected pathogen has a varying antibiotic sensitivity, and when high morbidity or mortality rates may be associated with failure to initiate correct antimicrobial therapy promptly. Concurrent administration of two or more antimicrobial agents may also be justified to obtain synergistic effects (enterococcal endocarditis), to treat infections likely due to multiple organisms (peritonitis following a ruptured viscus), and to prevent emergence of resistant forms of the primary infecting organism (tuberculosis). The indiscriminate use of multiple antimicrobial drugs should be avoided because of the expense, toxicity, and higher incidence of secondary infections with resistant organisms. In general, the simultaneous use of bacteriostatic and bactericidal drugs should be avoided.

C. Duration of therapy

1. The duration of antimicrobial therapy varies with the type of infection and the response to treatment, but drug administration should rarely be discontinued sooner than 3–5 days after the patient becomes afebrile.

2. Follow-up cultures should be obtained to assess the effectiveness of therapy. Changes in the normal flora are to be expected, but they do not require treatment unless there is evidence of tissue invasion.

3. After the acute illness has subsided ambulation should be encouraged to avoid the complications of prolonged bed rest. Weakness and easy fatigability may persist for many weeks after a severe viral or bacterial infection.

D. Failure of therapy to eradicate infection suggests incorrect diagnosis, inadequate supportive care and/or antibiotics, complications of the original infection, secondary infection, presence of some underlying disease process, or drug fever. Each of these possibilities should be evaluated.

E. Corticosteroids Patients receiving corticosteroids or who have recently discontinued them after prolonged therapy should be managed during acute sepsis as patients with adrenal insufficiency (see section on acute adrenal crisis in Chapter 17). Peripheral vascular collapse occurring with infection is probably an indication for massive corticosteroid dosage (e.g., hydrocortisone 1–2 gm/day). In general, the deleterious effects of steroids on containment of infections tends to weigh against their use.

F. Mechanisms of antimicrobial excretion; therapy in patients with renal insufficiency Antimicrobials excreted primarily in the bile are lincomycin, erythromycin, chlortetracycline, oleandomycin, and novobiocin. Ampicillin, penicillinase-resistant penicillins, and tetracyclines other than chlortetracycline undergo significant excretion in both bile and urine. Chloramphenicol, cephalothin, sulfonamides, isoniazid, and para-aminosalicylic acid are excreted primarily in the urine after significant inactivation.

The following antimicrobials are excreted primarily in the urine: streptomycin, kanamycin, polymyxin B, colistin, vancomycin, cephaloridine, penicillinase-sensitive penicillins, nitrofurantoin, and nalidixic acid. Dosage of these drugs and the tetracyclines (except chlortetracycline) should be reduced when renal function is less than 25% of normal; the penicillins and nalidixic acid are possible exceptions because of their low order of toxicity, but caution in patients with reduced renal function is justified (see Chapter 3). Assays for serum levels of the therapeutic agent can be utilized as a guide to therapy.

II. PNEUMONIA accounts for about 10% of admissions to medical wards, and it remains one of the leading causes of death during productive years of life. Since numerous bacteria, viruses, mycoplasma, and fungi can cause pneumonia, the clinical presentation may occur in many different forms. Moreover, many noninfectious processes may mimic pneumonia. Pneumonia must be considered in any patient with fever and a pulmonary infiltrate, but atelectasis, pulmonary infarct, pulmonary edema, alveolar proteinosis, granulomatous diseases, carcinoma, and aspiration or inhalation of toxic substances may be very difficult to distinguish from pneumonia caused by microorganisms.

A. Diagnosis

1. Sputum examination An adequate sputum specimen should be obtained for gross and microscopic examination. Administration of fluids intravenously, aerosolization of humidified air or warmed saline, and endotracheal or transtracheal aspiration are measures that may be helpful for collection of an adequate specimen.

a) The sputum in bacterial pneumonia is usually thick, purulent, and rusty or diffusely bloody, as opposed to the thinner, more serous, rarely blood-streaked sputum associated with viral pneumonia. A particularly sticky, gelatinous, bloody sputum is suggestive of klebsiella pneumonia or Type III pneumococcal pneumonia.

b) The gram-stained sputum smear commonly reveals PMN leukocytes and sheets of gram-positive diplococci, usually in pairs or short chains. The presence of 30% or more of gram-negative bacilli or gram-positive cocci resembling staphylococci suggests that these organisms may be the cause of the penumonia.

2. **Cultures** of sputum, blood, pleural fluid, and cerebrospinal fluid should be obtained when indicated. Best results are obtained when the specimens are plated on the ward or inoculated on standard transport media. Cultures of blood taken during the acute phases of illness are of special diagnostic reliability when positive, and should be obtained from each patient. From 10–30% of patients with pneumococcal pneumonia can be shown to have bacteremia if two cultures are obtained prior to therapy.

3. **Roentgenograms** of the chest are not diagnostic of bacterial pneumonia but usually show a segmental or homogeneous lobar density. Occasionally auscultatory signs are apparent before radiologic changes in early pneumonia. Abscess formation is rare in pneumococcal pneumonia, but is more common in klebsiella and staphylococcal pneumonia. Empyema occurs in about 1% and pleural effusion occurs in about 5% of cases.

B. **Management** Two principal questions should be answered before treatment of pneumonia is begun. What is the probable infecting pathogen? Is there a complication such as empyema, arthritis, meningitis, pulmonary abscess, or azotemia?

1. **Antibiotic therapy**

a) **Pneumococcal and streptococcal pneumonia** In uncomplicated cases the drug of choice is penicillin in doses of 0.6–1.2 million units per day intramuscularly. Oral penicillin has been used effectively, but its absorption from the gastrointestinal tract is less predictable in the acutely ill patient. Doses larger than 2.4 million units of PCN daily are attended by a higher rate of superinfection (*J.A.M.A.* 186:987, 1963). Erythromycin (2 gm per day) or a tetracycline (2 gm per day) may be used in patients allergic to penicillin. Rare instances of tetracycline-resistant pneumococci have been noted. Treatment should continue for at least a week, and until the patient has remained afebrile for 2–3 days.

b) **Staphylococcal pneumonia** Since about one-third of staphylococcal infections acquired outside of hospitals are caused by organisms resistant to PCN, as are the majority of hospital-acquired staphylococcal infections, initial treatment should include a penicillinase-resistant PCN such as methicillin (8–12 gm/day) or oxacillin (4–8 gm/day parenterally). If studies indicate that the staphylococcus is sensitive to PCN G, it is reasonable to substitute this less expensive and highly efficacious drug in a dose of 4 to 6 million units per day. Treatment of staphylococcal pneumonia should be continued for a minimum of 3–4 weeks in most instances.

c) **Klebsiella pneumonia** may be treated with a combination of kanamycin (1–1.5 gm/day) and cephalothin (6–12 gm/day). Treatment should be prolonged; it is wise to continue until no further radiographic improvement is occurring.

d) **Hemophilus pneumonia** may be treated with ampicillin, chloramphenicol, streptomycin, or tetracycline.

e) **Mycoplasma pneumoniae** infections will respond to erythromycin and tetracyclines.

2. **Changes in therapy** Any decision to change or add additional antibiotics must depend on the culture results, antibiotic sensitivities of the organism, and the clinical course. It is not rare for fever to fall slowly over a 7-day period, nor is it uncommon for a secondary rise in temperature to occur despite continued clinical improvement. The above are not indications for a change in antimicrobial therapy; rather repeat cultures and clinical reevaluation are indicated to exclude complications that do require a change in antibiotics. Continued temperature elevation may be associated with a sterile pleural effusion (which should be examined to exclude an empyema), drug fever, superinfection, or other complications.

C. **General therapeutic measures** The use of expectorants and antitussive agents is discussed in Chapter 8. Narcotics may be required to control paroxysms of cough or pleuritic pain but should be used cautiously, since they may depress respiration and hinder the clearance of secretions. Although pleuritic pain is difficult to relieve, ethyl chloride spray or intercostal nerve block may be tried when the pain is severe; chest binders should not be used. Adequate fluids should be administered and humidification provided with a steam or cold-water vaporizer.

Oxygen should be administered to patients with cyanosis and dyspnea; oxygen masks should not be used, however, because they interfere with coughing. Hiccups may be due to gastric dilatation; if the latter is excluded, administration of mild sedatives or chlorpromazine 25 mg QID may terminate the attack. Gastric dilatation and paralytic ileus are not uncommon accompaniments of pneumonia, particularly if the diaphragmatic pleura is irritated. Enemas may be sufficient in mild cases; neostigmine 0.25–0.50 mg subcutaneously may also be of help. Continuous gastric aspiration may be necessary if abdominal distention is significant.

D. **Complications** Empyemas require drainage either by repeated thoracenteses or by chest tube with closed drainage. The insertion of a chest tube is often required if the empyema is thick. Antibiotics, which should be given in large dosage, usually diffuse well into the serous cavities. Streptokinase-streptodornase (Varidase) 200,000 and 50,000 units respectively, dissolved in 20–50 ml saline may be injected into the pleural space in order to liquefy tenacious, purulent, fibrinous secretions; injection into several locations may be necessary when a loculated empyema is present. The liquefied material should be withdrawn 12–24 hours later. Although febrile reactions occur frequently and hypersensitivity phenomena occasionally, the incidence of serious adverse effects of the enzymes is low (see Chapter 8).

Endocarditis and meningitis are discussed in other sections of the Manual. Purulent pericarditis is rare; pericardiocentesis and occasionally surgery are necessary for cases not subsiding rapidly after appropriate antibiotic administration.

III. **URINARY TRACT INFECTIONS** (UTI) are a major medical problem because of their frequency, occasional resistance to treatment, and proneness to relapse and reinfection. The majority of patients with urinary tract infection are unaware of its presence (asymptomatic bacteriuria). Many different pathogens can infect tissues and fluids of the urinary system, but *E. coli* is far the most common pathogen. Other microorganisms that can be found include enterococci, proteus, pseudomonas and *Aerobacter aerogenes*. Infections with pseudomonas and proteus species usually follow the use of urinary catheters or other instruments in the bladder. Staphylococci are a rare cause of urinary tract infections. The probable source of infecting bacteria is the intestinal tract, and pathogens usually gain access to the urinary tract by passing retrograde through the urethra and bladder.

The prevalence of urinary tract infections in females rises from childbearing age to about age 60 years; these infections are rare in men below age 50 years. Obstructive lesions, instrumentation, and neurogenic bladder dysfunction are clearly associated with a higher incidence of urinary tract infections.

A. **Diagnosis**

1. **Microscopic examination** of an unspun clean-voided midstream urine specimen in acute pyelonephritis usually reveals numerous leukocytes occurring singly, in clumps, and in casts. If bacteria are seen on the uncentrifuged specimen with methylene blue or gram stain, at least 10^5 bacteria per milliliter are usually present.

2. **Culture** of the urine is the most important diagnostic procedure. A properly collected and promptly plated clean-voided midstream urine specimen (CVS) that yields 10^5 or more bacteria per milliliter on quantitative culture is usually diagnostic of a UTI and carries an 80% likelihood that a second CVS will give a similar count. *Follow-up cultures must be obtained at some time after treatment to test for persistence of bacteriuria.*

B. **Treatment** For proper treatment the organism should be identified and antibiotic susceptibility studies performed. The ideal chemotherapeutic approach is to employ a form of treatment which is capable of bactericidal action. The urinary levels of the various antibacterial drugs are important: they represent the concentration of the antibiotic in the medulla of the kidney. Any patient with recurrent or resistant urinary tract infection should have a thorough urologic investigation.

Because of the great variability in susceptibility to antimicrobial drugs, even within the same species, general rules are not applicable regarding antimicrobial therapy for this diverse group of organisms. The best results are obtained by employing the therapy suited to the microbes isolated from the individual patient. Suggested antimicrobial agents for initiating therapy in an acute episode before the culture and sensitivity studies are available include the following:

1. **Ampicillin** 500 mg administered every 6 hours.

2. **Penicillin-G** 800,000 units administered every 6 hours effects an average urine concentration of 100 μgm per ml; it is safe and worthy of trial.

3. **Tetracycline** 1 to 2 gm/day by mouth in divided dosage. Reduced dosage is required with a GFR of less than 50 ml/minute.

4. **Sulfisoxazole** 4 to 6 gm/day by mouth in divided dosage. Reduced dosage is required in renal failure.

For **resistant bacteria,** polymyxin B 1.0 to 1.5 mg/kg, colistin 2.5 to 5.0 mg/kg, kanamycin 15 mg/kg, or cephalothin 0.5 gm every 6 hours may be effective. Combination of penicillinase-resistant PCN (methicillin) with hydrolyzable PCN has recently been used in the treatment of UTI due to gram-negative bacilli. The semisynthetic PCN combines with penicillinase produced by these bacilli, thus increasing the antibacterial effectiveness of PCN G. Although prolonged treatment of a UTI has been advocated, some controlled studies (*New Eng. J. Med.* 275:70, 1966) have not demonstrated any significant benefit over conventional courses of 10–14 days. Only about 20–30% of patients with chronic infections remain free from significant bacteriuria after cessation of treatment, regardless of the type or duration of chemotherapy. Some recurrences are due to the same species and strain of microorganism that was present before therapy (relapse), whereas in others a new pathogen appears (reinfection). The prognosis may be more favorable among patients in whom recurrences are due to relapse; thus a more prolonged chemotherapeutic trial (6 weeks) is warranted in these patients. Reinfection of the elderly who have normal renal function should probably be treated with short courses of antibiotics and limited to periods during which the patients are symptomatic.

C. **Prevention** Urinary tract infections are the most frequent hospital-acquired infections. At times a urinary catheter is indispensable for therapy, but the indication for its use should be especially clear. When an indwelling urinary catheter must be used the following measures are recommended.

1. **Continuous irrigation** of the bladder through a triple-lumen catheter with a solution of 40 mg neomycin and 20 mg polymyxin per liter of normal saline reduces the incidence of catheter-associated urinary tract infections, bacteremia, and death. One lumen of the catheter is connected with closed sterile drainage, another with the balloon, and the third with a continuous inflow of antibacterial solution (40 ml/hour).

2. **Closed urinary drainage** system with a disposable, heavy-duty, plastic sterile bag and spigot attachment to permit semipermanent use is also efficacious. The catheters are not irrigated unless obstruction is suspected. Bags may be drained at 8-hour intervals, with care not to contaminate the mouth of the spigot.

3. After the catheter is removed a urine culture must be obtained, and treatment instituted for significant bacteriuria.

IV. **MENINGITIS** Meningeal inflammation is most often secondary to bacterial, viral, or fungal infections of the meninges, but sterile meningitis may be due to infections in tissues adjacent to the meninges (e.g., sinuses, middle ear), trauma, neoplastic disease, and subarachnoid hemorrhage.

The character of the cerebrospinal fluid (CSF) provides information of major importance in differential diagnosis. Neutrophilic pleocytosis, decreased CSF sugar concentration, and elevated CSF protein concentration, the classical accompaniments of bacterial meningitis, are most often associated in adults with infections caused by pneumococci, meningococci, tubercle bacilli, gram-negative bacilli, and cryptococci; *H. influenzae* meningitis, a frequent type of meningitis in children, is rare in adults. *In patients with suspected bacterial meningitis rapid completion of diagnostic procedures and initiation of therapy within 1 hour of admission are of utmost importance.*

A. Diagnostic measures

1. **Lumbar puncture** should be performed with a small-gauge needle and the CSF removed slowly.

    a) Because of the fastidiousness of meningococci, warmed culture media should be plated directly at the bedside. Blood, nasal swab, and aspirate of skin lesions should be handled similarly. Cultures should be incubated both aerobically and anaerobically, and antibiotic sensitivities should be determined.

    b) After the CSF has been cultured, cell and differential counts should be performed and gram-stained smears of the centrifuged sediment examined. Acid-fast stains and India ink preparations should also be examined, especially when the etiology of the meningitis is not apparent.

    c) If no organisms can be demonstrated on stained smear, repeat smears can be made aseptically from the CSF culture after 8–12 hours of incubation.

    d) CSF protein and sugar concentration and a blood sugar drawn 30 minutes before the LP should be measured. If viral meningitis is a possibility, specimens of CSF and blood should be stored at 4°C for study.

2. **Roentgenograms** of the chest and skull should be obtained to detect the source of infection or evidence of skull fracture.

B. Antibiotic therapy   Antibiotics must be given parenterally in high dosage.

1. **Initiation of therapy**   The choice of antimicrobial is governed by the morphology of the organisms on stained smear of the CSF. No organisms will be found in about 40% of cases, often because of previous antibiotic therapy. When bacterial meningitis is a reasonable possibility, antibiotics should be administered until a bacterial infection can be excluded. **The following broad-coverage regimens are suggested:**

    a) **Ampicillin** 150 mg/kg/day IM or IV in 6 divided doses or continuous IV infusion.

    b) **Aqueous PCN** 2 million units every 2 hours IM or IV or comparable doses by continuous IV infusion and **chloramphenicol** 50–75 mg/kg/day IM or IV in 4 divided doses or continuous IV infusion.

2. **Intrathecal administration**   In general, antibiotics need not be administered intrathecally except in the treatment of meningitis due to gram-negative bacilli and staphylococci. Some observers believe that penicillin should also be given intrathecally whenever the CSF is particularly purulent (as may occur in meningococcal or pneumococcal meningitis); 30,000 units crystalline PCN G are

dissolved in 10 ml isotonic saline and injected at the rate of 1 ml/min once daily after comparable amounts of CSF have been withdrawn.

3. **Therapy for specific infections**

   a) **Pneumococcus** PCN G should be given IM or IV in a dosage of 20–30 million units daily. Therapy should be continued for 14 days. Patients allergic to PCN may be given chloramphenicol 50–75 mg/kg/day or erythromycin 1 gm IV every 6 hours. Erythromycin is suspended in 50–100 ml saline and infused as rapidly as possible; addition of hydrocortisone 5–10 mg to each bottle will reduce the severe irritative effects of erythromycin on the vein.

   Simultaneous administration of a bacteriostatic antibiotic (tetracycline or chloramphenicol) with penicillin may antagonize the bactericidal action of penicillin in pneumococcal meningitis, and it is wise not to administer the drugs concurrently once the etiologic agent is known.

   b) **Meningococcus** PCN G 1–2 million units IM or IV every 2 hours or 10–20 million units/day by constant infusion. Therapy should be continued for 5 days after the patient is afebrile. Sulfonamides should not be given alone because of the presence of sulfonamide-resistant meningococci. Patients allergic to PCN should be given a sulfonamide (sulfadiazine or sulfisoxazole 5 gm in 1000 ml Ringer's-lactate infused IV as rapidly as possible, followed by 1 gm IV every 4 hours), and erythromycin 1 gm IV every 6 hours.

   Hypotension, purpura, and rapid clinical deterioration may occur in up to 40% of patients. Recent evidence suggests that these manifestations may be due to a myocarditis. Recommended management of hypotension can be found in Chapter 17. Corticosteroids probably do not favorably influence the mortality rate associated with fulminant meningococcemia. Patients with meningococcal meningitis are not infectious after the first 24 hours of therapy, and isolation procedures may be discontinued. Other cases or carriers among the patient's primary and secondary family members should be sought. Administration of 1–2 gm sulfadiazine will reduce the carrier rate for sensitive strains only; no effective prophylaxis is available for sulfonamide-resistant meningococci.

   c) **Hemophilus** Although in vitro sensitivity studies show that the organisms are usually sensitive to a number of antibiotics, ampicillin 150 mg/kg/day in 6 divided doses or chloramphenicol 50–75 mg/kg/day in 4 divided doses are the drugs generally believed to be most effective. The dose of chloramphenicol may be reduced to 2–3 gm/day after 5–7 days. In older age groups meningitis due to this organism are usually associated with head injury; surgery upon the sinuses, tonsils, or adenoids; spinal anesthesia; or such infections as sinusitis or penumonia.

   d) **Staphylococcus** Staphylococcal meningitis should be treated initially as if due to a penicillin-resistant strain. Methicillin 12–20 gm daily should be administered IV; crystalline PCN 20–30 million units/day should be administered concurrently until the ability of the staphylococcus to produce penicillinase is known.

Because methicillin does not enter the spinal fluid readily, intrathecal administration of methicillin 20–25 mg daily or bacitracin 5000–10,000 units daily constitutes an important part of the initial therapy. In patients allergic to PCN either vancomycin or erythromycin with chloramphenicol may be substituted.

Although the staphylococcus causes only about 4% of cases of meningitis, the mortality rate is high. Staphylococcal meningitis is one of the most difficult forms to treat, and usually develops from focal abscesses or by extension from infection of the middle ear or mastoid.

e) **Other gram-negative bacilli** In most cases the diagnosis is based on the extrameningeal focus of infection and the finding of gram-negative bacilli in the spinal fluid sediment. Until antibiotic sensitivity studies are complete, the selection of an antimicrobial is empirical. Chloramphenicol (streptomycin and a sulfonamide may be included) should be used as previously outlined. Treatment may be changed if the response is poor and if in vitro sensitivity tests indicate resistance to chloramphenicol. PCN G 40–60 million units/day has been used successfully in treating meningitis due to gram-negative bacilli resistant to other antibiotics. Meningitis caused by pseudomonas species may occur after spinal anesthesia, neurosurgical procedures, or urinary tract infection. Colistin IM or polymyxin B IV in standard dosage plus intrathecal administration of polymyxin B (2–4 mg daily dissolved in 10 ml isotonic saline and injected over a 10-minute period after removal of 10 ml CSF) is required.

f) **Others** Meningitis due to beta-hemolytic streptococci may be treated in the same manner as pneumococcal meningitis. Diphtheroids in the CSF are almost surely *Listeria monocytogenes*, for which tetracyclines are most effective. *Mima polymorpha* is resistant to PCN, and it must be differentiated from *Neisseria meningitidis*; tetracycline should be included in the therapeutic regimen. The management of meningitis due to *M. tuberculosis* and fungal organisms is described in subsequent sections.

4. **General measures** Particular attention must be given to maintenance of adequate hydration, electrolyte balance, and patency of airway. Deeply comatose patients may require tracheal intubation or occasionally tracheostomy. Diphenylhydantoin and barbiturates should be given parenterally for convulsions.

V. **BACTERIAL ENDOCARDITIS (BE)** is a microbial infection of the heart valves or of the endocardium in proximity to congenital heart defects. The infection may pursue a fulminant or prolonged course and is fatal unless treated. Microorganisms of low pathogenicity are often associated with a subacute course, whereas the course of BE due to microorganisms of high pathogenicity is often acute.

BE occurs most commonly in persons with preexisting heart disease without congestive heart failure or atrial fibrillation. Fever is the single most frequent sign of BE. Embolization is a characteristic feature and occurs most commonly to the spleen and kidney. Petechiae are the most common dermal manifestations. In the average case ABE (acute bacterial endocarditis) has been present for 2–3 weeks before the diagnosis is made, whereas SBE (subacute bacterial endocarditis) has been present an average of 3 months.

A. Blood cultures The causative organism should be isolated, if possible, and antibiotic sensitivities determined. Blood cultures are positive in 85% of cases; 4–6 cultures of 10 ml blood taken at intervals are usually adequate to demonstrate bacteremia, if present. Cultures may be temporally negative or delayed in growth in patients who have received inadequate or inappropriate antibiotic therapy. If ABE is suspected, blood cultures should be obtained rapidly at 30-minute intervals and treatment initiated. If SBE is present, rapid initiation of treatment is not necessary and cultures can be obtained over a 48-hour period.

B. Treatment is most often successful when begun early, when effective bactericidal antimicrobial therapy is used, and when therapy is continued for a long time. Selection of effective antibiotic therapy depends on the performance of tube-dilution sensitivity tests, or when the organism has not been isolated, the knowledge of the probable infecting organism and its antibiotic sensitivity.

   1. Alpha-hemolytic streptococci cause about 50% of cases of BE and 75% of cases of SBE. Streptococci of the microaerophilic' (13%) and anaerobic (3%) types are less frequent. All of these organisms are almost uniformly very sensitive to PCN. A recovery rate of 90% should be attained.

     a) Penicillin G: Penicillin 5 million units should be administered daily for 4 weeks. The penicillin may be administered IM in divided doses every 3 or 4 hours or IV by continuous infusion. Despite some favorable results, the oral route of therapy or a 2-week course of therapy cannot be recommended at present.

     b) Vancomycin, lincomycin, or erythromycin and streptomycin can be used as alternative antimicrobials in the patient allergic to penicillin.

   2. S. fecalis (enterococci) are implicated in about 10% of cases of BE and are often the cause of BE in older men and in women after abortion or endometritis. Combination of penicillin with streptomycin is frequently synergistic against these bacteria and is the treatment of choice. Serum of patients under treatment should exhibit bactericidal activity in a dilution of 1:8 or greater to assure adequate activity in vivo. From a therapeutic standpoint, all streptococci resistant to 0.5 unit or more of PCN G per milliliter should be considered in the class with enterococci, regardless of their biochemical and physiologic characteristics. The survival rate is 75–85%.

     a) Penicillin G 6–20 million units a day and streptomycin 0.5–1.0 gm twice a day should be administered for a minimum of 4 weeks. High doses of penicillin may be required, depending on the results of serum bactericidal activity during treatment. Eighth-nerve toxicity due to streptomycin is a recognized hazard, especially in older persons and in patients with impaired renal function. Probenecid should not be substituted for adequate doses of penicillin.

     b) No satisfactory alternative for penicillin is available for treatment of enterococcal endocarditis in patients allergic to penicillin. Skin testing and attempted hyposensitization to penicillin with the aid of a clinical immunologist are indicated.

3. **Staphylococci** cause about 23% of cases of BE and 50% of cases of ABE. *S. aureus* is a frequent cause of tricuspid or pulmonary valve endocarditis, particularly in drug addicts. Staphylococci are the most commonly implicated pathogens in prosthetic cardiac valve infections. The survival rate of patients with staphylococcal endocarditis is about 50%.

   a) Methicillin 8–16 gm a day should be administered parenterally for 6 weeks. Methicillin is unstable in acid solutions and should not be given by continuous IV drip unless the suspending medium is brought to pH 7.0. If the staphylococcus is sensitive to PCN G, this antibiotic should be given rather than methicillin, in a dose of 6–12 million units a day for 6 weeks.

   b) Vancomycin can be used as an alternative antibiotic in patients allergic to penicillin.

4. **Pneumococci and group A streptococci** cause 1–5% of cases of BE. PCN G 3–6 million units a day should be administered parenterally for 4 weeks.

5. **Gram-negative bacilli** are an increasingly common cause of BE, particularly in patients with prosthetic cardiac valves. Cures of prosthetic valve infection are rare. Successful therapy depends on antibiotic tube-dilution studies of the offending organism. Removal of the infected prosthesis with long-term suppressive antibiotic therapy should be strongly considered in patients with a poor response.

C. **Response to therapy** The institution of appropriate antibiotic therapy frequently leads to defervescence and increase in sense of well-being within 3–7 days. A low-grade fever may be present in about 12% of cases through the entire period of therapy. Drug fever may occasionally supervene and complicate the febrile course. Cessation of all therapy for 72 hours is not hazardous in SBE and may identify readily such a drug reaction. When BE recurs, it usually develops within 4 weeks after treatment stops. Temperature and blood cultures should be followed during this time on an outpatient basis.

D. **Prophylaxis** Since patients with rheumatic and congenital heart disease are especially vulnerable to BE, such patients should be protected with antibiotics whenever transient bacteremia is apt to occur. Antibiotics should be given before and after minor operative procedures (such as tonsillectomy, dental extraction or manipulation, GU procedures such as cystoscopy, and cardiac catheterizations), and to pregnant women at time of delivery.

   Procaine PCN and aqueous PCN, 600,000 units of each, should be given 1 hour before the procedure; and procaine PCN 600,000 units IM each day for 2 days afterward. PCN may be given orally; phenoxymethyl PCN is given in a dosage of 400,000 units QID on the day of, and 2 days after the procedure. In addition, aqueous PCN 600,000 units should be given 1 hour before the surgical procedure.

VI.   ENTERIC INFECTIONS

A. **Typhoid fever** Following ingestion of *Salmonella typhosa* man develops prolonged remittent fever, rose spots, splenomegaly, lymphadenopathy, or intestinal manifestations. Transmission occurs when water, milk, or food are contaminated by infected feces from patients or carriers. At the present time, fewer than 500 cases are reported annually in the United States, and a continuing downward trend can be expected. Laboratory diagnosis is made by the presence of leukopenia, isolation of *S. typhosa* from the blood, feces, or urine, and the demonstration of a rising titer of flagelle (H) and somatic (O) antibody.

1. **Specific therapy** Chloramphenicol, the drug of choice, is administered in doses of 50 mg/kg/day in 4 divided doses until the temperature is normal, then reduced to 30 mg/kg/day. Patients usually are afebrile in 3–5 days. Ampicillin is also effective; the dose is 1 gm every 6–8 hours administered IM for 2 weeks.

2. **Corticosteroids** In severely ill patients or patients showing no clinical response to antibiotics, prednisone 40–60 mg in 4 divided doses for 3 days, may be employed.

3. **Supportive therapy** Bed rest extending into early convalescence is essential. Laxatives and promiscuous use of enemas may induce intestinal perforation or hemorrhage. The use of salicylates is discouraged because some patients are unusually sensitive to their antipyretic effect; hypothermia and cardiovascular collapse may result after small doses.

4. **Complications** Intestinal hemorrhage occurs in 10–20% of patients, usually during the second or third week. Intestinal perforation occurs in 3% of patients. Relapses occur about two weeks after cessation of antibiotic therapy in 5–15% of patients.

5. **Carriers** About 10% of patients recovering from typhoid fever excrete organisms in their stool for long periods of time. Patients should be informed of the significance of this fact and instructed to avoid occupations (especially food handling) in which there is danger of spreading infection. Public health authorities should be notified.

   Removal of a diseased gallbladder results in termination of the chronic carrier state in about 85% of cases. Ampicillin 6 gm/day orally in 4 divided doses for 6 weeks combined with probenecid will apparently terminate the carrier state in most patients with normal gallbladder function. Chloramphenicol is not effective and should not be used.

B. **Other salmonella infections** More than 800 different serologic types of the genus Salmonella have been identified. There is a striking variation in the pathogenicity of the various serotypes, but almost all can produce human disease. Infections take the form of acute gastroenteritis, enteric or paratyphoid fever, bacteremia, and localized infections ranging from osteomyelitis to endocarditis. Patients with sickle-cell anemia are particularly susceptible to salmonellosis, especially osteomyelitis. Infection is almost always acquired by the oral route, usually by ingestion of contaminated food or drink. *Salmonella typhimurium* is the most prevalent type throughout the world. Diagnosis depends on isolation of the causative organism. Agglutination tests as performed in the usual clinical laboratory are not very helpful.

   1. **Treatment** of salmonella gastroenteritis is supportive. Dehydration should be corrected by the parenteral administration of fluids.

There is no convincing evidence that antimicrobial drugs alter the course of salmonella gastroenteritis. Chloramphenicol, 3 gm/day, is the antibiotic of choice in systemic infections. Ampicillin is also effective.

2. **Carriers**   The carrier state will spontaneously cease in 1 to 2 months in the vast majority of individuals. Antimicrobial therapy is usually not indicated in transient carriers of salmonella species.

C. **Bacillary dysentery (shigella infections)**   More than 10,000 cases of shigellosis were reported during 1966. With rare exceptions, human infections take the form of fever, abdominal pain, and diarrhea. The convalescent or asymptomatic carrier is the principal reservoir of the disease and transmission is by the fecal-oral route. The diagnosis is made by isolating the organism from stool cultures. These cultures are best obtained by swabbing the rectal mucosa. **Treatment:** Although sulfa drugs are widely used, the general emergence of sulfonamide-resistant organisms makes them no longer the drug of choice. Supportive therapy including rehydration is of utmost importance. Antibiotics may be used in severe infections or when bacteremia is suspected. Antibiotic disk sensitivity should be performed for proper selection of antimicrobial therapy. Ampicillin, tetracycline, and chloramphenicol may be tried in doses of 1–2 gm daily.

VII. **ANTIBIOTIC THERAPY IN SEPSIS OF UNKNOWN ETIOLOGY**   The early institution of appropriate antimicrobial therapy is essential for successful treatment of bacteremia. When the nature of the etiologic agent cannot be deduced from clinical findings and bacteriologic results are not readily available, a combination of bactericidal antibiotics seems most reasonable.

A penicillin, a polymyxin, and kanamycin are an effective combination of antibiotics for treatment of severe unidentified sepsis, since about 90% of gram-negative bacilli and essentially all clinically important gram-positive cocci are sensitive to this combination. Cephalothin is used as the penicillin-type of antibiotic in the combination because of its certain activity against almost all coagulase-positive staphylococci and other gram-positive cocci. Colistin is important because it is the best available antibiotic for pseudomonas strains. Kanamycin is included because of its efficacy against klebsiella-aerobacter and many strains of proteus. All three of these antibiotics are bactericidal, and antagonism has not been demonstrated. *It must be emphasized that this combination is an emergency or stopgap treatment and should be modified or simplified as soon as clinical and bacteriologic results permit.* If the infection does not respond within 5–7 days, therapy should be stopped and the diagnosis or sensitivity of the invading organism reassessed.

1. **Dosage in patients without renal impairment**

a) **Cephalothin**   6–12 gm per day administered IM or IV

b) **Colistin**   Sodium colistimethate 2.5–5.0 mg/kg body weight/day administered IM. Polymyxin B 1.5–2.5 mg/kg body weight administered IV may be substituted when intramuscular injections are not desirable, as in coagulation disorders or in the presence of severe neutropenia.

c) **Kanamycin**   15 mg/kg/day administered IM; IV administration should be avoided when possible. The dose of kanamycin and colistin should be reduced in patients with a creatinine clearance of less than 50–70 ml/min.

2. Approximate dosage in patients with renal impairment Because of the potential nephrotoxicity and ototoxicity of this regimen renal function should be monitored frequently and the dose modified accordingly. The creatinine clearance is a more reliable test of renal function than is the blood urea nitrogen, but the BUN is usually used initially as an indicator of renal function in patients with severe sepsis. Approximate dosage modification in patients with impaired renal function as measured by the BUN is shown in Table 9-4.

TABLE 9-4. Dosage Modification in Patients with Impaired Renal Function

Blood Urea Nitrogen	Sodium Colistimethate Dosage (Intramuscular)	Kanamycin Sulfate Dosage
Normal	2.5 mg/kg every 12 hrs	7.5 mg/kg every 8–12 hrs
20–50 mg/100 ml	2.5 mg/kg every 18 hrs	7.5 mg/kg every 12 hrs
50–100 mg/100 ml	2.5 mg/kg every 24 hrs	7.5 mg/kg every 24 hrs
> 100 mg/100 ml	2.5 mg/kg every 48 hrs	7.5 mg/kg every 48 hrs
Anuria		
	2.5 mg/kg every 4 days; measure serum activity before giving more; dialysis has negligible effect upon serum concentration	7.5 mg/kg every 4 days; measure serum activity before giving more; dialysis lowers serum concentration

VIII. VENEREAL DISEASES

A. Gonorrhea is a common bacterial disease of man characterized by a purulent inflammation of the mucosa of the genital tract. Man is the only reservoir, and transmission occurs almost exclusively by sexual contact. The usual incubation period is 2–8 days. Complications of infection include tenosynovitis, arthritis, papulopustular hemorrhagic rash, endocarditis, perihepatitis, and abscesses of internal organs. Both sexes, particularly females, may be asymptomatic carriers of the gonococcus.

1. Diagnosis A gram-stained smear usually shows intracellular gram-negative diplococci and is probably the best single diagnostic aid in gonococcal infections. The culture should be plated rapidly, preferably at the bedside, on any of several available commercial media and placed in a candle jar at 37°C. The gonococcus is distinguished from other neisseria species by its ability to ferment only glucose. Immunofluorescent techniques are valuable diagnostically, if available.

2. Treatment of acute infection Procaine PCN 2.4 million units IM gives a 98% cure rate in males. Females should probably receive 4.8 million units IM. For patients allergic to PCN, tetracycline 1.5 gm in a single dose may be substituted. The proportion of strains of gonococci acquiring relative resistance to penicillin is increasing throughout the world. Larger doses of antibiotics may be required in some areas.

Gonococcal arthritis may be treated with procaine PCN 5 million units parenterally for 7–14 days. Restoration of muscle strength and joint mobility in these patients is important. The synovial cavity should be tapped dry to relieve pressure and remove purulent material.

Gonococcal endocarditis may be treated with aqueous PCN 4–10 million units daily administered parenterally for 4–6 weeks, though the optimum dose is unknown.

Appropriate surgical procedures for localized suppurations, urethral strictures, and scarring of female internal genitalia are important. Treatment should also be given to sexual contacts. Public health authorities should be notified.

B. Syphilis The incubation period for a clinically apparent primary lesion (hard chancre) is usually 3–6 weeks. Manifestations of secondary lues may appear 2–12 weeks later and may occur several times during subsequent years. An appreciable number of persons may fail to have recognizable primary or secondary lesions.

Both primary and secondary syphilitic lesions are infectious; diagnosis may be made most readily by dark-field examination of fluid expressed from the lesions. Tertiary lues may become clinically manifest several years later in 50% or less of untreated patients; 25% of untreated cases appear to undergo spontaneous biologic cure.

1. Serologic tests for syphilis are of major importance in diagnosis but present difficulties in interpretation because many reactive serologic tests are reported in nonsyphilitic patients.

a) Nontreponemal tests The older tests for syphilis reagin (such as the Kolmer or VDRL) require a minimum of 1–3 weeks from onset of infection to give a positive result and are usually positive once secondary lesions develop; reagin titers tend to parallel disease activity. These tests, though practical and widely available, are not specific for syphilis; biologic false positive (BFP) tests may occur in nonsyphilitic diseases (e.g., infectious mononucleosis, primary atypical pneumonia) or chronically in more than 2% of the population in association with a variety of diseases, particularly autoimmune disorders.

b) Treponemal tests The new tests that measure treponemal antibodies have more specificity, although they too have definite limitations. They are of greatest value in helping to distinguish between BFP and truly reactive reagin tests for syphilis and to establish a correct diagnosis in patients with clinical evidence of syphilis (especially late syphilis) but with nonreactive blood and spinal fluid reagin tests.

The **fluorescent treponemal antibody test (FTA)**, particularly with the absorption technique (FTA-ABS tests), and *Treponema pallidum* immobilization test (TPI) are the most specific; refinements in technique have improved the sensitivity and specificity of the former, but the latter remains expensive and laborious. The Reiter protein complement fixation test (RPCF) initially thought to serve as a satisfactory substitute for the TPI test, has been shown to have a low correlation with the TPI test in those patients in whom serologic confirmation is most needed, i.e., those patients with a reactive reagin test and no clinical evidence of syphilis.

c) A practical regimen for diagnosing latent syphilis might use the

VDRL test as a screening procedure; a nonreactive result can be accepted as evidence for the absence of syphilis in patients with neither history nor clinical findings of the disease. A positive VDRL in the absence of clinical evidence of syphilis should be confirmed with an FTA-ABS to exclude a BFP reaction. Likewise, an FTA-ABS is indicated in those patients with history and physical findings compatible with syphilis in whom the VDRL is negative.

2. Treatment

a) **Primary, secondary, and latent syphilis with negative spinal fluid examination** may be treated with procaine PCN 600,000 units IM every day for 8 consecutive days or with benzathine PCN 2.4 million units IM on two occasions one week apart. Although lesser amounts of penicillin have been used successfully, the relapse rate is probably increased above the 2% level in primary syphilis and the 5–10% level in later forms.

Patients allergic to penicillin may be given tetracycline 500 mg QID for 15 days or erythromycin 500 mg QID for 20 days.

All patients with latent syphilis should have a CSF examination prior to therapy or should be treated as if they have neurosyphilis. Serologic tests should be performed at 3–6-month intervals and a CSF examination at one year; failure of treatment to effect a significant decline in serum reagin titer by the end of one year indicates a need for retreatment.

b) **Late syphilis** (cardiovascular, neural, late benign tertiary syphilis) should be treated with benzathine PCN 2.4 million units IM once weekly for 4 weeks or procaine PCN 600,000 units IM once daily for a total of 6–9 million units. Both duration of therapy and total PCN dosage are of importance; no benefit has been demonstrated from more than 10 million units of penicillin with treatment schedules as outlined above.

Tetracycline and erythromycin have not been adequately evaluated in late syphilis. Current recommendations are to use the same daily dose as for primary syphilis and doubling the duration of therapy.

c) **Pregnant women with a positive serology** should be treated unless it is known with certainty that adequate treatment has been carried out in the past and that the positive serology represents seroresistance, i.e., a fixed or slowly decreasing titer.

d) **The Jarisch-Herxheimer reaction,** attributed to breakdown products of killed treponemata, is characterized by fever associated with edema and inflammation about syphilitic lesions. The reaction occurs to some extent in the majority of patients, beginning several hours after initiation of therapy and lasting from 2 hours to 2 days. No specific therapy is indicated.

IX. MISCELLANEOUS DISEASES

A. **Brucellosis**   The diagnosis is made by agglutination test and isolation of the organism from cultures of blood, bone marrow, or abscess material. Treatment is with tetracycline 0.5 gm every 6 hours for 21 days. This schedule may be repeated if relapse occurs. In severe infections, streptomycin 1–2 gm daily IM for 14 days is administered in addition to the tetracycline therapy. Some authors believe that prednisone 20 mg every 8 hours should be used to reduce the toxic effects of endotoxin.

B. Tularemia The diagnosis is made by skin test, agglutination test, and isolation of the organism from infected material. Treatment is with streptomycin 0.5–1.0 gm every 12 hours for 10 days. The tetracycline antibiotics and chloramphenicol are also effective, but relapses may be more frequent.

C. Staphylococcus enterocolitis The diagnosis is made by the presence of diarrhea and a positive smear or culture of the stool for staphylococci. Vancomycin 0.5 gm orally every 4 to 6 hours for 3 to 5 days is the drug of choice.

X.   TUBERCULOSIS

A. General comments All evidence indicates that the initial choice of therapy frequently determines success or failure in the treatment of tuberculosis. Documentation of the diagnosis must include isolation of the organism in addition to smears and/or biopsy of appropriate material. It is important that the isolates be identified and antimicrobial sensitivity studies performed. Drug resistance is usually observed in patients who have had previous treatment but occasionally may be encountered in patients who never have had therapy. In addition, infections with atypical mycobacteria and systemic mycoses may mimic tuberculosis in all respects.

The treatment of tuberculosis is a chronic process requiring patience and understanding by the patient and the physician. Regular follow-up examinations and chest roentgenograms are necessary for the remainder of the patient's life. Treatment must be tailored to each patient's needs. Bed rest is necessary for those patients who are acutely ill, but others may be allowed up without detriment to therapy. Patients with active disease should be hospitalized during initiation of therapy so that they may be isolated during the most infectious stage of their disease, observed for toxic reactions to drugs, and evaluated in reference to need for surgery. Subsequent management may be at home if the clinical condition permits and if proper isolation techniques can be carried out. The presence of small children in the home is a contraindication to home management. Members of the patient's family and close contacts should have chest roentgenograms and purified protein derivative (PPD) skin tests.

B. Antituberculous drugs

1. Isoniazid (INH) is the most effective antituberculous drug available and should be administered initially as a part of every therapeutic regimen. The drug diffuses rapidly, even into cells, and is quickly absorbed from the GI tract. Peak blood levels of 0.5–4.0 μg/ml occur 1–2 hours after administration of an oral dose and fall 50% or more by 6 hours. Unaltered drug and its conjugates are excreted in the urine. Acetylation and thus inactivation of isoniazid occurs at a variable, genetically determined rate. Although slow acetylators may develop peripheral neuritis slightly more often and gain a slightly more rapid therapeutic effect than rapid acetylators, this variation is not of significance in clinical practice.

The **usual dose** is 5–6 mg/kg body weight/day but 10 mg/kg body weight/day may be given for the first 3–4 weeks of treatment of severe infection (meningitis, tuberculous pneumonia, or miliary tuberculosis).

Administered in conventional doses (5 mg/kg/day) isoniazid is virtually free from untoward reactions. The main adverse effect is a peripheral neuritis that results from the ability of the drug to produce a pyridoxine deficiency. This effect is uncommon at conventional doses unless malnutrition is present. At higher doses, however, it is much more common. In such cases pyridoxine 100 mg daily should be given concurrently to protect against the neuritis. Although pyridoxine may partially antagonize the antimicrobial action, it probably does not adversely influence therapeutic effectiveness. Mild cerebral effects such as slight euphoria, elevation of mood, and, occasionally, impairment of judgment and memory have been reported. Toxic psychosis is a rare manifestation of the drug which pyridoxine does not prevent. Hypersensitivity reactions manifested by fever, rash, liver function abnormality, and jaundice are rare.

2. **Streptomycin** is the next most effective of the primary antituberculous drugs. It is a strongly basic amine compound with toxicity for the cells of the vestibular and cochlear end organs and the kidney. Age is an important consideration in selecting the dose of daily streptomycin in initial therapy. Generally the dose should not exceed 1.0 gm per day. For patients over age 50, doses exceeding 0.5 gm per day should be used with extreme care. If considerations of age and status of renal function are borne in mind, and if administration of the drug is discontinued with onset of dizziness, vertigo, or unsteady gait, serious toxic effects will be minimized. The duration of daily streptomycin therapy should be limited to the first 6–12 weeks and the drug should be discontinued sooner if toxic reactions occur. Toxic reactions are discussed in preceding sections of this chapter.

3. **Para-aminosalicylic acid (PAS)** is a weak antituberculous drug which is not bactericidal for the organism. It is important in the treatment of tuberculosis because of its ability to prevent or delay development of resistance to INH and streptomycin and is always given in combination with these or other agents, never alone. It is rapidly absorbed from the GI tract and quickly excreted in the urine. The metabolism of PAS involves acetylation, and by competing with INH for this pathway PAS will raise the level of active INH in the serum. The **usual dose** is 8–12 gm/day in divided doses. The drug is a gastric irritant frequently causing anorexia, nausea, vomiting, bloating, and diarrhea. Interruption of therapy, reduction in dose, change to the calcium, potassium, or sodium salt or PAS-resin combination, or administration of the total daily dose at one time may help the patient accept the medication. It may also be administered with meals and at bedtime with a snack. **Side effects** of PAS may cause so much discomfort, however, that some patients will refuse to continue it in any form. Hypersensitivity reactions occasionally occur, usually after 3–4 weeks of therapy, and are manifested by fever, skin rash, eosinophilia, lymph node enlargement, and hepatitis.

4. **Other drugs,** often termed secondary drugs, should never be used in primary therapy. However, they may become necessary when

patients show progression of disease after an adequate trial of therapy, existence of in vitro resistance of the tubercle bacilli accompanied by evidence of therapeutic failure by primary drugs, and inability to tolerate the primary drugs. The use of the secondary drugs is limited by their toxicity, a low order of antibacterial activity, and the rapid emergence of resistant strains if sputum conversion is not rapidly attained. If a secondary drug is needed it should be used in combination with one or more of the primary drugs; this combination always includes INH and if necessary an additional secondary drug. The following list is not inclusive, and new drugs are being developed and tested.

a) **Ethambutol (Myambutol)** Dose 25 mg/kg once daily for 60 days reduced to a single dose of 15 mg/kg daily thereafter. Primary toxicity is retrobulbar optic neuritis which is dose-related and reversible.

b) **Ethionamide** Dose 500–1000 mg daily. Demonstrates GI intolerance and liver toxicity.

c) **Pyrazinamide** Dose 30–50 mg/kg daily. Demonstrates liver toxicity in 3–5% of patients and emergence of resistant organisms within 5–8 weeks.

d) **Cycloserine** Dose 500–2000 mg daily. Low doses may cause somnolence and muscle twitching, while doses above 1000 mg may cause convulsions.

e) **Viomycin** Dose 1 gm intramuscularly daily. Toxicity at this dose level is infrequent but includes eighth nerve and electrolyte imbalance.

f) **Kanamycin** Dose 1 gm intramuscularly daily. Toxic for eighth nerve and kidneys.

5. **Corticosteroid therapy** for tuberculosis is controversial and the only clear indication for its use is adrenal insufficiency. Effective antituberculous chemotherapy prevents dissemination of tuberculous infection in patients treated with the hormone. More rapid radiographic clearing of pneumonic infiltrates may occur, but there is no benefit in terms of cavity closure or sputum conversion. High-dose corticosteroids have been recommended for a short period of time when the objective is to smother overwhelming toxicity (miliary tuberculosis), or, hopefully, to preserve functioning pulmonary tissue; to prevent disabling sequelae such as pleural and pericardial fibrosis; and to prevent an intraspinal block.

C. **Surgery** Although most tuberculosis can be treated effectively with chemotherapy, treatment of those patients with such manifestations as large necrotic foci, thick-walled cavities, and positive sputum after six months of therapy may be facilitated by surgical resection. Management of the open-negative cavity remains controversial; many observers believe that such cavities should be resected if the patient is a good surgical risk.

D. **Treatment programs**

1. Prophylactic antituberculous therapy is indicated for children 8 years of age or less who are tuberculin-positive and patients who are recent converters from tuberculin-negative to tuberculin-positive status. INH plus PAS is the drug regimen of choice and

treatment should be continued for 18–24 months. Patients who are to receive long-term corticosteroid therapy should be given INH concurrently if their tuberculin skin test is positive, if recent or remote contact is suspected, and if there is risk of more than chance contact with tuberculosis in the future. Patients with sarcoidosis and Hodgkin's disease should receive INH in conjunction with long-term steroid therapy regardless of the results of PPD skin tests.

2. Statistically, all studies have shown that the combination of streptomycin daily and INH is as good as streptomycin-INH-PAS for previously untreated cases; the combination of INH and PAS is a close second. Pulmonary tuberculosis with or without cavity formation should be treated initially with adequate doses of INH and PAS. INH and streptomycin should be given for the treatment of tuberculous pneumonia, tuberculosis meningitis, miliary tuberculosis, and other types of extrapulmonary tuberculosis. If the patient is acutely ill, maximum doses of INH (10 mg/kg body weight/day) should be given initially. The INH may be given intramuscularly, 1.7 mg/kg every 8 hours, to comatose patients. Streptomycin therapy should be limited to the first 6–12 weeks and discontinued earlier if toxic reactions occur. If the response has been favorable, PAS should be substituted and treatment continued for a minimum of 24 months. In some patients therapy must be continued for a lifetime. Those patients whose disease becomes reactivated after it had been previously arrested with chemotherapy may respond to retreatment with the primary drugs.

3. Patients who fail to benefit from primary chemotherapy, with or without demonstration of in vitro resistance, present special problems. These patients frequently have extensive cavitary disease, poor host factors, unrelated medical problems, and are in an older age group. They must be treated in a hospital, since careful discipline and observation for toxicity to the secondary drugs is necessary. INH at 5 mg/kg body weight/day should be given in spite of possible resistance of the organism; its administration prevents back-mutation of drug-resistant organisms and possibly prevents progression of drug-resistant disease. Streptomycin and PAS are to be used only if the organisms show in vitro susceptibility. Use at least one of the secondary drugs to which the organisms are susceptible or to which the patient has never been exposed. If the organisms are resistant to all three of the primary drugs, use two or three of the secondary drugs. If successful, the combination of drugs should be continued for at least one year after achieving a noninfectious state, and INH should be continued indefinitely. Surgical intervention must be considered early in these patients.

4. Adjustments in drugs or their dosage in any of the treatment programs will depend on the clinical response, improvement in x-ray findings, disappearance of organisms, evidence of toxicity, etc.

E. **Atypical (unclassified) mycobacteria** may cause disease clinically, radiologically, and histologically indistinguishable from tuberculosis, or may be recovered from patients with no apparent disease. These organisms have been divided into four groups: Group I, the photochromogens; Group II, the scotochromogens; Group III, the nonphotochromogens; and Group IV, the rapid growers. Pulmonary infections may be caused by Group I photochromogen, *M. kansasii*, and the Group III nonphotochromogen, Battey bacillus. Cervical adenitis has been caused by Group I, II, and III organisms. "Swimming pool granuloma" may be caused by *M. balnei*, a photochromogen, and *M. ulcerans*, a nonphotochromogen. The course of the disease produced by atypical mycobacteria is often chronic and indolent. Evidence suggests that patients with active atypical mycobacterial infections are not a source of infection to others.

Accurate laboratory identification of the organism and drug sensitivity testing are of utmost importance. The atypical mycobacteria are generally more resistant to INH, streptomycin, and PAS than is *M. tuberculosis*, but these drugs should be used in initial therapy until results of drug sensitivity studies are available. Some investigations have shown that approximately 45% of Group I and II infections will respond to therapy with the primary drugs. One of the puzzling features of photochromogen diseases has been the lack of correlation of the sputum conversion with the results of in vitro susceptibility. The secondary drugs may be helpful in the treatment of these infections. Early surgical intervention often plays an important role in management of patients with atypical mycobacterial infections.

XI. SYSTEMIC MYCOSES

A. General comments   Histoplasmosis, coccidioidomycosis, North American blastomycosis, and nocardiosis frequently cause pulmonary disease and may result in disseminated disease, including meningitis and endocarditis, particularly in patients with some other debilitating illness. The diagnosis requires microscopic examination and culture of appropriate specimens, including biopsies. With histoplasmosis and coccidioidomycosis the complement-fixation antibody test is a useful diagnostic aid. The histoplasmin and coccidioidin skin tests may be helpful adjuncts in diagnosis. Positive skin tests may affect the antibody test and should be placed after obtaining serum. The antibody and skin test are not reliable for diagnosis of blastomycosis.

B. Treatment

    1. Amphotericin B is the drug of choice for histoplasmosis, coccidioidomycosis, North American blastomycosis, and cryptococcosis. The drug has no significant antibacterial activity and its only known mechanism of action is to bind sterols in the cell wall. It must be given intravenously; administration of 0.65 mg/kg body weight/day yields peak blood levels of approximately 0.5–3.5 µg/ml. The drug is excreted slowly in the urine, and blood levels 20 hours following administration may be in the range of 0.5–1.5 µg/ml. Cerebrospinal fluid concentration of the drug is 2–3.3% of the blood concentration. Intrathecal therapy should be reserved for those patients with severe or relapsed central nervous system infection. Some authorities prefer intracisternal or intraventricular administration, particularly in the case of adhesive arachnoiditis with block.

        a) Dosage and administration   Therapy with amphotericin B must be tailored to the ability of the patient to tolerate the drug. The outline given may have to be altered for each specific individual. Treatment should be initiated with 1 mg amphotericin B dissolved in 250 ml 5% D/W (precipitation will occur in saline) and infused IV over 2–6 hours. The dosage should be raised to 5 mg in 500 ml 5% D/W on the second day and 10 mg in 500 ml 5% D/W on the third day. The amount should then be increased by 10-mg increments daily until on the seventh day 50 mg in 500 ml 5% D/W is given. Then the 50-mg dose may be given three days each week, usually Monday, Wednesday, and Friday. Each infusion should run approximately 6 hours and the bottle should be protected from light during administration. To aid in preserving veins and preventing thrombophlebitis, heparin 1200–6000 units (10–50 mg) should be added to each bottle and scalp-vein sets should be used in infusion. To relieve side effects such as nausea, vomiting, chills, fever, and headache, aspirin 0.6–0.9 gm and chlorpromazine 25 mg may be given prior to each infusion. Hydrocortisone succinate 25 mg may be added to each bottle, if necessary, to alleviate these distressing symptoms. The duration of treatment varies with the type and severity of infection. For blastomycosis and histoplasmosis 2–3 gm may be adequate. However, adequate treatment of coccidioidomycosis may require 5 gm. Total doses of greater than 5 gm should be avoided if at all possible because of irreversible renal damage. With severe or relapsed CNS infections the usual intrathecal dose of 0.5–1.0 mg daily should be administered by barbotage according to directions supplied with the drug.

b) Adverse effects Thrombophlebitis, fever, chills, headache, nausea, and vomiting may occur is as many as 80% of patients receiving the drug, but these effects can usually be controlled by the measures described above. Renal toxicity is the most serious side effect and appears to be dosage-related. Transient azotemia occurs in almost all patients. Decreased concentrating ability, hematuria, proteinuria, and cylindruria may also occur. A urine specimen, BUN, and serum creatinine should be checked at least weekly. Evidence of increasing renal impairment will necessitate reduction in dosage or brief discontinuation of therapy. If treatment is discontinued for a week or more, therapy should be resumed with an initial dosage of 5 mg and increased as previously described. Although a mild degree of permanent renal damage may occur in many of the patients who receive amphotericin B, it is usually not clinically significant unless the total dosage has exceeded 5.0 gm or underlying renal disease is present.

2. Blastomycosis Although amphotericin B is the preferred drug, some investigators use 2-hydroxystilbamidine initially and reserve amphotericin B for those cases that are not responsive. The dose of 2-hydroxystilbamidine is 225 mg daily, dissolved in 200 ml 5% D/W and infused IV; protect the solution from the light. The drug is stored in the liver and kidneys, and impaired function of these organs is a relative contraindication to administration of the drug.

3. Actinomycosis Penicillin, the drug of choice, should be given in a dosage of 10 million units daily IM or IV for two weeks. Treatment may then be continued with an oral preparation given in a dosage of 1–2 million units per day for 3 months or until the lesions appear inactive for at least 1 month. Tetracycline, streptomycin, chloramphenicol, and sulfonamides also have been used successfully in treatment. Surgical excision of localized lesions may be helpful.

4. **Nocardiosis**   Sulfonamides and streptomycin have been effective in treatment. Sulfadiazine should be given in a dosage sufficient to maintain blood levels of 9–12 mg/100 ml. This usually requires 6–8 gm daily. Treatment should be continued for 3–6 months, or longer if necessary. Chloramphenicol and tetracycline also have been used with success, but penicillin is ineffective.

5. **Sportrichosis**   Iodides are quite effective in treatment; saturated solution of potassium iodide (SSKI) is the drug of choice for cutaneous and lymphatic forms. Therapy may be initiated with 1 ml TID and increased by 0.5–1.0 ml/day until a daily dose of 9–12 ml is reached. Treatment should be continued for 2–3 weeks after all lesions have healed. Amphotericin B should be used for patients with bone and joint involvement, disseminated sportrichosis, or iodine sensitivity.

I. **VIRAL HEPATITIS** Viral hepatitis may be due to the virus of either infectious or serum hepatitis but, in general, treatment of the two can be considered simultaneously. Although infectious hepatitis is frequently an incapacitating illness requiring a period of prolonged convalescence, the immediate fatality rate is only about 0.2%, and progression to chronic liver disease is apparently unusual. Serum hepatitis is frequently more severe and has a higher fatality rate than infectious hepatitis; both diseases are more serious in "high risk groups" such as teenage girls, pregnant and postmenopausal women, elderly individuals, and patients with underlying debilitating diseases. Because the course of the disease is so variable it is impossible to outline a standard program for treatment; basic principles involved are diet and restriction of physical activity.

A. All patients should be hospitalized initially. Reduction of physical activity may thus be enforced and adequate caloric intake ensured. Serial evaluation of liver function may facilitate early recognition of complications. Liver-function tests, particularly the serum bilirubin and transaminases, should be obtained at least once or twice weekly during the acute stage of the illness.

B. Measures to prevent spread of infection

    1. Intestinal (stool) isolation should be carried out for the first 2–3 weeks of the clinical illness in patients with infectious hepatitis. Although almost all patients begin to excrete the virus in their stool shortly before the onset of symptoms, and occasional patients do so for many months after the acute phase of the illness has subsided, it is generally accepted that most patients do not excrete the virus for longer than three weeks or so after the illness becomes clinically apparent; intestinal isolation for a longer period is neither practical nor necessary.

    2. Disposable needles and syringes, if available, should be used for patients with infectious or serum hepatitis. Otherwise, all equipment used for injection of medication or withdrawal of blood must be carefully autoclaved. Blood tubes sent to the laboratory should be labeled clearly as being from hepatitis patients. Patients must be warned never to be a blood donor in the future (although most carriers have not had clinically recognized hepatitis).

    3. Gamma globulin

        a) For persons exposed to infectious hepatitis Gamma globulin should be given to close contacts of patients, particularly members of their family. The presently recommended dose of

0.01–0.03 ml/pound body weight probably permits the development of active-passive immunity. Pregnant females are often given a larger dose, 0.06 ml/pound body weight. The duration of partial protection after the administration of gamma globulin, though dosage-dependent, has been estimated to range from 4 to 8 weeks. Once the illness has become clinically apparent its administration is of no value in reducing the severity of the disease.

b) **For persons exposed to serum hepatitis**   Unfortunately, most exposure to serum hepatitis occurs unknowingly; transfusion of blood containing the virus is probably the major mode of transmission. Because carriers cannot be detected and eliminated as blood donors, it has been suggested that gamma globulin be administered to all recipients of blood transfusions, in order to reduce the incidence of posttransfusion hepatitis. One published study (*New Eng. J. Med.* 273:59, 1965) concluded that the administration of 10 ml gamma globulin in the week after blood transfusion and again one month later will prevent about 75% of the cases of icteric posttransfusion hepatitis. However, the dose required is impractically large, considering the available supplies of gamma globulin, and data are relatively limited. Further studies will be necessary to clarify the role of gamma globulin in prophylaxis of serum hepatitis.

C. **Diet and vitamins**   Many patients will lose 5–10 pounds during the acute phase of the illness; anorexia, nausea, and vomiting may be serious problems.

1. A high-protein, high-calorie diet should be prescribed (3000 calories, 100–125 gm protein for the average-sized patient). Because anorexia, a significant problem in the early stages of the disease, is often less in the morning and worse later during the day, breakfast should be the largest meal; frequent small feedings rather than two subsequent large meals during the rest of the day are preferred. When anorexia is unusually severe or prolonged it may be necessary to administer supplemental calories intravenously or orally through a feeding tube.

2. Levels of carbohydrate and fat may be governed by the patient's desire; restriction of fat to 80 gm per day or less will occasionally reduce the nausea and abdominal bloating which may occur early in the disease.

3. Protein in amounts larger than 100–125 gm daily has no therapeutic advantage. (Protein restriction will be required when hepatic coma is impending.)

4. Caloric intake should be restricted during the convalescent phase if excessive weight gain occurs.

5. Vitamins should be given to malnourished and markedly anorectic patients; though often used routinely, they are probably of little therapeutic advantage in the average patient. Patients who develop bleeding from severe hypoprothrombinemia may be given vitamin K parenterally, although little benefit occurs when hepatocellular disease is severe.

6. Alcohol should not be consumed for the first six months after the illness is contracted.

D. Bed rest Considerable controversy exists over the exact amount of bed rest required during the acute stage of the illness. Most patients who are acutely ill prefer to remain in bed; as they feel better they may be allowed bathroom privileges and ambulatory activity in their room, except for a 90-minute period of bed rest after meals. After the bilirubin has dropped to 1.5 mg/100 ml, and the BSP to less than 10% retention in 45 minutes, gradually increasing ambulatory activity may be allowed for seven days; the patient may then return to work for half-days if strenuous activity is not required. If the BSP retention, transaminase level, and serum bilirubin levels at the end of one week of this program remain normal or continue to improve, full activity may be resumed by the end of the second week. A somewhat more conservative regimen with less rapid restoration of full activity is suggested for such high-risk groups as elderly patients, teenage girls, and pregnant and postmenopausal women.

E. Corticosteroids Although administration of corticosteroids may increase appetite and sense of well-being, diminish the bilirubin value, and decrease the periportal inflammatory reaction, most observers agree there is no adequately controlled evidence that steroid therapy alters the degree of liver necrosis or accelerates the rate of healing; there is no indication for routine use of corticosteroids in the usual case of hepatitis. They may be of value in rare cases of fulminant hepatitis associated with a rapidly deteriorating course, in hepatic coma or hepatic precoma associated with acute viral hepatitis, in subacute or chronic active hepatitis, which may have some features of lupus erythematosus, and occasionally in prolonged or relapsing cases. Initial dosages should be in the range of 40–60 mg/day of prednisone (or equivalent amounts of other preparations).

After a beneficial response has occurred, steroid dosage should be tapered over a 6–8-week period, then discontinued as a rule. Most observers agree, however, that steroid administration should be continued indefinitely for patients with chronic active hepatitis; the appropriate dosage is the smallest dose that will prevent a flare-up of the disease (as manifested by abnormalities of liver-function tests).

F. Follow-up after hospitalization Careful follow-up is mandatory. Laboratory and physical examinations after discharge should be performed at 1, 2, 4, 8, 16, 26, and 52 weeks if the patient's course has been satisfactory, or until all laboratory results have returned to normal.

G. Relapse occurs in about 10% of patients and is suggested by the recurrence of any of the above laboratory abnormalities, particularly if persistent. Treatment as in the earliest stages of the illness should be reinstituted. The prognosis is generally good, as only 3–5% of those patients with prolonged or relapsing hepatitis have evidence of active liver disease after one year. In any prolonged case the possibility of other types of hepatic disease must be considered.

H. Acute yellow atrophy is a rare but very severe form of viral hepatitis with a high mortality. It is marked by the development of hepatic precoma or coma, ascites, and/or impairment of coagulation. Intravenous administration of very large doses of corticosteroids, equivalent to 500–1000 mg/day of hydrocortisone, has been recommended. Recently, several reports have indicated that multiple exchange transfusions using fresh whole blood have been a successful form of treatment in some instances. Attention to meticulous detail is an absolute prerequisite for such a heroic and complicated therapeutic measure. The reader should consult the articles published on this subject for specific details of the procedures used (*New Eng. J. Med.* 274:473, 497, 1966; *J.A.M.A.* 202:267, 1967).

II. **CIRRHOSIS** may be of several morphologic forms, but the same general principles apply to each type.

A. Diet and vitamins

1. A moderately high-protein, high-calorie diet should be prescribed; better nutritional status alone may be accompanied by clinical and laboratory evidence of improvement in many patients with mild to moderate nutritional cirrhosis. Bedfast patients should be given at least 1900 cal/day (80 gm protein), sedentary patients 2500 cal (100 gm protein), and ambulatory patients 3000 cal (100–125 gm protein) if the clinical status does not preclude administration of large amounts of protein. Patients with severe hepatic insufficiency or portacaval shunts may develop hepatic coma when given large amounts of protein; the risk of precipitating coma may be minimized by limiting protein intake to 40 gm/day initially, and then increasing every 2–3 days. About half the calories should be supplied as carbohydrate. Acutely ill hospitalized patients may require supplemental feedings parenterally or orally (through a small flexible feeding tube). Salt restriction is indicated when fluid retention occurs.

2. Multivitamin preparations should be given to all patients; absorption of the fat-soluble vitamins A, D, E, and K, may be particularly impaired. Brief courses of vitamin K should be given parenterally when the prothrombin level is significantly depressed; even though hepatocellular disease is severe, a slight response may occur. Macrocytic anemia may be associated with either vitamin B_{12} or folic acid deficiency; the diagnosis and management are discussed in Chapter 12.

B. Rest Bed rest is indicated when fever, infection, marked constitutional symptoms, or deteriorating liver-function tests occur. As the patient improves, ambulatory activity should be slowly increased.

C. Alcohol Complete abstinence is recommended. Ingestion of small amounts of alcohol by the cirrhotic patient may produce acute fatty changes in the liver, and, occasionally, hypoglycemia.

D. Sedation Sedatives and narcotics that are metabolized in the liver (e.g., morphine, short-acting barbiturates), and drugs that occasionally produce intrahepatic cholestasis (e.g., phenothiazines) should be given cautiously in reduced dosage, if at all. Chlordiazepoxide, antihistamines (e.g., diphenhydramine), and paraldehyde may be used cautiously as daytime sedatives and bedtime hypnotics, if required.

E. Corticosteroids are not indicated in the usual case of cirrhosis. They may be clinically beneficial (by stimulating appetite, occasionally reducing pruritus in primary and secondary biliary cirrhosis, and facilitating diuresis) in a few situations, such as postnecrotic cirrhosis and "lupoid" or chronic active hepatitis with a progressive course, but available data do not confirm that their administration favorably influences the natural history of the disease.

F. **Cholestyramine (Cuemid),** a bile-acid sequestrant resin, may dramatically reduce pruritus in patients with liver disease and retention of bile salts (e.g., primary biliary cirrhosis or drug-induced cholestatic hepatitis). Although the pruritus associated with extrahepatic biliary obstruction may also lessen, surgical correction, when possible, is the obvious treatment of choice.

The usual dose is 4 gm mixed with fruit juices or applesauce, TID–QID. Toxicity is negligible, although large doses may induce steatorrhea and hypoprothrombinemia; more common side effects include nausea, and diarrhea or constipation. Because Cuemid is a chloride form of anion-exchange resin, hyperchloremic acidosis may rarely follow its prolonged administration.

III. **HEPATIC COMA** is frequently a terminal complication of advanced liver disease. The biochemical abnormalities responsible are not known, but many studies suggest that the clinical manifestations may result from disordered cerebral metabolism induced by the accumulation of significant amounts of nitrogenous substances, particularly ammonia, normally removed from the circulation by the liver. The gastrointestinal tract is the most important site of production of ammonia, which is formed from ingested ammonium salts or the action of bacterial ureases on protein; however, the kidney may also contribute significant amounts in certain circumstances (e.g., following administration of acetazolamide or thiazides, or in renal failure). Normally, ammonia is rapidly removed from the portal venous system and converted to urea by the liver, and little is present in the systemic circulation. However, with impairment of hepatic function or development of significant portal-system collateral channels, large amounts of ammonia may accumulate.

Theoretically, ammonia can interfere with cerebral metabolism by two mechanisms: (1) ammonia combines with alpha-ketoglutarate to form glutamic acid, thus removing an important link in the Krebs citric-acid cycle and reducing aerobic glycolysis in the brain; (2) ammonia combines with glutamic acid (normally present in high concentration in the brain and capable of supporting oxidative phosphorylation), forming glutamine, which is inactive.

However, the failure to demonstrate an elevated arterial ammonia concentration in all patients with hepatic coma suggests that other poorly defined derangements in intermediary cerebral metabolism, or effects of other toxic substances, may play a significant role in the pathogenesis.

A. **Precipitating factors** The most important factors which may precipitate hepatic coma are listed below. **Remember:** The usual tests of liver function may be of little help in predicting hepatic coma, which may develop in patients with minimally abnormal values.

1. Progressive hepatocellular disease unassociated with any acute insult to the liver.

2. Increased sources of blood ammonia: azotemia; high-protein diet; gastrointestinal bleeding; following administration of ammonium chloride, carbonic-anhydrase inhibitors, or thiazides.

3. Infections, hypotension or shock, general anesthesia, minor surgi-

cal procedures, paracentesis, dehydration, acute alcoholism, hypokalemia, alkalosis, administration of narcotics or sedatives.

4. Portacaval shunt operations, especially if dietary protein is not restricted postoperatively.

B. Clinical manifestations include disturbances in mental state (euphoria or depression early, then confusion, drowsiness, inappropriate behavior), flapping tremor (asterixis), hyperreflexia, EEG abnormalities (characterized by paroxysms of bilaterally synchronous, symmetrical, high-voltage slow waves in the delta range), and, finally, coma. Characteristic of hepatic coma is its tendency to fluctuate, particularly in the early stages; the longer and deeper the coma, the less is the likelihood for spontaneous variations or a favorable response to therapy. Treatment, therefore, should be started early, directed both at controlling coma and eliminating the precipitating causes.

C. Treatment Therapeutic measures considered important by most experts are discussed below; treatment is directed, for the most part, at reducing intestinal production of ammonia and decreasing the blood concentration of ammonia. It is difficult to assess the efficacy of therapy because the clinical manifestations of hepatic coma may fluctuate so widely.

1. Gastrointestinal bleeding, when present, should be arrested as quickly as possible. Blood should be removed from the intestinal tract: If upper GI bleeding is active, constant gastric aspiration should be started; if bleeding has ceased, a cathartic should be administered. Enemas may also be of value.

2. Administration of drugs containing ammonium or amino compounds, or those known to precipitate coma should be stopped.

3. Dietary protein should be reduced to nearly zero (initially), and adequate calories, preferably 1600–2000 calories daily, provided. A low-protein tube feeding, when required, may be made by mixing 2000 ml 10% glucose and 200 ml Lipomul or heavy cream. When tube feedings cannot be given, at least 500 calories/day should be given parenterally (thus decreasing endogenous protein breakdown by as much as 90%); 1000 ml 20% D/W will provide 800 calories. Multivitamins should be given orally or parenterally.

If clinical improvement occurs after several days of treatment, 20–40 gm/day of protein may be allowed in the diet, with increments of 10–20 gm every 2–4 days, if tolerated.

4. Administration of antibiotics will decrease intestinal bacteria. Neomycin 4–6 gm/day or paromomycin (Humatin) 50–75 mg/kg body weight/day may be given orally in divided dosage; tetracycline or other broad-spectrum antibiotics may be given orally or parenterally in the usual dosage. Prolonged administration of neomycin may be complicated by development of a malabsorption syndrome or staphylococcal enteritis; although only small amounts are absorbed, toxic blood levels may accrue if renal impairment is present.

Neomycin may be given by enema; 1–2 gm are added to 100–200 ml saline and administered twice daily as a retention enema.

5. Arginine and glutamic acid are often given with the rationale of "inactivating" or "removing" excess ammonia, but clinical responses in hepatic coma or precoma are not impressive in many instances. Carefully controlled clinical studies do not confirm that administration of arginine and glutamic acid is of unquestioned benefit; responses are seen most often when coma has been precipitated by an excessive ammonia load (e.g., GI bleeding, ammonium chloride ingestion, etc.).

Arginine, an important component in the ornithine or urea cycle, may be reduced in severe liver disease, thus producing a rate-limiting step in ammonia removal and urea synthesis; it is administered to increase utilization of ammonia in the urea cycle. Similarly, glutamic acid is given to increase utilization of ammonia in forming glutamine.

Glutamic acid may be given orally, 30–40 gm daily in divided dosage; monosodium glutamate may be administered orally or IV, 33 gm/day, but unfortunately it provides a large amount of sodium; L-arginine may be given orally, 20–40 gm daily, in divided dosage. Arginine glutamate (Modumate) is a neutral preparation, without sodium, containing 13.5 gm arginine and 12 gm glutamic acid in each 100 ml; 100–200 ml may be diluted in 500–1000 ml 5% or 10% D/W and infused BID–TID.

6. Other measures of importance

a) Any infection should be treated promptly with appropriate antibiotics.

b) Electrolyte abnormalities, especially hypokalemia, should be corrected. Hyponatremia is usually dilutional in nature and best treated by restricting water; rare cases associated with true sodium deficiency may require administration of hypertonic saline. When contraction of ECF volume, associated with oliguria and increasing azotemia, occurs, cautious expansion may be tried; synthetic ECF may be given, or human serum albumin administered IV in a dose of 25–50 gm, but sudden expansion of intravascular volume and pulmonary edema are hazards. If blood loss occurs, fresh blood should be transfused cautiously.

c) Corticosteroids are of little to no benefit when given to cirrhotic patients with hepatic coma.

IV. ASCITES AND EDEMA

A. Salt restriction Limitation of dietary sodium is the most important measure; no more than 500 mg sodium (1.3 gm salt) daily should be allowed at first. On occasion rigid restriction to 250 mg sodium/day will be necessary, but such diets are unpalatable and restricted in protein; to supply adequate protein, powdered protein supplements of a low-sodium milk, such as Lonalac, should be given. When diuresis has occurred, more sodium, e.g., 750–1000 mg daily, may be allowed cautiously.

B. Fluids Most patients with severe liver disease have impaired free-water excretion. When vigorous diuresis is being attempted, fluids should be limited to 1500 ml/day, or less, to preclude development of dilutional hyponatremia.

C. Diuretics The general use of diuretics is discussed in Chapter 5. Despite their value, numerous complications may follow their administration; severe electrolyte abnormalities are the most frequent and serious, particularly since such abnormalities in cirrhotic patients may precipitate hepatic coma. Experimentation is often necessary to determine the optimal diuretic program; a thorough understanding of the mechanism of action of the various preparations will allow one to outline better an intelligent and effective program. Patients undergoing sustained diuresis should not lose more than 10–15 pounds per week.

1. **Mercurial diuretics** may be given once or twice weekly at first; they are relatively safe. Their effectiveness may be enhanced by the prior administration of a chloride load. L-lysine (or arginine) monohydrochloride is preferable to ammonium chloride as the acidifying agent in order to avoid administration of large amounts of ammonium.

2. **Thiazide diuretics** are also effective, but the hypokalemia and increased blood ammonia concentrations following their administration may play a role in precipitating hepatic coma in patients with severe hepatic insufficiency; they must be given cautiously, and usually with potassium supplements. Concurrent administration of a thiazide and spironolactone or triamterene is often much more effective in inducing a prolonged diuresis than is administration of any of the drugs individually; the latter two are usually of little value when given alone. An additional benefit of combined therapy is the protection against hypokalemia; indeed, hyperkalemia may develop, and the serum potassium concentration should be measured frequently.

3. **Corticosteroids,** which increase free-water clearance, may be beneficial when hyponatremia is severe and the ECF volume markedly expanded; they may be given in addition to the diuretics discussed above. Some steroid analogs (e.g., methylprednisolone, triamcinolone, and dexamethasone) may induce saliuresis as well as increased free-water clearance. Steroids are usually given for 7–10 days in moderately large dosage (e.g., 40–60 mg/day of prednisone, or equivalent amounts of other preparations), then abruptly discontinued. Diuresis may not accompany their administration but often begins shortly after their withdrawal.

4. **Ethacrynic acid** may induce a brisk diuresis in cirrhotic patients with severe anasarca not responsive to other measures. Although the drug is an exceedingly effective diuretic, numerous electrolyte abnormalities may follow its administration; its use is discussed in the section on diuretics in Chapter 5.

5. **Furosemide** is a potent diuretic with a very rapid onset of action and brief duration of peak activity. Like ethacrynic acid, furosemide may often produce a diuresis when other agents have failed but careful attention must be paid to the possible development of water and electrolyte imbalance. Furosemide is given initially in a dose of 40 mg, then with increments of 40 mg until the desired effect is obtained. For further details see Chapter 5.

D. **Paracentesis** should be performed only for diagnostic purposes or when pressure symptoms caused by marked abdominal distention are severe; only sufficient fluid to alleviate discomfort should be removed. Complications include infection, hemorrhage, and, following removal of large amounts of ascitic fluid, electrolyte abnormalities, contraction of intravascular volume, hypotension, oliguria, azotemia, and occasionally hepatic coma. Protein depletion follows repeated paracenteses.

E. **Salt-free albumin,** 25 gm daily IV for 3–5 days, may initiate diuresis in occasional patients, even if marked hypoalbuminemia is not a problem. Sudden expansion of intravascular volume and pulmonary edema are hazards, however; the albumin must be administered slowly, and the venous pressure checked frequently. Benefits are seldom long-lasting, but occasionally a protracted diuresis is initiated.

F. **Portacaval anastomosis** has been an effective surgical treatment for intractable ascites. Results are occasionally striking, but criteria for patient selection are not defined, the operative mortality is great (about 40–50%), and a high incidence of complications (portal-systemic encephalopathy, persistent hypoalbuminemia, and ankle edema) may occur. Other surgical procedures which have been recommended include peritoneal-caval shunts and thoracic duct cannulation, but experience is limited.

V. **ESOPHAGEAL VARICES** Management of asymptomatic varices in the cirrhotic patient remains controversial; management of bleeding esophageal varices remains difficult and unsatisfactory. In one series of cirrhotic patients with varices, 35% died of liver failure secondary to hemorrhage and 15% died of exsanguination from varices (34% in the series of the Boston Inter-Hospital Liver Group). Of those who died as a result of hemorrhage, 71% did so during their first major bleeding episode, 20% during the second hemorrhage, and 7% during the third.

In a cirrhotic patient with massive upper gastrointestinal bleeding, it should not be assumed that hemorrhage is from esophageal varices; the incidence of bleeding from gastritis and duodenal ulcer is high in patients with cirrhosis. Appropriate diagnostic measures should be carried out when the patient's condition permits; if these cannot be performed immediately it is often wise to proceed with esophageal tamponade. The management of an acutely bleeding patient is described below.

A. **Replace blood** (See also the section on acute bleeding in Chapter 11.) Keep in mind the susceptibility of the cirrhotic patient to vascular overload and pulmonary edema. Use fresh blood, if possible, because it is lower in ammonia content than stored blood and may provide coagulation factors that are diminished in patients with severe liver disease.

B. **Administer vitamin K,** (phytonadione) IM, or IV slowly, in a dosage of 25–50 mg.

C. **Control bleeding** It is important to stop the bleeding as quickly as possible, not only to reduce transfusion requirements, but to prevent accumulation of large amounts of blood in the GI tract, which may precipitate hepatic coma.

1. **Ice-water lavage** of the stomach or gastric hypothermia may reduce bleeding temporarily.

2. **Vasopressin,** 20 units diluted in 100 ml 5% D/W and infused IV over a 10-minute period, will reduce portal pressure and may permit hemostasis; administration may be repeated at 3–4-hour intervals. The beneficial effects are attributable to splanchnic

vasoconstriction; coronary artery constriction also occurs, however, and the drug should not be given to patients with heart disease.

3. **Esophageal tamponade**   The Sengstaken triple-lumen tube or some variant is used. When it is properly applied, hemorrhage may be controlled in most patients despite the dangers associated with its use; careful attention must be given to details that seem minor.

a) Check balloons by trial inflation to detect leaks (best seen with balloons submerged in water).

b) Elevate the head of the bed slightly unless the patient is in shock.

c) Pass the tube through the nose if possible (discomfort is less, the use of the headguard is facilitated, and the patient will be able to talk, swallow, etc.). Topical anesthesia in the nose and pharynx may facilitate passage of the tube but is usually unnecessary. Tie a small-caliber tube along the upper tubing of the apparatus; this tube may be used for constant suctioning of secretions which tend to accumulate above the balloons and may be aspirated by the comatose patient.

d) Pass the tube to the 50-cm mark and inflate the gastric balloon with 150 ml air; apply at least double ties to prevent slow air leaks.

e) Draw the gastric balloon up gently against the cardia and fix the position of the tube against the nose or mouth with a sponge-rubber pad or split soft rubber ball secured to the tube with adhesive tape. Apply 1–2 pounds traction to the tube; an overhead bar and pulley system may be used, but many observers feel that this is dangerous and prefer attachment of the tubes to a baseball catcher's mask placed on the patient's head. A Kulick-Rousselot face mask-manometer-pressure alarm system, if available, may prove useful. The face mask is more comfortable than other improvised apparatus, the pressure in the gastric balloon may be regulated, pressure in the esophageal balloon may be constantly visualized on the manometer, and an alarm sounds if pull on the gastric balloon is lost or pressure in the esophageal balloon decreases.

f) When gastric tamponade is achieved lavage the stomach with ice water until clear and try to determine the site of bleeding; it may be unnecessary to inflate the esophageal balloon. Suction the stomach continuously.

g) Inflate the esophageal balloon, if bleeding persists, to 30–45 mm Hg, maintaining accurate pressure with an aneroid manometer and pumping bulb.

h) If bleeding fails to slow, inflate the gastric balloon to 400 ml, or consider either fluoroscopy (to check position of the tube) or administration of a water-soluble contrast medium to determine other sources of bleeding (if the patient's clinical condition permits).

i) If bleeding is controlled, drop the esophageal balloon pressure by decrements of 5 mm Hg to that level which will just control bleeding.

j) The patient must be attended constantly. Scissors should be attached to the end of the bed so that the tube may be cut immediately and the balloons allowed to deflate if displacement into the posterior pharynx occurs (asphyxiation may occur quickly).

k) Deflate the esophageal balloon for 5 minutes every 6–8 hours.

l) Tamponade should be maintained for 48 hours; then the tube is deflated and return of gastric aspirate used to determine whether bleeding recurs. If bleeding continues, the balloons may be reinflated for another 48 hours, but acute ulcerative esophagitis may occur with prolonged tamponade, and it may be preferable to perform some type of shunting procedure instead, if the patient's condition permits.

m) If no bleeding occurs within 24 hours after deflation, the tube may be removed and oral feeding of liquids begun.

n) During the period of tamponade, nutrition must be provided parenterally or tube feedings given through the stomach tube. Fluid and electrolyte balance must be maintained.

4. Emergency surgery Numerous procedures may be performed, but those most frequently done include portacaval shunts (see next section), esophagogastric resection, or ligation of esophageal varices. This subject is controversial. Some believe that transthoracic transesophageal suture of bleeding esophageal varices is the most effective emergency procedure for control of massive hemorrhage. The mortality, however, is about 30% or more, and protection against recurrent bleeding lasts only several months so that some shunting procedure usually must be performed subsequently. Thoracic duct cannulation may occasionally reduce bleeding from varices significantly, but experience is limited.

VI. SHUNT SURGERY Splenorenal or portacaval shunts may be performed in a variety of circumstances. Before operation, either in advance or in the operating room, splenoportagrams should be performed in order to elucidate the diameter, course, and patency of the splenic and portal veins, and any anomalous connections which might exist. When the portal vein is thrombosed or when hypersplenism is marked and splenectomy is indicated, splenorenal shunts are usually performed. In other situations, portacaval shunts are done; they have less tendency to undergo thrombosis and are more effective in reducing portal pressure and preventing hemorrhage from esophageal varices. Portacaval shunts may be constructed as end-to-side, side-to-side, or double-barreled anastomoses. A detailed discussion of indications for operation, operative mortality, selection of patients, and efficacy in prolonging survival is beyond the scope of this Manual; statistics vary from series to series, depending on patient selection and skill of the surgeon, and data from carefully controlled prospective studies are not available. A few general comments may be made, however.

A. Emergency portacaval shunt for treatment of bleeding esophageal varices carries a mortality of 25–50%. Unfortunately, patients with portal hypertension (secondary to intrahepatic disease) and difficult-to-control bleeding usually have the poorest liver function; the decision to operate cannot be based on definitive criteria.

B. Portacaval shunts may be performed electively for patients who have bled. The main contraindication to surgery is a changing clinical status; the procedure should be deferred until the clinical condition and laboratory studies are relatively stable. Patients with serum albumin less than 3.0 gm/100 ml, bilirubin greater than 3.0 mg/100 ml, ascites, previous episode of coma, or poor general condition (marked wasting, many spider angiomata, etc.) have a mortality rate approximating 50%, but in others with minimal to moderate impairment of hepatic function the immediate operative mortality is 10–15%. Although the status of liver function is not improved postoperatively, and the mortality of the underlying disease is not changed, the incidence of recurrent bleeding from esophageal varices is strikingly reduced; therefore, many experts recommend portacaval anastomosis after the first episode of bleeding for patients with minimal or moderate impairment of liver function. Portal-systemic encephalopathy may be a complication of surgery; the incidence is about 5–15%. The selection preoperatively of patients liable to develop neuropsychiatric changes is very difficult. The mental impairment may be incapacitating; administration of low-protein diet and antibiotics may decrease the severity; colectomy or ileosigmoidostomy has been beneficial in some patients.

C. Elective performance of a portacaval shunt in patients with demonstrable esophageal varices from which bleeding has not occurred cannot be recommended. Although the incidence of hemorrhage is decreased, the long-term survival does not appear to be improved.

VII. DRUG-INDUCED AND TOXIC LIVER DISEASE

A. **Toxic hepatitis** Liver injury may follow exposure to various chemicals or the administration of certain drugs. True hepatotoxins all have certain features in common—each produces a characteristic histologic pattern of liver damage; all persons exposed to the hepatotoxic agent develop liver damage if the dose is sufficient; the severity of damage is proportional to the dose; and similar reactions may be induced in experimental animals. Numerous mechanisms may explain the pathogenesis of liver injury, but the uniformity of the biochemical findings in the liver after exposure to many structurally different hepatotoxins suggests that the chain of events leading to necrosis follows a common pathway.

The more common hepatotoxins include hydrocarbons such as chloroform and carbon tetrachloride, arsenical compounds, phosphorus, and trinitrotoluene.

Treatment is supportive. If the patient is seen immediately after ingestion, the agent should be removed from the gastrointestinal tract (gastric lavage; cathartics). If clinical manifestations of liver disease appear, management is similar to that described for viral hepatitis. Administration of choline or corticosteroids is not of proved benefit; antibiotics, according to some observers, may prevent further damage by secondary bacterial infections.

B. **Drug-induced hepatitis** In contrast to the pattern of liver damage occurring after exposure to true hepatotoxins, most drugs affecting the liver produce features characteristic of a hypersensitivity reaction—the morphologic picture is variable; liver injury occurs sporadically in only a small number of people (often those with a history of other allergies or previous treatment with the offending drug);

liver injury occurs only in man and is not reproducible in experimental animals; the severity of the hepatic lesion is not correlated with the size of the dose; the latent period between exposure and development of manifestations is highly variable; and other manifestations of hypersensitivity (e.g., fever, rash, arthralgias, eosinophilia, etc.) are frequently present in association.

The predominant clinical, laboratory, and pathologic findings are those of cholestasis or hepatocellular damage; varying degrees of both may occur. Certain drugs, such as sulfonamides, may cause either type of liver damage. Fatalities are very uncommon; rarely, cirrhosis may develop as a late complication. Although abnormalities in liver function usually disappear promptly, severe disease simulating extrahepatic biliary obstruction may take several months to clear. The diagnosis of drug-induced liver damage may be difficult to establish, especially when the period between drug ingestion and development of hepatic injury is long; liver biopsy may not differentiate between intrahepatic cholestasis and extrahepatic obstruction, and a prolonged period of observation may be necessary to aid in establishing the diagnosis.

Table 10-1 lists selected drugs known to cause hepatitis; many more have been incriminated, and complete lists may be found in standard sources.

TABLE 10-1.   Selected Drugs Inducing Hepatitis

Drug (or class of drugs)	Comment
Phenothiazines	Usual picture is cholestatic hepatitis; incidence is less than 1%, but more than 25% of patients may have anicteric reactions manifested by elevations of serum alkaline phosphatase and transaminases
Monoamine oxidase inhibitors	Hepatocellular injury predominantly
Iminodibenzyl derivatives	Cholestatic hepatitis predominantly
Phenylbutazone	Hepatocellular injury
Probenecid	Hepatocellular injury
Diphenylhydantoin	Generalized hypersensitivity reaction with hepatic involvement
Phenobarbital	Generalized hypersensitivity reaction with hepatic involvement
Isoniazid	Generalized hypersensitivity reaction with hepatic involvement; reactions occur only, as a rule, when the drug is administered concurrently with a sensitizing agent, such as para-aminosalicylic acid
Para-aminosalicylic acid	Generalized hypersensitivity reaction with hepatic involvement
Pyrazinamide	Hepatocellular injury
Methimazole	Cholestatic hepatitis
Propylthiouracil	Hepatocellular injury

TABLE 10-1 (*Continued*)

Drug (or class of drugs)	Comment
Sulfonylureas	Cholestatic hepatitis; very rarely hepatocellular injury. Significant percentage of patients may have asymptomatic elevation of serum alkaline phosphatase levels, questionably related to administration of the drug
Sulfonamides	Hypersensitivity reaction with hepatitis; rarely hepatocellular injury
Novobiocin	Generalized hypersensitivity reaction with hepatitis is rare; not uncommon, however, is drug-induced elevation of unconjugated bilirubin level
Erythromycin estolate (Ilosone)	Cholestatic hepatitis
Tetracyclines	Therapeutic doses of chlortetracycline and oxytetracycline often produce fine fatty vacuolization of hepatic parenchyma, reversible after cessation of therapy, and of no clinical importance. Large IV doses of tetracyclines may cause severe and fatal hepatic failure especially in pregnant women near term (see Chapter 9, Antibiotics and Infectious Diseases).
Methyltestosterone (and all of the 17α-alkyl substituted testosterone derivatives, e.g., norethandrolone, methandrostenolone, etc.)	These compounds produce an unusual form of cholestatic hepatitis. Jaundice is never accompanied by clinical signs of hypersensitivity or histologic evidence of an inflammatory reaction in the liver, features usually seen in most other forms of drug-induced cholestatic hepatitis
	BSP retention is common, even in absence of cholestatic hepatitis
	The progestational agents, similarly substituted on the 17 position, are commonly used as oral contraceptives, and may rarely produce similar abnormalities
Fluothane (Halothane)	Some observers have reported the development of subacute hepatic necrosis after administration of fluothane anesthesia, but whether or not the fluothane per se induces hepatic damage has not been clarified; current data are controversial

Treatment is supportive. The suspected drug (or drugs) should be withdrawn and not administered again, although occasional patients may tolerate it subsequently; structurally similar drugs should be given cautiously, if at all. Severe pruritus may be controlled with cholestyramine. Corticosteroids may be given to patients with severe drug-induced hepatitis not responding to drug withdrawal and simple supportive measures, but their efficacy in producing beneficial effects has not been established. Other measures, supportive in nature, are similar to those recommended for the treatment of viral hepatitis.

PEPTIC ULCER

Therapy of a peptic ulcer has two main purposes, relief of symptoms and maximal healing of the ulcer. Treatment has included (1) admission to hospital, (2) antacids, (3) regulation of diet, (4) anticholinergic drugs, (5) cessation of smoking, (6) irradiation. Of these various measures, only cessation of smoking and admission to the hospital have been shown to improve the course of gastric ulcer, but none of these measures statistically influences the course of duodenal ulcer. Gastroenterologists disagree as to which forms of therapy are most efficacious and how prolonged the therapy should be. Difficulty in assessing the role of antacids and anticholinergic drugs has arisen because the dose of many preparations has not been adequate to produce effective neutralization of gastric juice or to inhibit gastric secretion.

I. **DUODENAL ULCER** The most reliable guide to effective therapy of uncomplicated duodenal ulcer is the relief of pain. The administration of medications (such as corticosteroids, ACTH, salicylates, reserpine, phenylbutazone, indomethacin) known to precipitate peptic ulceration or to cause bleeding or reactivation of ulcers should be discontinued if possible. Physicians must be alert to detect diseases such as hyperparathyroidism, cirrhosis, pancreatic islet-cell tumors, polycythemia vera, pseudoxanthoma elasticum, etc., in which an increased incidence of ulcer has been reported.

A. **Diet** Regulation of diet has been a traditional form of therapy for duodenal ulcer with patients advised to take "bland" foods with a predominance of milk and carbohydrates. The available evidence suggests that special diets with extensive restrictions are of little real value in achieving symptomatic relief or in preventing relapses of duodenal ulcer. The timing of meals is probably much more important than the foods per se. There is much less fluctuation in intragastric pH when a diet of the patient's own selection is fed at 2-hour intervals instead of 4-hour intervals. In addition, a meal may prolong the duration of action of antacids given one hour after eating. On this basis patients have been advised to have a midmorning, midafternoon, and midevening snack in addition to the three main meals. Interval feedings should be employed in conjunction with decreased meal size so that the total caloric intake is not raised. Many gastroenterologists, however, feel that an antacid can be substituted for the interval feedings with equal effectiveness. Detailed advice need not be given concerning foods to be taken or avoided, although the patient should be advised to avoid those foods which have been found to intensify pain. Caffeine-containing beverages (coffee, tea, and carbonated cola drinks) are perhaps best avoided because of their association with increased gastric secretion.

Milk and milk-containing drinks have been ritualistically included in peptic ulcer therapy. There is no real evidence that milk is better than any other protein-containing food in neutralizing gastric acid. Recent studies suggest that frequent milk feedings in fact result in higher gastric acidity than is present when patients eat the same food without milk therapy. The incidence of arteriosclerotic heart disease is 14% higher in white male ulcer patients treated with emphasis on diets rich in milk and milk products as compared to white male patients in the general population (*J. Michigan Med. Soc.* 59:1693, 1960). There seems, therefore, to be no justification in substituting milk for antacids in the treatment of peptic ulcer.

B. Alcohol and tobacco Alcohol should be avoided, since it stimulates gastric-acid secretion and irritates the mucosa; of more importance, as a rule, are the irregular dietary patterns and decreased food ingestion that often accompany alcohol consumption. Smoking should be stopped because it may interfere with the healing of a peptic ulcer and help to maintain its chronicity (*Lancet* 1:657, 1958). In some patients it will be necessary to allow a few cigarettes each day.

C. Sedatives Administration of sedatives has not been shown to produce remission or prevent further symptoms. However, mild sedatives (e.g., phenobarbital 15–30 mg QID) may be beneficial in a selected minority of patients with excessive anxiety, nervous tension, or insomnia.

D. Antacids are the mainstay of drug therapy in duodenal ulcer. Their purpose is to neutralize gastric hydrochloric acid and maintain the pH of the gastric contents above 5, well above the pH optimum for pepsin (1.7 pH). Timing and frequency of the administration is of crucial importance in the efficacy of these agents. When administered shortly after meals, antacids are ineffective and exert little neutralizing effect beyond that of the meal itself. To be effective antacids should be given during those periods when ingested food no longer exerts a buffering action upon gastric secretion. The main factor determining the duration of antacid effect is the rate of gastric emptying which is usually completed within the brief interval of 30 to 40 minutes. Therefore to give maximum neutralization of gastric contents, antacids should be given at hourly intervals between meals.

1. Antacid preparations (Table 11-1)

a) Calcium carbonate powder is the most effective antacid and by far the least expensive. The usual dose is 2 gm (one-half teaspoonful) in one-third glass of water (or 2 Tums tablets). Constipation may ensue; it can be relieved by substituting magnesium hydroxide (milk of magnesia) once or twice daily. Calcium carbonate is partially absorbed; if it is administered in very large doses, or with milk and cream, hypercalcemia may occur in certain patients. Serum calcium concentration should be checked after initiation of therapy. The addition of glycine to $CaCO_3$ (Titralac) has been claimed to supplement the buffering effects; such preparations have not been shown to be more beneficial than others.

b) Aluminum hydroxide preparations are moderately effective in reducing the gastric acidity (i.e., concentration of acid of gastric contents) and are nonabsorbable but frequently cause constipation. Addition of magnesium hydroxide or magnesium trisilicate decreases the tendency toward constipation. The usual dose is 15 ml.

c) **Magnesium hydroxide** preparations (e.g., milk of magnesia, which contains 8% magnesium hydroxide) are also moderately effective in reducing gastric acidity but frequently result in diarrhea. The usual dose is 15 ml.

d) **Aluminum or magnesium hydroxide tablets** are less effective than liquid preparations in neutralizing stomach contents. Calcium carbonate tablets (Tums) may be used when the patient is away from home and cannot take the liquid. Tablets should be chewed thoroughly before swallowing.

2. **Dosage schedule** In intensive antacid therapy for the initial heal-ing of duodenal ulcer, antacids in effective doses should be given every hour while the patient is awake; during the night, antacids should be given every 2 hours. In addition a mild sedative is bene-ficial at night to ensure return to sleep when the patient is so frequently awakened. Unfortunately there is no definite guide to the optimum length of time for administration of antacids. Two weeks after symptomatic relief has occurred the frequency of

TABLE 11-1. Antacid Preparations

Compound	Trade Name	Dose	Na+ Content (mg/ dose)	PO$_4$ Added	pH Produced in 150 ml 0.1N HCl
Aluminum hydroxide suspension	Amphojel	15 ml	18	No	3.8
Aluminum hydroxide with magnesium trisilicate	Gelusil	15 ml	22	7.2 mg CaPO$_4$/ dose	3.5
Aluminum hydroxide with magnesium hydroxide	Aludrox	15 ml	18	No	4.3
	Creamalin	15 ml	83	No	3.9
	Maalox	15 ml	16	No	5.8
	Mylanta*	10 ml	9	No	4.5
Aluminum carbonate gel	Basaljel	15 ml	9	No	4.2
Calcium carbonate		2 gm	0	No	5.3
Calcium carbonate with glycine	Titralac	5 ml	18	No	5.4
Calcium carbonate, magnesium carbonate, and magnesium trisilicate	Tums or Dicarbosil	2 tabs.	0	No	7.6
Magnesium hydroxide	Milk of magnesia	15 ml	0	No	9.1

*Also contains simethicone.

nocturnal administration of antacids can be reduced to every 4 hours. This regimen should be continued for 6–8 weeks beyond cessation of symptoms and then antacids may be discontinued. Recurrence rates are probably not altered by continued antacid therapy.

3. Problems of antacid therapy

a) Most antacids contain sodium (see Table 11-1) and if large quantities are given to patients with congestive heart failure or renal insufficiency, allowances must be made for the significant quantities of Na^+ that may be administered.

b) Aluminum-hydroxide-containing antacids bind and prevent absorption of orally administered antibiotics. When given simultaneously with or shortly before or after the antibiotic, blood levels may be decreased by as much as 70–90%. Antacids and antibiotics should not be administered within one hour of each other.

c) Milk-alkali syndrome Following ingestion of large quantities of soluble alkali (e.g., calcium carbonate 30–40 gm/day) with or without the ingestion of milk and cream (particularly when there is associated vomiting or impaired renal function), hypercalcemia, alkalosis, and azotemia may develop. If therapy is continued, further deterioration of renal function and nephrocalcinosis may occur. The symptoms (nausea, vomiting, constipation, anorexia, headache, mental confusion, weakness, polydipsia, polyuria) usually appear within a week after starting antacid therapy; severe manifestations are believed to occur only in patients with underlying renal disease. Administration of the antacid and milk should be stopped, nonabsorbable alkali substituted, and adequate fluid intake ensured. The chemical abnormalities can be corrected, and permanent renal damage is unlikely. Hyperparathyroidism must be excluded.

E. Anticholinergic drugs These compounds interfere with the transmission of nerve impulses mediated by acetylcholine at the neuroeffector junctions of postganglionic cholinergic nerves. In the dosage range used for the treatment of peptic ulcer they partially inhibit vagal stimulation and may reduce volume of gastric secretion, but they will not reduce the acid concentration of gastric juice secreted. In reducing the rate of gastric emptying, they may facilitate the neutralization of gastric contents by food and antacids.

Pepsin and mucus output are not significantly inhibited, and antral stasis may be associated with prolongation of the antral phase of acid secretion. In the fasting state anticholinergics are effective in reducing the volume of gastric secretion, but their depressant effect on meal-stimulated gastric acid production is controversial. Even in high doses none of the anticholinergics has a pharmacologic effect equivalent to the effect of surgical vagotomy. Several of these agents may have a more selective action on the stomach than does atropine.

1. The drugs may be effective in reducing gastric acid secretion when administered parenterally, less so when given orally. There is little evidence that they decrease the incidence of complications, although some patients experience relief of pain. Proof of benefit in asymptomatic or mildly symptomatic patients with duodenal ulcer is lacking.

2. Individual variation in response is marked. Dosage is inadequate for effective reduction of gastric secretion if no side effects are apparent; therefore, dosage should be increased until minor side effects, such as dryness of the mouth or blurred vision, are present. Drugs that inhibit both gastric-acid secretion and smooth-muscle motility include **propantheline bromide (Pro-Banthine)** and **isopropamide iodide (Darbid)**; usual dosage for Pro-Banthine is 15 mg TID and 30 mg HS; usual dosage for Darbid is 5–10 mg every 12 hours. Pro-Banthine should be administered with meals, since the effective dose is not obtained until 1 hour after administration; giving anticholinergics with meals allows the maximal therapeutic dose to be achieved after gastric emptying has occurred, when the pH would be falling to low levels.

3. **Side effects** include dry mouth, blurred vision and difficulty in accommodating, urinary hesitancy, constipation, headache, dizziness, weakness, tremors, nausea, vomiting, heartburn, flushing of the face, palpitations, and, more rarely, mental confusion. Severe side effects necessitate discontinuing the drug.

4. Anticholinergics should not be used in patients who have peptic esophagitis, hiatus hernia, gastric ulcer, cardiospasm, pyloric obstruction, recent hemorrhage, glaucoma, bladder-neck obstruction (acute urinary retention may develop), or severe coronary artery disease (the resultant tachycardia may result in decreased cardiac output). They should also be avoided prior to surgery or gastrointestinal x-ray examinations.

F. **Radiation therapy** In certain patients who fail to respond to conventional medical management and who are poor surgical risks, gastric irradiation is valuable therapy. Its efficacy depends upon decreasing gastric acidity by destruction of parietal cells. Approximately 10% of irradiated patients obtain transient achlorhydria and about 40% reduce acid production to half of the original level. Such changes do not occur for several weeks, but they can be maintained for weeks or months. However, ulcers have recurred in 46% of patients given radiation therapy.

G. **Gastric freezing** Although the procedure of gastric freezing is relatively safe and is sometimes associated with temporary reduction of pain, there is no evidence that gastric freezing accomplishes physiologic or therapeutic effects beyond those of placebo treatment. Major complications include GI bleeding and gastric ulceration.

H. **Recurrences** More than 50% of patients with duodenal ulcer will have at least one recurrence of the acute active ulcer during the five years following initial diagnosis. The recurrence rate decreases with time. The frequency and severity of recurrences may be reduced by a program that includes thorough treatment of the initial lesion, careful subsequent supervision regarding avoidance of alcohol, tobacco, and medications known to be associated with reactivation of ulcers, and resumption of a strict ulcer regimen whenever symptoms suggestive of reactivation occur.

II. COMPLICATIONS OF DUODENAL ULCER AND THEIR MANAGEMENT

A. **Refractory pain** Most patients with gastric or duodenal ulcers will be free of pain within two weeks after therapy has been started. Although failure to respond may be due to inadequate therapy because the patient does not follow the recommended program, persistent pain may indicate partial pyloric obstruction, penetration, or confined perforation of the ulcer. If pain persists the patient should be hospitalized in addition to the reinstitution of the intensive therapeutic program described above. Continuous gastric aspiration for 48 hours may afford relief of symptoms.

For patients who have not had relief from a course of intensive medical therapy as described above, surgical intervention should be considered strongly. For patients who obtain fair relief of symptoms while hospitalized but do poorly outside the hospital, the decision to recommend surgery becomes more difficult. Severe emotional disturbances or neurotic patterns weigh against recommendation of an operative procedure, as does previous difficulty in maintaining normal body weight. Factors that may influence a positive decision include a history of previous perforation or hemorrhage, presence of some degree of obstruction, location of the ulcer in the pyloric channel or postbulbar area, and inability to work because of symptoms.

B. Pyloric obstruction may be caused by spasm, inflammation, or edema adjacent to an active ulcer, or by fibrosis and scarring due to an old ulcer; a high degree of pyloric obstruction may exist with few symptoms. A patient who has 150 ml or more gastric contents on aspiration after an overnight fast has some degree of pyloric obstruction. A trial of medical management for 4–7 days is indicated in all instances, since most patients with obstruction secondary to spasm, edema, or inflammation will be relieved without surgical intervention. If the obstruction (as determined by repetitive measurements of gastric retention; see below) is not relieved by several days of intensive therapy, surgery is indicated.

The regimen for management of acute obstruction is as follows:

1. Gastric lavage with an Ewald tube is necessary to remove retained undigested material that would otherwise block the smaller indwelling Levin tube which is passed after lavage in order to maintain gastric suction.

2. Continuous gastric aspiration is maintained for 48 hours.

3. The tube is clamped on the morning of the third day, and the patient is fed 200 ml of water; 2 hours later the gastric residual is determined.

   a) If the residual is greater than 50 ml, gastric emptying is not satisfactory and continuous aspiration should be resumed for another 36 hours.

   b) If the residual is less than 50 ml, the tube is reclamped and feedings of clear liquids are continued at 2-hour intervals.

4. Gastric residual is again measured at 8 o'clock the following morning.

   a) If it is greater than 150 ml, the regimen of feeding and aspiration should be continued.

   b) When the overnight residual is less than 150 ml, the tube may be removed. The diet is gradually increased as tolerated from clear fluids to include soft foods. Antacids should be administered as soon as the continuous gastric aspiration is discontinued.

5. Gastric aspirations at 8 a.m. and 10 p.m. (2 hours after the last feeding) should continue in order to evaluate progress and determine the tolerance for oral feedings.

6. On the sixth or seventh day, if progress (as measured by tolerance to increasing quantities of food) has been satisfactory, the usual ulcer regimen may be started.

7. During restriction of oral fluids, electrolyte and fluid balance must be maintained with parenteral fluids. Vitamins should be added to the IV fluids. Inadequate replacement of electrolytes during continuous gastric aspiration will lead to the development of hypokalemia, hypochloremia, and alkalosis. The normal concentration in gastric juice of sodium is 20–80 mEq/L, of potassium 5–20 mEq/L, and of chloride 100–150 mEq/L.

8. Anticholinergic drugs should not be administered when gastric obstruction is present because they decrease gastric emptying rates.

C. **Perforation** Acute perforation of a gastric or duodenal ulcer is an urgent indication for operation. A simple closure of the perforation is usually performed, although a subtotal gastrectomy may be indicated on occasion. Medical management (constant gastric aspiration, fluid therapy, and large doses of antibiotics) has been advocated for patients who are seen 24 hours after perforation is presumed to have occurred or who are poor operative risks because of complicating illnesses. However, difficulties are encountered in maintaining proper position and patency of the tube and assessing closure of the perforation. Surgery may be necessary subsequently, and the preoperative condition of the patient will be less satisfactory than initially. For these reasons, operation is recommended as the initial treatment of perforated duodenal ulcer for any patient in whom there is no overriding contraindication.

D. **Acute bleeding** Significant GI bleeding occurs in about 15–20% of hospitalized patients with peptic ulcer. When a patient with known duodenal ulcer presents with massive GI bleeding, the ulcer is the most likely source; when massive GI bleeding occurs in a patient without previous history, the likelihood of duodenal ulcer as the source is 75–80%, but bleeding may be from esophageal varices, gastric ulcer, gastritis, hiatus hernia, etc.

To determine the origin of GI bleeding, immediate diagnostic study (esophagoscopy, gastroscopy, upper GI roentgenograms) has been recommended by some observers. At the Washington University Medical Center an upper GI series may be performed while the patient is still bleeding if he is not in shock; emergency endoscopy may then be done by arrangement with the Gastroenterology Division. If it seems likely that bleeding is from esophageal varices, a Sengstaken tube may be inserted initially. In all patients, including those with melena only, a stomach tube should be passed to empty the stomach, to test for gastric acidity, to ascertain whether or not pyloric obstruction is present, and to determine whether the bleeding is in the upper GI tract. In order to detect occult liver disease in a bleeding patient, bromsulfalein excretion should be measured. Although a negative test is good evidence against liver disease, it should be emphasized that abnormal results may be found in patients with severe bleeding and a normal liver, especially in older patients.

1. **General measures**

   a) The patient must be kept in bed.

   b) Mild sedatives may be given, but phenothiazine drugs, anticholinergic agents and narcotics should be avoided.

   c) Iced-saline lavage of the stomach or gastric cooling may serve to slow or halt bleeding temporarily. If iced-saline lavage is employed, an Ewald tube is passed to a point just below the cardia of the stomach. Lavage with several liters of iced saline is carried out to remove blood clots and hopefully to diminish or temporarily stop active bleeding. Such procedures may be particularly beneficial in preparing patients for roentgenographic or endoscopic examinations and in controlling massive bleeding in patients too ill to withstand immediate operation.

   d) In treatment of a patient who has bled but apparently stopped before admission to the hospital, an acute ulcer regimen (see above) may be started as soon as nausea and vomiting have ceased; no other measures may be necessary, and transfusion may not be required. For massive hemorrhage with hypotension or shock, immediate transfusion as described below is necessary. In either case, an internist and surgeon together should follow the patient from the time of his appearance at the hospital.

2. **Treatment of blood loss: Initial measures**   The following principles provide guidance and are not an inflexible set of rules. Each patient must be evaluated individually.

   a) Any patient who is bleeding rapidly and shows evidence of vascular collapse requires transfusion as soon as possible. Blood rather than its substitutes should be given; it should be crossmatched and available within 20–30 minutes after the patient is first seen. In the meantime isotonic saline is administered intravenously through an 18-gauge needle. If the patient is already in serious shock, Type O Rh-negative blood with Witebsky substance added may be used. Nasal oxygen is an important temporary adjunct.

   b) In the usual patient with moderate to severe shock the transfusion may be started at an approximate rate of 500 ml every 15–30 minutes (thrombocytopenia and other coagulation defects may occur when large amounts of blood are administered within a short time); as soon as real improvement in the patient's blood pressure and pulse rate is noted the transfusion rate should be slowed. Although patients with rapid acute blood loss generally tolerate such rapid transfusion quite well, pulmonary edema is always a danger, especially in elderly patients, and care must be taken to avoid overloading the circulation (*follow the central venous pressure frequently* and attempt to maintain it below 150 mm of saline). If blood loss has been chronic and if the clinical condition permits, initial blood replacement should be at a slow rate.

3. The rate of bleeding is often very difficult to judge, but evaluation of the following will aid in determining the need for additional blood replacement.

   a) Vital signs and clinical state   Vital signs should be recorded every 15–30 minutes initially, with the patient supine and raised to 60–90° (if he is not in shock). Although the pulse and blood pressure occasionally may be poor indicators of a serious degree of hypovolemia, **additional blood replacement is generally required when:**

    i) the systolic blood pressure is less than 90–100 mm Hg in a previously normotensive individual, or significantly lowered in a patient with known hypertension.

    ii) there is significant fall in blood pressure or increase in heart rate (of 20–30 beats/minute) as the patient sits up.

    iii) there are continued signs and symptoms of acute blood loss, e.g., pallor; cold, clammy extremities; chilliness; restlessness; thirst; dyspnea; faintness.

b) Urine output should be measured frequently. If dehydration is not a consideration, inadequate urine volume may reflect inadequate blood replacement.

c) Hematocrit The hematocrit will not reflect accurately the volume of blood lost initially, but provides a more reliable index after 8–12 hours. It should be maintained at 30–35% except for older patients and those with pulmonary or cardiac disease, in whom it should be maintained at 35–40% since these patients poorly tolerate acute blood loss. One unit (500 ml) of blood raises the hematocrit 3–4%.

d) Continued blood loss Recurrent hematemesis, aspiration of large quantities of blood through a nasogastric tube, or frequent bloody stools (especially if bright red) show that active bleeding continues and further transfusion is necessary.

4. Three units of blood (1500 ml) should be ready at all times.

5. Treatment after acute bleeding has stopped When bleeding has stopped, shock has been treated adequately, and there is no immediate consideration of surgery, hourly feedings may be started. Antacids are given, but aluminum hydroxide may combine with the blood in the bowel and result in severe fecal impaction. Milk of magnesia is useful as both antacid and laxative. After 48 hours an acute ulcer regimen, as described previously, may be instituted.

6. Indications for operation No hard-and-fast rules govern the selection of patients for surgery. Each patient must be considered individually. In general the decision depends upon an evaluation of the surgical and medical skills available. If bleeding stops promptly with medical therapy most physicians do not operate. Massive recurrence or continuation of hemorrhage, however, is usually felt to indicate prompt surgical intervention. Age per se should not be regarded as an indication for or against operative intervention for bleeding. The presence of other factors may influence a decision for early, but not immediate, operation. These include presence of postbulbar ulceration, pyloric obstruction, and past history of GI bleeding. Many physicians are somewhat less conservative in dealing with elderly patients, who frequently have an increased incidence of complications. Many recommend operation for any elderly patient who has sustained one episode of GI bleeding.

III.   **GASTRIC ULCER**   Perhaps as many as 5%–10% of gastric ulcers are malignant; the differentiation of malignant from benign lesions may be difficult.

A. Evaluation of the patient

1. **Roentgenography**   X-ray diagnosis is correct in approximately 90% of the cases when a gastric ulcer is judged definitely benign or definitely malignant, but in many cases x-ray examination does not provide definitive information.

2. **Gastric cytology**   Carefully obtained specimens provide useful information; at the Washington University Medical Center between 1955 and 1965 the incidence of false negative gastric cytology interpretations was less than 2%; false positive results were even less frequent.

3. **Gastroscopy** may be performed if the ulcer is located in an area of the stomach that can be visualized through the gastroscope; the gastrocamera permits better observation of gastric lesions.

4. **Measurement of gastric acidity**   The **maximal histamine test** may provide useful information.

   a) **Method**   With the patient sitting (and preferably under fluoroscopic control), a Levin tube is passed to a depth of 55 cm (second tube mark opposite the teeth of the average patient). The Levin tube can be connected to a constant-suction pump at −10 cm H_2O, but hand aspiration at 5-minute intervals is preferred. All gastric aspirate is collected while the patient is lying on his left side and is constantly expectorating. After basal secretions are obtained for one hour, β-imidazole (Histalog) 100 mg is injected subcutaneously. If histamine acid phosphate, 0.04 mg/kg body weight, is used an antihistamine, tripelennamine (Pyribenzamine), 50 mg, is given IM 30 minutes before the histamine to attenuate the systemic effects of histamine (stimulating effects on gastric secretion are not altered). Following stimulation all gastric juice is collected for another hour. The volume is recorded, and the secreted acid measured by titration to pH 7.0 (or to pH 8 with phenolphthalein as indicator) with 0.1N NaOH.

   b) **Results and interpretation (see Table 11-2)**   The volume of gastric secretion is 150–250 ml/hr in normal subjects and is generally higher in those with duodenal ulcer. The range of acid secretion for normal men is 0.1–42.1 mEq/hr (mean 17.1); for women, 0.3–28.2 mEq/hr (mean 9.4). Patients with duodenal ulcer often secrete significantly more acid. Values of less than 11 mEq/hr for men or 5 mEq/hr for women generally exclude duodenal ulcer as a serious consideration. True achlorhydria in patients with gastric ulcer signifies that the lesion is almost certainly malignant. Because some degree of hydrochloric acid production occurs in many patients with malignant gastric ulcers, acid secretion in response to histamine stimulation does not exclude carcinoma.

5. **Therapeutic trial**   In some patients the above studies may be inconclusive; roentgenographic response to medical management may be the only way (aside from surgery) of differentiating the benign from the malignant gastric ulcer (see below). **Don't forget:**

TABLE 11-2.   Interpretation of Intubation Gastric Analysis*

One-hour basal acid output

< 2 mEq = Normal, gastric ulcer, gastric cancer

2–5 mEq = Normal, gastric ulcer, or duodenal ulcer

> 5 mEq = Duodenal ulcer

> 20 mEq = Zollinger-Ellison syndrome

One-hour maximum acid output

0 mEq = True achlorhydria, gastritis, or gastric cancer

< 6 mEq = Normal, gastric ulcer, gastric cancer

6–35 mEq = Normal, duodenal ulcer

35–60 mEq = High-normal secretor, duodenal ulcer, Z-E syndrome

> 60 mEq = Zollinger-Ellison syndrome

Ratio of basal acid output to maximum acid output

$< 20\%$ = Normal, gastric ulcer, gastric cancer

20%–40% = Gastric or duodenal ulcer

40%–60% = Duodenal ulcer, Zollinger-Ellison syndrome

$> 60\%$ = Zollinger-Ellison syndrome

*Modified from H. L. Segal (*J.A.M.A.* 196:655, 1966).

The symptoms of a gastric carcinoma may be entirely relieved by a medical program.

B. Treatment

1. **Hospitalization** is advised to ensure strict adherence to the therapeutic program. Furthermore, substantial evidence suggests that bed rest per se is a significant factor in promoting the healing of gastric ulcers. Aside from bed rest, the only other measure shown to have significant effect on the rate of healing of gastric ulcer is the cessation of cigarette smoking.

2. **Diet and antacid therapy** are described in the previous section on management of duodenal ulcers.

3. **Sedatives** may be given as described previously.

4. **Anticholinergic drugs**   Gastric retention and the consequent stimulation of gastric-acid secretion (mediated by the mucosal hormone gastrin) may be important factors in the genesis of gastric ulcers. Administration of anticholinergic drugs, which reduce gastric emptying, is therefore not recommended.

C. **Follow-up**   The upper GI roentgenogram should be repeated in 3 weeks. If the ulcer is reduced in size by 50% or more the roentgenograms are performed at 3-week intervals until healing is complete (usually within 6–8 weeks). Use of the gastrocamera for serial follow-up of gastric ulcers is a promising technique with many advantages over serial radiography. Failure to obtain a decrease in ulcer size within 3 weeks justifies immediate operation. Once healing has occurred it is not necessary, as a rule, to obtain subsequent GI roentgenograms; the indication for reexamination is recurrence of symptoms.

IV.   COMPLICATIONS FOLLOWING GASTRECTOMY   Several of the more important difficulties that may arise following gastrectomy are discussed below.

   A. Anemia   Macrocytic or hypochromic microcytic anemia may develop following gastrectomy.

      1. Iron-deficiency anemia is not uncommon following partial gastrectomy but may not become apparent until several years after the operation. The anemia may develop even though there are no apparent reasons such as menstrual or gastrointestinal blood loss or deficient intake. Experimental studies indicate that iron absorption is inadequate in these patients, but the basis for the defect is unknown. Treatment consists of administration of an oral iron preparation, taken before meals to ensure adequate absorption. If body-iron stores are depleted, it may be beneficial to administer parenteral iron.

      2. Megaloblastic anemia is due to deficiency of vitamin B_{12}. It is rare following partial gastrectomy because adequate intrinsic factor is available, but it will follow total gastrectomy. It is slow to appear because large quantities of vitamin B_{12} are stored in the body and daily requirements are small. The biologic half-time of vitamin B_{12} is about 1 year. Manifestations of deficiency probably do not occur until the body load of B_{12} falls to about 200 μg. Macrocytosis and neutrophil hypersegmentation are usually the first evidence (average time of appearance is 2½ years after operation); anemia usually is manifest by 4 years. Neurologic complications may develop. Treatment is the same as for pernicious anemia.

   B. Dumping syndromes   A variety of unpleasant symptoms (abdominal cramps, borborygmi, marked weakness, epigastric discomfort, nausea, sweating, dizziness, palpitations, tachycardia, diarrhea, fainting) may occur within 30 minutes after eating and are attributed to rapid passage of gastric and duodenal contents into the jejunum following subtotal gastrectomy. Therapy is accordingly directed at lessening the osmolarity of the intestinal contents (by reducing carbohydrate ingestion) and diminishing the volume of the feeding (by eliminating fluids). Patients should take small, frequent feedings throughout the day and postpone their beverage until 30–60 minutes after eating. The diet should be high in fat and protein but low in carbohydrate.

   Patients with a subtotal gastrectomy and symptoms of hypoglycemia two hours after eating are helped by similar measures.

   In those few patients who have severe, incapacitating dumping syndrome, alteration of the anastomosis may be beneficial.

   C. Malnutrition   Most patients who fail to regain lost weight or continue to lose weight after gastrectomy do not eat enough because they have less appetite or feel full more rapidly. In some people, however, high-calorie diets do not promote weight gain; studies of transit time of various foods through the small intestine and of fat absorption may reveal no abnormalities, and the reasons for the weight loss are not clearly defined. Treatment is unsatisfactory, although bile salt deconjugation by bacterial overgrowth in an afferent loop can be diminished by antibiotics (tetracycline, 250 mg QID), thereby enhancing fat absorption. Anabolic steroids are of questionable value.

ULCERATIVE COLITIS

Chronic ulcerative colitis is a disease of unknown etiology marked by a variable clinical course punctuated by remissions, exacerbations, and fulminant crises associated with numerous complications. Therapy is difficult—not only in management of the physical complaints but also in management of a patient who is often emotionally immature, demanding, hostile, and apprehensive. The treatment of moderate to severe ulcerative colitis of the relapsing-remitting type is discussed below, and acute fulminant disease in the section following.

I. **RELAPSING-REMITTING ULCERATIVE COLITIS** Most patients with mild disease may be managed outside the hospital, but hospitalization is often advantageous in allowing the physician to establish close rapport with the patient, investigate cautiously any aggravating emotional influences in the patient's environment, and plan an intensive therapeutic program which best suits the patient's needs.

   A. **Diet** An ad libitum, flexible, and palatable diet ensuring adequate calories (2500–3000 calories daily) and protein (125–150 gm daily), especially for patients who are debilitated or have an associated protein-losing enteropathy, must be encouraged. Restricted diets are of little therapeutic value and may indeed be harmful; calories are often inadequate, and unpalatability discourages patient cooperation.

   Foods known by the patient to cause abdominal cramping, diarrhea, or flatulence should always be excluded; milk or milk products not uncommonly cause such symptoms and may have to be restricted on the basis of an associated lactase deficiency or on a nonspecific "allergic" basis. Very acutely ill patients may prefer a liquid or soft diet, but as symptoms subside, almost any food may be tolerated.

   B. **Rest** The need for adequate rest must be stressed. A short rest period after meals may be important psychologically for some patients; all patients should be encouraged to have 7–10 hours of sleep at night.

   C. **Emotional support** The physician must maintain an understanding, sympathetic, interested, and reassuring relationship with the patient. Dependency needs of patients with ulcerative colitis are often marked, and frequently the physician is the only person who can lend the patient the emotional support required. Exacerbations of the disease can often be related to emotional upsets. Mild sedatives, as butabarbital or amobarbital (15–30 mg QID), may be helpful; occasionally tranquilizers such as chlordiazepoxide may aid in alleviating anxieties.

   D. **Anticholinergic drugs** are not particularly effective in relieving cramps or diarrhea, and individual response is highly variable. They may be of occasional benefit in relieving symptoms associated with an active gastrocolic reflex, but high dosage may result in intestinal atony or toxic megacolon.

   E. **Antidiarrheal drugs** are discussed in Chapter 1. Diphenoxylate (Lomotil), 5–25 mg daily in divided dosage, deodorized tincture of opium, 10 drops in a half-glass of water TID–QID, or codeine, 15–30 mg QID, for example, may provide symptomatic relief and reduce the frequency of bowel movements, but such agents must be administered cautiously in severe ulcerative colitis, for they may precipitate toxic megacolon. Opiates should be used only for brief periods of time to avoid the possibilities of addiction, paralytic ileus, or masked perforation.

F. Antibacterial drugs   Administration of antibacterial agents is generally of little benefit. However, several carefully controlled clinical studies point out the efficacy of a sulfa preparation, salicylazosulfapyridine (Azulfidine); almost two-thirds of patients note a favorable response, and relapses are much less frequent. Although the use of this drug is empiric (no studies have elucidated the mechanism of action), and the incidence of side effects is significant (occurring in approximately 15% of patients), most gastroenterologists consider the drug one of the mainstays of therapy.

1. Salicylazosulfapyridine (Azulfidine) is a diazo compound of salicylic acid and sulfapyridine, excreted primarily in the feces, but partially absorbed, distributed throughout the body (with a high affinity for connective tissue), and then excreted in the urine.

    a) Dosage and administration   The drug is supplied in 0.5-gm tablets and is best tolerated if initial dosage is graduated. For acutely ill patients with much cramping and bloody diarrhea, begin treatment with 0.5 gm QID (after meals and at bedtime), increasing over several days to 1.5 gm 4–6 times daily; the usual dose is 8–16 tablets daily. If nausea, headache, and dizziness are marked, dosage may be reduced by half for several days, then increased again slowly.

    Response (decrease in number of stools, bloody mucus, abdominal cramping, and fever) often occurs in several days; sigmoidoscopic appearance of the colon may improve after 7–14 days. As healing occurs the dosage is gradually reduced (over several months) to maintenance of 0.5 gm QID.

    Most observers have continued maintenance therapy for 12 months or longer, noting prevention of relapses or a reduction in their frequency, duration, and severity.

    b) Side effects occur in about 15% of patients, a somewhat higher incidence than with other sulfonamides. Most common are headache, nausea, and vomiting, which may subside spontaneously or require a reduction in dosage. Less common are allergic reactions (fever, skin rash) or hematologic and renal complications; these are described in the section on sulfonamides in Chapter 9.

2. Other sulfonamides   Sulfa preparations other than Azulfidine have been used, but available evidence suggests that they are of little clinical benefit.

3. Other antibiotics   Patients allergic to sulfonamides may be treated with furazolidone (Furoxone) 100 mg QID for brief periods of time. Penicillin, ampicillin, and broad-spectrum antibiotics should be given, when indicated, for the treatment of purulent complications (perirectal abscesses, fistulas, etc.); they are of no benefit in the uncomplicated case of ulcerative colitis, and their prolonged administration may aggravate the basic disease, especially if staphylococcal or monilial enterocolitis should occur.

G. Corticosteroids and ACTH   Corticosteroids and ACTH are useful adjuncts to more conservative measures; though not curative, they may induce a rapid remission or marked decrease in clinical manifestations in severely ill patients. They are indicated for the treatment of patients with critical illness; with severe, chronic progressive disease not responsive to other measures; or with marked systemic manifestations as iridocyclitis, myocarditis, and erythema nodosum. Steroids should be used in conjunction with the other general measures described previously.

Corticosteroid preparations available, schedules for administration, and side effects are detailed in the formal discussion of cortisone and analogs in Chapter 16. Their use in ulcerative colitis is discussed below.

1. **Oral and parenteral steroids** The initial dose should be 10–15 mg of prednisone (or an equivalent amount of other preparations) QID. This dosage is continued for 3–6 weeks depending upon the clinical response; when diarrhea lessens, blood disappears from the stool, and sigmoidoscopic appearance of the colon begins to improve significantly, dosage may be reduced to 30 mg daily over a 3–4-week period, and administration of Azulfidine begun. When both bowel function and sigmoidoscopic appearance of the colon are essentially normal, attempts should be made to discontinue steroid administration over a 2–3-month period by reducing dosage gradually. The possibility of relapse always remains, in spite of continued conservative measures and Azulfidine administration, and steroid therapy may have to be restarted. However, continued "maintenance doses" of corticosteroids are known to be ineffective and are discouraged. Concerted efforts should be made to discontinue these drugs as rapidly as the clinical response allows. As noted in Chapter 16, it is sometimes possible to administer an entire 48-hour dose once every other day without loss of therapeutic benefit.

Steroids may be given parenterally to patients too ill to take them orally and to those with rapid intestinal transport and possible malabsorption. Rapidly effective preparations (succinate or phosphate salts) should be used, the initial dose of hydrocortisone succinate, for example, being 60–80 mg IM every 6 hours.

2. **Rectal steroids** Corticosteroids may be administered intrarectally in solution or in suppository form, primarily for the treatment of disease involving the rectum (ulcerative proctitis).

Steroid enemas may be given once or twice daily; they are prepared conveniently by placing the appropriate amount of steroid in an empty plastic enema "squeeze" bottle (such as a Fleet enema container), and adding 30–60 ml tap water; the enema should be administered with the patient in the left lateral position. The usual dosage is 100 mg of hydrocortisone succinate (or phosphate), 50 mg of prednisone, or 40 mg of methylprednisolone. Systemic absorption occurs to a variable degree. Commercial products specifically prepared for administration as a retention enema are available utilizing methylprednisolone acetate, which is relatively insoluble in aqueous media and produces little systemic absorption. Such preparations are usually administered for 2–3 weeks.

H. **Additional measures** Other important measures include administration of multivitamins to debilitated or malnourished patients, and oral or parenteral iron to those who develop iron-deficiency anemia. Transfusions may be necessary for those patients who have had marked blood loss from the colon. Barium enemas should be performed cautiously for fear of inducing a flare-up of the disease; they probably should not be performed at all in severely ill patients because of the risk of perforation. Finally, do not forget that on rare occasions persons using large amounts of cathartics may present a clinical picture indistinguishable from that of chronic ulcerative colitis.

II.   ACUTE FULMINANT ULCERATIVE COLITIS   Approximately 5–10% of patients with ulcerative colitis develop an acute fulminant phase (either as first attack or relapse) with severe diarrhea and abdominal pain, hemorrhage from the colon, fever, sepsis, marked toxicity, electrolyte abnormalities, dehydration, and complications such as perforation, peritonitis, pericolitis, and toxic megacolon. The last, one of the most severe complications of ulcerative colitis and associated with a high mortality, is characterized by marked abdominal distention and decreased or absent bowel sounds because of loss of contractility and extreme dilatation involving a bowel segment or the entire colon; the clinical picture may mimic bowel obstruction. The following measures are important.

A. Give nothing by mouth; start nasogastric suction to prevent further bowel distention (especially important if toxic megacolon has developed).

B. Give large amounts of appropriate electrolyte-containing fluids intravenously. Patients are often severely dehydrated because of the profuse diarrhea and may require 4–5 liters of fluid during the first 24 hours. The commonest electrolyte abnormality is hypokalemia, and large amounts of potassium may be required. Electrolytes must be determined frequently. Transfusions of blood should be given as required.

C. Give antibiotics parenterally; ampicillin, cephalothin, etc., may be selected.

D. Give large doses of corticosteroids as previously described.

E. Do not use anticholinergic drugs; administer narcotics, if required, sparingly. (Both these agents may contribute to flaccid paralysis of the colon.)

F. Surgery   Those acutely ill patients not responding to intensive medical therapy within 7–10 days must be considered for operation, the procedure of choice usually being a colectomy and ileostomy. It is preferable to avoid surgery, if possible, but occasionally the severity of the situation and the inability to exclude one or multiple perforations of the colon preclude waiting and necessitate immediate operation, despite the risks. A more detailed discussion of types of operations and indications for surgery is beyond the scope of this Manual.

ACUTE PANCREATITIS

I.   GENERAL COMMENTS   Acute pancreatitis is a medical problem commonly presenting difficulties in diagnosis and treatment. Symptoms may vary from mild upper abdominal discomfort to severe abdominal pain associated with physical findings indistinguishable from those seen in other acute intra-abdominal conditions. Elevation of the serum amylase is not specific for pancreatitis, and in certain clinical situations suggesting perforated viscus, mesenteric vascular occlusion, etc., exploratory laparotomy may be indicated. Although every possible effort should be made to avoid abdominal surgery in acute pancreatitis, operation per se is not usually associated with an increased mortality as long as the pancreas itself is not manipulated.

II.   TREATMENT   Acute pancreatitis is associated with higher morbidity and mortality rates than any other common nonmalignant disease of the gastrointestinal tract; much can be done to reduce the intensity and duration of an acute attack. The aims of therapy are to relieve pain, to treat shock, to replace fluid and electrolytes, to correct disturbances in carbohydrate metabolism, to suppress pancreatic secretions, and to prevent secondary infection.

A. Relief of pain   Pain usually decreases in severity after 48 hours, reflecting a reduction in the acute inflammatory process; persisting pain, especially if associated with a continued elevation of the serum amylase concentration or an abdominal mass, may indicate the development of a pancreatic pseudocyst.

1. Narcotics   Large doses are often required to relieve severe pain, even though opiates may produce spasm of the biliary-pancreatic ducts and sphincter of Oddi. Meperidine is the drug of choice and may be given IM in a dosage of 100–150 mg every 3–4 hours.

2. Antispasmodics   Amyl nitrite, nitroglycerin, papaverine, and anticholinergic drugs have been tried in attempts to reduce spasm of the ducts or sphincter of Oddi; they are not usually of significant clinical benefit, even though most patients are given anticholinergic agents (e.g., atropine or propantheline) routinely for the reasons discussed below.

B. Correction of hypovolemia and shock   Hypovolemia occurs in cases of acute pancreatitis. Shock is often associated with severe disease. The fluid losses are similar in magnitude to those seen in severe burns, and, indeed, the process may be considered a form of retroperitoneal burn. Adequate fluids must be given IV to maintain the extracellular fluid volume. Measurement of the central venous pressure provides information helpful in determining the amount of fluid necessary for volume repletion. It is often necessary to give 2–3 liters synthetic ECF or lactate-Ringer's solution rapidly when the patient is first seen. Most electrolyte-containing solutions should contain added potassium, 40 mEq/L (to replace potassium lost through nasogastric suction or secretion into dilated atonic bowel), unless oliguria or anuria is present.

Should hypovolemic shock occur, whole blood or plasma should be given in preference to dextran or electrolyte solutions.

C. Decrease in pancreatic secretion   The production of pancreatic proteolytic enzymes (which contribute to continuing inflammation) may be decreased by reducing the stimuli to pancreatic secretion.

1. NPO order   This eliminates the chief stimulus to the secretion of pancreozymin, secreted in response to the presence of food in the duodenum.

2. Nasogastric suction   Removal of hydrochloric acid from the stomach prevents the release of secretin; gastric distention, which may accompany an associated adynamic ileus, is prevented. Nasogastric suction should be continued for at least 24 hours after complete relief of pain (usually 2–3 days); premature reintroduction of food may precipitate a relapse.

3. **Anticholinergic drugs** may also aid in reduction of pancreatic secretion by suppression of vagus mechanisms and should be given in full dosage if used.

D. Other measures

1. **Electrolyte replacement,** as discussed above, may become a complex problem because of losses in emesis or gastric suction, paralytic ileus, and exudation into the peritoneal cavity. Lactic acidosis may occur if shock is present, and hyperkalemia may become significant if there is marked tissue breakdown in face of oliguria. Serum electrolytes and urine output should be measured frequently.

2. **Calcium gluconate** (10 ml of 10% solution) should be given IV as often as necessary to correct neuromuscular irritability or tetany associated with hypocalcemia secondary to deposition of calcium soaps in the pancreas and surrounding tissues; large amounts may be required. A serum calcium level below 7 mg/100 ml is an ominous prognostic sign.

3. **Antibiotics,** particularly ampicillin or cephalothin, may be given in severe cases of acute pancreatitis. Although their routine use is controversial, many observers rationalize that the likelihood of secondary infection or abscess formation is significant enough in severely ill patients to warrant their administration. Either chlortetracycline or oxytetracycline, both of which are concentrated and excreted in the bile, may be used.

4. **Insulin** may be required if marked hyperglycemia occurs. Patients with acute pancreatitis are often sensitive to insulin; small doses of crystalline insulin at 6-hourly intervals are preferable to the long-acting preparations.

5. **Drugs of unproved benefit** include corticosteroids and trypsin inhibitors. Steroids may reduce pancreatic inflammation experimentally, but clinically they are of little benefit; they may be given in large dosage if severe shock occurs. The trypsin inhibitor, Trasylol, prepared from bovine parotid glands, and claimed as beneficial in acute pancreatitis by preventing pancreatic autodigestion by trypsin, cannot be recommended because evidence to date fails to show that it has any clinical benefit.

E. Management of the recovery phase

After the patient has responded favorably to treatment of the acute phase, usually on or about the sixth day, treatment may include small amounts of clear fat-free liquids, anticholinergics administered parenterally or orally in full therapeutic doses, nonabsorbable antacids every hour, and supplemental fluids and electrolytes IV. Recurrent manifestations of pancreatitis require immediate reinstitution of nasogastric secretion. After recovery from an acute attack, x-ray studies frequently show nonvisualization of the gallbladder for 4–6 weeks following pancreatitis. The roentgenographic examination of the gallbladder must therefore be repeated at a later date if visualization fails to occur following the acute episode.

12. Anemia and
Bleeding Disorders

ANEMIA

Precise diagnosis is required for the intelligent and effective management of the patient with anemia. Documentation of the anemia by measurement of hemoglobin concentration, hematocrit or red cell count; determination of the red cell constants; and measurement of the reticulocyte count (best expressed as the absolute reticulocyte count, normal being approximately 25,000–75,000 per cu mm) can be provided by almost any laboratory. Of unparalleled value in the prompt initial evaluation of anemia by the physician himself is a careful look at the patient's blood film. After such an examination, more complex studies will often be indicated to confirm the diagnosis, to quantitate the extent of the deficit already surmised by the physician and to plan a rational mode of treatment. The alternative approach—the unthinking administration of "shotgun" therapy—cannot be too strongly deplored for a number of reasons:

1. The diagnosis of a single deficiency will be missed, precluding specific, often inexpensive treatment.

2. The diagnosis of nondeficiency states (e.g., hemolytic anemia) will be overlooked and appropriate therapy delayed.

3. The patient may even be harmed (e.g., use of folate-containing oral preparations alone in pernicious anemia).

I. DEFICIENCY AND HYPOPROLIFERATIVE STATES

A. Iron-deficiency anemia

1. In severe iron deficiency the red blood cells are microcytic (MCV < 80 cu μ) and hypochromic (MCHC < 30%); the serum iron is less than 40 μg/100 ml; the total iron-binding capacity is increased to levels usually above 400 μg/100 ml; the iron-binding protein is less than 10% saturated with iron; and no stainable iron can be found in the marrow. Milder degrees of iron deficiency, however, are more difficult to recognize. As deficiency develops, iron stores first decrease, reflected by diminished, then absent, stainable hemosiderin in the marrow; the serum-iron concentration falls and transferrin levels increase (with consequent reduction of transferrin saturation to 15% or lower); sideroblasts disappear from the marrow with concomitant development of mild normochromic normocytic anemia; and only then do hypochromic microcytic anemia and severe tissue-iron deficiency occur. The most sensitive studies for the diagnosis of early or mild iron deficiency, therefore,

are iron stain of the bone marrow and determination of the percentage saturation of transferrin.

The body of a normal adult contains approximately 2–6 gm of iron, 60–75% of which is present in circulating hemoglobin, 20–30% in hemosiderin and ferritin iron stores and the remainder in myoglobin, cellular enzymes, and transferrin. Iron assimilation normally balances iron loss; if iron absorption ceases and excretion continues (up to 1 mg/day for men and postmenopausal women), 6–8 years must elapse before the development of significant anemia. That occurs only with very inadequate diets, or in patients with various malabsorption syndromes; in the absence of these abnormalities iron-deficiency anemia develops because of excessive loss of iron or hemoglobin. The most common causes are excessive menstrual blood flow and multiple pregnancies in the female; when these are not pertinent considerations, careful studies should be carried out to determine the source of blood loss, usually from the gastrointestinal tract.

2. **Treatment** The optimal daily dose should provide enough iron to support a maximal hemoglobin increase in a patient with iron-deficiency anemia, i.e., 0.3 gm/100 ml blood/day (15 gm/blood volume of 5 liters). Because of persistence of hypochromia and microcytosis during therapy, the response is best followed by measurement of hemoglobin concentration rather than hematocrit or red cell count. Since hemoglobin contains 0.34% iron, absorption of 50 mg iron/day would be required. Assuming that 20% of an oral dose of a ferrous iron preparation is absorbed, the total daily dose should provide 200–250 mg of elemental iron. Administration of oral iron should be continued for 4–6 months after the hemoglobin level has returned to normal in order also to replenish the depleted body stores of iron. The total amount required can be calculated: if a patient initially has 5 gm hemoglobin/100 ml, then 9 gm/100 ml will be required to increase the level to a normal value of about 14 gm/100 ml. With a blood volume of 5 liters, a total of 450 gm of hemoglobin must be synthesized, requiring about 1.5 gm iron (450×0.0034). Allowing an additional 0.5–1.0 gm for storage iron, a total of 2.0–2.5 gm iron must be supplied to correct the deficiency. Because of the markedly variable absorption of oral iron, these calculations pertain only to parenteral iron; oral administration must be continued empirically for some months (see above).

a) **Oral administration** Ferrous salts are preferred because they are more efficiently absorbed. Recommended iron preparations are listed in Table 12-1. Gastrointestinal effects of nausea and diarrhea may be minimized by giving the tablets after meals (although absorption may be impaired) and initiating therapy with one tablet on the first day, two on the second, etc. Patients should be told that the stools will become black. Although the guaiac test for occult blood in the stool is not affected by iron salts, other tests (e.g., orthotoluidine) may give false positive reactions. Only confusion and added expense can result from dispensing iron preparations that contain vitamins, other minerals, liver extract, etc. Nor is there any indication for iron prepared in slow-release pellets; these may be suboptimally absorbed because the proximal small bowel, where iron is absorbed, is bypassed.

TABLE 12-1. Recommended Oral Iron Preparations

Preparation	Size Tablet (gm)	Iron Content per Tablet %	Iron Content per Tablet mg Fe	Acceptable Adult Dose (Tablets/Day)
Ferrous sulfate, $7H_2O$	0.32	20	60	4
Ferrous sulfate, exsiccated	0.20	29	60	4
Ferrous gluconate	0.32	12	40	5 or 6
Ferrous fumarate	0.20	33	66	4
	0.32	33	105	2 or 3
Ferroglycine sulfate	0.25	16	40	5 or 6

b) Parenteral administration Parenteral iron therapy is more expensive than oral, more uncomfortable, more dangerous (fatal reactions continue to be reported), and sometimes disfiguring because of skin staining after IM injection; in addition, the response is not significantly faster than with oral preparations. Parenteral administration, therefore, should be reserved exclusively for those patients who are unable to tolerate or absorb adequate amounts of orally administered iron, e.g., those with malabsorption syndromes, ulcerative colitis, regional ileitis, colostomy, ileostomy, or intestinal shunts; those with chronic blood loss extensive enough that iron therapy by the oral route alone does not suffice (e.g., hereditary hemorrhagic telangiectasia, severe menorrhagia); and those who are unable to tolerate oral iron preparations (less than 5% of patients).

The dose of iron to be injected may be calculated from the table in the package insert or by the following formula (with Hb expressed in grams):

$$(\text{Normal Hb} - \text{Initial Hb}) \times 0.255 = $$
grams iron to be administered

i) Iron-dextran (Imferon) is a complex of ferric hydroxide and low-molecular-weight dextran supplied as a dark brown solution, pH 6.0, containing 50 mg Fe/ml for deep IM injection in the buttocks. In order to prevent staining of superficial tissues a Z-track injection technique must be utilized and separate needles used for withdrawing the medication from the vial and for injection. After the amount to be given is calculated (see above), a test dose (0.25 ml) is injected the first day followed by 2.0–5.0 ml daily until the total dose has been administered. It is wise not to give more than 2.0 ml in one injection site. Adverse reactions include local pain and tissue staining at the injection site, headaches, fever, arthralgias, nausea, vomiting, urticaria, back pain, and, rarely, anaphylaxis and death; hemosiderosis may occur with excessive dosage. Sarcomas at injection sites have been reported in animals but not in humans.

ii) Dextriferron (Astrafer) is a complex of ferric hydroxide and partially hydrolyzed dextrin containing 20 mg Fe/ml (pH

7.3). It is given intravenously. The starting dose of 1.5 ml (30 mg) is increased by daily increments of 1.0–1.5 ml until a maximum of 5 ml is injected each day. Toxic reactions are similar to those for Imferon but occur more frequently.

iii) Jectofer is an iron-sorbitol-citric acid complex stabilized with dextrin, pH 7.2–7.9, containing 50 mg Fe/ml for IM injection. The usual daily dose is 2.0 ml. Reactions are similar to those for other preparations; in addition, dizziness, flushing, genitourinary irritation, and transient alterations in taste perception have been reported. Patients excrete about 20–30% of an injected dose in the urine, which may turn black on standing. The total dose should be increased by 20–30% to correct for this loss.

3. Acute iron toxicity   The ubiquity of iron preparations demands that the physician be prepared to deal with acute intoxication, almost exclusively in children. Of greatest importance in prevention of iron poisoning in children is the warning of mothers for whom iron is prescribed to keep the tablets out of the reach of toddlers. The rapid progression of symptoms—severe gastrointestinal upset, shock, acidosis, coma, and death—in as short a period as four hours requires prompt treatment by: (a) gastric lavage with 1% $NaHCO_3$; (b) gastric instillation of 5–8 gm deferoxamine in 50 ml distilled water; (c) 1–2 gm deferoxamine every 3–4 hours given intramuscularly (1 gm/L can be given intravenously at a maximum rate of 15 ml/kg body weight/hr if shock is present); and (d) appropriate supportive therapy for gastrointestinal hemorrhage, acidosis, and shock.

B. Megaloblastic anemias

1. Diagnosis   Megaloblastic anemias are most commonly due to deficiency of vitamin B_{12}, folic acid, or both. Differentiation of pernicious anemia from other megaloblastic anemias is particularly important, since therapy with vitamin B_{12} must be continued for life, and since partial correction of the hematologic abnormalities of pernicious anemia may occur following administration of folic acid while neurologic damage progresses and occasionally becomes irreversible. Clinical features of megaloblastic anemias and laboratory studies helpful in differential diagnosis are reviewed in standard sources. More commonly, measurement of serum B_{12} and folic acid levels should be carried out. On occasion, however, evaluation of the response to therapeutic trials of folic acid or vitamin B_{12} is necessary to arrive at a definitive diagnosis. This procedure involves a control period on a diet low in vitamin B_{12} and folate. The Schilling test should be delayed until completion of the therapeutic trial. Patients suspected of vitamin B_{12} deficiency should be given 1–2 µg vitamin B_{12} IM daily for 10 days (some observers use slightly larger doses); those suspected of folate deficiency should be given 50–200 µg folic acid IM daily for 10 days. The reticulocyte response should be measured daily. Patients whose deficiency is predominantly in vitamin B_{12} will respond to this small dose of B_{12} but not to folate; those whose deficiency is predominantly in folic acid will respond to the small dose of folate but not to B_{12}. After the differentiation has been made, therapeutic doses of the appropriate agent should be administered. As an alternative to the differential therapeutic trial, blood for folate and vitamin B_{12} determinations may be drawn and treatment begun immediately as described for the patient with pernicious anemia in relapse.

Recently, increasing consideration has been given to the possibility that nonhematologic manifestations of deficiency of B_{12} or folic acid (e.g., behavioral abnormalities in the aged and fetal wastage in the woman of childbearing age) may characterize a large pool of deficient but not yet anemic patients.

2. Treatment of pernicious anemia

a) Vitamin B_{12} (cyanocobalamin or hydroxycobalamin); dosage and administration The minimum daily requirement probably lies in the range of 0.1–1.0 µg, but therapy must eventually restore the depleted total body load of 4 mg or more. When cyanocobalamin is administered, as much as 75–85% of a single 200–1000 µg dose may be lost in the urine; because the loss is only 50% with hydroxycobalamin, the latter is the preparation of choice. Initial therapy consists of 100 µg **IM** every other day for 2 weeks, then monthly for the lifetime of the patient; because of the safety and low cost of the vitamin, many physicians will use as much as 1000 µg per injection.

Oral B_{12}-intrinsic factor preparations are not recommended, since most patients become refractory. Liver extracts are no longer used.

b) Response to therapy Within 8 hours after specific treatment is started, the bone marrow begins a transformation from megaloblastic to normoblastic morphology; this change is often complete within 48 hours. Serum bilirubin, lactic dehydrogenase, and iron concentration fall rapidly; indeed, the latter may fall to subnormal levels (the diagnosis of concomitant iron deficiency, however, requires the demonstration of persistent hypoferremia or diminished marrow-iron stores after several weeks of therapy). Reticulocytosis begins on the second or third day and is maximal on the fourth to twelfth day. Symptomatic improvement may occur within 1–3 days. During the period of reticulocytosis there may be significant expansion of the plasma volume as well as of the red-cell mass, so that hypervolemia may precipitate congestive heart failure in the patient with diminished cardiac reserve. The red blood cell count begins to rise after the peak reticulocytosis, reaching normal 4–8 weeks after the initiation of therapy.

3. Treatment of folic-acid deficiency anemias Folic-acid (pteroylglutamic acid) deficiency may be due to dietary inadequacy, impaired small-bowel absorption (e.g., steatorrhea, regional ileitis, extensive small-bowel resection, etc.), increased requirement (e.g., pregnancy, chronic hemolysis), or interference with utilization (as in alcoholism or therapy with antimetabolites or diphenylhydantoin). The minimum daily requirement of folic acid is probably around 50 µg, rising tenfold in the pregnant female; deficiency begins to be manifest after one month of folate deprivation, followed by full-blown megaloblastic anemia after 3–4 months. After vitamin B_{12} deficiency is excluded, patients with folate deficiency may be treated with a maintenance dose of 5 mg/day orally. Therapy must be continued indefinitely for patients with malabsorption or dietary inadequacy; 6 months of treatment is adequate for the megaloblastic anemia of pregnancy.

C. Certain anemias may also result from the deficiency or impaired utilization of specific substances (e.g., pyridoxine, vitamin E, ascorbic acid, etc.) probably necessary for maintenance of normal hemoglobin values. Although anemia is seen in patients diagnosed as having scurvy, concomitant folic acid deficiency secondary to dietary inadequacy is probably responsible.

D. Bone marrow failure exists when less than a normal number of erythrocytes is delivered to the peripheral blood (absolute marrow failure) or the marrow does not increase its production as much as would a normal marrow in response to a similar stimulus such as hemolysis or blood loss (relative marrow failure). The anemias of bone marrow failure may be divided into two major categories: (a) congenital (Fanconi's anemia) and idiopathic acquired bone marrow failure, where no antecedent cause is recognized, and (b) secondary marrow hypoproliferation, associated with renal disease, neoplasms, endocrinopathies, "collagen" diseases, myeloproliferative disorders, various hemolytic states, and exposure to ionizing radiation or chemical agents.

The anemia is generally normocytic but may be macrocytic; pancytopenia is often present, although pure red-cell aplasia may occur. The bone marrow may be morphologically hypoplastic, normocellular, or hypercellular, the last frequently associated with the presence of ringed sideroblasts on iron stain of the marrow.

Before anemia is accepted as "refractory" by some authorities, absolute or relative deficiency state is excluded by therapeutic trials with iron, vitamin B_{12}, folic acid (with or without ascorbic acid), liver extract, B-complex vitamins, pyridoxine (in pharmacologic doses), and thyroid. If the anemia is truly refractory, certain general principles of management, outlined below, are important. It should be apparent that associated failure of leukocyte and platelet production considerably worsens the prognosis.

1. Recognition and removal of the cause A careful history of exposure to chemicals and drugs should be obtained. The patient's home and place of business should be searched carefully for possible offending agents, and the patient must be instructed to avoid all potentially toxic chemicals and drugs insofar as possible.

2. Transfusions should be administered only when necessary, so that complications such as hepatitis, hemosiderosis, and isoimmunization are minimized. Chronic anemia is generally tolerated well, and transfusion is usually not necessary unless the hemoglobin concentration falls below 6–7 gm/100 ml or the patient has distressing symptoms such as angina pectoris or congestive heart failure at a higher hemoglobin concentration. Cross-matching, including direct and indirect Coombs' tests, should be done with extreme care, since sensitization to minor blood groups may occur after repeated transfusions. Buffy-coat-poor or washed red blood cells are of value in minimizing the distressing isoimmune reactions to leukocyte, platelet, or serum-protein antigens in the donor blood.

3. Treatment of infection and hemorrhage Infections should be treated vigorously with appropriate antibiotics, but prophylactic administration of antibiotics should be discouraged. Hemorrhagic manifestations, usually due to thrombocytopenia, are often difficult to control; but reduction in bleeding may follow transfusion of platelet concentrates or, occasionally, administration of corticosteroids (e.g., prednisone 10–20 mg daily).

4. **Corticosteroids** Remissions following the treatment of "refractory anemias" with corticosteroids are uncommon; nonetheless, a reasonable trial of therapy (prednisone 40–80 mg daily for 4 weeks) is justified in all cases; if no benefit is obtained dosage should be tapered and therapy discontinued (except see **3** above).

5. **Androgens (anabolic steroids)** One cannot predict which patients will respond to androgens; favorable responses may occur in as many as 60% of children, but results in adults are less encouraging. Nonetheless, a trial of therapy is worthwhile, since the incidence of spontaneous remissions is low and results with other forms of therapy are disappointing. As with corticosteroids the rationale for administration of androgenic agents is primarily empiric. An adequate trial of therapy should last 3–4 months, and the dosage administered should be large (e.g., testosterone enanthate 200–600 mg IM weekly; fluoxymesterone 30–40 mg/day orally; or equivalent doses of other preparations; injections are best avoided in leukopenic or thrombocytopenic patients). Virilizing side effects are not uncommon; rarely, cholestatic jaundice may occur. Anabolic steroids and glucocorticoids may be administered concurrently.

6. **Splenectomy** Precise criteria for selection of patients for splenectomy do not exist. A beneficial effect is more likely when there is shortened red-cell survival (with or without significant erythrocyte sequestration in the spleen), splenomegaly, at least partial response to administration of corticosteroids, and evidence of some bone marrow activity rather than complete aplasia.

7. **General measures** Appropriate measures should be taken to prevent bleeding and infection in the patient with pancytopenia. Toothbrushes should be soft and used gently. The stools should be kept soft, and only the softest tissues used in cleansing the perineum. Medications should be given orally whenever possible. When needle punctures are necessary, the skin should be prepared with iodine or similar antiseptics. Prophylactic isolation (reverse isolation) should be considered for hospitalized patients.

E. **Myelofibrosis** No specific treatment is available, but in general the guidelines of therapy for bone marrow failure may be followed. Blood transfusions should be given when necessary to control the anemia. Anabolic steroids may be of transient benefit in some patients, especially those with residual marrow and effective erythropoiesis, as established by ferrokinetic measurements. However, increased spleen size, hyperuricemia, and fluid retention are not uncommon with androgens. Corticosteroids may be of value when there is a hemolytic component of the anemia or when thrombocytopenia is severe.

When massive splenomegaly and severe anemia coexist it is often difficult, even with measurement of ^{51}Cr-tagged red blood cell survival and ferrokinetic studies, to determine whether myeloid metaplasia in the spleen is contributing to overall hematopoiesis at a greater rate than the rate at which the hypersplenism is causing blood destruction. Some patients have improved significantly (as manifested by reduction in spleen size, amelioration of symptoms related to hypermetabolism, and decrease in transfusion requirements) following a course of therapy with busulfan. The doses of busulfan are lower than those given in chronic myelocytic leukemia, however, since leukopenia is easily produced. Some patients have benefited transiently from irradiation of the spleen; this must be administered cautiously in small doses to minimize the risk of persistent and refractory resultant pancytopenia. Carefully planned splenectomy may be considered in patients who have significant hemolysis, who have had a favorable response to corticosteroids, and who have, as is almost always the case, evidence on isotope studies of hematopoiesis elsewhere than in the spleen. The risks of rebound thrombocytosis must be considered; they may be decreased with myelosuppressive drugs and/or heparin anticoagulation.

II. ABNORMAL RED BLOOD CELL DESTRUCTION—HEMOLYTIC ANEMIAS
Increased rates of red blood cell destruction occur in many disorders. If the shortening of erythrocyte survival is not too great and the bone marrow is able to compensate by producing more cells, red-cell counts may remain normal. Anemia results when the hemolytic process is more severe and/or the bone marrow production of erythrocytes cannot keep pace. Hemolytic disorders may be due to intracorpuscular defects of the red cell (often hereditary), to a wide variety of extracorpuscular influences (e.g., drugs, antibodies, dyssplenism, etc.) or to a combination of the two types of abnormalities. Definition of the type of hemolytic anemia is essential for effective management.

A. Intracorpuscular defects

   1. **Hereditary spherocytosis** is characterized by spherocytic erythrocytes and increased osmotic fragility and autohemolysis of the red cells. Abnormalities in the permeability of the cell to cations, heightened glycolytic rate, and membrane lipid abnormalities probably contribute to the accelerated splenic destruction of the red cells. The anemia can be cured permanently by splenectomy, although the red blood cell defect persists. Splenectomy may be justified even though patients have neither anemia nor jaundice, for complications such as cholelithiasis, short stature, and leg ulcers may be avoided. Severe aplastic crises may occur, but usually no specific therapy other than blood transfusions is required; recovery occurs in about 10 days; splenectomy should then be performed. A search for cholelithiasis prior to splenectomy is important; cholecystectomy may be performed at time of splenectomy, if indicated.

   2. **Hereditary nonspherocytic hemolytic anemias** constitute a group of disorders caused by a variety of specific, genetically determined biochemical defects of red cells. The enzymatic defects recognized to date include most of the steps in the Embden-Meyerhof glycolytic pathway, many of the steps in the hexose-monophosphate shunt pathway (especially glucose-6-phosphate dehydrogenase [G6PD] and 6-phosphogluconic dehydrogenase) and the related reaction catalyzed by glutathione reductase. In addition, glutathione deficiency has also been described. The most common disease in these groups is G6PD deficiency, present as an X-chromosome-linked trait in 13% of American Negroes. Exposure to any one of

TABLE 12-2.   Drugs That Produce Hemolysis in Patients with G6PD Deficiency

Analgesics (acetanilid, aspirin, phenacetin, etc.)

Antimalarials (chloroquine, primaquine, quinine, etc.) and congeners (quinidine, gin-and-tonic)

Chloramphenicol

Dimercaprol

Methylene blue

Naphthalene

Nitrofurans (nitrofurantoin, furazolidine, etc.)

Para-aminosalicylic acid

Phenylhydrazine

Probenecid

Sulfonamides

Sulfones

Trinitrotoluene

Water-soluble vitamin K analogs

a large number of drugs or even febrile disease states result in a self-limited hemolysis of older red cells. The drugs that have been implicated in hemolysis are included in Table 12-2. In addition, fava beans, infectious hepatitis, and other acute and chronic illnesses have been implicated. In the less commonly affected Caucasian, the hemizygous male may have more severe, and occasionally fatal, hemolytic episodes; and even the heterozygous female may be clinically affected. It should be noted that in the midst of a hemolytic episode and a brisk reticulocytosis, the diagnosis may be masked by the relatively high enzyme activity of the young cells. Hemolysis of transfused blood from a G6PD-deficient donor may be seen in a transfusion recipient taking, for example, a sulfonamide.

In contrast to the predictably good response to splenectomy in hereditary spherocytosis, the anemia of pyruvate kinase deficiency is only partially corrected by splenectomy. Splenectomy is useless in G6PD deficiency and related hexose-monophosphate shunt pathway defects.

3. Sickle-cell anemia   There is no specific therapy; complications of the disease must be treated as they arise. Maintenance of adequate hemoglobin levels and tissue oxygenation, however, may reduce the incidence of certain complications. The frequency of crises may be reduced in some patients by partial exchange transfusions given at about six-week intervals to maintain the population of normal red blood cells at 15–40%. However, a prolonged program of such exchange is seldom practicable. Healing of leg ulcers may be accelerated and hematuria may cease after transfusions and bed rest. During painful crises analgesics should be given as required; nasal oxygen should be administered intermittently (so as not to depress erythropoiesis) ; and fluid balance must be maintained; excessive narcosis should be avoided, since the resultant respiratory depression and hypoxia may augment intravascular sickling. There is no evidence that transfusion of blood decreases the duration of a painful crisis, which usually subsides in less than one week. Aplastic crises are less common than painful crises; they usually occur in children and may be fatal. Marrow function usually returns within several days, but aplasia may persist as long as 2–3 weeks. During this interval transfusions should be administered as required. Frequent aplastic crises in a patient with sickle-cell disease or increased requirements for transfusion should suggest the possibility of concomitant folic acid depletion; 5 mg folic acid daily may be given for prophylactic therapy.

Certain infections, particularly salmonella osteomyelitis or septicemia, occur with increased frequency in patients with sickle-cell disease and should be treated vigorously. Surgery for such complications as cholelithiasis, priapism, etc., is associated with an increased morbidity and mortality; the importance of carefully administered anesthesia and maintenance of oxygenation cannot be overemphasized. Pregnancy is associated with a higher maternal and fetal mortality rate than in normal women; pregnant patients must be followed closely and, ideally, transfused to a hematocrit of 35% three weeks before delivery. Genetic counseling is important.

4. **The thalassemias** are characterized by an underproduction of normally occurring globin chains of hemoglobin, by "ineffective erythropoiesis," and by accelerated extramedullary destruction of red cells. No specific therapy is available for thalassemia major; therapy is unnecessary for most patients with thalassemia minor or intermedia. Survival to early adulthood has been reported in patients with thalassemia major whose complications are managed with extreme care. Transfusions are given as needed to avoid the major symptoms of anemia, but they should be given sparingly to minimize iron overload. Medications containing iron should be carefully avoided. The value of therapy of the cardiac and hepatic manifestations of hemosiderosis with iron-chelating drugs remains to be established. Congestive heart failure and cardiac arrhythmias, often due to hemosiderosis, should be managed appropriately. Serious infections are common and must be promptly recognized and adequately treated. The possibility of secondary folic acid deficiency should be kept in mind. Splenectomy may be beneficial when evidence of marked hypersplenism and increasing transfusion requirements are present; this operation should be deferred past early childhood because of the probably increased susceptibility of children to severe bacterial infections after splenectomy. Although patients with thalassemia major may have episodes of severe abdominal pain of unknown causation mimicking an acute surgical abdomen, surgical intervention should be avoided, if possible, because of the increased morbidity and mortality.

5. **Paroxysmal nocturnal hemoglobinuria** Therapeutic measures of importance are directed at prevention and management of the three major complications, i.e., thrombosis, infection, and aplastic and/or hemolytic crises. Infusion of 1000 ml of 6% low-molecular-weight dextran may be helpful in controlling hemolysis as an initial measure during crises, but hemorrhagic manifestations may occur after repeated use. When transfusions are required, packed red blood cells carefully washed with saline should be used, since

plasma may cause massive hemolysis by mechanisms not clear. Splenectomy is seldom of value in controlling the disease but may be beneficial when massive splenomegaly and hypersplenism are present; postsplenectomy thrombocytosis, however, will increase the tendency to thrombosis. Oral administration of androgens (e.g., fluoxymesterone, 20–30 mg daily) may be beneficial by stimulating erythropoiesis and, perhaps, reducing hemolysis. Anticoagulation with a coumarin derivative may decrease the incidence of thrombotic complications, but heparin administration probably should be avoided because this drug may increase hemolysis. Corticosteroids have not been demonstrated to be of value.

Because of the loss of hemoglobin and hemosiderin in the urine, patients may become iron-deficient. Iron should then be given if deficiency is clearly established, although such therapy may transiently increase hemolysis.

B. Extracorpuscular abnormalities

1. **Hemolytic anemias with autoantibodies (autoimmune hemolytic anemia, AHA)** Included in this category are a heterogeneous group of disorders characterized by the presence on the surface of the patient's red cells (and/or in his serum) of one or more immune globulins that are detectable by a positive reaction with antihuman globulin (Coombs') serum. The anemia may be subdivided into symptomatic (secondary) AHA or idiopathic AHA. Symptomatic AHA includes those cases in which the anemia is secondary to an identifiable underlying disease or therapy (neoplastic hematopoietic disorders such as chronic lymphocytic leukemia; collagen diseases; drugs such as penicillin and methyldopa; and miscellaneous conditions such as carcinoma, sarcoid, primary atypical pneumonia, infectious mononucleosis, ovarian cysts, etc.); idiopathic AHA comprises the 20–70% of cases in which no underlying disease or associated disorder can be demonstrated.

The coating globulins most commonly are 7S "incomplete" gamma globulins reacting with red cells at body temperature, 37°C (warm antibodies), or 19S macroglobulins reacting optimally at 4–10°C (cold antibodies); the latter may occur as agglutinins (in association with primary atypical pneumonia or chronic cold hemagglutinin disease) or as hemolysins (in paroxysmal cold hemoglobinuria). Patients with cold antibodies tend to respond less well to administration of corticosteroids or splenectomy; they should avoid exposure to low temperatures.

Therapy in symptomatic AHA should be directed at control of the underlying disease process, although more specific measures, as described below, may become necessary. Therapy in idiopathic AHA should be specifically directed at decreasing the rate of red blood cell destruction.

a) **Corticosteroids** are the drugs of choice. Initial dosage, though determined by the severity of the hemolytic process, is usually in the range of 60–100 mg prednisone daily. Therapy should be continued for 1–3 weeks before it is decided that steroids will not be of benefit. If remission occurs, the corticosteroid dosage should be reduced slowly over a 6–8-week period, then discontinued or kept at the minimum dosage necessary to maintain that remission, optimally at a level of 10 mg or less of prednisone per day to avoid complications of therapy. Prolonged therapy may be required; on occasion small doses of corticosteroids must be administered indefinitely. Approximately 65–70% of patients (particularly those with warm antibodies) given adequate dosage of steroids will have a complete (though often transient) remission; 15% show no benefit and the remainder have a partial response. ACTH has no advantages over glucocorticoids.

b) **Splenectomy** should be considered for patients who are not benefited by corticosteroids or who require high-dosage corticosteroids (e.g., prednisone greater than 10–20 mg daily) for 6 months or longer in order to maintain control of the disease. Splenectomy is more likely to be of benefit when warm rather than cold antibodies are present. The value of measurement of splenic uptake of ^{51}Cr-labeled red cells and of spleen size in predicting response to splenectomy has been questioned in a recent comprehensive study. Transient improvement is common after splenectomy; the operation carries a small but significant risk. About 50% of patients have a permanent remission. In nonresponders to splenectomy resumption of steroid therapy may be of value.

c) **Immunosuppressive drugs** Agents that suppress antibody formation (e.g., 6-mercaptopurine, azathioprine, cyclophosphamide, thioguanine, nitrogen mustard, chlorambucil) may rarely be beneficial in the treatment of AHA that persists after corticosteroid therapy and splenectomy; their use is discussed in Chapter 13.

d) **Blood transfusions** should be avoided if possible; benefits from transfusion is transient because of rapid destruction of transfused cells. Typing and cross-matching may become extremely difficult; minor-blood-group sensitization is not uncommon and may aggravate the hemolytic process; and, finally, tissue-iron overload may occur with repeated transfusions.

2. **Acquired hemolytic anemia without autoantibodies (Coombs' negative)** Management is directed at recognition and treatment of the underlying or associated disease.

Malaria and bartonellosis, which cause hemolytic anemia by direct parasitic infestation of the erythrocyte, may be recognized by examination of the peripheral blood or bone marrow; treatment of either disease cures the hemolytic anemia. Cold agglutinins may appear in as many as 90% of patients with severe primary atypical pneumonia, but severe hemolytic anemia is a rare concomitant; if hemolysis does occur it is usually self-limiting, but on occasion corticosteroids may be required for control; rarely, transfusion of blood prewarmed to 37°C is necessary. The hemolytic anemia occasionally associated with infectious mononucleosis also is transient and self-limiting, but when severe may require treatment with corticosteroids. Acute hemolytic episodes may also occur in association with infections due to *Clostridium welchii, Vibrio comma,* and rarely other bacteria. Paroxysmal cold hemoglobinuria may be idiopathic or occur in association with syphilis.

A variety of chemical agents and drugs may also cause hemolysis in normal individuals; therapy is nonspecific and consists mainly of preventing further exposure to the offending agent. On occasion, chelating agents may be beneficial, as for example the administration of versenate for the treatment of patients with lead poisoning. Hemolytic anemias may also be caused by physical injury (severe burns, heart prostheses, or scarred heart valves), or occur in association with a wide variety of diseases (neoplasms, lymphomas, renal disease, etc.) ; therapy should be supportive and directed to treatment of the primary disease.

III. **ANEMIAS ASSOCIATED WITH SPECIFIC DISEASE STATES** The anemia of **infection** is usually normocytic and normochromic. Impaired erythrocyte production combined with decreased erythrocyte survival and diminished reutilization of iron from hemoglobin catabolism are the underlying mechanisms of this anemia. It does not respond to the administration of iron or other hematinic agents, but hemoglobin values usually return to normal after adequate treatment of the underlying disease.

Many factors may play a role in the anemia associated with **chronic liver disease.** Red blood cell constants are usually macrocytic; leukopenia and thrombocytopenia may also occur if congestive splenomegaly leads to functional hypersplenism. Both diminished production and excessive destruction of red blood cells may contribute to the anemia. Occult loss of blood in the stool is common, and iron deficiency may complicate the picture. Folic acid deficiency frequently plays a role in the pathogenesis of the anemia, usually in malnourished alcoholic patients with cirrhosis.

Anemia is a constant finding in patients with **chronic renal insufficiency** and azotemia; erythrokinetic studies usually show both accelerated destruction and diminished production of erythrocytes. Red blood cell constants are usually normochromic and normocytic. Acute hemolytic episodes may rarely occur. No specific therapy is available, although those few patients who have an associated iron deficiency may benefit from iron. Response to folic acid has been reported in the occasional patient with megaloblastic anemia, especially after hemodialysis.

The anemia associated with **rheumatoid arthritis** is either hypochromic or normochromic, and normocytic; an increased rate of red blood cell destruction, diminished capacity of the bone marrow to meet the increased demand, and defective utilization of iron in erythropoiesis may all play a role in pathogenesis. No specific therapy is available except splenectomy for hypersplenism in Felty's syndrome.

The anemia of **malignancy** is similar to the anemia associated with infection; other mechanisms which may contribute, however, include blood loss, invasion of bone marrow by malignant cells, hemolysis, and rarely folic acid deficiency. No satisfactory therapy is available, although the anemia may respond with successful treatment of the underlying disease process. Transfusions should be given as required. From 25–60% of patients with **myxedema** may have an anemia, usually mild, morphologically macrocytic or normocytic, and most often normochromic. Red blood cell production is decreased, and the anemia responds slowly to the administration of thyroid. Associated deficiencies of iron and vitamin B_{12} are not uncommon; these respond to the usual therapy.

During **pregnancy** the hemoglobin concentration begins to decrease after the eighth week of gestation and becomes stationary between the sixteenth and twenty-second weeks; this mild physiologic "anemia" of pregnancy occurs because plasma volume increases to a greater degree than does the total red blood cell volume. More severe anemias (hemoglobin less than 10 gm/100 ml) are usually hypochromic and microcytic, and reflect iron deficiency. The prophylactic administration of iron (40 mg/day) during pregnancy usually prevents serious anemia and is widely recommended. Megaloblastic anemia of pregnancy is less common than iron deficiency in this country and responds to the administration of folic acid, 5 mg daily.

IV.   BLOOD TRANSFUSION

A.   Indications

1. **Acute blood loss** is the most important indication for transfusion of whole blood to restore the blood volume after massive bleeding. Following acute blood loss the hemoglobin or hematocrit value will not accurately reflect the degree of blood loss until fluid shifts occur.

2. **Hypoplastic anemia or bone marrow failure**   Transfusions of packed red blood cells should be given in order to maintain the hemoglobin concentration at a level that permits adequate organ perfusion and reasonable freedom from symptoms (usually 6–8 gm/100 ml). The hemoglobin level need not be restored completely to normal. The bleeding manifestations of concomitant thrombocytopenia may be brought under control with administration of platelet concentrates.

3. **Hemolytic anemia**   In general, transfusions should be avoided whenever possible. If the patient becomes symptomatic from a rapid fall in hemoglobin concentration associated with an acute hemolytic episode or temporary bone marrow hypoplasia, transfusion with packed red blood cells will be necessary.

4. **Other specific indications**   Healing of leg ulcers in patients with **sickle-cell anemia** may be promoted by restoring the hemoglobin value nearly to normal in conjunction with bed rest and local wound care. Patients with **severe renal insufficiency** maintain optimal renal plasma flow when the hematocrit is kept between 22% and 27%. Transfusion is also indicated when severe anemia causes or aggravates such symptoms as cerebrovascular insufficiency or angina pectoris. Fresh normal whole blood or plasma may be used as a source of deficient coagulation factors such as fibrinogen, prothrombin, and factors V and VIII; the other, more stable factors are found in stored blood as well.

B.   Complications and dangers

1. **Cardiac failure**   Patients with borderline cardiac compensation should be given blood cautiously through a venous pressure set; monitoring the central venous pressure may avert difficulty. Packed red blood cells rather than whole blood should be given. It is usually advisable to digitalize such patients before transfusion.

2. **Febrile reactions**   Many febrile reactions are produced by antibodies to leukocytes and less often to platelets or plasma proteins in patients who have received multiple transfusions. Reactions often may be prevented by removing the plasma and the buffy coat after the red blood cells have sedimented. For patients who have had severe reactions it may be advisable to sediment the erythrocytes in dextran and then remove the leukocyte-rich plasma. Administration of an antihistamine usually does not prevent these febrile reactions. Febrile reactions may also result from contamination of transfusion equipment with pyrogenic material.

3. **Allergic reactions,** as manifested by urticaria, are relatively common, but asthma and vascular collapse are rare. Administration of an antihistamine, e.g., diphenhydramine (Benadryl), 50 mg orally prior to transfusion may prevent or lessen the severity of such reactions.

4. **Bacterial contamination** of blood is extremely rare in modern blood banks, but this complication produces severe reactions with high mortality rates. If such a reaction is suspected the transfusion should be stopped immediately; the remaining donor blood should be examined under the microscope (after gram-staining) and cultured at 4°, 20°, and 37°C. Appropriate antibiotics and supportive care for shock, etc., should be given.

5. **Transmission of disease** At least 0.5% of patients transfused with 1000 ml or more will develop clinically apparent viral hepatitis. The reported incidence of posttransfusion hepatitis varies and depends on numerous factors including the number of transfusions given, the source of the blood (e.g., professional donor vs. family member), the completeness of follow-up, and whether anicteric as as well as icteric cases are discovered. The reported incidence of anicteric cases has been as high as 87 cases per 1000 units of blood transfused. Pooled plasma and plasma fractions multiply the risks of infection with hepatitis virus.

   Syphilis, malaria, and brucellosis are rarely transmitted by blood transfusion.

6. **Citrate intoxication** is extremely rare. It may occur in infants receiving exchange transfusions and in normal adults given more than 2000 ml citrated blood rapidly (in 30 minutes or less); adults with severe liver disease or undergoing operations under hypothermia may develop citrate intoxication with smaller amounts of blood. The clinical manifestations resemble those of hypocalcemia. If more than 2000 ml of blood must be given rapidly, 10 ml 10% calcium gluconate should be injected IV into a different vein for each subsequent 1000 ml blood transfused.

7. **Excessive bleeding** that follows massive transfusion, exchange transfusion, or extracorporeal circulation is in part related to the decrease in number of competent circulating platelets, with variable additional defects in the coagulation mechanism.

8. **Potassium intoxication** Normally, red blood cells contain 100 mEq of potassium per liter (of packed red cells); plasma contains 4–5 mEq/L. When whole blood has been stored for 10 days, the K+ concentration in the plasma is 15 mEq/L and after 28 days it is about 30 mEq/L. To minimize red blood cell destruction and potassium release when transfusions must be given to patients with hyperkalemia or renal insufficiency, fresh blood or blood stored less than 5 days should be given.

9. **Transfusion hemosiderosis** A large number of transfusions given to a patient who is not bleeding will lead to accumulation of large stores of iron, since each unit of blood contains 200–250 mg iron.

10. **Air embolism** is very rare with the widespread use of plastic bags for blood administration but may occur on exposure of veins for cannulation. Normal adults may tolerate as much as 200 ml air IV, but for seriously ill patients as little as 10 ml air may be fatal. A

patient sustaining venous air embolism should be placed in a head-down, feet-up position on his left side.

11. **Hemolytic transfusion reactions** are serious; diagnosis and therapy must be prompt. When such a reaction is suspected, the transfusion should be stopped and the following investigative and therapeutic measures carried out.

a) Clinical manifestations of intravascular hemolysis:

   i) Phase I (immediate) symptoms, which usually begin after 50 ml or less of blood have been given, include a throbbing headache, severe lumbar pain (almost pathognomonic), precordial pain, dyspnea, anxiety, and restlessness. Hemolytic reactions may occur, however, with few or no symptoms, especially in obtunded or anesthetized patients. Objective signs include flushed face, then cyanosis; distended neck veins; initial slowing of the pulse followed by a rapid and thready beat; diaphoresis; cold, clammy skin; and then profound shock, usually within an hour. Bleeding may follow disseminated intravascular coagulation, presumably from release of erythrocytic thromboplastic substances.

   ii) Phase II (interval) For an interval of several hours to days the patient appears symptomatically improved. Objectively, however, there is hemoglobinemia, hemoglobinuria, and occasionally jaundice. Oliguria or anuria may supervene.

   iii) Phase III (acute renal failure) This is not an invariable concomitant of intravascular hemolysis and may reflect prior renal disease or a period of hypotension or acidosis, as well as hemoglobinuria. If proper therapy is instituted patients may survive acute renal failure. Management is discussed in Chapter 3.

b) Investigative procedures

   i) Save the remaining donor blood for further testing.

   ii) Draw a sample of venous blood from the patient. These two samples can then be used for regrouping and a search for a hemolytic antibody by direct and indirect Coombs' test.

   iii) Attempt to demonstrate hemolysis by obtaining a venous blood sample from the patient's opposite arm. Use a large needle and allow the blood to flow freely into a versene or liquid citrate (prothrombin time) tube. After gentle centrifugation the plasma may be examined by hand spectroscopy or quantitative methods for the presence of free hemoglobin. If more than 6 hours have elapsed before the sample is drawn, increased bilirubin and methemalbumin and decreased or absent haptoglobin levels may be measured.

c) Treatment

   i) Immediate If there is any doubt about symptoms suggestive of transfusion reaction, stop the blood at once without awaiting development of further symptoms.

   ii) Phase I If hypotension develops, give adequate amounts of compatible blood (after a blood sample has been obtained for the studies previously outlined) or other fluids in order to restore the circulating blood volume. Vasopressor drugs should be used if necessary, but they will be poorly effective if hypovolemia is a major problem. Infusions of mannitol (as described in Chapter 3) have been used by some observers in an attempt to prevent the development of renal failure.

- iii) **Phase II** In the presence of oliguria it is important to limit fluid intake to insensible losses plus other fluid output. Do not give fluids, either orally or parenterally, that contain potassium. Maintain adequate nutrition and electrolyte balance, but do not "push fluids" in an attempt to force damaged kidneys to function.
- iv) **Phase III** The management of acute renal failure is discussed in Chapter 3.

C. Emergency transfusions There is seldom enough delay in typing and cross-matching to warrant the administration of possibly incompatible blood; the administration of saline or plasma expanders, such as dextran, while blood is being prepared offers less danger than the administration of unselected Type O Rh-negative (universal donor) blood to which has been added Witebsky A and B substances (to absorb A and B agglutinins). Witebsky substance does not absorb all antibodies, and dangerous hemolytic reactions may still occur—for example, the incomplete (IgG) anti-A which is often found in high titer in persons previously treated with antisera such as antitetanus serum is not absorbed by Witebsky A substance.

In rare situations, as in acute blood loss with severe shock, it may be necessary to transfuse the patient before proper cross-matching can be done. If that is the case, O-negative blood of measured low titers of anti-A and anti-B can be used. Such blood is available in many blood banks for this use. If just a few units are to be given it is not necessary to add Witebsky A and B substances; however, when many units of blood must be given, these substances should be used, with the reservations noted in the previous paragraph. After a patient has been given many units of O-negative blood, it may be preferable to continue his transfusions during that episode with O-negative blood; switching to A blood, for example, if the recipient is found to be type A, might result in hemolysis of the A blood by the anti-A antibodies added during the O-negative blood transfusions.

It is also possible, if the recipient is a male or a postmenopausal female who is known never to have had blood transfusions in the past, to use O-positive blood in a similar fashion as described above. Although some hemolysis may occur after a number of days (if the recipient should be Rh negative) because of production of anti-Rh antibody, such hemolysis is relatively minor and not life-threatening.

In circumstances where the recipient's blood type is known but there is no time for cross-matching, or the less common type B or AB blood is unavailable immediately, uncrossmatched Rh negative blood may be given, subject to the reservations noted above, according to the following scheme:

Recipient	Donor
O	O
B	O (with B substance added)
A	A
AB	A (with B substance added)

If B substance is unavailable, Witebsky A and B substance can be used, with the knowledge that elevated anti-A titers will be induced in the type-B recipients.

BLEEDING DISORDERS

The diagnostic label "bleeding disorder" both frightens the patient and alarms the physician. A clear picture of the related physiologic systems that maintain the normal balance between hemorrhage and thrombosis is shrouded in complexity. While the necessary complete characterization of a problem of disordered hemostasis requires the skills of a specialized and frequently not readily available laboratory, the initial formulation of the problem and appropriate immediate therapeutic maneuvers can be made by the thoughtful physician backed by a reliable clinical laboratory. The purpose of this section is twofold: to outline the nature and interpretation of studies that can be carried out as part of the initial work-up and to discuss briefly the most common bleeding disorders, their diagnosis, and their immediate therapy. The details of the extensive investigations that should eventually be done to confirm the initial impression and the long-term management of these difficult and often protracted clinical situations are presented in the many excellent standard texts of bleeding disorders.

I. CLINICAL STUDIES

A. History The following details of the bleeding should be ascertained:

1. The date of onset of any bleeding problems and the details of previous bleeding episodes (or, equally significant, their absence despite surgical procedures, etc.). Onset of clinical bleeding in adult life does not preclude a congenital defect in coagulation.

2. Family history of bleeding disorders.

3. Associated medical history—e.g., underlying diseases (uremia, cirrhosis, malignant disease, collagen disorders, etc.), drugs, transfusions, etc.

4. Type of bleeding: For example, the characteristic (though by no means invariable) picture of bleeding secondary to a congenital clotting factor deficiency includes spontaneous bleeding into deep tissues (joints, muscles, viscera, CNS) and severe but delayed hemorrhage postoperatively. Vascular and platelet diseases, on the other hand, most often present with spontaneous bleeding into the skin, mucous membranes, and from cuts and venipunctures.

B. Laboratory studies

1. **Bleeding time** The Ivy method should be used; bleeding for longer than 7–10 minutes suggests a disorder of platelet number or function or of capillary integrity.

2. **Platelet count** A quantitative measure by direct count using phase-contrast microscopy should be carried out.

3. **Prothrombin time** In this test, tissue thromboplastin (usually a brain extract) is added to plasma to measure the integrity of the so-called "extrinsic" clotting system (Fig. 12-1).

4. **Partial thromboplastin time** This test is performed in a manner similar to the prothrombin time, except an "incomplete" thromboplastin (cephalin) is substituted for the whole brain extract.

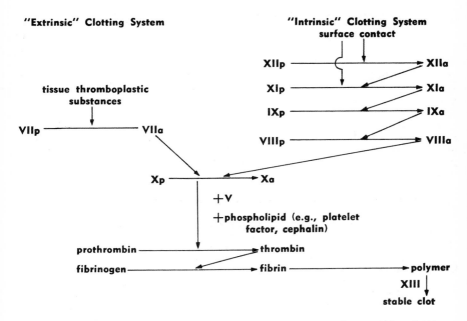

Fig. 12-1. *p* represents precursor or inactive form of the clotting factor; *a* represents the active form. Calcium ion is required at a number of steps in both the "intrinsic" and "extrinsic" clotting sequences.

Kaolin is usually added to the test system in order to ensure complete activation of the "contact" factors (XI and XII). These modifications allow assay of the "intrinsic" clotting system (see Fig. 12-1).

5. **Measurement of fibrinogen** is important in the increasingly commonly recognized states of consumption coagulopathy and enhanced fibrinolysis (see below).

   a) **Fi test** A simple slide agglutination test that will allow recognition of fibrinogen levels below 100 mg/100 ml (normal 250–400) by the absence of agglutination is available.

   b) **Thrombin time** The addition of standardized amounts of commercial thrombin to plasma will cause clotting within a period of time inversely related to the fibrinogen concentration of the plasma. Both tests can give spurious values, however, in the presence of fibrinogen breakdown products resulting from heightened fibrinolysis.

6. **Fibrinolysis** can be assessed by the time taken for the clot formed in whole blood or in the thrombin-time tubes to lyse at 37°C. Dissolution of the clot in several hours indicates clinically important fibrinolysis.

7. Detection of circulating anticoagulants This test should be made a part of every bleeding disorder evaluation. Most simply, a 1:1 mixture of the patient's plasma and normal plasma can be used in the prothrombin time, partial thromboplastin time, or thrombin time. The 50% concentration of normal plasma is adequate to correct for any factor deficiencies in the patient's plasma yet will not sufficiently dilute circulating anticoagulants to correct the tests.

Note: Of the clinically encountered bleeding disorders, only factor XIII deficiency would not be recognized by one or more of the above tests. Once these tests had indicated the correct diagnostic category, the appropriate factor assays or other detailed studies should be carried out by a specialized clotting laboratory. The results of the above tests in specific deficiency states are given in Table 12-3.

II. CLASSIFICATION OF CLINICAL BLEEDING DISORDERS

A. Congenital clotting factor deficiencies Table 12-4 describes the properties of the individual factors and the characteristics of their deficiency states. As noted, the clinical expression of these disorders is variable. Common to the clotting factors is their participation in reinforcing the platelet plug initially formed at bleeding sites. In their absence, therefore, late bleeding after surgical or other types of trauma and injury may be expected, for the fragile platelet plug will be unable to progress to a permanent clot. Specialized features of the individual deficiency states are described in the standard texts. Therapy can be achieved by fresh whole blood or plasma, or fresh frozen plasma if the exact defect is unknown (see Table 12-3). If the patient is a known classical hemophiliac (factor VIII deficiency), however, the use of cryoprecipitate is indicated, for by using this readily available concentrate a large amount of factor VIII can be delivered in a small volume. To prepare cryoprecipitate, fresh whole blood is centrifuged in the cold, and the plasma is drawn off and rapidly frozen within the plastic bag by packing the container in crushed CO_2 snow (Dry Ice) for 10–15 minutes until the plasma is frozen. Thawing is then allowed in the refrigerator (approximately 4°C) for 18–24 hours. The plastic bag is then spun for 15 minutes at 2000 g in a refrigerated centrifuge, the supernatant plasma removed, and the precipitate-containing bag stored in the freezer. For use, 10 ml sterile citrated saline (commercially available) is used to dissolve the precipitate, and the solution is administered intravenously. A filter set is commonly employed for administration because of the persistence of undissolved material in the solution, although this does diminish the net yield of AHG in the concentrate. Protective levels of factor VIII (i.e., a concentration greater than 20% of normal in the patient's blood during most of the day) can be achieved in the adult hemophiliac by the rapid initial infusion of 15–30 bags of reconstituted cryoprecipitate followed by maintenance infusion of 10–15 bags rapidly twice daily for 1 to 1½ weeks in the case of severe bleeding or after surgical procedures. Relatively minor bleeding (small cuts, etc.) can be controlled by less vigorous therapy.

Vascular hemophilia (von Willebrand's disease) represents a special case of an inherited deficiency state. In this common disorder there is a dual defect: platelet adhesiveness is reduced (accounting for the prolonged bleeding time) and factor VIII levels are low, usually in

TABLE 12-3. Results of Laboratory Tests in Hereditary Deficiency States

Factor	Synonyms	Prothrombin Time	Partial Thromboplastin Time	Thrombin Time	Bleeding Time
I	Fibrinogen	P	P	P	N
II	Prothrombin	P	P	N	N
V	Proaccelerin, labile factor	P	P	N	N
VII	Proconvertin, stable factor	P	N	N	N
VIII	Antihemophilic factor (AHF)	N	P	N	N
IX	Christmas factor, plasma thromboplastin component (PTC)	N	P	N	N
X	Stuart (-Prower) factor	P	P	N	N
XI	Plasma thromboplastin antecedent (PTA)	N	P	N	N
XII	Hageman factor	N	P	N	N
XIII	Fibrin-stabilizing factor (FSF)	N	N	N	N
Vascular hemophilia (von Willebrand's disease)		N	P or N	N	P
Platelet deficiency (quantitative or qualitative)		N	N	N	P

P, prolonged; N, normal.

Factor V deficiency cannot be distinguished by these tests from prothrombin deficiency, but the latter is exceptionally rare as a congenital defect.

Deficiency of factors VIII, IX, XI, and XII cannot be differentiated by these tests. The last is almost never associated with spontaneous bleeding; the first three can all be corrected with fresh blood or plasma or fresh frozen plasma if the past history or family history does not allow differentiation among the disorders (see Table 12-4).

TABLE 12-4. Characteristics of Clotting Factors and Hereditary Deficiency States

Factor	In Vivo Half Life (hrs)	Inheritance Pattern	Present in Bank Plasma	Concentrate Available	Clinical Characteristics of Inherited Deficiency§
I	100	Autosomal recessive	Yes	Yes*	Severe postoperative but rarely spontaneous bleeding
II	50–72	Autosomal recessive	Yes	Yes†	Variable bleeding picture
V	20–40	Autosomal recessive	No	No	Mild spontaneous bleeding (epistaxis and menorrhagia) and postoperative bleeding
VII	4–6	Autosomal recessive	Yes	Yes†	May present as severe spontaneous or postoperative bleeding
VIII	10–20	Sex-linked recessive	No	Yes‡	Mild to severe spontaneous (especially joint, muscle, viscera, CNS) and postoperative bleeding
IX	25–30	Sex-linked recessive	Yes	Yes†	Same as VIII
X	25–50'	Autosomal recessive	Yes	Yes†	Moderate to severe spontaneous and postoperative bleeding
XI	40–80	Autosomal recessive	Yes	No	Seldom severe spontaneous bleeding (bruising, menorrhagia)

XII	50	Autosomal recessive	Yes	No	Very rarely significant clinical bleeding (traumatic or postoperative only)
XIII	100–150	Autosomal recessive	Yes	No	May be severe, especially spontaneous CNS and postnatal umbilical bleeding
Vascular hemophilia (von Willebrand's disease)	?	Autosomal dominant	See text	—	Common disorder; most often mild with bruising, mucosal hemorrhage and menorrhagia; may mimic hemophilia clinically

* Commercial fibrinogen concentrate available.

† These factors can be concentrated in a chromatographically separable fraction of fresh plasma (see *New Eng. J. Med.* 273:667, 1965).

‡ Present in commercial fibrinogen concentrate but preferably administered as a concentrate prepared from fresh plasma by cryo-precipitation (see text).

§ The commonest clinical manifestations are tabulated; however, variability in presentation prevents reliable identification of a specific deficiency state from the clinical picture alone.

the range of 5% to 15% of normal. Clinical bleeding correlates with the severity of the factor VIII deficiency, and initial therapy is similar to that of the hemophiliac, though less factor VIII is usually required. Unique to von Willebrand's disease, however, is the slow rise in factor VIII level seen after the infusion of normal (or even classical hemophilic!) bank plasma, which is itself devoid of factor VIII. Probably the plasma supplies some missing ingredient that allows the patient with von Willebrand's disease to synthesize his own factor VIII. The clinical importance of this observation is that in the bleeding patient with this disorder, factor VIII concentrate is required initially to control bleeding; if, however, the patient receives bank plasma as well on admission, he will no longer need precious cryoprecipitate after 24 hours and can be managed by the daily transfusion of several units of bank plasma.

B. Acquired deficiency states

1. **Deficiency of the vitamin K-dependent factors (II, VII, IX, X)** This state should be considered in the bleeding patient with disease of the hepatobiliary system or with intestinal malabsorption, and in the patient using coumarin or indanedione anticoagulants. Therapy with vitamin K_1 should be effective in all these conditions except those associated with hepatocellular dysfunction, in which case the liver is often unable to respond to vitamin K. In this situation replacement therapy may be effective. The patient with liver disease may, however, bleed for a number of reasons (thrombocytopenia, abnormalities of the fibrinolytic system, consumption coagulopathy, deficiency of one or more clotting factors). Therapy that corrects only one defect may therefore be inadequate to halt clinical bleeding.

2. **Consumption coagulopathy and fibrinolysis** An increasing number of clinical situations are being recognized in which severe bleeding is associated with low concentrations of one or more of the following: platelets, fibrinogen, prothrombin, and factors V and VIII. Common to all these clotting components is that they are the only ones used up (or consumed) in the process of coagulation. Therefore, despite the fact that thrombi are frequently absent both clinically and pathologically, the disorder characterized by the combined deficiency of the above factors is described as consumption coagulopathy (or intravascular coagulation). Diagnosis of the state is made difficult because all the factors may not be depressed at any given moment. For example, rebound elevation of factor VIII may be seen while the platelet count is still low. Moreover, the fibrinolytic system is often active in the consumption coagulopathies, and differentiation from isolated fibrinolysis is frequently impossible. The diagnosis is further complicated by the fact that fibrinolysis, without concomitant consumption coagulopathy, can cause proteolysis of fibrinogen and factors V and VIII. The lowered platelet count and very low level of fibrinogen are the two most helpful distinguishing features of consumption coagulopathy.

   a) **The clinical settings** in which consumption coagulopathy has been described include infections (meningococcemia, gram-negative sepsis, malaria, Rocky Mountain spotted fever), malignant diseases (carcinomatosis, acute granulocytic leukemia), obstetric complications (abruptio placentae, retained dead fetus, amniotic fluid embolism, septic abortion), cirrhosis, hemolytic anemia, snakebite, large-vessel clotting (venous thromboses, Kasabach-Merritt syndrome), drug therapy (ristocetin), operations and postoperatively (especially pulmonary surgery or the use of extracorporeal circulation), heatstroke, and probably in a poorly understood group of diseases that include thrombotic thrombocytopenia purpura, the hemolytic-uremic syndrome, and purpura fulminans.

b) **The treatment of bleeding episodes** in such cases is difficult and largely empirical. In situations in which the duration of the presumed stimulus to activation of the clotting system is limited, as in obstetric complications, fresh whole blood may tide the patient over the hemorrhage. In other cases in which the consumption coagulopathy is uncomplicated by concomitant fibrinolysis, the use of heparin alone is effective. Fibrinolytic states without evidence of consumption coagulopathy may be treated with antifibrinolytic agents such as epsilon-aminocaproic acid (EACA) or Trasylol. In the all too common situation in which both fibrinolysis and consumption coagulopathy seem to be present or cannot be differentiated, the patient should be treated first with heparin and then with an antifibrinolytic agent. Use of the agents in reverse order, or the employment of EACA alone, may block compensatory fibrinolysis and allow intravascular coagulation to proceed unchecked with disastrous consequences. The cessation of bleeding may be hastened, once heparinization has been achieved, by replacement of the depleted factors by infusing fresh plasma or whole blood or commercial fibrinogen concentrates.

3. **Thrombocytopenia** Acquired thrombocytopenia is considerably more common than either congenital thrombocytopenia or the rare qualitative defects in platelet function without thrombocytopenia. Lowered platelet counts can be either idiopathic or secondary to such conditions as liver disease with hypersplenism (or other causes of splenomegaly), infiltrative or hypoplastic bone marrow diseases, infections (viral, bacterial, and protozoan), systemic lupus erythematosus and related diseases, massive transfusion with stored bank blood, and drugs (quinine and congeners such as found in gin-and-tonic, barbiturates, sulfonamides, and such related compounds as thiazide diuretics and others). Clinically, purpura, ecchymosis, bleeding into the hollow viscera, and central nervous system hemorrhage may be seen.

Therapy should be directed toward the underlying disorder, if one is present. In idiopathic thrombocytopenic purpura, common in females and persons under 40 years of age, the likelihood of spontaneous remission varies inversely with age at onset. Adults may be given a trial of prednisone, 40–60 mg/day, for up to 3–4 weeks. If a response is obtained withdraw the drug gradually, watching carefully for recrudesence of the thrombocytopenia. If no response is achieved or if exacerbation is seen when corticosteroids are withdrawn, splenectomy may be considered. The patient who is asymptomatic or who has only modest reduction of platelet count will probably not require surgery. However, if the patient is one of the 50% who do not respond permanently to corticosteroids, if he does not have a spontaneous remission within 3–6 months, or if he has persistent or severe bleeding, splenectomy should be performed. Occasionally a patient refractory to steroids preoperatively and persistently thrombocytopenic after splenectomy will respond to a course of prednisone after surgery. The rare case of persistent thrombocytopenia on prednisone with remission after withdrawal of the steroid should be kept in mind.

4. **Circulating anticoagulants** Included in the broad category of naturally occurring circulating anticoagulants are the following:

   a) **Clotting inhibitors in systemic lupus erythematosus** These inhibitors, rarely associated with significant bleeding, may be detected by prolongation of the prothrombin time and the partial thromboplastin time, with positive results in the tests for anticoagulant as described above. The anticoagulant may disappear when the patient is treated with corticosteroids. The exact site at which the clotting sequence is inhibited is not clear.

   b) **Antithrombins** This class of anticoagulant is seen in a number of situations, most important of which are the various states associated with fibrinogenolysis or with hypergammaglobulinemia (e.g., rheumatoid arthritis) or dysgammaglobulinemia (e.g., multiple myeloma). The thrombin, prothrombin, and partial thromboplastin times are prolonged and the patient may respond to corticosteroid or antineoplastic therapy directed at the underlying disorder.

   c) **Inhibitors of specific clotting factors**

      i) Antifactor VIII in hemophiliacs may be recognized when a typical bleeding episode fails to respond to factor VIII therapy. In such grave situations, avoiding the use of factor VIII and reliance on local hemostatic measures to halt bleeding and the use of washed red cells to replace blood loss may result, over a period of time, in lowering of the antifactor VIII titer to the point at which cryoprecipitate is again effective. Very rarely, exchange transfusion or corticosteroid therapy is effective in reducing the level of inhibitor. Too commonly, however, the presence of antifactor VIII leads to the death of the patient.

      ii) Antifactor VIII may appear spontaneously in females 1–12 months postpartum; the anticoagulant may disappear after months to years. Antifactor VIII is also rarely seen in patients with allergic reactions, elderly people, and patients with carcinomatosis. Presentation may be as visceral hemorrhage. The anticoagulant frequently disappears spontaneously but may lead to fatal bleeding.

      iii) Very rarely, inhibitors of transfused replacement factors may be seen in the other congenital deficiency states, such as Christmas disease (factor IX deficiency). As in classical hemophilia, the results of treatment of bleeding in the presence of the anticoagulant are discouraging.

The rapid development of chemotherapeutic agents for malignant diseases has resulted in a significant increase in the responsibilities of the internist for treatment of neoplasms. Although there has been a marked increase in the biochemical and therapeutic investigation of neoplastic diseases, the desired goal has not yet been achieved; but progress has been steady and there have been encouraging clinical trials. Since the field of chemotherapy is rapidly changing as new investigational drugs are added to the therapeutic regimens, no attempt is made to review comprehensively all the available agents; instead, the clinical use of a few well-accepted drugs is outlined in the following section. In the second section, the basic chemotherapeutic approach to certain more common neoplasms is discussed. A section on the principles of chemotherapy follows the description of the available agents.

AVAILABLE AGENTS

I. **ALKYLATING AGENTS** denote compounds that are capable of replacing a hydrogen atom in another molecule with an alkyl radical, thus combining chemically with certain nucleophilic metabolically important groups (e.g., amino, phosphate, sulfhydryl, hydroxyl, imidazole, carboxyl). These agents have a capacity to interfere with mitosis, produce chromosomal damage and mutation (hence the term *radiomimetics*), suppress normal immune responses, and inhibit tumors by virtue of cytotoxicity. These agents can be divided into the nitrogen mustards, the ethylenimines, and the alkyl sulfonates.

A. **Nitrogen mustards** The parent compound, mechlorethamine, is a powerful surface vesicant that must be given intravenously. Various modifications of the molecule have been made in attempts to change its avidity for various tissues, decrease its toxicity, and allow its oral administration.

1. **Mechlorethamine (HN2, nitrogen mustard, Mustargen HCl)**, the first of the nitrogen mustards, has been more widely studied than any of its congeners.

a) **Clinical indications** The drug is most useful in disseminated Hodgkin's disease. It may be used with or without radiation therapy when systemic manifestations are present or when radiation is not feasible. The drug is highly effective in providing relief from tumor compression of vital structures such as the trachea, superior vena cava, and the spinal cord. Other lymphomas and myeloproliferative diseases may respond satisfactorily, but more effective therapy is available for these disorders. Occasional palliation has been observed in carcinoma of lungs, ovary, breast, and kidney and in testicular tumors.

b) Absorption, metabolism, and excretion Mechlorethamine can be absorbed from either the alimentary tract or parenteral sites of administration, but severe local reactions preclude its use except by intravenous route. Within minutes after administration, mechlorethamine undergoes chemical transformation and combines with either water or reactive compounds of tissue cells. Urinary excretion of drug is less than 0.01%.

c) Dosage and administration Mechlorethamine is supplied in powder form in 20-ml vials containing 10 mg of drug. A fresh solution of the drug should be prepared before each administration by adding 10 ml of sterile distilled water; it should be injected immediately by intravenous route only (see below). A usual course of therapy with mechlorethamine consists of administration of a total dose of 0.4 mg/kg body weight. Although this total dose may be given in two or four daily consecutive injections, a single administration may be preferred; the therapeutic response is equal and the patient is spared the side effects for 2–4 days.

For systemic therapy the drug must be given IV; extreme care must be taken to avoid extravasation. The solution must be injected into the tubing of a rapidly flowing intravenous transfusion (5% D/W or normal saline); this technique not only reduces the chances of extravasation but also lowers the concentration of the drug at the site of injection. The rate of injection is unimportant, provided only a few minutes are taken for injection. To avoid nausea and vomiting, an antiemetic (chlorpromazine 25 mg) and sedative (amobarbital 90 mg) may be given half an hour prior to mustard administration (usually at bedtime).

A dose of 10–20 mg (independent of body weight) may be used intracavitarily (pleural, peritoneal, or pericardial cavity), following drainage of fluid. Chylous effusions respond poorly. (For proper mode of administration see Serous Effusions, in the section Treatment of Specific Diseases.)

d) Toxicity If the drug comes in contact with the skin or mucous membranes, these areas should be treated immediately with 2% sodium thiocyanate solution (which neutralizes HN2 activity) and copious quantities of water. Nausea, vomiting, diarrhea, anorexia, weakness, maculopapular dermatitis, and rarely mucosal ulceration of the GI tract or thrombophlebitis in the injected vein may occur. Granulocytopenia and thrombocytopenia are maximal two weeks after administration; recovery requires 4–6 weeks. Rarely, the hemoglobin level may be decreased at a somewhat later date. The drug is contraindicated during pregnancy, especially in the first trimester, since fetal abnormalities have been produced in mammalian experiments.

2. Chlorambucil (Leukeran)

a) Clinical indications The greatest clinical usefulness of chlorambucil is in chronic lymphocytic leukemia, although beneficial results have been obtained in Hodgkin's disease, other lymphomas, and some cases of ovarian tumor, testicular tumors, multiple myeloma, and primary macroglobulinemia.

b) **Absorption, metabolism, and excretion** Oral absorption is adequate and reliable. Information regarding metabolism and excretion is still incomplete.

c) **Dosage and administration** Chlorambucil is available in 2-mg tablets for oral administration. The standard initial dosage is 0.1–0.2 mg/kg body weight in a single daily dose before breakfast for 3–6 weeks. Blood counts must be followed weekly. With fall in total leukocyte count or clinical improvement, the dosage is reduced to maintenance (usually 2 mg daily or 6–8 mg twice a week before breakfast).

d) **Toxicity** Bone marrow depression is usually rapidly reversible; great care must be exercised, however, in the treatment of patients with hypoplastic marrow and the "packed marrow syndrome" of chronic lymphocytic leukemia, or those being given concomitant x-ray therapy. Mild GI upset occurs occasionally; hepatotoxicity, exfoliative dermatitis, and allergic febrile reactions are rare.

3. **Cyclophosphamide (Cytoxan)** is inactive in vitro; hydrolysis by tissue enzymes (phosphamidases and phosphatases) results in the release of an active compound. Since activity of these enzymes is high in tumors and low in megakaryocytes, a platelet-sparing effect might be expected, and has indeed been reported.

   a) **Clinical indications** The spectrum of activity of cyclophosphamide is comparable to that of nitrogen mustard; good results in Hodgkin's disease and other lymphomas have been confirmed. Beneficial results have been obtained in multiple myeloma, chronic lymphocytic leukemia, and acute lymphoblastic leukemia of childhood. Temporary palliative effects have been reported in bronchogenic carcinoma, ovarian malignancies, and neuroblastoma.

   b) **Absorption, metabolism, and excretion** Cyclophosphamide is well absorbed orally. The drug is probably activated in blood, liver, or both. Urine and fecal excretion after oral ingestion accounts for about 40–50% of the ingested dose.

   c) **Dosage and administration** Cyclophosphamide is supplied in 50-mg tablets and as a powder (100 or 200 mg) in sterile vials (which should be kept refrigerated to preserve activity). Various dosage schedules have been tried, but optimal regimens have not yet been established. The drug can be given orally, IV, IM, intrapleurally, intraperitoneally, and sometimes directly into tumors. The drug is usually given orally or IV. For relatively susceptible neoplasms (e.g., leukemia and lymphoma) 2–3 mg/kg/day (100–200 mg daily) may be given either IV or orally. For relatively resistant neoplasms (solid tumors), initial doses range from 4 to 8 mg/kg/day for 5–7 days, followed by a maintenance dose of 50–200 mg/day orally, or 5 mg/kg IV twice weekly. Continuation of therapy and maintenance dosage depend on the response and the total leukocyte count, which should remain in the range of 2000–5000/cu mm.

   d) **Toxicity** is primarily hematologic, leukopenia being the main indication for dosage reduction or discontinuance of therapy; thrombocytopenia is less common than with mechlorethamine. Reversible alopecia, usually after 3 weeks or more of treatment, occurs in about 30% of patients; nausea, vomiting, dizziness, hepatotoxicity, and mucosal ulcerations may occur. Transverse ridging of the nails and greater skin pigmentation have been reported. Sterile chemical cystitis is not uncommon and may present as a profound hemorrhagic cystitis in 20–30% of patients. The frequency of this complication has caused some observers to limit use of the drug, even though the cystitis usually subsides spontaneously (occasionally it is necessary to discontinue therapy temporarily).

4. **Melphalan** is the phenylalanine derivative of nitrogen mustard. The L-isomer is more effective than the D-isomer (medphalan) and is marketed as Alkeran.

   a) **Indications**   Melphalan is useful in the treatment of multiple myeloma. Available evidence suggests that about one-third of patients with multiple myeloma show favorable response to oral administration of the drug. In a variety of other neoplastic conditions (e.g., melanoma, seminoma, malignant lymphoma, and ovarian carcinoma) its use may be precluded by substantial bone marrow toxicity.

   b) **Absorption, metabolism, and excretion**   Melphalan is well absorbed when given orally but can be used intravenously. The drug probably remains active in the blood for 6 hours and is slowly metabolized.

   c) **Dosage and administration**   Melphalan is supplied in 2-mg tablets. No drug regimen has been established, but usually 6–8 mg/day is given for 10–14 days. Administration is then discontinued for 3–6 weeks; blood counts should be followed carefully and a maintenance dose of 2 mg or less is started when white blood cell and platelet counts begin to rise. An alternate regimen is to administer 0.15 mg/kg body weight daily for 7 days. This course is followed by a rest period until the nadir of bone marrow suppression is reached; then maintenance with 1–3 mg daily is continued to keep the white blood cell count between 3000 and 3500/cu mm.

   d) **Toxicity** is similar to that of other alkylating agents, but thrombocytopenia seems to be more common. Nausea and vomiting are infrequent; alopecia does not occur; hepatic and renal toxicity have not yet been reported. The drug should not be used concurrently with other cytotoxic agents or radiation.

B. **Ethylenimines** are not extensively used anymore, partly because of severe and unpredictable toxicity and partly due to availability of better therapeutic agents. A brief summary of these compounds is included, however.

   1. **Triethylene melamine (TEM)** has been used primarily for the treatment of Hodgkin's disease, other lymphomas, and chronic lymphocytic leukemia that cannot be treated with other alkylating agents; on rare occasions it has been used for treatment of chronic granulocytic leukemia and polycythemia vera. Toxic effects on the bone marrow are unpredictable and severe, however, and the other nitrogen mustard preparations and derivatives are safer and of equal effectiveness. The drug should be given by an experienced chemotherapist.

2. **Triethylene thiophosphoramide (Thiotepa)** has been of most benefit in the treatment of advanced carcinoma of the ovary and it may be considered as an adjunct to surgery for treatment of carcinoma of the breast; it may be used with limited effectiveness in lymphomas, malignant melanoma, and carcinoma of the lung or bladder.

C. Alkyl sulfonates (busulfan) (Myleran)

1. **Clinical indications** Busulfan is the most useful of the chemical agents available for the treatment of chronic granulocytic leukemia; in many clinics its administration is regarded as the initial treatment of choice. A temporary remission occurs in the majority of patients; certainly symptoms are relieved, and the course of the disease is probably prolonged. Beneficial results have also been reported in polycythemia vera and myeloid metaplasia; the thrombocytosis occurring in these diseases may be especially well controlled.

2. **Absorption, metabolism, and excretion** Busulfan is well absorbed after oral administration. Within minutes the drug is metabolized to methanesulfonic acid and is excreted by the kidneys.

3. **Dosage and preparations** Busulfan is supplied in 2-mg tablets. For chronic granulocytic leukemia a single daily dose of 4–8 mg is given orally and continued until the leukocyte count, determined weekly, falls to 50% of its original level, when dosage should be reduced. The drug should be discontinued if leukocyte count falls below 10,000/cu mm. The rate of decline in leukocyte count is usually proportional to the dosage used. The time required for production of a remission depends on the height of the original leukocyte level, the count being halved about every 3 weeks. The patient's sense of well-being returns, granulocytic elements in both blood and bone marrow return to normal or near normal levels, the enlarged liver and spleen decrease in size, and the anemia and thrombocytopenia tend to be corrected. Remissions may persist as long as 2 years. In some clinics maintenance doses of 2 mg/day or 6–8 mg one day each week are given in the hope of prolonging the remission; whether this procedure is effective is still unconfirmed.

   When the initial WBC is normal or low, and when busulfan is employed for the treatment of polycythemia vera or myeloid metaplasia, the same dosage schedule is followed, but one must proceed with caution to avoid serious bone marrow depression. Treatment should be stopped if the white blood cell count falls below 3000/cu mm or the platelet count below 50,000/cu mm.

4. **Toxicity,** other than the myelosuppressive effect, includes the following: generalized skin pigmentation, anhidrosis, alopecia, nausea, vomiting, diarrhea, cheilosis, glossitis, impotence, sterility, amenorrhea, gynecomastia, hyperuricemia (and renal damage), cytologic dysplasia, and pulmonary fibrosis. The drug has been used without ill effects during pregnancy, but fetal malformations have been reported to occur, and its use should be avoided during the first trimester.

II. **ANTIMETABOLITES** A large and heterogeneous group of analogs and derivatives of biologically important compounds (ranging from amino-acid analogs and antivitamins to halogenated purines and pyrimidines) has been tested for antitumor properties. They interfere with the synthesis of essential cell components by competing with the natural substrates for the enzyme involved, or by contributing to the synthesis of unnatural cell constituents. In general, they have their greatest toxicity in tissues which are metabolically very active.

A. Folic acid antagonists These compounds differ from folic acid only by subtle alterations in structure; they compete for and very avidly combine with the intracellular enzyme, folic reductase, thereby interfering with the synthesis of tetrahydrofolic acid (THF), which is a coenzyme important in a variety of metabolic transformations necessary for DNA synthesis. Folinic acid (citrovorum factor), a metabolic intermediate, may counteract the effects of the folic acid antagonist if given parenterally immediately following administration of the antimetabolite. **Methotrexate** (formerly amethopterin) is the folic acid antagonist most widely used. Aminopterin and dichloro derivatives used earlier have been replaced by methotrexate.

1. **Clinical indications** Methotrexate is a very useful drug in the management of acute leukemia in children. Remission rates up to 47% have been reported. Methotrexate has established its value in curative treatment of choriocarcinoma in females; results in male choriocarcinoma are poor. Beneficial results have been reported in mycosis fungoides and carcinoma of the breast, pharynx, and testis (in combination with other drugs). The drug has been used in psoriasis and as an immunosuppressive agent.

2. **Absorption, metabolism, and excretion** Methotrexate is readily absorbed from the alimentary tract but may be given parenterally. From 40% to 50% of a small dose and up to 90% of a larger dose is excreted unchanged in the urine in 48 hours, a major portion of it during the first 8 hours. The drug is poorly transported across the blood-brain barrier. The drug retained in the body is primarily bound to folate reductase.

3. **Dosage and administration** Methotrexate is provided in 2.5-mg tablets and in powder form 5 or 50 mg in sterile vials. The daily oral dose is 2.5–5.0 mg/day for children and 2.5–10.0 mg/day for adults. The biologic effects of the daily single dose may be quite different from divided doses administered every 6–12 hours. The drug should be started at lower range and continued for 3–4 weeks. If remission or toxicity appears during this period, the drug is discontinued for a few days and restarted at a lower dose. If remission and/or toxicity is not evident, the drug should be administered at a higher level.

   In choriocarcinoma, intensive treatment should be employed, and 10–30 mg methotrexate may be used daily for 5 days. It is imperative that methotrexate be given to the maximum tolerance level, since complete remissions or cures up to 5 years or longer have been reported. **Warning:** Since the drug is excreted by the kidneys, the dosage should be reduced in the presence of renal insufficiency, and the patients should be watched very carefully for signs of toxicity.

   Special uses Intrathecal administration for meningeal leukemia (0.8 mg/kg every other day for 4 doses) with concomitant parenteral folinic acid therapy 3 to 6 mg IM (to minimize or prevent systemic toxicity) has resulted in impressive results in infants and children. Temporary benefit has been achieved after intra-arterial perfusion of localized surgically incurable solid tumors, particularly tumors of the head, neck and pelvis, and melanoma.

4. **Toxicity** consists primarily of bone marrow depression, oral and gastrointestinal mucosal ulceration and hemorrhage, and alopecia. In case of inadvertent overdosage, 3–6 mg of folinic acid should be given within 4 hours of methotrexate administration.

B. **Purine analogs**   6-mercaptopurine (6-MP) is the most widely used; other compounds such as 6-thioguanine, 6-chloropurine, 2,6-diaminopurine, and 8-azaguanine have no demonstrable superiority. 6-MP probably exerts its action by inhibiting the synthesis of DNA and other essential compounds either by prevention of purine incorporation into DNA or by the utilization of 6-MP to form an unnatural DNA.

1. **6-mercaptopurine (Purinethol)**

   a) **Clinical indications**   The drug, effective primarily in the treatment of acute lymphocytic leukemia, may also be used in other acute leukemias. For acute lymphocytic leukemia remission after the first course of therapy may be expected in approximately 35% of children and 15% of adults. The 90% one-year mortality rate (for untreated children) may be reduced to 50%, but a statistically significant improvement does not occur in adults. This drug is not indicated in the treatment of chronic lymphocytic leukemia, Hodgkin's disease, or solid tumors.

   b) **Absorption, metabolism, and excretion**   6-mercaptopurine is readily absorbed from the GI tract without any damage to intestinal mucosa. The drug is rapidly metabolized (a half-life of about 90 minutes) and excreted by the kidneys in its changed form. Degradation of the drug by xanthine oxidase is markedly inhibited in the presence of allopurinol.

   c) **Dosage and administration**   6-mercaptopurine is available in 50-mg tablets. The dosage is 2.5 mg/kg/day (150–250 mg/day) given in one dose. Therapy is continued for 4–6 weeks, or until hematologic or clinical improvement occurs; maintenance therapy may be continued in a dosage range of 50–100 mg/day. Dosage should be reduced to about 25% of the original dose in patients receiving allopurinol concurrently.

   d) **Toxicity** consists primarily of bone marrow depression. Nausea, vomiting, and anorexia occur in 25% of patients; stomatitis and diarrhea are less common. Reversible cholestatic jaundice, hepatic necrosis, hyperuricemia, dermatitis, and drug fever have also been reported.

2. **Azathioprine (Imuran)**, a 6-MP derivative, has been used in the treatment of autoimmune diseases such as idiopathic thrombocytopenic purpura, autoimmune hemolytic anemia, systemic lupus erythematosus, and in the nephrotic syndrome, but experience is very limited at the present time. The drug offers no advantages over 6-MP in the treatment of leukemia. The oral dosage for immunosuppressive therapy is 2–4 mg/kg body weight daily.

C. **Pyrimidine analogs**   These compounds interfere with pyrimidine conversion to nucleic acid. The antitumor properties of various compounds, including 6-azauracil, 2-thiouracil, and 5-fluoro-2'-deoxyuridine, have been tested, but the most effective and widely used of those which are clinically available is **5-fluorouracil (5-FU)**.

1. **5-Fluorouracil (5-FU)**

   a) Clinical indications   5-FU can be of considerable palliative value in gastrointestinal, ovarian, and breast neoplasm. Beneficial response has been reported in 30% of the cases and may be quite dramatic in some cases. The response in leukemia, lymphoma, carcinoma of the lungs, pancreas and prostate is poor.

   b) Absorption, metabolism, and excretion   The drug is usually administered intravenously, since degradation of 5-FU is rapid by oral route. Most of the drug is converted into CO_2 and urea, mostly in the liver. About 10% of the injected dose is excreted by the kidneys.

   c) Dosage and administration   5-FU is available in 10-ml ampules containing 500 mg. The recommended dose for an average patient is 15 mg/kg/day for 5 days. If no toxicity appears, then 7.5 mg/kg/day may be given on alternate days for 4 additional doses. (No more than 1 gm/day should be given.) In severely sick patients or patients with evidence of hematopoietic, renal, or liver dysfunction, no more than 4 doses should be administered, for severe toxicity may occur. The first course should always be given in the hospital under close supervision.

   d) Toxicity   The earliest symptoms to appear are anorexia and nausea, followed by stomatitis and diarrhea, at which point therapy should be stopped. Stomatitis may develop as a white, patchy membrane, resulting in ulceration and necrosis. Bone marrow depression may begin as early as the second or third day or as late as the third week. The nadir of bone marrow depression is usually reached by the tenth to the fourteenth day after the first dose. Alopecia, nail changes, dermatitis, and increased pigmentation of the skin have been reported.

III.   **VINCA ALKALOIDS**   Although four different alkaloids have been fractionated, only vinblastine and vincristine have received wide clinical trial and will be discussed in this section. The mechanism of action of vinca alkaloids is not known but probably occurs at the metaphase stage of mitotic division of neoplastic cells.

Vinblastine is absorbed erratically from the gastrointestinal tract and is associated with GI toxicity. The vinca alkaloids are cleared rapidly from the blood and are excreted primarily (90%) by the liver into the biliary tract. Any obstruction in bile flow results in greater toxicity of these drugs.

A. Vinblastine (Velban) is recommended for treatment of Hodgkin's disease and choriocarcinoma. The efficacy of vinblastine in Hodgkin's disease approaches that of nitrogen mustard, and some oncologists believe this drug to be equal or better than mustards. Vinblastine is effective in lymphomas when resistance to akylating agents has developed. The value of vinblastine in female choriocarcinoma is significant because response has been noted after the disease had become refractory to methotrexate.

The drug is supplied in 10-mg vials. The usual dose in Hodgkin's disease is 0.1 mg/kg body weight as the first single dose and then 0.15 mg/kg/week thereafter. Main toxicity is bone marrow depression, which occurs from the fourth to the tenth day after administration of drug. Other toxic effects include neurologic manifestations such as paresthesias, loss of deep tendon reflexes, and more rarely headaches, convulsion, atonic lens, and urinary retention. These complications, however, are seen rarely with the recommended dose in the absence of biliary obstruction. Transient alopecia has been reported.

B. Vincristine (Oncovin) has a spectrum of clinical activity that is similar to that of vinblastine but with certain differences. Vincristine is most useful in acute leukemia of childhood, and is comparable to corticosteroids or antimetabolites in efficacy. It has been employed in the treatment of lymphocytic lymphosarcoma with good results. Since vincristine has less myelosuppressive activity, it may be more desirable in the presence of pancytopenia.

Vincristine is available in vials of 1 mg or 5 mg. The initial dose is 0.01 mg/kg intravenously. If no toxicity ensues then the dose is increased by 0.01 mg/kg/week until toxicity appears or response is achieved. Adult patients with lymphoma will usually respond to 0.02–0.05 mg/kg/week, but children may require higher doses up to 0.1 mg/kg/week. The toxicity is mainly neurologic and can be severe and irreversible. Paresthesias, loss of deep tendon reflexes, neuritic pain, muscle weakness (manifested by foot drop and inability to walk), hoarseness, ptosis, and diplopia are common. Severe neurologic manifestation may be avoided by cessation of therapy or reduction of dosage on the earliest symptoms of tingling and paresthesias. Severe constipation resulting in obstruction and abdominal pain has been reported and can be prevented by prophylactic use of laxatives. Alopecia may occur in 20% of patients but frequently is reversible even if administration of the drug is continued.

IV. HORMONES

A. Corticosteroids are of great value in the treatment of the autoimmune hemolytic anemia associated with chronic lymphocytic leukemia and lymphomas. The "packed marrow syndrome" of chronic lymphocytic leukemia, with associated thrombocytopenia and severe anemia, may respond either to moderate daily doses (prednisone 20–40 mg/day) or to large doses at weekly intervals (e.g., prednisone 100–200 mg once weekly), with or without concomitant administration of chlorambucil. In acute lymphocytic leukemia and the acute leukemic phase of lymphosarcoma, corticosteroids may be the treatment of choice, either with or without concomitant 6-MP therapy. Most hematologists agree that steroids are of little or no benefit in other forms of acute leukemia, and some believe that they are contraindicated in chronic granulocytic leukemia. In combination with melphalan or chlorambucil, steroid administration may result in both subjective (bone pain, appetite, etc.) and objective (plasma proteins, anemia, etc.) improvement in a small percentage of patients with multiple myeloma. Corticosteroids may be used in the treatment of early mycosis fungoides, and for metastatic breast cancer (after other measures such as androgens, estrogens, oophorectomy, etc., have been tried); a second or third remission may be induced in as many as 40% of patients, according to some authors. Steroids may be used as a last-resort palliative therapy in metastatic prostatic cancer.

B. Androgens (e.g., testosterone propionate 150–300 mg IM weekly) are useful, usually after oophorectomy, in the treatment of metastatic breast cancer in women who are premenopausal or less than 5 years postmenopausal. Halotestin 30 mg orally daily may be used instead of intramuscular preparations.

C. **Estrogens** (e.g., stilbestrol 5–15 mg/day orally) are the hormones of choice in the treatment of metastatic breast carcinoma in women more than 5 years postmenopausal. In metastatic prostatic carcinoma the drug is given in similar dosage, preferably after orchiectomy if symptoms appear.

D. **Progestational agents** (e.g., progesterone or hydroxyprogesterone caproate 150–1000 mg IM weekly) have been reported to induce objective remission, occasionally prolonged, in patients with far-advanced carcinoma of the endometrium.

V. **ANTIBIOTICS** Certain antibiotics too toxic to be used clinically for their antimicrobial effects have been found to inhibit the growth of tumor cells. Of the agents available, such as actinomycin C, mitomycin C, puromycin, streptovitacin A, mithramycin, streptonigrin, and dactinomycin, the last has been most widely used clinically. **Dactinomycin** (actinomycin D) (Cosmegen) has proved most effective in the treatment of tumors of mesodermal origin in children, particularly Wilms's tumor; rhabdomyosarcoma and Ewing's sarcoma may also respond satisfactorily. The drug is more effective when used in conjunction with irradiation therapy; synergistic effects seem to occur. Experience with other agents is more limited, but mithramycin has been reported to induce objective regression of disseminated testicular tumors (especially embryonal), and streptonigrin to be of benefit in the treatment of mycosis fungoides and certain lymphomas. More detailed comments about these agents are beyond the scope of this Manual.

VI. **MISCELLANEOUS AGENTS** **Urethane,** an anesthetic agent with oncolytic effects, has been used with variable results in the treatment of multiple myeloma. Because of generally poor responses, occasionally fatal side effects, and the development of more effective drugs (such as melphalan), it is not widely used. **Deacetylmethylcolchicine (Demecolcin, Colcemid)** and other derivatives of the alkaloid colchicine cause metaphase arrest and have been used in the treatment of leukemia. **O,p′DDD,** which causes involutional changes in the adrenal cortex, has been used successfully in the treatment of metastatic adrenocortical carcinoma.

VII. **RADIOACTIVE ISOTOPES** A discussion of the use of radioactive isotopes in the treatment of malignant disease is beyond the scope of this Manual; the use of radioactive phosphorus is discussed in the section on polycythemia vera.

PRINCIPLES OF CHEMOTHERAPY

Chemotherapy is one of three major methods available for treating malignant neoplasms, the other two being surgery and ionizing radiation. Since "cures" are few in disseminated cancer, it is mandatory that treatment be directed to adequate control of the disease. Chemotherapy can fill this role adequately when surgery and radiation are impractical. An aggressive utilization of chemotherapy may result in relief of symptoms, regression of tumor, rehabilitation, and longer survival. Because of these potentialities, patients should be given the benefit of a full therapeutic program. Before a decision is made to treat a patient with these agents, he must be evaluated as follows:

1. **Diagnosis** Since various chemotherapeutic agents have a specific activity against a single type of cancer, it is essential that every attempt be made to establish the site of origin and the morphologic type of malignancy. Administration of an antineoplastic agent is fraught with hazards and should not be undertaken until the nature of the disease is verified.

2. **Selection of a patient** Chemotherapy may be initiated at the earliest signs of metastatic disease, especially in susceptible tumors. As the disease progresses, the patient may decompensate, and chemotherapy dosage may have to be modified. Well nourished, ambulatory, and otherwise healthy patients are best suited for chemotherapy; if one agent fails to control the disease, there may be time to use another drug. The critically ill, moribund patient is not an ideal candidate for chemotherapy; the risk of complications is greatly increased.

3. **Selection of chemotherapeutic agents** To select expertly the best chemotherapeutic agent for a patient, one must be thoroughly aware of the effects and side effects of a drug. A potentially cytotoxic drug in a pancytopenic patient may be extremely hazardous. A chemotherapeutic agent does not have to produce systemic toxicity to achieve antitumor effect; however, side effects must occur if maximum response is desired. The physician must consider the harmful effects of the drug on a patient if no tumor response is obtained. One may try a combination of agents to achieve synergetic antitumor effects and counteract side effects.

4. **Supportive therapy** During chemotherapy, every attempt should be made to relieve distressful symptoms. Anemia should be treated adequately and blood transfusions given, if necessary. The administration of corticosteroids may be helpful in stimulating erythropoiesis and reducing inflammation and edema around the tumor. Secondary infections should be treated promptly and adequately. Any unexplainable alteration in the course of the disease should alert the physician to the possibility of a second disease process. **Allopurinol** (100 mg TID) may be administered to avoid uric acid nephropathy. **Caution:** The dose of 6-MP or Imuran should be reduced to about 25% of the original dose if allopurinol is administered concomitantly.

TREATMENT OF SPECIFIC DISEASES

I. **LEUKEMIAS** The general principles guiding therapy in the leukemias include attempts to induce morphologic changes approaching normal in the bone marrow and peripheral blood; prevention and control of hemorrhage and infections; antianemia measures; and most important, maintenance of an asymptomatic ambulatory state outside the hospital.

A. **Acute granulocytic** and **acute monocytic leukemia** are approached therapeutically as one disease. They occur primarily in adults, in contrast to acute lymphocytic leukemia, and the prognosis and prospects for remission are less good. Patients who have leukopenia when first seen generally have a better prognosis.

In the last 4 years the chemotherapy of acute granulocytic and acute monocytic leukemias has undergone a major change. Since the introduction of combination chemotherapy (e.g., VAMP, described below), remission can be achieved in about 70% of adults. The toxicity is substantial, and intensive supportive therapy including transfusion of red blood cells and platelets may be required. This program has been modified to induce remissions by vincristine-prednisone alone (this combination being optimum). In spite of the higher remission rate, the use of combination therapy has been limited due to its toxicity. The most commonly used agent is 6-mercaptopurine to which corticosteroids are added in case of leukopenia and thrombocytopenia.

Remissions are usually short-lived, and relapses occur invariably. Unfortunately, none of the chemotherapeutic agents is very effective in maintaining a remission. Cytosine arabinoside, a new drug under investigation, appears to be as effective as VAMP but has significant bone marrow toxicity.

1. **Dosage and administration for induction of remission** are as follows:

   a) **6-MP alone,** 2.5 mg/kg/day in a single dose orally for at least 4 weeks or until remission or toxicity appears.

   b) **6-MP + prednisone** Prednisone 0.5–1.5 mg/kg/day orally in divided doses is used in addition to 6-MP. Some hematologists are reluctant to use prednisone initially because it seems to cause rapid deterioration in a few instances.

   c) **Vincristine + prednisone**
   Vincristine 25–50 μg/kg/week IV
   Prednisone 2–5 mg/kg/day orally
   The drugs are continued until remission or toxicity appears. Prednisone is reduced rapidly to smaller doses after 4 weeks.

   d) **VAMP**

   Vincristine 25 μg/kg/week IV

   Methotrexate 2.5 mg/day orally

   6-MP 1.25 mg/kg/day orally

   Prednisone 1.0 mg/kg/day orally

   All the drugs are begun simultaneously and should be continued for 6 weeks or until remission or toxicity appears. If toxicity can be ascribed to a single drug, that agent is discontinued or dosage is reduced. Once remission is achieved, additional courses of therapy may be given in early relapse. The effectiveness of this regimen is not well established.

2. **Maintenance of remission** Various attempts at maintenance of remission have been only partially successful. Some hematologists have repeated the induction courses prophylactically during remission but the results have been disappointing. Methotrexate 30 mg/sq M/twice a week administered IM during remission increases the maintenance period significantly in childhood leukemia, but no such beneficial effects have been noted in adults.*

B. **Acute lymphocytic leukemia** is the commonest form of leukemia in children; the prognosis and response to therapy are better than in the above. Corticosteroids and vincristine, the drugs of choice, may be expected to induce first remissions in 70–90% of cases. 6-MP or methotrexate may induce second, third, or even fourth remissions;

*See Appendix II.

in combination with adequate supportive therapy median survival may be extended to one year or more. The treatment of the acute leukemic phase of lymphosarcoma is similar to that of acute lymphocytic leukemia.

C. **Meningeal leukemia** is more common in childhood acute lymphocytic leukemia but occurs in all types and all age groups. Once a patient develops meningeal leukemia, it may behave independently of the bone marrow status; the patient may develop acute exacerbation of meningeal leukemia while in bone marrow remission.

Since most of the drugs (except BCNU) do not cross the blood-brain barrier, the treatment is administered by the intrathecal route. BCNU (bis-β-chloroethyl nitrosourea, an investigational drug) crosses the blood-brain barrier, but it is doubtful that effective cerebrospinal fluid levels can be achieved by the systemic route. Methotrexate 0.8 mg/kg administered intrathecally every other day for 4 doses is the preferred treatment. Folinic acid (citrovorum factor) should be given parenterally if no systemic effects are desired. It is doubtful whether the prophylactic intrathecal administration of methotrexate in meningeal leukemias in remission is valuable. A new agent now being investigated, cytosine arabinoside, used intrathecally is also effective. Radiation therapy to the craniospinal axis has been employed but is only transiently effective and not very practical.

D. **Chronic granulocytic leukemia,** in its early stages, responds with great regularity to therapy, and the median survival may be increased from approximately 29 months (in untreated patients) to as long as 44 months (in patients treated with busulfan). Splenic irradiation may be the initial preferred treatment, particularly in patients with pronounced splenomegaly. Busulfan is the chemotherapeutic agent of choice, but in resistant cases 6-MP may be used instead; leukocytosis and white-cell immaturity may be effectively controlled, although effects are usually transient. Administration of corticosteroids may cause an exacerbation of the disease, and many authorities believe their use is contraindicated. Blastic crises are treated as acute granulocytic leukemias, but remissions are rare; 6-MP is the most commonly used drug.

E. **Chronic lymphocytic leukemia,** an extremely variable disease which may be quite benign and slowly progressive, often requires no therapy for long periods of time, especially in elderly patients; in other patients it may be rapidly fatal, however. Chlorambucil is the chemotherapeutic agent of choice, but TEM, mechlorethamine, and corticosteroids may be used in special situations. Irradiation may be valuable for the treatment of enlarged lymph nodes which are uncomfortable or unsightly. The packed-marrow syndrome may respond to corticosteroids, as described previously, with or without concomitant chlorambucil administration. The autoimmune hemolytic anemia which complicates approximately 10% of cases of chronic lymphocytic leukemia responds well to corticosteroids. Hypersplenism, which is not uncommon, responds to splenectomy and less satisfactorily to splenic irradiation.

II. LYMPHOMAS

A. **Hodgkin's disease** is a fairly common neoplasm with a reported death rate of 17 per 1,000,000 in the United States. Hodgkin's disease accounts for 40% of all lymphomas. The diagnosis rests upon the presence of Reed-Sternberg cells in biopsy material (usually a lymph node biopsy). The prognosis and treatment of this neoplasm depend on the extent of involvement; consequently, a uniform classification (listed below) has been adopted.

Stage I   Disease limited to one node-bearing area

Stage II-1   Disease limited to two contiguous node-bearing areas on the same side of the diaphragm

Stage II-2   Disease in more than two node-bearing areas or in two noncontiguous areas on the same side of the diaphragm

Stage III   Disease on both sides of the diaphragm but limited to involvement of the lymph nodes, spleen, and Waldeyer's ring

Stage IV   Involvement of the bone marrow, lung parenchyma, pleura, liver, bone, skin, kidneys, gastrointestinal tract, or any tissue or organ other than the lymph nodes, spleen, or Waldeyer's ring

All stages are subclassified **A** or **B** to indicate the absence or presence, respectively, of any of the following documented, otherwise unexplained symptoms: fever, night sweats, pruritus, or weight loss greater than 10% of normal body weight.

Lymphangiography should be performed on all patients before they can be classified as stage I or II to exclude retroperitoneal lymph node involvement. This added information is important, since in stage I definitely and in stage II in all probability, a "cure" can be achieved, and treatment is an all-out effort to achieve normal life span. In stages III and IV the treatment is directed mainly to control of the disease, though many radiotherapists and chemotherapists are challenging this pessimistic view. The following treatments are available:

1. **Stages I and II** Radiation therapy is the treatment of choice for stages I and II Hodgkin's disease. A course of intensive, extended-field supravoltage radiotherapy should be administered by an experienced radiotherapist and must include all adjacent node-bearing areas. In selected cases chemotherapy may be used in an emergency situation or in the control of systemic toxicity as an adjuvant to radiotherapy but never as a substitute.

2. **Stages III and IV** The aim of treatment in these stages of the disease is to control the disease adequately and enable a patient to continue a productive and normal life. Some radiotherapists believe that even in stage III it is possible to achieve prolonged remission in a majority of cases, but the available data are not convincing. Chemotherapy should be the treatment in these patients; radiation therapy may be used for localized disease areas. Prior treatment and duration of disease have an adverse effect on response to chemotherapy.

   a) **Mechlorethamine** has been the most effective chemotherapeutic agent. The total dose of 0.4 mg/kg per course is tolerated by most patients and produces tumor regression in over 60% of the patients. The drug is contraindicated in patients with marked leukopenia and/or thrombocytopenia. The results are often poor in previously treated patients.

b) **Vinblastine** has shown marked effectiveness in Hodgkin's disease and is at least as effective as nitrogen mustard. Given intravenously in dosage of 0.1–0.2 mg/kg/week (adjusted to leukocyte count), it may produce a response in over 80% of patients. At least 6 weeks should be allowed to achieve maximum antitumor effect. Because of its slow action, this drug is not suited for emergency treatment. The results are poor in previously treated patients.

c) **Chlorambucil,** another alkylating agent, is inferior to mechlorethamine (in rapidity of action and tumor response). This drug is best suited for maintaining remissions produced by other agents because of the ease of administration and less pronounced toxicity. The usual maintenance dose is 2–4 mg daily and is adjusted to leukocyte count.

d) **Cyclophosphamide** has been used widely in Hodgkin's disease. Though it may occasionally produce a remission in a patient resistant to other alkylating agents, it is generally less effective than vinblastine and mechlorethamine.

e) **Corticosteroids** are indicated in patients with systemic toxicity and/or patients with anemia, leukopenia, or thrombocytopenia. Prednisone is effective in only 20–30% of the patients, but in special circumstances (e.g., hemolytic anemia) may be the only suitable agent. Although as much as 1 mg/kg/day may be necessary, dosage in the range of 20–30 mg per day is usually effective.

f) **Combination therapy** Enough data are now available to indicate that combination chemotherapy is more effective than any single agent. The dosage has been reduced to eliminate serious toxicity, and advantage is derived from synergic antitumor effects of various agents. In one study (*Ann. Int. Med.* 67:424, 1967), combination therapy produced complete remissions in 85% of all cases and in 80% of stages II and III patients. A 14-day course of therapy is used alternatively with a 14-day rest period or longer if toxicity persists. The drugs used are as follows:*

Prednisone	60 mg/sq **M**	day 1–14	PO
Cyclophosphamide	600 mg/sq **M**	day 1, 7	IV
Methotrexate	30 mg/sq **M**	day 4, 8, 12	IV
Vincristine	1.2 mg/sq **M**	day 1, 7	IV

g) **Methylhydrazine and streptonigrin** may be of some value, but the available data are insufficient for evaluation.

3. **Treatment of special complications**

a) **Neurologic involvement** Spinal cord involvement occurs in 5–10% of patients with Hodgkin's disease. Early recognition is important, since adequate therapy instituted at any time before development of complete paraplegia is rewarded with satisfactory responses in a high percentage of cases. Radicular pain pattern, elevated spinal fluid proteins, and myelograms may uncover the disease process long before neurologic deficits become manifested. In these cases radiation therapy to the compressed area of the

*See Appendix II.

spinal cord may be the sole treatment. In progressive neurologic syndromes, it is wise to administer a course of mechlorethamine before starting radiation therapy. If, however, weakness is rapidly progressive or there is a progression of neurologic deficits in spite of mechlorethamine administration, emergency laminectomy is indicated.

b) Serous effusions can be a cause of much distress to a patient and constitute a difficult problem. Various approaches have been tried, but none is very effective. Chylous effusions respond poorly to all measures (probably because of obstruction of the thoracic duct). Mechlorethamine has been instilled in the pleural cavity in doses of 15–20 mg. The best response is obtained by partial drainage of fluid before HN2 instillation, allowing ½ hour for the drug to start a reaction and then draining the remaining fluid over the next 36 hours. Radiophosphorus or colloidal gold has not produced significantly better results. Recently Atabrine has been used in doses of 100–200 mg daily intracavitarily for 4–5 days with occasional good response.

B. Reticulum-cell sarcoma   Treatment is similar to that for Hodgkin's disease. Cyclophosphamide seems to produce better response, but remissions tend to be of shorter duration. Radiotherapy is effective for control of localized tumor masses, but the results of intensive radiotherapy are not yet impressive. Some cases respond dramatically to the administration of vincristine, but the remission is usually short lived.

C. Lymphocytic lymphosarcoma   Chlorambucil is the chemotherapeutic agent most commonly used. The response to treatment is slightly better than in reticulum-cell sarcoma. Prednisone may induce remission in a significant number of patients. The duration of remissions is short; the tumor becomes resistant to therapy and may transform terminally into leukemia.

III.   **MULTIPLE MYELOMA** is characterized by malignant plasma-cell proliferation, monoclonal gammapathy, progressive anemia, osteolytic lesions of the bones, and hypercalcemia. Every patient does not present all the features of the disease; the symptoms and signs vary in severity. Some hematologists are reluctant to treat asymptomatic patients, since the available therapy is effective in only 30–50% of the patients and the toxicity may be substantial. Others treat their patients soon after diagnosis to control the disease before systemic toxicity appears which may limit the chemotherapy.

Of the available agents melphalan has been credited with the best results. More than 50% of the patients show objective response. The usual regimen is to administer 6–8 mg/day orally for 10–14 days, followed by a rest period until the nadir of bone marrow suppression is reached (usually 3 weeks later), after which a maintenance dose of 2 mg or less is prescribed to keep the leukocyte count between 3000 and 4000/cu mm. The limiting factor is thrombocytopenia, which can be very severe. (For a recent review see *Blood* 30:74, 1967.)

Cyclophosphamide is also effective, but is probably less effective than melphalan. The toxicity of Cytoxan is less marked, and this agent may be used in relatively asymptomatic patients. Data presently available are insufficient to draw any conclusion about long-term effects of cyclophosphamide in multiple myeloma. The usual regimen is to administer 200 mg orally per day initially until leukocyte count falls to 2500–3000/cu mm, then discontinue the drug temporarily and restart at a maintenance dose of 50–100 mg daily orally.

Corticosteroids are usually effective in toxic patients. Prednisone may stimulate bone marrow regeneration, lower hypercalcemia, and produce a sense of well-being. There is no conclusive evidence that steroids possess any antimyeloma activity. Usual dose is 30 mg orally daily. Testosterone 400 mg IM weekly is advocated to enhance erythropoiesis and myelopoiesis.

Sodium fluoride in the dosage of 50 mg TID ½ hour before meals has been effective in relieving bone pain. The available data are too meager to interpret the long-term effects of fluorides. Local radiotherapy is singularly effective in relieving bone pain and reducing extraosseous tumor masses. Usually 1000 to 1500 rads are a sufficient dose.

Ambulation and hydration are perhaps the two most significant supportive measures. Dehydration must be avoided.

IV. POLYCYTHEMIA VERA Phlebotomy whenever the hematocrit rises above 55% may suffice as the only treatment for younger patients or those who do not have severe thrombocytosis; myelosuppressive therapy is generally indicated for older patients or those who have a marked elevation of the platelet count. Radioactive phosphorus, P^{32}, is usually used when a panmyelopathy is present; 3.5–5.0 mc may be given IV. Dosage should not be repeated for at least three months. Busulfan may be used for the control of thrombocytosis; some hematologists advocate chlorambucil for this purpose.

The increasing incidence of acute leukemia in polycythemia vera patients treated with P^{32} may be due either to prolonged survival or to a leukemogenic effect of P^{32}. Splenic irradiation may be given to relieve the discomfort of an extremely enlarged spleen, but splenectomy is contraindicated because of the resultant thrombocytosis which frequently develops.

V. SOLID TUMORS A comprehensive review of the chemotherapy of solid tumors is beyond the scope of this Manual; however, a brief description of common carcinomas is included.

A. Carcinoma of the breast is the most common neoplasm of the female; of all women treated adequately (by surgery and radiation), 45% will develop metastatic disease and require palliative therapy.

1. Premenopausal women

a) Castration (oophorectomy) is indicated for disseminated disease only and should not be employed for prophylactic treatment.

b) Androgenic hormones are used next after castration. The response is poor (20–30%), and these drugs should never supplant castration in the premenopausal patient. The most satisfactory response is obtained in patients with painful osseous metastases. 2-alpha-methyl dihydrotestosterone propionate (100 mg IM 3 times weekly) is somewhat less virilizing than other preparations. Other side effects include fluid retention, hypercalcemia, and a transient flare-up of pain.

c) Adrenalectomy may be performed if castration has produced objective improvement. Fifty percent may respond, but the patients must be selected very carefully because of the necessity of corticosteroid replacement. Hypophysectomy may produce equally good results.

d) **Cytotoxic therapy** is used when hormonal therapy is not effective. The following agents are occasionally effective: nitrogen mustard, 5-FU, cyclophosphamide, and vinblastine.

e) **Radiotherapy** is very effective for localized tumor areas and can relieve pain satisfactorily.

2. **Postmenopausal women** (at least 5 years postmenopause)

a) **Estrogen** is effective in 40–50% of patients. Hepatic and cerebral metastases respond poorly. The following compounds are available: Premarin (10 mg TID), ethinylestradiol (1 mg TID), diethylstilbestrol (5 mg TID). The side effects include fluid retention, uterine bleeding, stress incontinence, and hypercalcemia (which manifests during the first few days of therapy).

b) If and when estrogen therapy fails the treatment as described in premenopausal patients is followed.

B. **Carcinoma of the lung** responds poorly to chemotherapy. The remission rate is low, and duration of remission tends to be short. Surgical resection in stage I, and possibly in stage II, and radiotherapy subsequently comprise the first line of treatment. In disseminated disease alkylating agents (e.g., nitrogen mustard and cyclophosphamide) and methotrexate may produce remissions in 10% of the patients.

C. **Carcinoma of the prostate**

1. **Orchiectomy** is generally accepted as the most important and effective step in the control of prostatic cancer. Favorable responses are observed in about 70% of the cases and may be maintained from a few months to several years.

2. **Estrogen** is usually administered as prophylactic maintenance therapy after castration. Usually diethylstilbestrol (1–5 mg daily) is used, but in patients not castrated, or unresponsive, as much as 15–25 mg/day may be used. Some oncologists suggest that estrogen may be used only after symptomatic metastases occur.

3. **Radiotherapy** may be used locally to control pain and tumor masses.

D. **Gastrointestinal cancer** The only drug that has been useful in carcinoma of gastrointestinal origin is 5-fluorouracil (5-FU). A remission rate of 15–20% can be achieved in metastatic colorectal, gastric, pancreatic, and biliary neoplasms (in that order). The dosage and mode of administration have been outlined in the section Agents Available, earlier in this chapter.

14. Thyroid Disease

I. **THYROID FUNCTION TESTS** A diagnosis of thyroid disease is frequently made on the basis of history and physical findings, but laboratory tests confirm the diagnosis and assess efficacy of therapy. More importantly, they may establish a definitive diagnosis in patients with a confusing clinical picture. A number of newer tests provide significant information in certain situations, but the most reliable tests are the PBI and RAI uptake. Although their values are affected by many nonthyroidal diseases and drugs, most difficulties in interpretation occur when the patient has previously received iodides or organic iodine dyes, which elevate the PBI and depress the RAI uptake for varying periods of time. The duration of effect of the more important compounds on the PBI and RAI uptake are listed below. In general, the PBI becomes valid sooner than the RAI uptake.

A. Iodides Although inorganic iodides are rapidly excreted, they may affect the PBI and RAI uptake for four weeks or more. If they have been administered for long periods of time, their effects may persist as long as six months. Cutaneous application of iodides may also transiently affect these tests; Darbid and Tuss-Ornade, which contain iodide salts, may exert effects for longer periods of time. Thyroxine determination by column chromatography can be used when iodides are present.

B. Organic iodine compounds

    1. Short duration of effect Aqueous intravascular or pyelographic dyes such as Diodrast, Urokon, Hippuran, Hypaque, Renografin, or Conray. The PBI is generally valid after 2 weeks and the RAI uptake after 4 weeks.

    2. Medium duration of effect Cholecystographic dyes such as Telepaque, Cholografin, Priodax; iodinated drugs such as Diodoquin and Vioform. The PBI may be valid after 3 months, but not usually until 6 months. RAI values are generally valid after 4–6 months.

    3. Long duration of effect Lipiodol and Pantopaque (used for myelography and bronchography) and Ethiodol (used for lymphangiography) affect the PBI and RAI uptake for 1–5 years or longer. The cholecystographic dye, Teridax, used many years ago, has been known to influence the PBI for 25 years or longer.

C. Thyroid, thyroxine, triiodothyronine Each grain of desiccated thyroid raises the PBI about 2 µg/100 ml; the equivalent dose of levothyroxine (0.1 mg) has a somewhat more marked effect. Both drugs depress the RAI uptake. Triiodothyronine depresses both the PBI and RAI uptake in normal subjects, and does not increase the PBI appreciably when used in the treatment of hypothyroidism.

D. Alterations in thyroid-hormone-binding proteins Over 99.9% of plasma thyroxine is bound to three serum proteins—thyroid-binding globulin (60%), prealbumin (30%), and albumin (10%). Stimuli which increase TBG concentration, such as estrogens (including oral contraceptives and pregnancy) elevate the PBI. Conversely, androgens, large doses of salicylates, Dilantin, and protein-losing states will lower PBI values. When abnormalities of thyroid-hormone binding are present, tests that are helpful in interpretation of the PBI include: the resin or red cell ^{131}I-T_3 (triiodothyronine) uptake, RAI uptake, and serum "free" (unbound) thyroxine concentration.

II. HYPERTHYROIDISM

A. General comments Hyperthyroidism is manifested by signs of hypermetabolism and hyperactivity of the autonomic nervous system. Etiologies include: diffuse toxic goiter, exogenous overingestion of thyroxine, functioning thyroid adenoma, "toxic" nodular goiter, and rarely thyroid carcinoma and choriocarcinoma. In diffuse toxic goiter (Graves' disease), excessive thyroid stimulation is ascribed to long-acting thyroid stimulator (LATS), a 7S IgG globulin found in the plasma of 50–80% of such patients. These patients uniquely may develop pretibial myxedema and ophthalmopathy.

B. General principles of management

1. Hospitalization Patients may be treated outside the hospital except for those with severe thyroxicosis, impending "thyroid storm," or cardiac complications.

2. Sedation Because of overactivity, irritability, and other nervous system symptoms, sedation is an important adjunct in therapy. Phenobarbital (30–60 mg QID) is useful. When symptoms of autonomic nervous system overactivity predominate, reserpine (1–2.5 mg daily in single or divided dosage) to effect adrenergic depletion, or the sympatholytic agent guanethidine (50–150 mg daily) are recommended. Hypotension may occur, particularly with guanethidine, although hyperthyroid patients tolerate larger doses than do euthyroid subjects.

3. Diet The diet should be balanced and sufficient in caloric value to permit restoration of lost weight. Multivitamin supplementation is suggested because of increased requirements.

4. Arrhythmias and congestive heart failure Hyperthyroidism may cause heart failure or arrhythmias, especially in elderly persons in whom the cardiac symptoms may be the only overt manifestation of the disease. Between 15% and 40% (percentage decreasing with age) of hyperthyroid patients with cardiac involvement do not have underlying organic heart disease. Digitalis is indicated even though adequate control of the cardiac abnormalities may occur only with return to the euthyroid state. The dosage of digitalis required is frequently larger than usual.

C. Choice of therapy Specific treatment may be medical (administration of antithyroid drugs or radioactive iodine) or surgical. Factors that influence the choice include age of the patient, size and type of gland (nodular or diffuse), severity of the illness, presence of complicating disease, pregnancy, and the extent to which the patient can cooperate with a prolonged medical regimen.

1. Children and adolescents with hyperthyroidism usually respond well to antithyroid drugs; long-term administration (one year or more) of such drugs is the initial therapy of choice according to many observers in a cooperative and reliable patient. For patients not suited to close observation over a long period, surgery is advised. The recurrence rate after completion of therapy is about 50%.

2. During pregnancy the response to antithyroid drugs and thyroidectomy is equally good. Some experts administer levothyroxine concurrently with antithyroid drugs or after surgery to ensure adequate fetal hormone and thus prevent the development of large fetal goiters or fetal hypothyroidism. RAI should not be given, for the fetal thyroid takes up significant amounts of RAI by the twelfth week of gestation.

3. RAI is the therapy of choice for patients who are poor surgical risks, for patients with postoperative recurrence of hyperthyroidism, and generally for patients over the age of 40. Many physicians have been lowering the age limits for the use of RAI, however, and some groups are treating patients in their twenties with RAI. The treatment of juvenile hyperthyroidism with RAI, however, has been associated with the later development of thyroid nodules, and recent studies have shown effects of RAI on leukocyte chromosomes; the significance of these findings is unclear at present.

4. Large goiters (whether diffuse or multinodular) producing compression symptoms should be removed.

D. Specific antithyroid drugs

1. **Iodine** Therapeutic doses of iodine (in hyperthyroid patients) inhibit thyroxine synthesis and release, cause involutional changes in the thyroid cells, and decrease thyroid vascularity. Patients may note subjective improvement within 24 hours and continue to improve for 10–14 days; after this period of maximum response the clinical condition may remain static, or, more likely, the symptomatology and the BMR will slowly increase. The initial response parallels the thyroxine-decay curve, supporting the concept that iodine inhibits thyroidal thyroxine release. This response pattern, characteristic of diffuse toxic goiters, is not usually seen in patients with toxic nodular goiters.

   a) **Preparations and dosage** The preparation of choice is saturated solution of potassium iodide (SSKI). The usual dose is 5 drops TID in a half-glass of water, providing 750 mg iodine daily, a dose far in excess of that necessary for maximum response; it is almost tasteless. Lugol's solution (10% KI and 5% iodine) should not be used because it is exceedingly distasteful.

   b) **Indications**

   i) The prime use of iodine is in preparing patients for surgery; after a course of antithyroid drugs has produced euthyroidism, SSKI is given for 10–14 days before surgery

to reduce vascularity of the gland and cause involutional changes in the thyroid follicular epithelium.

ii) Iodine may be used in combination with antithyroid drugs after treatment with RAI to bring about more rapid control of hyperthyroidism.

iii) Hyperthyroid crises.

iv) Iodine should not be used in conjunction with potassium perchlorate because the agents are competitive, and the iodine overcomes the perchlorate-induced block with resultant exacerbation of the hyperthyroidism.

c) **Toxic reactions**   Chronic iodine toxicity is not infrequent. The most common manifestation is an acneiform skin rash. Other symptoms often begin in the upper respiratory tract with sneezing, rhinorrhea, cough, or sore throat; headache, painful swelling of the salivary glands, pancreatitis, diarrhea, vomiting, and fever may also occur. Less common are hypersensitivity reactions with angioneurotic edema, exfoliative dermatitis, and hypersensitivity angiitis. The dosage is important in determining the severity of the reaction, even when it is of a hypersensitivity type; doses less than those precipitating the reaction may be taken for prolonged periods without further trouble.

2. **Thiourea derivatives** are used for definitive treatment of hyperthyroidism, for preparing thyrotoxic patients for thyroidectomy, occasionally for controlling the disease in the period after RAI administration when radiation effects have not yet become manifest. These drugs have no effect on iodine trapping, but prevent conversion of iodide to iodinated tyrosines by blocking organification of iodide; they also inhibit the coupling of iodotyrosines to form thyroxine, and propylthiouracil interferes with the peripheral deiodination and actions of thyroxine. Eighty percent of each dose is absorbed from the GI tract within 2 hours; significant blood levels occur within 15 minutes and disappear rapidly. Effective serum concentrations can be maintained with evenly spaced doses every 6–8 hours.

a) **Preparations and dosage**   Several compounds are available, but only two described below are used widely in this country.

i) **Propylthiouracil**   The average starting dose is 100–150 mg every 6–8 hours, but may be as high as 1.0 gm daily. If the patient responds, reduce to 300–400 mg daily after 5–6 weeks, to 150–300 mg daily after 8 weeks, then to maintenance doses of 100–200 mg daily after 6–8 months. Therapy is continued for 12–18 months to complete the course.

ii) **Methimazole (Tapazole)**   The average starting dose is 10 mg every 6 to 8 hours; after 5–6 weeks reduce to 25–30 mg daily; after 8 weeks reduce to 15–20 mg daily; after 6–8 months reduce to 5–10 mg daily for 12–18 months to complete the course of therapy.

b) The above dosage schedules provide guidelines, but patients with hyperthyroidism vary in the severity of their disease and clinical response; dosage of antithyroid drugs must be adjusted, as required, to maintain euthyroidism during the course of therapy.

c) The drugs are usually given in evenly divided doses (at least every 8 hours) to maintain effective blood levels. Although the necessity for evenly spaced doses has frequently been stressed, one report (*New Eng. J. Med.* 272:888, 1965) suggests that a single dose of propylthiouracil or methimazole is effective in inducing or maintaining a remission. Current data are too limited to recommend this treatment schedule as the one of choice.

d) Continuance of therapy and dosage schedule are dictated by clinical response. Among patients who showed no response by the sixth week of therapy, more than 90% were not taking the drug as directed, or the dosage was inadequate.

e) Patients with very large or multinodular goiters may require 2–4 times the dosage listed above.

f) **Results of therapy**   The therapeutic response is usually linear with time and unrelated to the severity of the disease; best guides to response are the clinical course, BMR, and PBI. Persistent remission after completion of the full course of therapy, as described above, may be achieved in about 50% of patients with toxic diffuse goiter. Of the patients who relapse, 70% will do so within 2 months after discontinuing therapy.

T_3 suppression tests of ^{131}I uptake after 6 months of treatment have been used to recognize patients prone to relapse after discontinuation of therapy. Those patients who exhibit greater than 50% suppressibility are likely to sustain a remission after antithyroid treatment, whereas those who fail to show suppression of uptake after T_3 require close follow-up and probably therapy with RAI or surgery (*Lancet* 2:1041, 1967).

g) **Toxic reactions**   There is no significant difference between the side effects of propylthiouracil and of methimazole when they are given in equivalent dosage.

  i) Skin rashes in 3–5% of patients, fever in 1–3%, and rarely, arthralgias, diarrhea, hypoprothrombinemia, and cholestatic jaundice.

  ii) Granulocytopenia occurs in 5% of patients, with the highest incidence in the first few months of treatment. Since the appearance of granulocytopenia seems dosage-related, it often becomes milder and of no clinical importance if the dosage of the drug is significantly reduced. If the white blood cell count falls below 3000/cu mm and the granulocytes below 40%, however, administration of antithyroid drugs should be discontinued. Routine periodic leukocyte counts cannot be relied upon to foreshadow agranulocytosis, because that complication is usually sudden in onset.

  iii) Agranulocytosis occurs in less than 0.5% of patients; it most often develops during the first course of therapy between the third and seventh weeks. The prognosis is relatively good (80% recovery) if the drug is withdrawn immediately and any infection is promptly treated; the granulocytes usually reappear within 5–8 days. Once this reaction has occurred to any of the thiouracils, other methods of treatment probably should be used, although one can often employ another antithyroid drug without difficulty.

3. Potassium perchlorate blocks iodide trapping by the thyroid. Though not widely used, it is efficient, inexpensive, and especially useful for patients who cannot take thiouracils. The usual dose is 250 mg QID. Initial reports noted a low incidence of mild side effects, primarily gastritis, but more recently a few serious reactions, notably aplastic anemia, have been described.

E. Radioactive iodine ^{131}I is the therapy of choice for most cases of hyperthyroidism in adults. The physical half-life of ^{131}I is 8 days; the therapeutic results are produced primarily by beta particles (90%) and to a very small extent by gamma rays. Radioiodine is concentrated by the thyroid gland, and destroying radiation is delivered to the acinar tissue; RAI exerts 50% of its effect within 8 days, 85% within 30 days, and, generally, maximal effects in 60–70 days.

1. Dosage The dose of ^{131}I must be individualized and is usually estimated from the thyroid gland size (as determined by palpation and/or thyroid scans) and the 24-hour RAI uptake. The usual dose is 100–150 μc RAI/gm estimated thyroid weight; larger doses are needed for toxic nodular goiters. The total curative dose for most patients with diffuse toxic goiters is 5–12 mc; some nodular glands may require 20–50 mc. Recently a lower dosage of ^{131}I, utilized in 116 patients (80 μc ^{131}I per estimated gram of thyroid), resulted in a reduction in permanent hypothyroidism from 33% to 6%; return to a euthyroid state required four months in 77% of the patients studied (*New Eng. J. Med.* 277:559, 1967).

2. Regimen for radiotherapy Certain considerations pertaining to use of ^{131}I are listed below.

a) Since the effects of ^{131}I therapy are slow, very ill or "poor risk" patients with severe complicating heart disease may be given antithyroid drugs for 2–3 weeks before administration of RAI; the drugs are discontinued 4 days before RAI is given.

b) Mild transient exacerbation of symptoms may occur 5–10 days after RAI therapy; these symptoms are due to follicular damage, with spillage of increased amounts of thyroxine and triiodothyronine into the circulation. Treatment is with sedation; antithyroid drugs are of no help.

c) Patients taking anticoagulant drugs may very rarely bleed into the thyroid. The prothrombin level should be above 20%; no other precautions are necessary.

d) At the end of 8 weeks, patients showing no response may have the initial dose of RAI repeated; those showing moderate improvement may be given half the initial dose; those with marked improvement should be reevaluated in another 4–6 weeks, since additional therapy may not be required.

e) Some authorities feel that levothyroxine (0.1–0.2 mg daily) should be given routinely after RAI therapy (see below).

3. Results of therapy

a) Thyrotoxicosis can be cured with a sufficient dose of RAI in essentially all patients. About 65% of patients treated with current regimens have been cured with one dose. Eight to 10 weeks are required for a patient with diffuse toxic goiter to reach euthyroidism and 12–14 weeks or longer for a patient with nodular toxic goiter. Most diffuse toxic goiters will decrease significantly after RAI, but the change in size of nodular glands is unpredictable and often slight. Therapeutic failures, usually a reflection of inadequate dosage, occur in less than 5% of patients.

b) Permanent hypothyroidism occurs in 7–10% of patients during the first year following therapy. Recent statistics indicate that an additional 3% of patients develop hypothyroidism each succeeding year for 7–10 years, so that half or more of patients given carefully calculated doses of RAI may eventually become hypothyroid. The high incidence of this complication, initially unsuspected, and the insidious manner in which the symptoms may develop (often resulting in a significant delay before the patient seeks medical attention) have been used as arguments by some against the use of RAI for the treatment of hyperthyroidism. Most experts, however, do not feel that one should be dissuaded from using RAI, but point out the importance of lifetime follow-up for all patients treated with it.

c) Hypoparathyroidism has been reported after the administration of large doses of RAI for the induction of hypothyroidism in patients with heart disease; this complication is rare.

4. **Late effects of irradiation** An increased incidence of carcinoma of the thyroid has been reported in individuals who have received external irradiation to the neck during childhood. The incidence of carcinoma of the thyroid does not appear to be increased by RAI treatment in the adult. To evaluate RAI effects upon the incidence of leukemia, a large cooperative study involving 22,000 patients treated with ^{131}I was begun in 1961. No differences in leukemia incidence rates have been demonstrated between patients treated with ^{131}I and those treated with surgery.

F. **Thyroidectomy** Operations should not be performed until a course of antithyroid therapy has resulted in euthyroidism. Antithyroid drugs are given for 6–8 weeks or longer, if necessary, until the patient is euthyroid; iodides are then given concurrently for the two weeks prior to surgery to reduce the vascularity of the thyroid gland and increase its firmness. With such preparation for operation, the incidence of postoperative thyroid storm has been almost eliminated.

Complications of surgery

1. Recurrence of hyperthyroidism is noted in 5–15% of patients, usually within 36 months. Additional surgery is not recommended because the procedure is technically more difficult and associated with a significantly higher percentage of complications; such patients should be treated with RAI, as a rule.

2. The operative mortality is 0.2–0.5% usually because of bleeding into the neck, inadequate preoperative therapy and resultant thyroid storm, or excessive administration of antithyroid drugs preoperatively, resulting in hypothyroidism. In most recent series, almost all operative deaths have been associated with hypothyroidism.

3. Paralysis of one vocal cord (due to interruption of the recurrent laryngeal nerve) occurs in about 1% of patients; paralysis is serious if bilateral. Function of both vocal cords should be determined before surgery.

4. Permanent myxedema occurs in 2–10% of patients; transient hypothyroidism occurs more frequently.

5. Frank tetany may appear within 1–7 days postoperatively (rarely at longer intervals) and is usually temporary; the incidence of permanent hypoparathyroidism is about 1%. These patients should be treated as described in the section on hypoparathyroidism. Three to six months after thyroidectomy, serum calcium and phosphorus determinations should be made on every patient, since hypoparathyroidism (with its important complication of rapidly progressive cataracts) can occur without overt clinical manifestations of hypocalcemia.

III. SEVERE MANIFESTATIONS OF THYROTOXICOSIS AND THEIR MANAGEMENT

A. Malignant exophthalmos   Medical treatment of progressive ophthalmopathy (exophthalmos, which may be accompanied by extraocular muscle weakness, chemosis, injection, and impairment of visual acuity) is at present unsatisfactory. Variability of the clinical course renders evaluation of treatment difficult. The pathogenesis is not known. One investigator has reported dramatic regression in eye changes following complete thyroidal ablation with repeated large doses of ^{131}I (> 100 mc), but this result has not been confirmed generally. Most authorities, however, agree that hyperthyroidism should be promptly controlled, since eye signs often improve as it subsides, and that posttreatment hypothyroidism should be avoided.

1. General measures   The eyes should be protected from wind and dust with the use of "artificial tears" (1% methylcellulose eyedrops) and perhaps temporary tarsorrhaphy. The patient should sleep with his head elevated.

2. Corticosteroids   For severe, rapidly progressive exophthalmos the patient should be hospitalized, and large doses of corticosteroids (80–100 mg of prednisone daily or an equivalent amount of other preparations) administered for 14 days. If improvement occurs, the dosage can be reduced gradually to the lowest effective maintenance level. If no improvement has occurred after 4 weeks, corticosteroid therapy should be discontinued. For less severe cases of exophthalmos, outpatient treatment with smaller doses of corticosteroids (20 mg prednisone daily) for about two weeks may bring about improvement, especially disappearance of chemosis. Corticosteroid maintenance therapy should be discontinued after 3–6 months.

3. Surgical decompression is necessary in severe cases, and the results are frequently gratifying. Objectives of the operation are to restore vision, to restore use of extraocular muscles and the ability to close the eyelids, to relieve increased orbital tension, and to attain a satisfactory cosmetic result. The most rewarding procedure to date is that described by Ogura (*Med. Clin. N. Amer.* 52:399, 1968), which consists of transantral decompression in which the ethmoid air cells are exenterated; the floor and medial wall of the orbit are then removed. This procedure avoids incisions on the face or scalp, surgical trauma of the already injured eye, and serious immediate or late postoperative complications. Removal of the lateral orbital wall (Moran operation) provides less satisfactory decompression, and removal of superior orbital plate (Naffziger operation) is a formidable procedure requiring entry into the cranial cavity.

B. **Thyroid storm or crisis** is a severe medical emergency which may occur spontaneously, or after surgery of any sort in an inadequately controlled thyrotoxic patient, but probably the commonest precipitating cause is infection.

1. **Manifestations** The diagnosis is made on the basis of the clinical findings, which include hyperpyrexia, tachycardia or cardiac arrhythmias, dehydration, dry skin, vomiting, diarrhea, extreme restlessness and delirium, followed by stupor, coma, and shock.

2. **Treatment** is directed against four features of the disease—increased release of thyroid hormones, thyroid hormone peripheral effects, failure of homeostatic mechanisms to compensate for demands imposed by severe thyrotoxicosis, and precipitating illness (*New Eng. J. Med.* 247:1252, 1966).

   a) For shock, vasopressor agents are given (see section on shock in Chapter 17).

   b) For hyperpyrexia: salicylates, hypothermic blanket, and phenothiazines. The hypothermic effect of phenothiazines is attributed to their central action on the thermoregulatory centers of the hypothalamus, their peripheral vasodilating action, and their capacity to prevent shivering. Large doses may be necessary, e.g., prochlorperazine 10–15 mg IM every 4 hours; severe hypotension may be a complication.

   c) Adequate fluids and electrolytes parenterally, adequate calories (preferably in the form of feedings through a stomach tube), and large doses of multivitamins.

   d) Nasal oxygen, or preferably oxygen tent with attached air conditioner.

   e) Reserpine 2.5 mg IM every 6–12 hours. Although hyperthyroid patients have less marked drops in blood pressure than do euthyroid individuals, severe hypotension may develop, especially in elderly patients, or those also receiving phenothiazines.
   Guanethidine may also be used for its sympatholytic effects; cardiovascular and neuromuscular manifestations of thyroid storm may be effectively controlled without the pronounced sedation produced by reserpine. Guanethidine 50 mg may be given orally every 12 hours; if no response is apparent, subsequent doses may be increased to 150 mg unless orthostatic hypotension occurs.

   f) Corticosteroids: Hydrocortisone succinate 400–600 mg/24 hours IV; an equivalent amount of other preparations may be used.

   g) Methimazole (or propylthiouracil in equivalent dosage) 30 mg immediately and 30 mg TID thereafter during the acute stage.

   h) Iodides: Sodium iodide should be added to parenteral fluids (2.0 gm/24 hours), or SSKI, 10–15 drops QID, may be given orally.

Administer each dose of iodides one hour after the administration of methimazole; iodides are therefore prevented from being incorporated into hormone stores within the gland.

i) As the patient responds, oral medications may be substituted for those which have been given parenterally. Following recovery from crisis, definitive antithyroid therapy should be carried out.

j) Heart failure should be treated with digitalis and diuretics.

IV.   HYPOTHYROIDISM Nongoitrous hypothyroidism may be primary or secondary to pituitary disease. Primary hypothyroidism may occur spontaneously or may follow thyroiditis, thyroidectomy, or administration of therapeutic doses of RAI. The objective of treatment is restoration of euthyroid status. Because many thyroid extract preparations are not standardized by a bioassay technique, because different lots may vary in potency and may deteriorate with long standing, and because synthetic levothyroxine is now widely available, predictable, and not significantly more expensive (10–20% more than thyroid extract depending on preparation and pharmacy), many observers feel that there is little indication for continued use of thyroid extract in the treatment of hypothyroidism. Sodium levothyroxine, usually referred to as thyroxine, is available as Synthroid (tablets of 0.025, 0.05, 0.1, 0.15, 0.2, and 0.3 mg) and Letter, a micronized preparation (tablets of 0.025, 0.05, 0.1, 0.2, 0.3, and 0.5 mg). Thyroxine 0.1 mg = thyroid extract 60 mg = triiodothyronine (T_3) (Cytomel) 25 µg. The usual replacement dose of thyroxine is 0.2–0.3 mg daily (= 120–180 mg thyroid extract).

A. Replacement therapy

1. Mildly hypothyroid patients can be begun directly on a schedule of 0.1–0.3 mg of levothyroxine (T_4) daily. Most patients require 0.2 mg/day for restoration of euthyroidism.

2. Severely myxedematous patients have traditionally been treated by a graduated schedule of hormone beginning with 0.025 mg daily which is doubled every several weeks. At present, most authorities feel that a full replacement regimen can be instituted immediately, except in those patients with a history of coronary artery disease, where the graduated program must be used. In the event that angina pectoris is precipitated, the dosage should be reduced. Recently a mixture of T_3 and T_4 has been proposed to provide "physiologic" replacement and PBI values corresponding to normal (*Ann. Intern. Med.* 90:67, 1967). There are no data, however, to support the need in man for T_3 as well as T_4 in replacement programs.

B. Myxedema coma is a rare condition manifested by unresponsiveness, hypothermia, hypotension, and hypoventilation. Mortality is appreciable, and parenteral therapy with thyroid hormone should be instituted rapidly. One schedule that resulted in reduction in mortality without serious sequelae involved the administration of 500 µg T_4 IV in a single injection (*Arch. Intern. Med.* 113:89, 1964). Oral (nasogastric tube) or IM T_3 (100–150 µg daily) has also been employed. In addition, supportive therapy may require tracheostomy with assisted ventilation, glucocorticoids, pressor agents, etc. Hypothermia should not be corrected rapidly.

V. THYROID NODULES

A. Multinodular goiters

1. Large multinodular goiters may result from specific metabolic defects (e.g., iodine deficiency, enzyme defects), or prolonged ingestion of iodides or goitrogens, but the majority are not associated with any readily diagnosable abnormality. Although the glands are usually benign and the patients euthyroid, these goiters occasionally harbor a carcinoma or cause thyrotoxicosis. When neither of these is a problem, therapy is required only for cosmetic reasons or compression symptoms.

2. For simple nontoxic multinodular glands, administration of thyroxine (0.2–0.3 mg daily) may halt further enlargement or cause involution of the gland and disappearance of the nodules.

3. For large glands causing compression symptoms or marked tracheal deviation, thyroidectomy is the treatment of choice. Following operation, thyroxine should be administered indefinitely in replacement dose to prevent recurrence of the goiter.

B. Solitary thyroid nodules
The management of single thyroid nodules remains controversial because of the great variation in the incidence of carcinoma reported in such nodules; the following generalities may be helpful.

1. Single nodules are described as "warm" or "cold" on scans of the thyroid. "Warm" nodules concentrate radioactive iodine in a degree equal to or greater than that of the surrounding gland; "cold" nodules concentrate less. The incidence of carcinoma in warm nodules is very low; "cold" nodules are more frequently malignant (4–25%, depending on the series and selection of patients).

   In either case, many observers would observe such nodules for a period of six months while the patient is receiving suppressive doses of thyroxine (0.2–0.3 mg daily); if the nodule fails to decrease in size, surgical removal would then be recommended. Other experts insist that such periods of observation are of no value and recommend immediate operation.

2. There is almost complete agreement, however, that solitary nodules should be removed immediately in the following situations:

   a) If the patient is less than 20 years of age; the evidence of malignancy is increased in young patients.

   b) If the nodule is unusually hard, greater than 2.0 cm in diameter, or rapidly growing.

VI. THYROIDITIS

A. Acute thyroiditis (subacute thyroiditis, de Quervain's thyroiditis, granulomatous thyroiditis)

1. **General comments** The etiology is unknown, but the disease is presumed by many to represent a viral infection of the thyroid gland. Clinical manifestations include moderate to severe local tenderness and pain in the thyroid, often asymmetrical, often radiating into the jaw or ear, and accompanied by chills, fever, sweats, and malaise. In severe cases transient hyperthyroidism may occur, due

to release of thyroid hormone from the inflamed gland. Symptoms may persist for months.

Laboratory studies usually show a low 24-hour RAI uptake, normal or elevated PBI; the sedimentation rate is usually elevated.

2. Treatment

   a) Aspirin is the drug of choice; when given in full dosage (3–4.8 gm daily), local and systemic symptoms are usually well controlled. Therapy should be continued until the patient has been asymptomatic for 4–6 weeks, then cautiously withdrawn. If symptoms recur, treatment is restarted.

   b) Thyroxine (0.2–0.3 mg daily) may be beneficial in shortening the course of the disease. It should not be given if the patient is hyperthyroid.

   c) Corticosteroids usually cause dramatic cessation of symptoms (often within 24 hours), but their use should be reserved for relatively severe cases because of the frequent exacerbation of symptoms (in 30–50% of patients) after therapy is discontinued. The usual initial dosage is 30–40 mg prednisone daily (or equivalent amount of other preparations); when symptoms have subsided for a week or so, dosage may be tapered slowly over a 3–4-week period and discontinued.

   d) Antithyroid drugs have no effect on the disease and should not be given. If symptoms of hyperthyroidism require treatment, sedatives and reserpine or guanethidine should be administered.

B. Hashimoto's thyroiditis (struma lymphomatosa) is thought to represent an autoimmune disorder because of the frequency with which antibodies to thyroglobulin and other thyroid antigens can be demonstrated; the precise etiology remains obscure. The disease is most common in middle-aged females; symptoms, which are minimal, often include gradual enlargement of the thyroid gland and manifestations of hypothyroidism; pain, fever, and other symptoms are rare (unless some other systemic disease is also present). Many observers believe that almost all cases of spontaneous primary myxedema in adults are a result of Hashimoto's thyroiditis. The only treatment required, as a rule, is the administration of thyroxine to those patients who develop hypothyroidism.

C. Suppurative thyroiditis is a rare disease, usually following septicemia or spread of infection from adjacent tissues. The causative organism should be identified, and appropriate antibiotics administered; surgical drainage may be required if localized abscess formation occurs.

VII. HYPOPARATHYROIDISM Hypoparathyroidism after treatment of thyrotoxicosis most frequently follows thyroidectomy, but may very rarely follow administration of very large doses of RAI used either to treat hyperthyroidism or to treat angina in the euthyroid patient. It does not occur after the use of antithyroid drugs. Hypoparathyroidism (either clinical or chemical) may occur in the immediate postoperative period. It may also appear months or years after thyroidectomy. All patients who have had thyroid surgery require determinations of the serum calcium and phosphorus postoperatively, and again in 3, 6, and 12 months, in order to detect clinically inapparent hypoparathyroidism.

A. If tetany appears in the postoperative period, 10% calcium gluconate

(10–30 ml) should be given IV until the tetany is controlled. Calcium chloride should not be used because thrombophlebitis and sloughing of soft tissues may occur if it is extravasated. Clinical signs of hypocalcemia and the serum calcium and phosphorus levels should be followed closely. The Sulkowitch urine test, though of limited value, generally indicates significant hypocalcemia if negative. Hypocalcemia may be present when the Sulkowitch test is positive, however, especially if the patient is receiving vitamin D.

B. If the tetany does not cease after IV administration of calcium gluconate, if it recurs, or if the serum calcium level remains low postoperatively, oral administration of calcium and/or vitamin D (depending upon the severity of the hypoparathyroidism) should be begun, and the serum calcium and phosphorus levels measured frequently in order to determine proper dosage. **Preparations:**

1. Vitamin D (e.g., Calciferol, Deltalin), 50,000-unit capsules. The maintenance dose is usually 50,000–150,000 units daily, but therapy should be initiated with 200,000 units daily. The response to vitamin D is not rapid; generally 7–10 days elapse before the serum calcium is raised significantly; effects persist at least several weeks after administration is stopped. Patients receiving long-term therapy with vitamin D should be observed closely for the development of hypercalcemia which, along with renal insufficiency, may occur insidiously and with few symptoms. Corticosteroids will rapidly reverse the hypercalcemia of vitamin D intoxication.

2. Crystalline dihydrotachysterol may be substituted for vitamin D; 1 mg approximates 3 mg (120,000 units) of vitamin D (Calciferol). Dihydrotachysterol possesses the advantage of shorter duration of action, thereby allowing more rapid dissipation of toxic effects (hypercalcemia). In a recent study, a maximum dose of 1 mg was sufficient to maintain the serum calcium, regardless of prior vitamin D dosage (*New Eng. J. Med.* 276:894, 1967). Commercial AT 10 (Hytakerol) does not give results comparable to those of *crystalline* dihydrotachysterol.

3. Calcium gluconate tablets (0.3 and 0.6 gm) and wafers (1.0 gm) contain approximately 10% calcium. The usual dose is 10–15 gm calcium gluconate daily. Calcium lactate powder (18.37% calcium) is available. Preparations containing phosphate should not be used.

15. Diabetes Mellitus

I. **GENERAL APPROACH TO THERAPY** Once the diagnosis of diabetes mellitus is made, selection of a proper diet becomes a necessary and basic part of any treatment program. Whether or not insulin or oral hypoglycemic agents will be required depends on the degree of control achieved by the diet; this is generally a reflection of the severity of the diabetes, the age of the patient at the onset of the disease, and the body weight. The patient who is less than 15 years of age when diabetes is contracted is considered a "juvenile diabetic." Many juvenile and some adult diabetic patients, especially those who are thin, are referred to as "brittle diabetics" because they are exceedingly unstable, so that small increments or decrements in insulin dosage may provoke severe hypoglycemia or ketosis. Most adult-onset diabetics are more stable in that slight changes in insulin dose do not alter diabetic control significantly; rapid and frequent development of ketoacidosis is distinctly less common.

A. **What constitutes adequate control of diabetes?** The aims of diabetic management include correction of the metabolic abnormalities with diet and drugs, attainment and maintenance of ideal body weight, and the prevention of complications associated with the disease. There has been gross disagreement as to how to achieve the last goal; i.e., how carefully should the chemical abnormalities be controlled? Severe retinopathy, nephropathy, and/or neuropathy may develop in any patient with diabetes, and may even be the presenting complaints. Nonetheless, careful control of diabetes may play a role in delaying the onset and progression of these complications. For most patients the achievement of good control is not incompatible with a relatively normal life.

B. **Which patients can be managed by diet alone?** A very high percentage of patients with adult-onset diabetes, obesity, and few symptoms can be managed solely with a low-calorie weight-reduction diet. Marked increase in carbohydrate (CHO) tolerance may occur as the excess weight is lost. Significant and persistent glycosuria continuing for 2–3 weeks after initiation of diet often reflects the patient's failure to follow the dietary regimen and indicates the need for more vigorous treatment by the addition of insulin or an oral hypoglycemic agent.

C. **Which patients can be controlled by oral hypoglycemic agents?** The sulfonylureas and phenformin provide initial satisfactory control in roughly two-thirds of the older patients who have adult-onset, stable diabetes of relatively short duration, and minimal or no insulin requirements. These drugs are unlikely to be effective in patients requiring more than 40 units of insulin per day but may be tried. The sulfonylureas are ineffective following pancreatectomy or in patients with juvenile or "brittle" diabetes, but in these latter patients the sulfonylureas or phenformin may be a useful adjunct to insulin. Neither the long-term effects of these drugs on the incidence of vascular and neurologic complications nor their effectiveness in the treatment of early diabetes or so-called prediabetes can be assessed at present.

D. Which patients require insulin? Insulin is required for juvenile or brittle diabetics, patients not responsive to diet and an oral hypoglycemic agent, and many mild diabetics (not ordinarily requiring insulin) during acute major stresses, as infection or surgery. Approximately 30–35% of diabetics require insulin regularly.

E. What laboratory procedures are of assistance in evaluation of diabetic control?

1. Urinary sugar

a) Spot tests Urines should be tested before meals and at bedtime (7 and 11 a.m., 4 and 9 p.m.) when multiple doses of regular insulin are being given, and during periods of insulin dosage changes, acute illness, or surgery. The bladder should be emptied 30 minutes before collection of the test sample. For patients outside the hospital the urine should be tested before breakfast and either one hour before supper or at bedtime, depending on the time of maximum action of the insulin preparation taken. For patients controlled with diet alone or oral hypoglycemic agents, urine may be tested once daily before breakfast. Tests 2–3 hours after meals, however, will be of value in determining the presence of significant fluctuations of blood sugar, provided that the renal threshold for glucose is not markedly elevated.

b) Fractional urines All urine is saved between 7–11 a.m., 11 a.m.–4 p.m., 4–9 p.m., and 9 p.m.–7 a.m.; the urine sugar test is performed on an aliquot of the total amount collected during each interval. These determinations are important during periods of final adjustment of insulin dosage when it is desirable to know whether there has been any glycosuria during the interval.

c) Quantitative tests Determination of the glucose concentration in the fractional specimens allows one to compute the number of grams of sugar spilled each 24 hours. Since qualitative measurements are occasionally misleading, quantitative values may be useful in evaluating the control of brittle diabetics.

d) Clinitest tablets are preferable to Tes-Tape and Clinistix because glycosuria is more accurately quantitated. The ease of use of test papers, however, is an important advantage for many patients, especially when they are away from home.

2. Urinary ketones should be checked with nitroprusside reagents, either tablets (Acetest) or strips (Ketostix), during acute illnesses or periods of 3–4+ glycosuria; this precaution is particularly important for unstable diabetics or in any patient who has ever been in ketoacidosis.

3. Blood sugar Initially, samples should be obtained during fasting,

2 hours after main meals, and at times of maximum effect of the insulin preparation given. If one obtains capillary (fingerstick) or arterial blood and measures the secreted urinary sugar at the same time, the renal threshold for glucose may be estimated. Blood sugars should always be obtained during suspected hypoglycemic reactions.

F. **What to tell the patient** The patient must be educated thoroughly regarding the technique of insulin injection, insulin refrigeration, types of insulin syringes, syringe care, diet calculation, urine testing, symptoms and treatment of hypoglycemia, significance of acute illnesses and ketonuria, and proper foot care. All patients should carry a diabetic card or "dog tag." A number of manuals which explain the nature and management of diabetes in simple terms are available. Of particular value are the *Lilly Diabetic Manual* and *Joslin's Diabetic Manual for the Patient.*

II. **DIET** Diet is the basis of all treatment of diabetes. Diet alone may correct the metabolic abnormalities; a stable dietary intake, essential for management with insulin or oral agents, does not preclude selection of varied, palatable, and nutritious meals.

A. **Diet orders** The total number of calories and grams of CHO, protein, and fat, the frequency and time of feedings, and the amount of CHO in grams to be given at each feeding should be specified.

B. **Diet calculation**

1. **The following factors are of importance:** patient's age, sex, activity, present and ideal body weight (IBW), and type of therapy (diet alone, hypoglycemic drugs, insulin). If insulin is required, the time of maximum action of the preparation used must be considered. A patient is much more likely to follow a diet based on his previous eating habits.

2. **Total calories**

   a) Give 30–35 cal/kg IBW for nonobese middle-aged men; give slightly less for women.

   b) Give 40–45 cal/kg IBW for the underweight or very active patient.

   c) Give 20–25 cal/kg IBW if weight reduction is necessary.

3. **Total CHO (4 cal/gm)** Provide 40% of total calories as CHO (easily calculated in grams by dividing total calories by 10). The division of CHO intake should be dictated by the patient's desires and type of therapy. Patients on diet alone or oral hypoglycemic drugs may have the CHO intake equally divided between the three major meals; a bedtime snack may be allowed. Patients receiving intermediate-acting insulins should have a relatively light breakfast and a midafternoon and/or bedtime feeding (15–20 gm CHO).

4. **Total protein (4 cal/gm)** Provide 20% of total calories as protein except when patients on high-calorie diets cannot afford the cost of this amount of protein. During pregnancy and lactation larger amounts are required.

5. **Total fat (9 cal/gm)** Give remainder of total calories (usually 40%) as fat. Approximately half the fat should be polyunsaturated

(liquid fats derived from vegetable sources; margarine rich in unsaturated fatty acids).

C. Dietary instructions   The physician and dietitian must make sure that the patient and members of his family understand the basis of the diet. Diet instruction should begin several days prior to discharge from the hospital. Many physicians can prescribe an appropriate diet, yet have little or no idea how this prescription will be translated into a set of instructions which the patient can follow easily whether at home or away.

1. Many hospitals plan meals using standard "exchange lists" adopted by the American Diabetes Association and the American Dietetic Association. In this plan, foods are divided into six groups (the exchange groups) ; each food of the particular group, in the portion stated, contains about the same amount of CHO, protein, or fat as any other food of that group. The patient is directed as to the number of exchanges to take from the various lists for the three main meals and between-meal snacks. The lists are composed as follows:

(1)   Milk (whole, dried, etc.) : 1 exchange $= 1$ cup whole milk

(2a)   Vegetables which need not be measured.

(2b)   Vegetables with 7 gm CHO content per exchange.

(3)   Fruits with 10 gm CHO content per exchange.

(4)   Breads, cereals, and starchy vegetables with 15 gm CHO content per exchange.

(5)   Major protein foods (fish, meat, eggs, cheese) : 1 protein exchange contains 7 gm protein.

(6)   Fat exchanges: Contain 5 gm fat (e.g., 1 tsp. butter) per exchange.

> Copies of the lists plus six standard meal plans (ranging from 1200 to 2600 cal) may be obtained from the American Diabetes Association, Inc., 1 E. 45th St., New York, N.Y. 10017, or the American Dietetic Association, 620 N. Michigan Ave., Chicago, Ill. 60611.

2. A different system is used at the Washington University Medical Center and seems preferred by patients because it allows somewhat greater flexibility in selection of the CHO quota of each meal. The patients are taught to compute the diet using common household measures (cup, tsp., tbsp.) and a set of food lists that expresses CHO in "teaspoons of sugar value," a unit equivalent to 4 gm of glucose. Foods are assigned to the various lists on the basis of their CHO content. The diet prescription lists the amount of protein and fat to be consumed at each meal (from lists similar to the protein and fat exchange lists described above) and then designates the teaspoons of sugar value allowed; the patient can choose fruit, vegetables, bread, or cereals from any of the lists to equal this value. Dietary instruction is essential in order to assure that the patient will select foods that are well balanced in vitamins and minerals.

D. Diabetic foods   A large number are available, especially water-packed fruits and vegetables, which are recommended on diabetic diets;

prices are 10–20% higher than for corresponding syrup-packed foods. Calorie-free carbonated drinks and certain candies are permissible, but some of the "diabetic" chocolates, cookies, etc., contain basic ingredients with significant food value, even though they are glucose-free; these cannot be consumed in addition to the diet but may be substituted for other foods. Most diabetic patients receive sufficiently liberal CHO allowances so that occasional small amounts of ice cream, etc., may be used. Satisfactory sugar substitutes are saccharin, and sodium or calcium cyclamate (Sucaryl).

E. **Vitamins** Supplemental multivitamins are desirable for patients with caloric intake of less than 1200, during periods of poor control, or in patients with malabsorption.

III. INSULIN

A. **Insulin preparations** Available preparations are listed in Table 15-1. Most commercial insulin is a mixture of beef and pork insulins.

TABLE 15-1. Insulin Preparations

Type of Insulin	Suspension	Effects Begin	Maximum Action	Duration of Effect (in hrs)
		(hrs after subcut. injection)		
Regular (crystalline)	Solution	¼	4–6	6–8
Semilente	Amorphous	½	4–6	12–16
Globin	Solution	2–3	6–10	12–18
NPH	Crystalline	3	8–12	18–24
Lente	30% amorphous and 70% crystalline	3	8–12	18–28
PZI	Amorphous	3–4	14–20	24–36
Ultralente	Crystalline	3–4	16–18	30–36

1. Insulin is available in dilutions of 40 units/ml (all syringes and labels are color-coded red) and 80 units/ml (color code is green), but more dilute or concentrated preparations can be obtained for special situations. When ordering insulin, specify the dilution and make sure that the syringe is calibrated in the same units.

2. **NPH and PZI** are both mixtures of zinc, protamine (a polypeptide), and insulin, but PZI contains a much greater ratio of protamine to insulin than does NPH. Therefore, regular and NPH may be mixed together in the same syringe (but not more than one unit regular insulin to each 4–5 units NPH) and given as one injection without greatly altering the spectrum of action of either; PZI and regular insulin must be given as separate injections if their individual effects are to be retained.

3. **Semilente and Ultralente insulins** are combinations of insulin, zinc, and acetate buffer, with pH changes determining their degree of solubility and hence their rate of absorption. The spectrum of

action is essentially the same as for regular and PZI, respectively. Lente insulin, a combination of 70% Ultralente and 30% Semilente, has much the same therapeutic properties as NPH. Since the Lente insulins contain no protamine, they are of value in the occasional patient allergic to protamine or its impurities. Regular insulin in large amounts should not be mixed with Lente insulin because the pH is altered and hence the predictability of its absorption, but a regular-to-Lente ratio of 1:5 may be tried.

B. Selection of preparation

1. **Regular insulin** is required during acidosis and other acute situations (e.g., severe infections, surgery) when the patient's food intake is variable. It is often used in combination with longer-acting insulins for routine management.

2. **Intermediate insulins** (especially NPH or Lente) when used alone and administered once daily 30–45 minutes before breakfast provide adequate control in most stable adult diabetics requiring less than 50 units/day.

   a) Many severe diabetics, however, are more easily regulated if 20–25% of the total daily NPH insulin is given before supper. This generalization is especially true if difficulty is experienced in maintaining relatively normal fasting blood sugar values without causing afternoon hypoglycemia.

   b) If morning hyperglycemia is a problem, decrease the CHO content of breakfast and add small amounts (5–15 units) of regular insulin to the morning dose of NPH (or add Semilente to Lente). This combination is particularly valuable for patients requiring moderately large doses of insulin.

3. **Long-acting insulins** used alone are rarely indicated; hypoglycemic reactions following their administration often occur during the sleeping hours and hence may be prolonged and severe.

C. Initiation of therapy

1. For new patients presenting with severe diabetes, administer regular insulin before each meal, giving 10–20 units for 4+ urine sugar, 10–15 units for 3+, 5–10 units for 2+, 0–5 units for 1+; response to therapy should be observed closely for several days and adjustment in insulin dosage made until the total daily requirements can be estimated moderately well. Then give instead one-half to two-thirds of this amount as a single dose of one of the intermediate preparations. Further adjustments in dosage and addition or substitution of another preparation may be necessary, and are indicated by the patient's "chemical" response.

2. For patients presenting with mild or moderate diabetes without significant ketosis, treatment may be started with an arbitrary amount (usually 10–15 units) of an intermediate preparation; further adjustments are made as dictated by response.

D. Adjustment of dosage

1. For patients receiving intermediate insulins, increments of 5 units may be made every day if moderate glycosuria persists throughout the day. If the patient is approaching control or is a brittle dia-

betic sensitive to insulin, increments should be limited to 2–4 units every second day.

2. If urinary or blood sugar values fluctuate markedly the cause may be incorrect measurement of insulin, faulty technique of injection, irregular dietary intake, or marked day-to-day changes in physical activity. Emotional stresses, particularly in juvenile diabetics, play a significant role in upsetting regulation. Resumption of adequate control requires relatively constant food intake and exercise.

3. **"Somogyi phenomenon"** This term is used to describe an uncommon state characterized by fluctuating degrees of glycosuria and hyperglycemia associated with ketonuria and apparently rising insulin requirements. This sequence of events is provoked by episodes of hypoglycemia which may not be recognized and which induce accelerated release of catecholamines, adrenal corticosteroids, and growth hormone, which oppose the effect of the injected insulin. This apparent worsening of the diabetic state is often treated by increasing the insulin dosage when in reality the diabetes can be brought back into a state of control by *decreasing* the insulin dose.

4. **The following factors increase insulin requirements:** weight gain, increased food intake, pregnancy, decreased exercise, hyperthyroidism, acute infections, hyperadrenocorticism, acromegaly, and treatment with drugs, as glucocorticoids, thyroid, epinephrine, and thiazide diuretics.

   a) During periods of decreased physical activity or mild infections, small increases in insulin dosage generally allow adequate control.

   b) During moderately severe infections, supplemental doses of regular insulin may be required at 4–6-hour intervals as indicated by urine tests.

   c) Severe infections with anorexia, vomiting, and ketosis necessitate hospitalization. Preferably, regular insulin alone (on a sliding scale) should be given until food intake and insulin requirements stabilize. Then the former diabetic regimen may be resumed.

5. **The following factors decrease insulin requirements:** weight reduction, decreased caloric intake, increased physical activity, advent of renal insufficiency, termination of treatment with the drugs mentioned above, hypothyroidism, hypoadrenocorticism, hypopituitarism, and recovery from hyperthyroidism, acute infections, or ketoacidosis. Juvenile diabetics not infrequently have a period of apparent recovery of islet-cell function after the disease first appears and before permanent diabetes develops. Changes in insulin requirements may occur rapidly; failure to recognize this development and to decrease insulin dosage accordingly (occasionally it may be possible to substitute tolbutamide or discontinue therapy entirely) may result in severe hypoglycemic reactions.

E. **Insulin administration during surgical procedures.** When a diabetic patient requires an operation, the following points should be kept in mind:

1. Ketosis and hypoglycemia must be avoided during the operative and postoperative periods.

2. Minor procedures generally require no great change in the diabetic regimen.

3. Elective major operations should be delayed until the diabetes is under good control. When a patient with severe acidosis requires an emergency operation, the procedure should be delayed several hours (if at all possible) until dehydration and acidosis are partially corrected.

4. If the patient takes insulin, it must be continued during surgery in a dose that approximates the usual daily requirements. If the patient takes oral hypoglycemic agents *small* doses of insulin instead are usually required during the operative and postoperative periods.

5. Adequate CHO in the form of IV 5–10% glucose (200–250 gm/day) should be supplied during and after operation until oral intake is reestablished.

6. Urinary and blood ketones should be checked every 6 hours on the day of operation and the first postoperative day. Urinary sugar tests may be difficult to interpret if large amounts of glucose are administered IV.

F. Reactions to insulin

1. **Hypoglycemia** Prolonged or repeated hypoglycemia may cause permanent brain damage or precipitate angina pectoris. Patients should be taught to recognize the symptoms and should carry mints or hard candy with them at all times. **Mild reactions** usually subside following ingestion of candy or orange juice. For **severe reactions** 20–30 ml of 50% glucose are given IV, followed by oral CHO or infusion of 5% glucose in order to prevent recurrent hypoglycemia. Brittle diabetics and the immediate family of these patients should be instructed in the use of **glucagon,** a polypeptide secreted by pancreatic alpha cells, which produces glycogenolysis and prompt release of glucose from the liver and may be used for the treatment of certain cases of insulin-induced hypoglycemia. It is indicated primarily when the patient cannot safely ingest glucose. Maximum effects occur in 10–15 minutes. The dose is 1–2 mg IM or subcutaneously and may be repeated once in 15 minutes.

2. **Skin reactions**

   a) Transient localized urticarial lesions usually occur during the first few weeks of therapy and later disappear. Generally no change in regimen is needed. However, deeper injection of insulin, administration of antihistamines, or change to another insulin preparation may be tried.

   b) Subcutaneous fibrosis results from repeated injection into the same area and may be avoided by rotating injection sites. Insulin is irregularly absorbed from these areas.

   c) Localized atrophy or hypertrophy of subcutaneous fat is unsightly but otherwise of no significance; the cause is unknown. Generally the fat deposits return to normal with time.

   d) Induration, necrosis, ulceration, infection, and scarring may follow intracutaneous injections.

3. Immunologic reactions

a) Insulin allergy Reactions may be mild and local or, very rarely, severe and general (urticaria, angioneurotic edema, anaphylactic shock). They may represent allergy to the protein (protamine) added to insulin, to tissue proteins of the animal source, or to the animal insulin itself. Further reactions may be prevented by switching to an insulin preparation without added protein (Lente) or by using insulin from a different animal.

b) Insulin resistance Some patients require very large doses of insulin (from 200 to thousands of units daily). In many instances this requirement can be related to the presence of insulin antibodies which bind large amounts of insulin. The insulin-resistant state may be transient or prolonged for years, and may end abruptly with the sudden development of hypoglycemia. Therapy is difficult. Porcine insulin, which more closely resembles human insulin (and is therefore less antigenic), may be substituted for the usual pork-beef mixtures. If insulin requirements do not drop, one may then consider dealanated insulin, which is prepared by carboxypeptidase hydrolysis of porcine insulin, resulting in the removal of the C-terminal alanine of the B chain. At present, this preparation can be obtained only by special request and is available in concentrations of 100 units/ml and 500 units/ml. The removal of the C-terminal alanine results in no loss of biologic activity but alters the antigenicity of the protein.

The most effective treatment is the administration of corticosteroids (usual initial dose is 40–60 mg/day of prednisone, for example); insulin requirements may drop dramatically and remain low, even following cessation of steroid therapy.

IV. ORAL HYPOGLYCEMIC AGENTS

A. Sulfonylureas These drugs stimulate insulin release from the pancreas; the resultant reduction in blood sugar is due chiefly to suppression of glucose release by the liver.

1. Preparations and dosage

a) Tolbutamide (Orinase) Available in 0.5-gm tablets. The usual starting dose is 0.5 gm BID. Dosage may be increased to 2.0 gm/day in order to achieve control, but larger doses are usually no more effective and cause increased side effects. If the patient is being switched from insulin, its administration may be discontinued abruptly if the daily dosage is less than 30 units. If larger amounts are being taken, the insulin dosage should be decreased 20–30% on the day tolbutamide administration is begun, and by similar decrements every 1–2 days as the patient responds. Tolbutamide has a half-life of 4–5 hours and should be given in divided dosage.

b) Chlorpropamide (Diabinese) Available in 0.1- and 0.25-gm tablets. The usual starting dose is 0.1 gm/day, and the maintenance dose is 0.2–0.5 gm/day; larger doses may result in profound hypoglycemia and should not be given. If the patient has been on insulin it should be tapered more rapidly than suggested for tolbutamide. Chlorpropamide has a half-life of 30–35 hours and need be given only once daily.

c) **Acetohexamide (Dymelor)**   Available in 0.25- and 0.5-gm tablets. The dosage range is 0.25–1.5 gm/day, given once daily. If control is not achieved with 1.5 gm/day, larger doses will not be more effective. Sustained hypoglycemia may occur because the half-life of acetohexamide is in excess of 6 hours, and metabolites of the drug, particularly hydroxyhexamide, are metabolically active (unlike those of tolbutamide, which will not induce hypoglycemia). Patients may be transferred from insulin as described for chlorpropamide.

d) **Tolazamide (Tolinase)**   Available in 0.1- and 0.25-gm tablets. The usual daily dosage is 300 mg or less, but as much as 1000 mg/day has been given to severe diabetics in order to achieve satisfactory control. Larger doses are generally not of further benefit. If the daily dosage of the drug is 500 mg or less it may be administered once daily; larger doses should be given in divided dosage twice daily. Therapy is usually initiated with 250–300 mg daily; patients being switched from insulin may be managed as discussed above.

Some metabolites of tolazamide have hypoglycemic activity, although they are less active than the parent compound. The drug is absorbed more slowly than either tolbutamide or chlorpropamide (peak blood levels occur in 4–8 hours after administration of a dose); the average biologic half-life is 7 hours.

2. **Response to therapy**   When patients are selected as described in the introductory section of this chapter, 65–70% will show an initial favorable response to tolbutamide. The remainder are "primary failures"—i.e., the response after four weeks of therapy is poor. The response rate is somewhat better with chlorpropamide; occasional patients not responsive to tolbutamide will respond to chlorpropamide (or acetohexamide or phenformin) or combinations of the drugs. The persistence of sustained hyperglycemia or the development of ketosis necessitates changing to insulin therapy. "Secondary failure" to tolbutamide, i.e., lack of responsiveness after satisfactory control for weeks or months, occurs in 5–30% of patients; some evidence suggests that this percentage increases with time. The incidence of unexplained drug failure is probably less than 5%; remaining failures are probably related to unwise initial selection of patients, poor adherence to diet, inadequate dosage, etc. As with primary failures, substitution of acetohexamide, chlorpropamide, or phenformin may give satisfactory control.

Tolazamide, the most recently available sulfonylurea preparation, is said to achieve adequate control in some diabetics not responsive to any of the other oral hypoglycemic agents, but data are still relatively limited. Administration of phenformin (e.g., 25 mg twice daily) concurrently with tolazamide may effect control of diabetes not adequately controlled by tolazamide alone.

3. **Side effects**   These are similar for all preparations, but more common with chlorpropamide (8%) than with tolbutamide (3%); the incidence of side effects with acetohexamide and tolazamide is relatively low.

a) Profound and sustained hypoglycemia may be produced by all agents, but is more common with chlorpropamide, probably because of its long half-life. However, even the hypoglycemia occurring in patients receiving tolbutamide may be protracted (despite tolbutamide's short half-life), lasting 24 hours or more; a varying degree of hypoglycemia may persist up to four days after withdrawal of the drug, despite administration of glucose in apparently adequate quantities. **Remember:** Patients experiencing severe hypoglycemia due to sulfonylureas may require large amounts of glucose for several days in order to maintain normal blood sugar levels.

b) Toxic reactions necessitate discontinuing the drugs in 1–3% of patients. These include anorexia, nausea, vomiting, abdominal pain, diarrhea; skin rashes (erythema, urticaria, photosensitivity, etc.); and hematopoietic effects, which include leukopenia, thrombocytopenia, and very rarely agranulocytosis. Hepatomegaly and abnormalities of the liver-function tests (especially elevation of alkaline phosphatase in patients receiving acetohexamide) may occur, but these are difficult to interpret in diabetics; cholestatic jaundice occurs rarely.

c) Marked flushing, accompanied by nausea, dyspnea, and palpitations, may occur in up to 10% of patients following ingestion of alcohol; this reaction is similar to that seen after Antabuse-and-alcohol ingestion and may often be prevented by ingestion of an antihistamine one hour before drinking alcoholic beverages. Histopathologic lesions of myocarditis and diffuse microgranulomas have been noted in autopsy studies of patients given tolbutamide, but no clinical correlation has been found, and the significance of these findings is unknown.

B. Phenethylbiguanide This drug is available as **phenformin (DBI).** Its exact mechanism of action remains unknown; experimentally, it inhibits certain enzymes involved in oxidative phosphorylation and enhances anaerobic glycolysis. Decreased hepatic gluconeogenesis and increased uptake of glucose by peripheral tissues occur. Mild elevations of serum lactate are frequently observed. In contrast to the sulfonylureas, phenformin does not cause hypoglycemia in normal individuals.

1. Preparations and dosage Phenformin is available as 25-mg tablets and 50-mg timed-disintegration capsules (DBI-TD). The duration of action of the tablets is about 4 hours. The capsules release about two-thirds of the drug in 4 hours and almost all within 8 hours; their total duration of action is about 12 hours. Therapy should be initiated with 25–50 mg daily and increased by 25–50 mg every 2–4 days. The usual maintenance dose is 100–150 mg/day; larger doses are rarely indicated. If the patient is being switched from insulin, the dosage of insulin should be decreased as described in the section on tolbutamide. The gastrointestinal side effects (see below) are common and often quite annoying, thus limiting patient acceptability of the drug.

2. Clinical use The indications for phenformin alone are similar to those for the sulfonylureas; however, the drug may be particularly useful in the following situations:

a) Secondary failures with sulfonylureas A moderate number of such patients, excluding those with severe diabetes, may be controlled by phenformin alone or in combination with a sulfonylurea.

b) Juvenile or brittle diabetes The combined use of phenformin and insulin, though controversial, may allow smoother control of the diabetes in unstable growth-onset diabetics or may make possible a reduction in insulin dosage (although this seems of little advantage for those patients who are well controlled on insulin alone).

3. Side effects

a) Early side effects, occurring within the first few days of treatment, are common and related to dosage; they include anorexia, nausea, vomiting, diarrhea, and metallic taste in the mouth; they may disappear with reduction in dosage and are less frequent with the timed-disintegration capsules.

b) Late reactions, appearing after several months of therapy in as many as 20% of patients, include lassitude, weakness, and weight loss; they usually reflect inadequate control of the diabetes and the necessity for insulin administration. No serious hepatic or hematopoietic toxicity has been reported.

c) Ketonuria and slight ketonemia are not infrequent despite relatively normal blood sugar values; ketoacidosis may occur, especially with mild stresses such as intercurrent infections. Ketonuria may disappear if the carbohydrate content of the diet is increased; severe ketosis usually indicates the need for insulin.

d) Minor elevation of the plasma lactate concentration occurs commonly in patients receiving the usual amounts of phenformin; this change reflects increased anaerobic glycolysis and is not usually of clinical significance. However, severe, and occasionally fatal, lactic acidosis may occur. It may develop suddenly in patients who have been receiving phenformin for periods of time without previous complications; it is most common in diabetics with renal insufficiency (who should be given the drug cautiously, if at all). The clinical picture is that of severe diabetic ketoacidosis, and indeed, the latter diagnosis may be made mistakenly after the demonstration of ketonuria. **Remember:** Ketonuria occurs commonly in patients taking phenformin, and, when present, should not dissuade one from suspecting lactic acidosis in the appropriate clinical setting; the diagnosis can be confirmed by demonstrating elevated serum concentrations of lactic acid and an elevated lactate-to-pyruvate ratio. Treatment of lactic acidosis is discussed in Chapter 2.

V. DIABETES AND PREGNANCY Almost every known complication of pregnancy occurs more frequently in diabetic mothers. Glucose tolerance decreases and insulin requirements rise during pregnancy, especially during the third trimester; insulin requirements drop rapidly postpartum. Special care must be taken to assure adequate protein intake (at least 100 gm/day), vitamin-mineral supplements, and avoidance of ketosis and excessive weight gain. Oral hypoglycemic agents should not be given during pregnancy; insulin should be used instead. Evidence in experimental animals suggests that tolbutamide may be teratogenic. Selection of optimal time and mode of delivery, and fetal complications are discussed in standard texts. In general, delivery should be accomplished by 36 or 37 weeks of pregnancy. Diabetic management during delivery is similar to that required during surgery.

DIABETIC ACIDOSIS

Diabetic ketoacidosis is a severe metabolic disturbance with clinical features due primarily to the accumulation of large amounts of glucose and beta-oxybutyric acids in the blood; lactic acid and free fatty acids may contribute to the acidosis. The recovery rate in diabetic acidosis is determined by the degree and duration of central nervous system dysfunction, the presence of shock, the degree of acidosis, the presence of complicating illnesses and the therapeutic skill of the physician. Therapy must be precise and requires strict attention to detail. The principles of therapy considered important by the Washington University Department of Medicine are detailed below.

I.   GENERAL COMMENTS

A. Clinical observations   Observe and record the blood pressure, pulse, rate and depth of respirations, mental status, and degree of hydration every 30 minutes. Urine output must be recorded as closely as possible. Catheterization is usually justified only in comatose patients.

B. Laboratory determinations   Follow urinary sugar and acetone every 30–60 minutes, plasma acetone every 2 hours, and blood sugar, CO_2, and serum $K+$ every 4–6 hours until recovery is well established. A BUN, hematocrit, and ECG should be done initially, and the ECG repeated every few hours (especially if serum $K+$ determinations are not feasible).

1. Measure plasma acetone undiluted and in 1:2 and 1:4 dilutions. Crush the Acetest tablet before using, because the intact tablet may not be adequately wetted by undiluted plasma and false negative readings may result.

2. In following urinary sugar, use glucose oxidase paper (Tes-Tape or Clinistix) if fructose has been administered; Clinitest tablets measure all urinary reducing substances and, because of fructosuria, may show strong positive reactions in the presence of hypoglycemia.

II.   TREATMENT PROGRAM

TREATMENT PROGRAM   Therapeutic goals are restoration of normal CHO, fat, and protein metabolism by administration of insulin; replacement of extracellular and intracellular fluids by administration of water and salt; prompt recognition and treatment of complications. If the patient is first seen outside the hospital with Kussmaul respiration and has 4+ urinary sugar and acetone, give 75 units regular insulin subcutaneously, transfer to the hospital, and proceed as outlined below.

A. Insulin   Most patients with acidosis are relatively refractory to the actions of insulin, and some may require huge doses. The patient with mild acidosis or simple ketosis, however, shows only slight resistance, and large doses of insulin should be avoided in order to preclude the development of hypoglycemia. As acidosis is corrected, sensitivity to insulin increases, and the dosage must be reduced markedly. Ketonemia and ketonuria may persist as the blood sugar falls; blood glucose must be measured frequently in order to prevent hypoglycemia as treatment progresses. The initial insulin dosage should be determined by the clinical status and degree of ketonuria and ketonemia. Do not wait for the blood sugar and CO_2 values; these results will be more useful in determining subsequent insulin dosage.

1. **Severe acidosis** Coma is profound, and plasma acetone is 4+ in a 1:2 or greater dilution. Give 200 units regular insulin subcutaneously and 100 units IV.

   a) Then give 75–100 units subcutaneously every hour until response (as determined by significant decrease in blood sugar, blood ketones, or glycosuria) is noted. However, if the initial CO_2 is reported as less than 5 mEq/L, give instead subsequent doses of 100–125 units subcutaneously every hour.

   b) When peripheral vascular collapse is present give one-half of each dose IV until shock is corrected.

2. **Moderate acidosis** Plasma acetone is 4+ in a 1:1 dilution, and hyperpnea is usually marked. Give 100–150 units regular insulin subcutaneously and 50–100 units IV, then 50–75 units subcutaneously every hour until response is noted.

3. **Mild acidosis** Plasma acetone is 4+ undiluted and less than 4+ or negative in further dilutions; the CO_2 is usually above 10 mEq/L. Give 100 units regular insulin subcutaneously, then 50 units every 2–3 hours until response is noted.

4. **Insulin dosage after response** When the plasma acetone is reduced to trace–1+ or the CO_2 rises above 15 mEq/L, start insulin every 4–6 hours, adjusting dosage on basis of the response.

B. **Fluids** Dehydration in severe acidosis is striking and correction may require administration of as much as 100 ml fluid/kg body weight during the first 24 hours. Hypotonic solutions should be used because of the plasma hypertonicity (each 100 mg glucose/100 ml blood equals 5.5 mOsm/L). Isotonic saline is undesirable because its chloride concentration exceeds that of the extracellular fluid (ECF) and the resultant hyperchloremia may aggravate the metabolic acidosis; fluids that are preferable include 0.45% (half-isotonic) saline, Ringer's, sodium bicarbonate, and lactate-Ringer's (if lactic acidosis is not a consideration). $NaHCO_3$ is commercially available in concentrations of 7.5% (approx. 45 mEq HCO_3^- per 50-ml ampule), 5% (approx. 300 mEq HCO_3^- per 500-ml bottle), and 1.4% (approx. 85 mEq HCO_3^- per 500-ml bottle).

Severe acidosis itself is harmful and should be corrected promptly by the initial administration of alkali; as a rule, not more than 250–300 mEq of bicarbonate or lactate should be given (in order to prevent significant alkalosis at a later stage of treatment). As a general rule of thumb, alkali administration probably should be stopped when venous bicarbonate levels approach 15 mEq/L. As therapy progresses and CHO is given as vehicle for free water, either glucose or fructose may be used.

1. For moderate or severe acidosis give 3.0–4.5 liters of fluid during the first 3–4 hours.

   a) Start with 1000–2000 ml 0.45% NaCl to which is added 88 mEq/L of $NaHCO_3$; **or** 1000–2000 ml 1/6 molar sodium lactate.

   b) Follow the above fluids with 2000–2500 ml lactate-Ringer's solution.

2. After the first 3–4 hours of treatment replace free water, CHO, and intracellular electrolytes.

   a) Continue IV fluids at a slower rate, giving 1000 ml every 3–4 hours.

b) Use 5% D/W with either 0.45% NaCl or lactate-Ringer's in a ratio of 1:1 or 1:2.

c) When urine sugar falls to 3+ or blood sugar below 250 mg/100 ml, 5% D/W must be given.

3. Diabetics with mild to moderate ketosis and no great elevation of blood sugar may be given glucose from the time therapy is started.

C. Supplemental potassium Hypokalemia, with muscular paralysis or weakness, cardiac arrhythmias, gastric atony, or intestinal ileus, may be fatal unless adequate potassium is administered. Potassium supplements should be given to most patients with adequate urine output beginning ordinarily 3–4 hours after initiation of therapy, sooner if the initial serum potassium was low or normal, if clinical evidence of hypokalemia is present, or if the blood sugar response to insulin is very rapid. From 100 to 200 mEq are usually required, but occasionally larger amounts will be necessary. Total body deficits of potassium are generally in the range of 5 mEq/kg body weight.

III. RECOVERY PHASE

A. Delay oral feedings of CHO and fluids until the patient can take them without risk of vomiting or gastric retention; continue supplemental potassium (orange juice and K-Triplex or KCl); do not discontinue IV fluids until it is apparent that oral feedings will be tolerated. Soft or liquid diets should be given initially; after 24–48 hours a regular diabetic diet may be given.

B. Known diabetics should be given one-half to two-thirds their previous dose of intermediate-acting insulin when a regular schedule is resumed; "new" diabetics may be given 10–20 units of an intermediate preparation. Supplemental regular insulin is given when required, and dosage adjustments are made as previously described.

IV. COMPLICATIONS

A. Shock

1. Hypotension prior to or early in the course of treatment is usually due to hypovolemia; the blood pressure usually returns to normal with restoration of the ECF volume, which should be monitored by central venous pressure (see Chapter 17).

2. When hypotension does not respond to the administration of adequate fluids, or when shock occurs later during the course of treatment, the cause is usually vasomotor instability with marked decrease in peripheral vascular resistance; the mechanism is unknown. This complication must be recognized promptly if therapy is to be effective. Blood pressure readings must be scrutinized carefully even though the patient appears to be doing well clinically and signs of peripheral vascular collapse are absent. If they start downward, treatment should be started immediately. It should be emphasized that *treating the blood pressure reading* is both proper and necessary in this situation, since CNS function may be altered by factors other than hypotension (ketonemia, acidosis), and since urinary output rarely is depressed because of the concomitant substantial solute diuresis (glycosuria). Treatment should consist of vasoconstrictor agents, since these have been shown to be effective in this situation. Marked reduction in peripheral vascular resistance and normal or increased cardiac output have been reported (*Clin. Sci.* 6:247, 1948); whether or not there is a *relative* deficit in cardiac output that might provide a rationale for the use of inotropic drugs is not established. (See Chapter 17 for proper dosage of vasopressors.)

B. **"Paradoxical" spinal-fluid acidosis** Clinical neurologic abnormalities in acidosis are better correlated with pH of cerebrospinal fluid (CSF) than with blood pH. Due to the rapid equilibration of gaseous CO_2 and the slower, active transport of bicarbonate across the blood-brain barrier, CSF pH may fall transiently during correction of arterial acid-base derangement (*New Eng. J. Med.* 277:605, 1967). The general absence of focal neurologic deficits in this situation will usually allow clinical differentiation from cerebrovascular accidents occurring during the course of diabetic acidosis. Onset of the CNS symptoms (5–10 hours after the start of therapy) suggests, and measurement of CSF pH, pCO_2, and HCO_3^- confirms, this diagnosis. **Specific therapy is prevention** and consists of judicious restraint regarding the amount and rapidity of infusion of parenteral bicarbonate. By this means, severe depression of CSF pH should be avoidable.

C. **Other complications,** usually iatrogenic, include hypernatremia and edema (following administration of isotonic rather than hypotonic solutions), pulmonary edema (following injudicious rapid administration of fluids to patients with congestive heart failure), hypoglycemia, and hypokalemia.

HYPEROSMOLAR NONKETOACIDOTIC DIABETIC COMA

Increasing attention has been paid in recent years to the syndrome of frank coma or milder degrees of CNS dysfunction in association with marked plasma hyperosmolarity but without significant ketoacidosis. Hyperglycemia, sometimes of monumental degree, and hypernatremia are the major factors in the production of the hyperosmolar state, but azotemia is also commonly present. Dehydration is usually extreme, and underlying vascular disease is common. Both diminished water intake and inadequate renal excretion of solute contribute. The complications of this syndrome include shock, acute tubular necrosis, vascular thromboses; CNS manifestations are felt to be the consequence of intracellular cerebral dehydration.

Treatment differs from that of the usual case of diabetic acidosis in that alkali is unnecessary, and fluid administration on a larger scale is usually required. The need for *hypotonic* fluid therapy is absolute, as administration of isotonic fluids will fail to correct the hyperosmolarity and may cause clinical deterioration or death. Early statements that insulin requirements are relatively small do not appear to have borne up as further experience with this syndrome has accumulated. Prognosis is grave, probably in part due to the advanced age and underlying vascular disease in most of the patients thus far reported; mortality has approached 50%.

Diseases of the joints are common and are responsible for much pain and disability; arthritis is second only to heart disease as a cause of chronic limitation of major activity. Although arthritis cripples a tremendous number of persons each year, it kills relatively few. No other group of diseases causes so much suffering to so many people for so long. Because of the large number of diseases that have symptoms or findings referable to the joints or adjacent tissues, classification of arthritic disorders has been difficult. One must differentiate carefully between "rheumatism" (which encompasses anything from vague muscle aches to deep bone pains), and true arthritis with objective findings. The American Rheumatism Association has published a primer on the rheumatic diseases which includes the official classification and critical review of pathophysiology of the diseases of the joints (*J.A.M.A.* 190:127, 425, 509, 741, 1964).

I. **RHEUMATOID ARTHRITIS** is a systemic disease of unknown etiology in which inflammatory changes occur throughout the connective tissue of the body. The onset is usually insidious; most characteristic is the morning stiffness, myalgia, arthralgia, and polyarthritis of the smaller joints of the hands and feet, with a tendency for symmetrical distribution after the disease has become established. The arthritis is produced by a chronic proliferative inflammation of the synovial membrane which may result in permanent damage to the articular cartilage and joint capsule. The course of the disease, in spite of unexplainable remissions and exacerbations, is progressive, leading to characteristic deformities and disability. Rheumatoid factor, if present, helps in establishing the diagnosis. While the natural history of the disease may not be significantly altered by the currently available therapy, much can be done to suppress inflammation, reduce pain, maintain function, and prevent deformity. Therapeutic measures should be directed at achieving maximum control of the disease at minimum risk.

A. **General measures**

1. **Emotional support** Because of the progressive nature of rheumatoid arthritis, chronic anxiety and depression frequently become the most incapacitating factors. An understanding of the patient's personality and emotional reaction to his illness should guide the physician in explaining candidly, in lay terms, the nature of the disease, its treatment, and the prognosis. Unshakable faith in the ability of the patient to cooperate and willingness to answer all questions honestly may do much to eradicate the misunderstanding that so often results in depression and disability. Sedatives or antidepressants may be used if tenseness or emotional unrest are real problems.

2. **Rest**   Systemic and articular rest are beneficial in most instances. Acutely ill patients should be hospitalized for complete bed rest; others require varying amounts of rest periods. Unduly fatiguing activity should be discouraged, but a regular program of exercise (see below) should be initiated. The feeling of stiffness that may follow a rest period should not influence the amount of rest; the stiffness is more apparent at the beginning but diminishes with continuation of the program. Unless the physician stresses the transient nature of this stiffness and the vital importance of rest, the patient may not cooperate.

Articular rest is accomplished by bed rest (in the case of weight-bearing joints) and may be further enhanced by appropriate support from splints. The purpose of splints is not only to provide rest but also to relieve spasm, thus reducing pain and deformities. They should be removable to allow the patient adequate ambulation and exercise of the affected extremities every day. These orthopedic supports should be worn especially during the sleeping hours when unguarded motion may be painful and involuntary flexion tends to increase. Good body posture may be maintained by the use of a firm mattress or bedboard. A footboard may be used to prevent foot drop.

3. **Physical therapy**   Intelligent use of physical therapy is one of the most valuable adjuncts in the management of rheumatoid arthritis. In acutely ill patients, passive-active exercises should be performed within the limits of pain from the very beginning of management. The duration and frequency of these exercises should be limited not by increase of pain during the exercise but by the pain that persists after the completion of exercise. Pain lasting more than an hour after exercise usually indicates that exercise was too vigorous and should be decreased in amount but not discontinued. Patients should be started on a program of exercises in the hospital under careful supervision and issued specific instructions for the type of exercise and its duration. As activity of the disease subsides, resistive exercises should be increased and continued at home indefinitely.

4. **Heat**   may be applied either locally or generally. Moist heat produces muscle relaxation and analgesia, and should be administered from 15-30 minutes before exercise. It may be achieved by moist applications or tub bath. Heat may increase pain in an acutely inflamed joint and should be used cautiously. Infrared lamp, diathermy, and ultrasound are contraindicated in inflamed joints and do not offer any particular advantage over a heat lamp or hot bath.

5. **Occupational therapy**   is an objective type of treatment to hasten the patient's recovery and contribute to his adjustment or hospitalization. Activities should be designed to meet the patient's physical and psychologic needs, thus providing physical and mental diversion. Occupational therapy may be employed long before active exercises are initiated and may contribute greatly to preserving or restoring morale, correcting bad posture in bed, and, above all, reducing the element of fear. It should be instituted early to allay anxiety and the dread of being hurt by any form of exercise. Occupational therapy should complement physical therapy; but one must be careful that the patient does not overwork.

6. **Intra-articular injection** of corticosteroids is only a temporary palliative measure and should be used only as an adjunct to the therapeutic program; the chief usefulness of the drugs is in improving
the joint function for physical therapy and orthopedic procedures. The more actively inflamed joints are best suited for this
treatment. The beneficial effect lasts from 1–3 weeks, but the joints
can be reinjected repeatedly without loss of therapeutic effect,
though subluxation and subchondral bone resorption have been
reported with multiple injections. Hydrocortisone acetate 25 mg
or triamcinolone hexacetonide 10–20 mg, depending upon the size
of the joint, may be used. One must make sure that the drug is
delivered into the synovial cavity to achieve a beneficial effect. In
some cases the pain and swelling may increase after injection, but
only transiently. Infection, though rare, is a real hazard. In larger
joints (knee joint), nitrogen mustard 1.0 mg may be used in addition to 25 mg hydrocortisone acetate to achieve prolonged effect,
though one must make sure of the intrasynovial delivery of the
drug. This combination is much more effective in the prolifera-
tively active joint. Larger dosage does not have any particular
benefit but may increase toxicity substantially. The intra-articular
injections of steroids are contraindicated in the presence of sepsis
or multiple joint involvement.

B. **Salicylates**   Aspirin is the most useful drug in the treatment of
rheumatoid arthritis. It is mildly anti-inflammatory as well as analgesic, and may suppress objective signs of joint inflammation remarkably well. Optimal effects are obtained by regular, not sporadic,
administration. The proper dose of aspirin or sodium salicylate is
that which provides maximum relief of musculoskeletal symptoms
without causing toxicity.

Most observers give large dosage initially; when toxic symptoms
develop, a slightly lower maintenance dose is chosen; therapy is continued more or less indefinitely.

The usual daily maintenance dose of aspirin is 4–6 gm (14–20
300-mg tablets given in divided dosage, e.g., 2 or 3 tablets every 3–4
hours) ; the minimum dose should be 12 tablets daily; some patients,
especially young adults, may tolerate up to 24 tablets daily. Gastric
distress may be minimized by administering aspirin with meals or a
snack; enteric-coated preparations do not entirely obviate the problem of epigastric discomfort and have the disadvantages of erratic
absorption and requirement for larger dosage to obtain corresponding
blood levels of salicylate. Rectal absorption is not complete. The blood
salicylate level has a dose-weight relationship, and a heavy person
requires increased amounts. Patients with rheumatoid arthritis have
lower blood aspirin levels as compared with controls, and those with
an active disease require higher doses of salicylates to maintain an
adequate blood level than those with an inactive disease. A brief
summary of the complications and toxicity is included in Figure 16-1;
for detailed discussion refer to Chapter 1.

Drugs such as propoxyphene and codeine offer little analgesia
beyond that of salicylates. For those patients whose arthritis is not
well relieved by physical measures (see above) and maximally tolerated doses of salicylates, no unanimity exists about which drugs to
add next; those used are gold salts, phenylbutazone, indomethacin,
antimalarials, and corticosteroids. They are discussed in the following sections. A few patients not benefited by the above measures

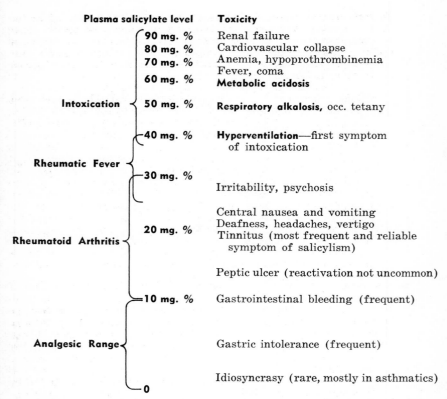

Fig. 16-1. Complications and Toxicity of Salicylate Therapy. (Adapted from Bayles and Tenckhoff, Exhibit, Amer. Med. Assn., Dec. 1958.)

have been given full doses of nitrogen mustard or antimetabolites such as azathioprine, but data are so limited at present that further discussion is not warranted.

C. Gold salts   Chrysotherapy is helpful in selected patients who have not improved with conservative measures. The mechanism of the action of gold salts is not known, though affected joints seem to retain gold salts selectively. The only therapeutic effect of gold is to suppress activity; thus it is useful in early active stages of the disease. Once irreparable damage has occurred, no benefits can be derived by use of gold as a "last resort" measure. Since the therapeutic effects of gold are not manifested for 2–4 months after institution of therapy and since corticosteroids are more potent compounds with rapid action, selection of the patient for gold therapy should be considered carefully. Gold therapy should never be the initial therapy in rheumatoid arthritis. Gold therapy is indicated in situations in which a young person continues to show signs of arthritic activity in spite of a good conservative program, especially in the presence of peptic ulcer, diabetes mellitus, tuberculosis, or other complications that prevent the use of corticosteroids. It may be the treatment of choice in patients who have developed side effects from prolonged steroid therapy, even though the beneficial effects may be less marked than corticosteroids. Almost 50% of patients improve significantly, but relapses are common after cessation of therapy, though repeated courses may be given.

1. **Preparations** are listed below. Gold sodium thiomalate and gold thioglucose are used most frequently. Although aqueous preparations may be given IV, they are almost always given IM; suspensions are given only IM.

Preparations	Water-soluble	Physical state	Au content (%)
Gold sodium thiosulfate	Yes	Aqueous solution	37
Gold sodium thiomalate (Myochrysine)	Yes	Aqueous solution	50
Gold thioglucose (Solganal)	Yes	Oil suspension	50
Gold calcium thiomalate	No	Oil suspension	50
Gold thioglucoanalide	No	Oil suspension	54

2. **Doses and administration** Since the therapeutic effects are directly proportional to the amount of gold retained in the body, prolonged courses have to be given. Initially, 10 mg is given, then 25 mg the next week, and 50 mg every week thereafter (provided the initial doses were well tolerated) for 16–20 weeks. Blood counts and urinalysis should be performed before each injection and the patient should be actively questioned for metallic taste and skin reactions including itching. If the patient has not shown any improvement after this amount of treatment, chrysotherapy is considered of no value and should be discontinued. If improvement has occurred, the treatment should be continued as maintenance therapy—50 mg at 2-week intervals may be given for 4 doses, at 3-week intervals for 4 doses, and usually once a month thereafter for years. Should a relapse occur when injections are given at 2–4-week intervals, resumption of weekly injections is advised for 6 or more weeks, depending on the response.

3. **Toxic effects** Toxicity is frequent (approximately 30% of patients). Since the drug is accumulated in the body and excreted slowly by the kidneys, it may be months before all signs of toxicity subside. Fortunately, 90% of the reactions are dermatitis and stomatitis, which are completely reversible after cessation of therapy; up to 5% are serious, irreversible, occasionally fatal reactions. Toxicity usually appears after 300 to 500 mg of gold have been injected.

   a) **Cutaneous** eruption is almost always preceded by pruritus for several days or even weeks. As a rule, dermatitis occurring without itching during gold therapy may not be due to drug toxicity. Erythema or mild rash may appear after 2 or 3 injections but usually subsides, and further therapy may be well tolerated. The severe skin reactions do not occur until after

300–400 mg of gold salts have been injected. These are photosensitivity reactions, varying from a localized lesion to exfoliative dermatitis, and respond well to corticosteroids. Alopecia is usually transient and regrowth is the rule.

b) **Gastrointestinal** Stomatitis frequently accompanies dermatitis but may appear without skin eruption. A metallic taste often precedes stomatitis. Ulcerative enterocolitis and toxic hepatitis are very rare.

c) **Renal** damage is rare, but may be severe. Lipoid nephrosis and membranous glomerulonephritis have been observed. Urinalysis must be done before each injection and further investigations performed if hematuria or proteinuria is significant.

d) **Hematologic** manifestations, though rare, may be fatal. Thrombocytopenic purpura, aplastic anemia, and agranulocytosis have been reported. Frequently eosinophilia may precede gold toxicity and suggests impending toxicity.

e) **Others,** including vasomotor reaction with generalized erythema, warmth, giddiness, and blurred vision, may occur during the early weeks, but are usually self-limiting. Peripheral neuropathy has also been reported.

D. **Phenylbutazone (Butazolidin)** and **oxyphenbutazone (Tandearil)** are drugs with analgesic, anti-inflammatory, and uricosuric properties. Their mechanism of action is not known. They are occasionally beneficial in rheumatoid arthritis (in the minority of cases, when articular manifestations develop rapidly), although quite effective in the relief of symptoms of gouty arthritis and ankylosing spondylitis. Their effect in rheumatoid arthritis is due to anti-inflammatory action, thus the drugs should not be used chronically as analgesics. Therapeutic effects should be evident in a week; if no response is noted in 7–10 days the drugs should be discontinued. Prolonged use and/or higher dosage results only in increased toxicity. Oxyphenbutazone appears to be less toxic than the parent drug but is also less effective. Both drugs have been largely discarded in the treatment of rheumatoid arthritis but may be effective occasionally in an active refractory case.

The **usual dose** of either drug is 100 mg TID–QID with meals (to lessen gastrointestinal irritation) ; larger doses are not more effective.

Toxic effects are frequent and are occasionally fatal. Many appear only after several weeks of therapy and seem related to the size of the daily dose. The most common are nausea, skin rash, and edema. Sodium and water retention may be marked, precipitating congestive heart failure, and the drug should be given cautiously, if at all, to elderly patients. Vomiting, diarrhea, stomatitis, epigastric distress, peptic ulcer, exfoliative dermatitis, toxic hepatitis, renal damage, vertigo, and generalized hypersensitivity reactions may occur.

Hematopoietic effects may be severe. Agranulocytosis, thrombocytopenia, anemia, leukemoid reactions, and occasionally aplastic anemia have been reported.

Pyrazolon compounds may inhibit degradation of tolbutamide, and patients receiving both drugs may require dosage reduction of tolbutamide in order to prevent severe hypoglycemic reactions. Similarly, both drugs may potentiate the effect of coumarin drugs, with the result of undue prolongation of the prothrombin time.

E. **Indomethacin (Indocin),** an arylacetic acid, is a nonsteroid compound
   with anti-inflammatory, antipyretic, and analgesic properties. The
   precise mechanism of action is not known. It is well absorbed from
   the gastrointestinal tract after oral administration; peak blood levels
   are reached in 1–2 hours and it is rapidly excreted in about 4 hours.
   Two-thirds of the drug is excreted through the kidneys and the
   dosage should be reduced in azotemic patients.

   1. **Indications** Indomethacin has been reported to be beneficial in
      reducing stiffness, joint swelling, and tenderness; relieving pain;
      and improving joint mobility. These benefits are greatest in gout,
      followed in decreasing order by ankylosing spondylitis, osteo-
      arthritis, and rheumatoid arthritis.

      Indomethacin, when used in therapeutic doses, produces good to
      excellent response in 25% of the cases of rheumatoid arthritis.
      Carefully controlled studies have clearly established that indo-
      methacin is not more effective than aspirin in the treatment of
      rheumatoid arthritis; its use should be restricted to patients who
      cannot tolerate aspirin. Which patients will respond to indometh-
      acin cannot be predicted; those who do respond often note im-
      provement within 24–48 hours, although therapy should be
      continued for 3–4 weeks before concluding that the drug is of no
      benefit.

      Indomethacin does not alter the basic disease process; eleva-
      tions in sedimentation rate and rheumatoid arthritis factor gen-
      erally persist. (A review of recent clinical trials appears in *Clin.
      Pharmacol. Ther.* 9:94, 1968.)

   2. **Dosage and administration** Dosage of indomethacin for patients
      with rheumatoid arthritis is usually 25 mg 2 or 3 times daily after
      meals. The daily dose may be increased to a total of 100 mg, but
      higher dosage is associated with a higher incidence of side effects
      (as high as 60–70% when the dose is 150–200 mg/day). Contrary
      to popular belief, the concurrent use of indomethacin does not help
      to reduce the corticosteroid requirements. The drug should not be
      given if safer drugs (e.g., salicylates) are effective in providing
      symptomatic relief.

   3. **Side effects** Initial studies with indomethacin were carried out
      with the drug in tablet form and in significantly higher dosage than
      now recommended; adverse side effects were reported in more
      than 50% of patients. With the use of capsules, side effects are
      reported in one-third of patients and about 20% of the patients
      cannot tolerate the drug.

      a) Headache, dizziness, and lightheadedness (the commonest side
         effects) occur in 20–40% of patients. They may subside
         spontaneously with continued administration of the drug;
         reduction in dosage or discontinuance of therapy is often neces-
         sary, however.

      b) Anorexia, nausea, or vomiting may occur in 20% of patients.
         Epigastric distress, also very common, may be lessened by
         administering the drug with meals. A number of reports indi-
         cate development or reactivation of duodenal or gastric ulcers
         after indomethacin administration, and massive fatal gastro-
         intestinal bleeding and perforation have occurred; occult
         gastrointestinal bleeding is not uncommon. Indomethacin is

contraindicated in patients with active peptic disease or a history of duodenal ulcer.

c) Other side effects include vertigo, tinnitus, somnolence, blurred vision, nervousness, trembling, occasional mental symptoms mimicking alcohol intoxication (e.g., giddiness, confusion, unsteadiness), diarrhea, stomatitis, pruritus, skin rashes, urticaria, and angioneurotic edema. Indomethacin may aggravate psychiatric disturbances, epilepsy, or parkinsonism. Increases in BUN (often transient) may occur; a few reports of leukopenia and abnormal liver-function tests (increase in alkaline phosphatase and transaminases; positive cephalin-cholesterol flocculation) have appeared. Corneal opacities, visual-field changes, and pallor of the optic disk have been reported.

F. Antimalarials Chloroquine (Aralen) and hydroxychloroquine (Plaquenil) may have a moderate, but significant, beneficial effect in many patients with rheumatoid arthritis. The mechanism of action is not known, though it seems that those patients who also manifest a positive LE phenomenon are most likely to achieve clinical benefit. Which patients will respond cannot be determined in advance.

1. **Chloroquine phosphate** is usually given as a 250-mg tablet daily at supper or at bedtime. If toxic effects appear, administration should be stopped and resumed at half-dose. **Hydroxychloroquine phosphate** is administered in doses of 200 mg twice a day initially. It is tolerated better than chloroquine and is claimed to have fewer side effects. These drugs should be given with caution with gold salts or phenylbutazone, and in patients with psoriasis, quinine sensitivity, or liver, kidney, or lung disease. Therapeutic response, if any, seldom occurs before 3–6 months of continuous therapy. Toxic effects, detailed below, occur in up to 50% of patients; the rare but serious ocular toxicity is considered by some physicians too great a risk to warrant use of the drug.

2. **Toxic manifestations** include skin rashes, GI symptoms (nausea, vomiting, anorexia, epigastric pain) in 15–20% of patients, and occasionally hyperpigmentation of the skin, alopecia, blanching of the hair, leukopenia, headache, mental confusion, toxic psychosis, neuromyopathy, bone marrow depression (very rare), and ocular lesions. **Ocular abnormalities** occur in more than half of patients and are of two primary types.

   a) About 50% of patients develop a keratopathy secondary to deposit of chloroquine in the cornea; although not strictly related to dosage or duration of therapy (occasionally detected as early as two weeks after initiation of therapy) it is more common in patients receiving larger doses for a long time. Most patients are asymptomatic, but some complain of blurred vision, halos around lights, or photophobia. The keratopathy is benign, with deposits disappearing within six months after cessation of therapy; there are no deleterious effects on visual acuity.

   b) Retinopathy, on the other hand, is a serious complication that may permanently impair vision. Although recently there has been controversy as to incidence, it is stated that 1:1000 or 2000 patients will develop retinal damage. The lesion is usually (but not always) related to length of therapy and dosage, most patients having received 500 mg or more of chloroquine daily for longer than one year. The pathogenesis is thought related to the accumulation of chloroquine in the melanin-containing tissues of the eye (which concentrate the drug). Symptoms include difficulty with distance vision, photophobia, problems with accommodation, and field defects such as pericentral negative scotomata and decreased peripheral vision. Objective changes in the retina and in vision may be determined at early stages by the ophthalmologist; patients receiving long-term chloroquine therapy should have a careful ophthalmologic examination (including central visual fields) every 3 months. Unfortunately, many of the tests currently employed to diagnose retinal pathology are not sufficiently sensitive to detect early injury; a more sensitive method has been described, involving determination of the visual threshold for a small retinal area (*Arch. Ophthal.* 75:171, 1966). Detection of retinopathy requires immediate cessation of therapy; unfortunately, significant progression of visual loss may continue for 1–2 years. **Caution:** Chloroquine poisoning in children is rapidly fatal, even with small amounts of the drug. No specific antidote is available; therefore patients should be warned to keep chloroquine out of the reach of children.

G. **Corticosteroids** Cortisone was first introduced for the treatment of rheumatoid arthritis in 1949 with the hope that a curative agent had been found; experience, however, has shown the striking limitations and hazards, in addition to benefits, associated with steroid therapy.

Steroids have been used for the treatment of numerous diseases other than rheumatoid arthritis. The following section, though containing many comments specific for rheumatoid arthritis, is the only formal discussion of steroids in the Manual, and the information relating to available preparations, administration, and side effects is of a general nature, applicable to the use of steroids in almost all situations.

1. **Indications** Corticosteroids do not alter the basic disease process in rheumatoid arthritis; beneficial effects are due to nonspecific anti-inflammatory actions and must be weighed against the many serious side effects associated with long-term administration. In view of these toxic effects, steroid administration should not be given until a careful survey for the presence of contraindications and infections has been completed, and should usually not be the initial treatment unless it is the only available therapeutic measure or unless systemic manifestations are severe.

Steroids may be considered for severely ill patients with high fever and marked toxicity, for those with rapidly progressive articular or systemic disease not manageable by the measures previously described, and for patients with unbearable pain requiring narcotics for relief.

2. **Preparations** See Table 16-1.

3. **Dosage** From the very beginning of therapy, attempts should be made to administer the smallest dose that will alleviate symptoms. The initial dose should be low, e.g., 10–20 mg of prednisone daily; gradual increments may be made until symptoms have been controlled, but remember that functional effectiveness is the primary goal of therapy, and it may be necessary to compromise at a dose that relieves symptoms only partially.

When a beneficial response has occurred, repeated efforts should be made to decrease dosage to an absolute minimum, desirably to less than 10 mg of prednisone daily. A daily dosage of 20–30 mg of prednisone, for example, may be reduced by 2.5 mg daily once or twice weekly. With the realization that rheumatoid arthritis may be a cyclic disease with occasional remissions, periodic attempts should be made to withdraw steroids entirely, even though the disease may flare into activity with tapering of dosage.

4. **Administration**   Prednisone is the most commonly used preparation; the anti-inflammatory effects of equivalent amounts of other analogs are similar. Although it has not been possible to reduce undesirable side effects of corticosteroids by modification of the steroid molecule, certain preparations tend to produce less salt retention (see Table 16-1); methylprednisolone, for example, may occasionally cause significant natriuresis. Triamcinolone has been reported to cause a higher incidence of myopathy and dexamethasone a more striking cushingoid appearance.

Steroids should be administered orally to patients on maintenance therapy; although depot preparations (usually acetate or acetonide suspensions) are available for IM injection, their use is generally to be discouraged. Succinate and phosphate salts of several preparations (e.g., hydrocortisone, methylprednisolone, dexamethasone) are available for use IV or IM; they exert their effects immediately and are used for urgent situations.

Steroids are generally administered in divided dosage 3 or 4 times daily, but recent study suggests that administration of the total daily dosage once each day is just as effective; there is no decrease in incidence of side effects, however. Other studies suggest that the total 48-hour amount of steroid may be given in a single dose every other day without a decrease in therapeutic efficacy, but with a reduction in incidence and severity of side effects and in degree of adrenal suppression. This concept remains somewhat controversial.

When corticosteroids are to be withdrawn after long-term administration, dosage should be tapered gradually over several weeks. Although the recovery of the adrenal cortex per se is rapid, that of the pituitary is delayed; thus ACTH administration is of little if any benefit during withdrawal. See paragraph j in the following discussion of side effects for the management of stress situations in the months following cessation of steroid therapy.

5. **Side effects**   Numerous undesirable effects are associated with prolonged corticosteroid administration; most are dosage-related.

   a) **Infections**   Corticosteroids may decrease resistance to infections; those ordinarily superficial or minor may become systemic and fulminating; quiescent diseases such as tuberculosis (see section on treatment of tuberculosis in Chapter 9 for comments about prophylactic administration of isoniazid), bronchiectasis, and pyelonephritis may be exacerbated or disseminated; and organisms usually considered nonpathogenic (including fungi) may cause serious systemic disease. Because the local and systemic signs and symptoms of infection may be masked, diagnosis and treatment are often delayed.

   b) **Mental reactions** range from mild irritability, euphoria, nervousness, and insomnia, to severe depression or organic psychosis

TABLE 16-1. Corticosteroid Preparations

U.S.P. Name	Structure of Synthetic Analog	Trade Names	Approx. Equiv. Dose (mg)	Anti-infl. Potency	Mineralocort. Potency	Usual Starting Dose (mg/day)
Hydrocortisone (cortisol)	—	—	20.0	1.0	1.0	80–120
Cortisone	—	—	25.0	0.8	1.0	100–150
Prednisone	delta-1-cortisone	Meticorten Deltasone	5.0	3.0–5.0	0.8	20–30
Prednisolone	delta-1-cortisol	Meticortelone Hydeltra Delta-Cortef	5.0	3.0–5.0	0.8	20–30
Triamcinolone	9-alpha fluoro-16-alpha-hydroxy-prednisolone	Aristocort Kenacort	4.0	5.0	0	16–24
Dexamethasone	9-alpha-fluoro-16-alpha-methyl-prednisolone	Decadron Deronil Gammacorten Hexadrol	0.75	20.0–30.0	0	3.0–4.5
Methylprednisolone	6-alpha-methyl-prednisolone	Medrol	4.0	5.0	0	16–24
Fluprednisolone	6-alpha fluoro-prednisolone	Alphadrol	1.5	15.0–20.0	0	6–9
Betamethasone	9-alpha fluoro-16-beta-methyl-prednisolone	Celestone	0.6	30.0–35.0	0	2.4–3.6
Paramethasone	6-alpha fluoro-16-alpha-methyl-prednisolone 21-acetate	Haldrone	2.0	10.0	0	8–12

(in about 5% of patients). Any significant change in mood or affect may herald more serious manifestations.

c) **Cushingoid cosmetic effects** include weight gain, redistribution of fat with central obesity and moon face, striae, ecchymoses, acne, and hirsutism. Although most of these disappear within several months after cessation of therapy, the hirsutism may be permanent.

d) **Peptic ulcers** (especially gastric) occur with increased frequency; their development appears more related to steroid dosage than to duration of therapy. Most patients taking corticosteroids should be given frequent feedings and antacids prophylactically.

e) **Osteoporosis** develops commonly in patients who have taken steroids for longer than six months, regardless of dosage. Compression fractures of the thoracic or lumbar vertebrae occur in 10–15% of patients (especially postmenopausal women) on prolonged therapy. Although administration of calcium salts and anabolic hormones should theoretically reduce the severity of this complication, their use prophylactically is of questionable value.

f) **Myopathy** Muscle weakness, and later, atrophy, may occur, with involvement particularly of proximal muscle groups in the shoulder and pelvic girdle; this complication is reported more commonly with triamcinolone than with other steroids. The myopathy usually, though not always, clears within 3–4 weeks after cessation of therapy.

g) **Diabetes mellitus** may be initiated or aggravated by steroids but is not a contraindication to therapy. Overt diabetics should be followed closely; occasional blood sugar and urine sugar determinations should be performed on all patients (especially those with a family history of diabetes).

h) **Sodium and water retention** and/or **hypokalemia** may cause difficulties in patients receiving large doses of cortisone or cortisol. Less of a problem occurs with the steroid analogs possessing minimal mineralocorticoid activity, and salt restriction or potassium supplementation is not usually necessary. unless large doses are being given.

i) **Other undesirable effects** include menstrual irregularities, increased perspiration, thrombophlebitis or other thrombotic complications, acute pancreatitis or pancreatic atrophy, nodular panniculitis (on withdrawal of steroids), aseptic necrosis of the femoral head, and necrotizing arteritis; this last complication is seen essentially in patients with rheumatoid arthritis and may be related to the underlying disease rather than the steroid therapy. Posterior subcapsular cataracts, usually bilateral, are reported in up to 40% of patients given moderate to high doses of steroids over a long duration (1–2 years or longer); the degree of lens opacity appears related to the steroid dosage. Although a few reports question the existence or incidence of steroid-induced cataracts, most data support the concept that steroid administration does, indeed, induce lenticular opacities. Pseudotumor cerebri, although rare, may occur in children following rapid reduction of steroid dosage or change to a different preparation; signs and symptoms may mimic those of a brain tumor. A temporary increase in steroid dosage is usually followed by a fall in the CSF pressure; recurrence may be prevented by tapering the dosage very gradually over several weeks.

j) **Adrenal insufficiency** Symptoms of hypoadrenalism may appear during severe stress (e.g., serious intercurrent illness or major surgery) in patients on maintenance doses of steroids or in the six months or so following their withdrawal. The degree of pituitary-adrenal unresponsiveness appears related to steroid dosage, schedule for administration (daily vs every 48 hours), and length of therapy. Although some studies suggest that the degree of pituitary-adrenal unresponsiveness in certain situations is less than previously thought (see, for example, *Ann. Intern. Med.* 61:11, 1964), most observers agree that patients on long-term steroid therapy undergoing general anesthesia and/ or major surgery should be given supplemental doses of steroids.

Cortisone acetate 100 mg should be given IM 24 hours before and again immediately preceding operation. During operation 100 mg hydrocortisone succinate or phosphate should be infused IV. Postoperatively steroid dosage may be tapered to the usual maintenance level over 2–5 days if there are no complications. (See additional comments in the section on adrenal crisis in the chapter on medical emergencies.)

II. **GOUT** is an inherited metabolic disorder of unknown etiology characterized by hyperuricemia, acute and recurrent or chronic arthritis, and deposits of urates in the joints, skin, and kidneys. In the development of primary gout, there are four stages to be considered, each requiring different management—asymptomatic hyperuricemia, acute gouty arthritis, interval phase, and chronic gouty arthritis. (A review of therapy appears in *Amer. J. Med. Sci.* 274:893, 1967.)

A. **Asymptomatic hyperuricemia** About 20–40% of male members of a family in which there is a male with gout will have hyperuricemia; the incidence of acute gouty attack in these patients is not known. Most physicians agree that a young hyperuricemic male (serum uric acid greater than 8.0 mg/100 ml) in a family with a gouty pedigree should be given uricosuric drugs. This regimen seems to provide protection against urate deposition, but the available data do not indicate any reduction in the incidence of acute arthritis. Asymptomatic subjects with family history of gout but normal serum uric acid generally do not need any treatment.

B. **Acute gouty arthritis** The first attack of arthritis usually occurs suddenly, most commonly in the fourth decade. About one-half of initial attacks involve the great toe; other sites of involvement are the instep, ankle, heel, knee, and other joints. The involved joint may swell markedly within a few hours and become hot, dusky red, and extremely tender. Response to treatment is markedly increased if therapy is initiated promptly.

1. **Pathogenesis** of acute gouty arthritis is not yet completely understood. The intra-articular deposition of monosodium urate mono-

hydrate microcrystals, usually but not always associated with hyperuricemia, is the initial event. This usually results in an inflammatory response and the urate crystals are phagocytized by leukocytes; the resultant metabolic activity causes increased lactate production and a drop in local pH which, in turn, leads to further crystallization of urates. The enigma of the cause of initial crystallization has not, as yet, been solved.

2. **Treatment** Colchicine is the drug most commonly used, but phenylbutazone and indomethacin are also exceedingly effective.

a) **Colchicine** is thought to act by inhibiting phagocytosis of urates by leukocytes, thus interrupting the cycle of further urate deposition and inflammation. The drug is not entirely specific for gout, since sarcoid arthritis and occasionally rheumatoid arthritis also respond. In prodromal stages of an acute gouty attack, administration of a few tablets may arrest the episode; in a full-blown attack, symptoms are usually relieved rapidly. **Dose** is one 0.5-mg tablet every hour until pain is relieved, GI side effects (nausea, vomiting, diarrhea) develop, or a total of 12–15 tablets have been given; 8–10 tablets are usually required to terminate an acute attack. If relief is delayed or symptoms recur, a second course may be given after 48 hours. Intravenously administered colchicine, also very effective, appears less likely to produce GI toxicity; the dose is 1.0 mg (diluted with 5–10 ml saline) initially, followed by 0.5 mg every 3–6 hours; the maximum dose should not exceed 3–4 mg. Care must be taken to ensure that the injection is made intravenously, as colchicine solution is irritating if injected outside the vein.

Side effects are primarily vomiting and diarrhea; they may be controlled with prochlorperazine and paregoric. Other toxic effects are rare, but hypersensitivity reactions, alopecia, and one case of vascular purpura have been reported.

b) **Phenylbutazone** is equally or slightly more effective in acute gout, generally free of serious toxicity when given in the dosage recommended, and often advantageous in that it does not cause the unpleasant GI reactions of colchicine. During the first 24 hours 600–800 mg are given (in divided dosage, every 4–6 hours); daily dosage is reduced gradually thereafter and therapy discontinued after 4–7 days. Phenylbutazone has been shown to be effective in some patients resistant to colchicine.

c) **Indomethacin** is also reported to be rapidly effective, although experience with this new agent is relatively limited and side effects are common. Dosage is 50 mg TID until all signs and symptoms subside.

d) **Other therapy** In fulminant cases corticosteroids may be considered, especially if response to conventional therapy is poor. Exacerbations tend to occur as dosage is being reduced and a maintenance dose of 0.5–1 mg colchicine is advised to avoid reactivation. The affected joint should be immobilized, and bed rest is advisable. Uricosuric agents should not be used during acute attacks, since they may cause flare-ups of the disease.

C. **Interval phase and chronic gouty arthritis** In some patients the second attack does not occur for many years, but the majority of patients develop recurrent attacks in increasing frequency and severity. The presence of tophi is pathognomonic of gout, but in the absence of tophi, hyperuricemia and a typical attack establishes the diagnosis. Because of extreme variability, it is not possible to formulate a uniform plan of therapy for all patients. The aim of treatment in this stage of the disease is to avoid any precipitating factors and to mitigate acute episodes. In patients who suffer from an occasional acute episode only, no daily treatment may be necessary; in severe progressive disease, colchicine may have to be added to uricosuric agents and the diet restricted. According to some authors allopurinol may be the mainstay of therapy in chronic gout.

1. **Diet** Since the availability of effective uricosuric drugs, rigid control of purine intake is seldom necessary. Dietary objectives include weight reduction to ideal body weight for the obese, and avoidance of high-purine foods (liver, kidney, sweetbreads, sardines, anchovies) and foods known by the patient to precipitate acute attacks. A high fluid intake will minimize the risk of uric acid calculi formation.

2. **Colchicine** Administration of maintenance doses of colchicine in small amounts (1–2 tablets daily) often reduces the frequency and severity of acute attacks of gout; some observers recommend colchicine alone for the patient who has only minimal elevation of the serum uric acid concentration. To lessen chances for development of an acute attack, colchicine also should be given just before and after surgery, during intercurrent illness, and during initiation of uricosuric therapy. Toxicity of prolonged administration of small doses of colchicine is negligible.

3. **Uricosuric drugs** These agents cause a marked increase in urinary excretion of uric acid by interfering with renal tubular reabsorption. They are remarkably effective in preventing and/or reversing disabling chronic tophaceous gout. They are indicated for patients who have demonstrable tophi, serum uric acid levels above 8 mg/100 ml, or frequent or severe attacks of gout despite colchicine prophylaxis. Although they may be relatively ineffective in the presence of renal insufficiency, azotemia per se is not a contraindication to their administration. During initiation of therapy acute attacks of gout may occur, or urate calculi may develop (secondary to marked uricosuria); the former may be minimized by concurrent administration of colchicine, the latter by maintaining a high fluid intake and alkalinizing the urine, and both by starting therapy with a small dose of the drug, and increasing this gradually. Therapy, once begun, should be continued indefinitely in most circumstances.

   a) **Probenecid (Benemid)** is the preferred drug for routine use. The usual dose is 0.5 gm 2–4 times daily as determined by changes in the serum uric acid, which should be maintained at near-normal levels. Therapy should be started with 0.5 gm daily, increasing to maintenance dosage over a 7-day period. Aspirin, which in small doses counteracts the effects of probenecid (and sulfinpyrazone as well), should not be given concurrently. Side effects are rare and include headache, GI upsets, flushing, and dizziness. Hypersensitivity reactions have been reported; occasionally reducing substances, not glucose, may appear in the urine, giving false-positive results with Clinitest tablets.

   b) **Sulfinpyrazone (Anturane)** is a potent drug; it may be effective in the face of renal insufficiency. Its effects and those of probenecid are additive. Therapy is usually begun with 50 mg BID; the usual maintenance dose is 100 mg QID with meals or milk (to reduce GI upsets). The most common side effects are upper GI disturbances and skin rash; the drug should be given cautiously to patients with a history of peptic ulcer. Salicylates should not be given concurrently.

c) **Other agents**   Aspirin is effective in doses of 5–6 gm daily, but most patients cannot tolerate this amount. When less than 3.0 gm daily is given urate retention and hyperuricemia occur. Acetohexamide, another uricosuric agent, may be useful in the presence of diabetes mellitus. Coumarin compounds are also uricosuric but are of no value clinically.

4. **Allopurinol (Zyloprim)** is 4-hydroxypyrazolo (3,4-d) pyrimidine (HPP), an isomer of hypoxanthine. Although clinical experience with the drug is still relatively limited, allopurinol appears to be very effective in the treatment of severe gout and relatively free of toxicity. The literature should be followed closely (a review by Rundles *et al.* appears in *Ann. Intern. Med.* 64:229, 1966).

a) **Mechanism of action**   Allopurinol inhibits the enzyme xanthine oxidase, thus suppressing the formation of uric acid from xanthine and hypoxanthine; evidence also suggests that de novo purine biosynthesis is reduced. The serum uric acid level begins to fall within 48 hours of administration of the drug and is maximally suppressed in 7–10 days; the fall is paralleled by a similar reduction in urinary uric acid excretion. The serum and urine concentrations of the oxypurines (xanthine and hypoxanthine) rise. Allopurinol is metabolized to alloxanthine, which also is an inhibitor of xanthine oxidase.

b) **Clinical use**   The clinical effects of allopurinol are dose- and time-related. To prevent an increased number of acute attacks of gout when therapy with allopurinol is initiated, other drugs (e.g., colchicine or uricosuric agents) which the patient may have been taking should be continued for several weeks, then tapered in dosage and discontinued, if desired. Although the incidence of acute attacks of gout may not decrease initially with this therapy, their frequency and severity subsequently decline. With continued administration of the proper dose of the drug, serum uric acid concentration may be maintained at normal or low levels, chronic tophaceous deposits may resolve, and the incidence of uric acid nephrolithiasis decreases strikingly (the formation of urinary uric acid stones virtually ceases). The drug may be effective in the presence of renal insufficiency unless unusually severe, and even then appreciable reduction in the serum uric acid levels may occur. Uricosuric drugs and uricosuric doses of aspirin may be given concurrently with allopurinol. Recent evidence indicates that tophi may resolve faster when allopurinol and a uricosuric agent are administered together than when either is used alone.

The drug is indicated for the treatment of primary gout that is unusually severe or is complicated by urate nephropathy or uric acid nephrolithiasis; it may be given to patients sensitive to probenecid. The drug is also useful in preventing the complications of hyperuricemia (particularly urate deposits in the kidney or uric acid stone formation) in patients with neoplastic disease (especially lymphomas and leukemia) given large doses of antimetabolites or steroids resulting in massive nucleoprotein breakdown. The drug should not be given to women of child-bearing age.

c) **Dosage** Allopurinol is supplied in 100-mg tablets. The usual daily dose required to reduce serum urate levels to normal in patients with mild disease is 200–300 mg (in divided dosage); patients with moderate to severe disease often require 400–600 mg/day, but up to 800–1000 mg daily may be given if necessary, particularly to patients with severe tophaceous disease.

d) **Side effects** reported to date are few. The most common is skin rash, but others that have been reported include diarrhea, abdominal pain, nausea, vomiting, drug fever, and, very rarely, leukopenia or elevation of liver enzymes. The chances for development of acute gouty attacks during initiation of therapy may be reduced by concurrent administration of colchicine or other uricosuric drugs, as previously noted. Although the solubility of xanthine in acid urine is similar to that of uric acid, an increased incidence of xanthine stones has not been reported to date.

D. **Secondary gout** may occur in a number of hematologic disorders associated with increased nucleoprotein breakdown; uric acid excretion may be markedly elevated, and the incidence of uric acid nephrolithiasis is increased. Acute hyperuricemia and severe renal insufficiency may be precipitated by administration of chemotherapeutic agents to patients with leukemia or lymphomas. The pathogenesis of uric acid nephropathy is related to intraluminal precipitation of uric acid in the distal tubules and collecting ducts, resulting in progressive obstruction of nephrons; factors influencing precipitation include the magnitude and duration of hyperuricemia, degree of hydration, and urinary pH.

Therapeutic measures of importance in prophylaxis of uric acid nephropathy include allopurinol, adequate hydration to ensure brisk urine flow, and alkalinization of urine to attain maximal uric acid solubility. Fluid intake should be 2–3 liters daily. Urine pH should be maintained at 7.0 or above by oral administration of $NaHCO_3$ (10–15 gm daily) and/or acetazolamide (0.5–1.0 gm daily); potassium supplementation (40–80 mEq daily) will usually be necessary to prevent hypokalemia when acetazolamide and/or $NaHCO_3$ is given.

Should acute uric acid nephropathy occur, fluids, $NaHCO_3$, and acetazolamide may be given IV if the patient is not oliguric. When oliguria is a problem, alkalinization of urine is difficult with acetazolamide alone, and administration of large quantities of fluid and sodium is contraindicated; in this circumstance diuresis may be initiated by cautious administration of an osmotic diuretic, such as mannitol, and subsequent urinary alkalinization achieved as described above. It is possible to prevent hyperuricemia by giving allopurinol routinely to patients with diseases producing secondary gout. If treatment with ionizing radiation or a cytotoxic drug is contemplated, it is advisable to start allopurinol concomitantly. **Remember:** The administration of allopurinol does not replace alkalinization of urine and adequate fluid intake.

III. **ANKYLOSING SPONDYLITIS** Marie-Strümpell disease is characterized by a progressive polyarthritis involving the sacroiliac joints and the spinal apophyseal joints and adjacent soft tissues; about 50% of patients have peripheral joint involvement indistinguishable from that of rheumatoid arthritis. Iritis occurs in 25–30% of patients, and aortitis or carditis in 1–4%; progressive aortic insufficiency may develop.

Principles of management are similar to those for rheumatoid arthritis. Flexion deformity must be avoided as far as possible by providing adequate relief of pain, a very firm flat bed without pillows under the head, and postural exercises designed to strengthen paraspinal muscles and increase breathing capacity. Activity requiring use of the extensor muscles of the back should be encouraged. A back brace is usually not indicated unless there is persistent pain and muscle spasm, or progressive postural deformity unrelieved by exercises.

Because daily postural exercise is the most important measure in a long-range therapeutic program, pain must be relieved; otherwise the patient will usually not perform the recommended exercises. Salicylates are the drug of choice; those not benefited should be given phenylbutazone (100 mg QID for 7–10 days, then maintenance dosage of 50–200 mg daily), which provides effective symptomatic relief in the majority of patients. Phenylbutazone may be given for months, if required, but dosage should be reduced to a minimum, since toxicity (as previously described) is usually dosage-related. Indomethacin is also reported to be quite effective.

Corticosteroids are of value, but, as in rheumatoid arthritis, they must be considered palliative, not curative, and a complement to other therapy, not a substitute. Other measures are more beneficial in relieving the usual symptoms, but steroids may be required for the treatment of rapidly progressive disease and systemic manifestations as carditis or iridocyclitis. The dosage is essentially the same as that used in rheumatoid arthritis.

Radiation therapy of symptomatic areas of the spine may reduce pain, stiffness, and tenderness in up to 75% of patients; effects appear in 3–6 weeks and may last for many months. The value of radiation in decreasing discomfort and disability must be weighed against the usual hazards associated with radiotherapy.

Gold salts are of no value in the treatment of rheumatoid spondylitis.

IV. **DEGENERATIVE JOINT DISEASE** Osteoarthritis is a progressive disease characterized by deterioration of articular cartilage, proliferation of juxta-articular bone, symptoms of joint pain on motion or weight bearing, and stiffness after periods of inactivity. Limitation of motion may occur secondary to muscle spasm; contractures or mechanical deformity of joints may develop. The disease may be severely disabling when major weight-bearing joints as the hip and knee are involved.

Therapeutic measures include reassurance that the disease will not be disabling (as a rule), sustained dosage of aspirin (2.4–3.6 gm daily), heat, avoidance of aggravating activity, and weight reduction for the obese. Exercise will help to prevent joint instability and muscle atrophy. Intra-articular injection of steroids may be of transient benefit when inflammation of a single large joint occurs. Phenylbutazone and indomethacin are also effective in decreasing symptoms; corticosteroids administered systemically are of little value. Surgical measures may be required when advanced disabling disease occurs in one or two large joints.

V.   **REITER'S SYNDROME**   The disease is characterized by urethritis, arthritis, and conjunctivitis; the course is acute, self-limited, and without residual, as a rule. The clinical course is not modified by the administration of corticosteroids, antibiotics, phenylbutazone, or aspirin. Therapy is nonspecific and symptomatic; arthritis is usually relieved best by aspirin. Local and/or systemic steroids may be required when uveitis or iritis is severe.

VI.   **PYOGENIC ARTHRITIS**   When acute bacterial arthritis is suspected, joint fluid must be obtained for bacteriologic study. Besides gram-positive cocci, enteric organisms, gonococci, and tubercle bacilli, a wide variety of organisms (brucella, hemophilus, listeria, mimaea species, etc.) may be the offending agents. Because many of these may be difficult to culture in vitro, culture media should be inoculated immediately and incubated both aerobically and anaerobically. When an organism is isolated, antibiotic sensitivity studies should be performed.

Basic therapeutic measures include immobilization of the affected joint in a position of function and administration of appropriate antibiotics in massive dosage. Concentrations of antibiotics in synovial fluid approach those of serum when there is synovial inflammation; intra-articular instillation of antibiotics is not required. Antibiotic therapy should be continued at high dose levels for 2–4 weeks depending on the organism, its antibiotic sensitivity, and clinical response of the affected joint.

Repeated joint aspirations are useful in providing symptomatic relief, in removing purulent material that may inhibit antibiotic effectiveness, in providing a means of following the therapeutic response, and most importantly, in preventing the destructive effects of pus on the cartilage matrix.

I. **SHOCK** is a complex physiologic state in which tissue perfusion is inadequate. The consequence is cellular injury. Although numerous specific etiologies have been identified, shock can be conveniently regarded as the result of one or a combination of three pathophysiologic events: loss of circulating blood volume (hypovolemic), heart failure (cardiogenic), loss of peripheral vascular resistance (neurogenic). A common cause of hypovolemic shock is gastrointestinal bleeding, but fluid loss from vomiting and/or diarrhea, trauma, burns, peritonitis, and pancreatitis is also common. Myocardial infarction is the most common cause of cardiogenic shock, but other cardiac causes of low output—arrhythmias, pericardial tamponade, pulmonary embolus—must be considered. Spinal-cord or brain-stem injury is the classic cause of neurogenic shock.

Classification of shock in terms of these three pathophysiologic events is an oversimplification of this complex state but is useful in guiding a rational approach to therapy. It is not wise to consider only one pathologic event in an individual patient, for shock is frequently caused by a combination of events. For instance, septic shock can be a combination of hypovolemia, heart failure, and loss of vascular resistance. Although most patients with myocardial infarction and shock have reduced cardiac output, some exhibit little abnormality of output and respond to expansion of intravascular volume. Some patients—diabetics, cirrhotics, patients with septic shock—have warm skin that may be associated with a low peripheral resistance.

The characteristic clinical manifestations of shock consist of pallor, cold and moist skin, collapsed peripheral veins, sluggish capillary filling, rapid "thready" pulse, decreased urine output, changes in mental state, and a fall in blood pressure. Acidosis is usually associated. When the necessary techniques are available, measurement of blood volume, cardiac output, peripheral resistance, and pH can be used to monitor treatment.

A. **Central venous pressure (CVP)** The true intrathoracic CVP is important both in diagnosing and treating shock. Cardiogenic and hypovolemic shock can usually be differentiated clinically by measuring the CVP. Elevated CVP means inadequacy of the heart as a pump, or circulatory overload. Low CVP indicates relative or absolute hypovolemia and the need to expand intravascular volume. A normal CVP may not accurately reflect the extent of hypovolemia or the extent of pump failure; a trial of rapid fluid administration may be necessary as a functional test of pump function and volume capacity. If the CVP remains normal despite volume expansion, hypovolemia represents a major component of shock; if CVP rises rapidly, the cardiogenic component of shock is playing a major role. The CVP is usually normal in neurogenic shock.

A hypovolemic component of shock should be considered and treated first in those patients with unexplained shock. If the CVP is low or normal, the circulating blood volume should be expanded until the CVP rises to approximately 150 mm saline. If shock persists, cardiogenic and neurogenic etiologies should be considered and treated appropriately.

The CVP is most easily measured by threading a long polyethylene catheter into the superior vena cava or right atrium via the median basilic vein. The catheter can be attached to a manometer and to intravenous fluids by a three-way stopcock. The manometer should be zeroed at the midchest level with the patient lying flat. The fluids being given intravenously can be used to fill the manometer, and by turning the stopcock the CVP can be measured. All intravenous catheters should be removed within 72 hours to avoid phlebitis and septicemia. If measurement of the CVP is still required, another vein must be used.

B. Drugs The drugs used in treating shock are primarily vasopressors, although vasodilators are currently of great interest and are strongly recommended by some authors. The action of these drugs is best understood by considering the alpha-beta concept, a pharmacologic concept introduced in 1948. Adrenergic receptors, alpha and beta, mediate the actions of sympathomimetic amines. Although these receptors have not been anatomically demonstrated, the physiologic concept of alpha and beta mediators is of practical value to the physician in directing drug therapy. Alpha receptors mediate vasoconstriction; beta receptors mediate vasodilatation and positive inotropic and chronotropic effects on the heart. Some drugs are alpha stimulators, some beta stimulators; many are both. A few drugs are alpha blockers; in general, these have the same hemodynamic actions as beta stimulators. Beta blocking drugs cause mild vasoconstriction and inhibit the positive inotropic and chronotropic adrenergic effects on the heart.

The mechanism of action, route of administration, and dosage of these vasoactive drugs are listed in Table 17-1. The choice of the proper drug is not always easy. The physician must try to select a drug that restores adequate perfusion to vital areas. Simply restoring blood pressure to normal may not do that, and in many cases the restoration of a normal blood pressure may be associated with a fall in tissue perfusion. Because adequate tissue perfusion is most important, investigators have recently stressed the use of vasodilators, both beta adrenergic stimulators and alpha adrenergic blockers, in an attempt to provide normal tissue perfusion. Because the literature is changing and growing so rapidly, it is difficult to recommend a drug of choice for all cases of shock. Ideally, the drug of choice would restore blood flow to vital areas without compromising blood pressure. The physician should choose his drugs with this goal in mind.

1. Isoproterenol (Isuprel), a beta adrenergic stimulator, raises cardiac output by increasing the rate and force of myocardial contraction, and increases tissue perfusion by decreasing total peripheral resistance; theoretically it is the ideal drug. Cardiac output is usually raised by the inotropic and chronotropic actions of the drug, but peripheral vasodilatory effects may be striking, and cardiac output may fall because of peripheral pooling of the effective blood volume; this change is usually reflected in a low central venous pressure. Therefore, central venous pressure must be monitored during isoproterenol administration, and intravenous fluid must be given fast enough to maintain a normal central venous pressure.

2. **Levarterenol (Levophed) and metaraminol (Aramine),** stimulators of both alpha and beta adrenergic receptors, have positive inotropic effects on the heart, but their major effect is mediated through alpha adrenergic receptors and results in marked vasoconstriction. Metaraminol releases norepinephrine from nerve endings rather than acting directly on receptors in vascular smooth muscle, and its effects may be blocked by catecholamine depletion. Cardiac output increases unless blood pressure is raised excessively; hypertension will add to the cardiac work load and will cause reflex bradycardia, which will reduce cardiac output. Therefore, an attempt should not be made to bring the blood pressure to preshock levels with these agents; a systolic pressure of 90–100 mm Hg is usually high enough to permit adequate tissue perfusion.

3. **Methoxamine (Vasoxyl) and phenylephrine (Neo-Synephrine),** alpha adrenergic stimulators, and **angiotensin (Hypertensin)** increase blood pressure by vasoconstriction only; cardiac output usually falls, and decreased tissue perfusion results. These agents have little place, if any, in the treatment of clinical shock other than neurogenic shock, but most patients with neurogenic shock will respond to volume expansion. However, these drugs are useful if shock is caused by a supraventricular tachycardia, for they will slow the sinus rate and prolong atrioventricular conduction by increasing vagotonic reflexes (see Chapter 6).

4. **Phentolamine (Regitine) and phenoxybenzamine (Dibenzyline),** alpha adrenergic blocking agents, counteract the vasoconstriction usually associated with shock, cause vasodilatation, and increase tissue perfusion providing that cardiac output is maintained. Results with these agents in the treatment of experimental shock, primarily endotoxin shock in dogs, have been favorable, and results with phenoxybenzamine in clinical shock have been encouraging. Adequate replacement of intravascular fluid volume is necessary. Phenoxybenzamine for parenteral use is available for investigational purposes only. The literature should be consulted for recent advances in the treatment of shock with alpha adrenergic blockers.

5. **Corticosteroids** may be of value in shock even in the absence of evidence of adrenal insufficiency. They increase cardiac output by a positive inotropic effect and also decrease peripheral resistance. Although unequivocal evidence of benefit is not available, several investigators have reported improvement in therapeutic results when steroids are used in pharmacologic doses. Short-term, high-dose steroid therapy does no harm and may be beneficial. Administration of 1.0 gm of hydrocortisone (or its synthetic equivalent) during the first hour and 500 mg every 6 hours during the initial 72 hours of treatment is recommended for the management of bacteremic shock.

C. Treatment of shock

1. **General measures** An adequate airway must be maintained and nasal oxygen 8–10 L/min administered. An intravenous catheter should be put in the superior vena cava or right atrium and fluids given intravenously until CVP is 150 mm saline; **expanding the**

intravascular volume is the most important therapeutic maneuver in treating shock. Blood pressure should be recorded often, and measurement of urine volume and assessment of mental function must be recorded frequently.

Measuring arterial pH is extremely helpful, for shock is frequently accompanied by acidosis requiring bicarbonate intravenously.

2. **Hypovolemic shock** should be suspected and treated in all patients in shock. These patients will usually have low CVPs, increased peripheral resistance, and reduced cardiac output secondary to poor venous return. Blood, plasma, synthetic ECF (see Chapter 2), isotonic saline, or occasionally dextran should be given as fast as possible; circulatory overload is rare if the CVP is maintained below 150 mm saline. The treatment of hemorrhagic shock is discussed in Chapter 11. Remember that hypovolemia often complicates cardiogenic, neurogenic, bacteremic, and anaphylactic shock. If the patient has not recovered when the CVP reaches 150 mm saline, other causes of shock should be considered and treated. **The importance of adequate volume expansion cannot be overemphasized.**

3. **Cardiogenic shock** is most often seen following myocardial infarction. It is usually associated with high CVP and increased peripheral resistance, although some patients exhibit normal or low CVPs and peripheral dilatation. The crux of the problem is usually reduction in cardiac contractility and cardiac output; therefore, the therapeutic aim is to increase cardiac output. Despite numerous studies there is no uniform, clinically safe, reliable way to achieve this aim. The following is a workable approach.

   a) **CVP should be measured;** if normal or low, fluids should be given intravenously. The CVP usually rises rapidly with relatively small infusions of fluid.

   b) **Isoproterenol (Isuprel)** increases cardiac output by its positive inotropic and chronotropic actions and also increases tissue perfusion by correcting the intense vasoconstriction usually associated with cardiogenic shock. Its main disadvantage is the increased incidence of cardiac arrhythmias; it should not be used if the heart rate is 120/min or higher. Ideally, the patient should be watched by continuous cardiac monitoring. The ultimate benefits and risks of isoproterenol in cardiogenic shock have not been completely evaluated. See Table 17-1 for dosage.

   c) **Metaraminol (Aramine) and levarterenol (Levophed)** are still the mainstays of therapy. In small doses they increase cardiac output with minimal vasoconstriction. With larger doses vascular resistance increases markedly and cardiac output usually falls. Systolic pressure should be maintained between 90 and 100 mm Hg, and no attempt should be made to bring blood pressure back to preshock levels, providing sensorium and urine flow are normal. Cardiac arrhythmias remain a significant hazard, especially in a failing heart; continuous cardiac monitoring is desirable. See Table 17-1 for dosage.

   d) **Digitalis glycosides** are indicated if congestive heart failure is clinically manifest. Theoretically, the increase in myocardial contractility and consequent increase in cardiac output offer distinct advantages. The benefits and risks of digitalis in

TABLE 17-1. Certain Vasoactive Drugs*

Generic Name (Trade Name)	Route and Dose			Comments
	Subcut.	IM	IV	
Isoproterenol (Isuprel)			1 mg (5 ml) in 500 ml 5% D/S or D/W by infusion	A beta adrenergic stimulator that increases cardiac output and decreases peripheral resistance. Rates of administration causing heart rates above 120 may predispose to cardiac arrhythmias
Metaraminol (Aramine)	2–10 mg	2–10 mg	0.5–5 mg by injection or 25–100 mg in 500 ml 5% D/W by infusion	Both an alpha and beta adrenergic stimulator with alpha stimulation predominantly. Increases peripheral resistance and cardiac output, providing reflex bradycardia is prevented
Levarterenol (Levophed)			4–8 mg (4–8 ml) in 1000 ml 5% D/S or D/W by infusion	Same action as metaraminol, but more potent

*This table is meant only to serve as a guide to dosage; dosage schedules must be tailored to the clinical situation.

clinical cardiogenic shock are not sufficiently documented to make an unequivocal statement for or against its routine use. If used, a rapid-acting preparation should be employed. For dosage see Table 5-2.

4. **The neurogenic component of shock** usually follows severe injury to the spinal cord which causes a loss in vasomotor tone; vasodilatation and hypotension result from the loss of peripheral vascular resistance. Vasodilatation also contributes to circulatory collapse in diabetic patients with ketoacidosis whose shock does not respond to expansion of intravascular volume. This form of shock may be the sole indication for strictly alpha adrenergic stimulators— methoxamine (Vasoxyl) and phenylephrine (Neo-Synephrine)— and the vasoconstrictor, angiotensin (Hypertensin). However, the circulating blood volume should be expanded, with frequent monitoring by CVP measurement. Moreover, shock associated with drugs causing central nervous system depression (i.e., barbiturates, narcotics, tranquilizers, etc.) has been shown to be a special form of hypovolemia and not due to vasomotor failure (*Amer. J. Med.* 38:853, 1965).

5. **Bacteremic shock** may be associated with increased, normal, or decreased cardiac output, CVP, blood volume, and peripheral resistance. The following scheme provides a useful approach to bacteremic shock and **may be used in any patient in shock of unknown etiology.** The antibiotics recommended for bacteremic shock are discussed in Chapter 9.

   a) Determine the CVP; if it is low, **expand intravascular volume** to bring the CVP to 150 mm.

   b) **Administer steroids;** use hydrocortisone, 1.0 gm (or equivalent) IV initially followed by 500 mg IV every 6 hours for 72 hours.

   c) **Administer a vasoactive amine if shock persists.** Isoproterenol (Isuprel) should be used first; however, if the patient remains warm and pink with strong pulse (i.e., no clinical evidence of vasoconstriction), metaraminol (Aramine) or levarterenol (Levophed) may be used. Maintain systolic pressure between 90 and 100 mm Hg; observe sensorium and urine output carefully. Never sacrifice tissue perfusion for the satisfaction of obtaining a normal blood pressure; a urine output of at least 30 ml per hour usually reflects adequate tissue perfusion.

6. **Anaphylactic shock** usually occurs after administration of drugs or therapeutic agents to which the patient has become sensitized. Epinephrine remains the drug of choice, although a recent study of the hemodynamics of anaphylactic shock in man indicates that shock is related to a loss of fluid from the intravascular compartment and may be corrected by restoring intravascular volume (Hanashiro and Weil, *Arch. Intern. Med.* 119:129, 1967). Bronchospasm and laryngeal edema, unusual in other types of shock, are characteristic hazards of anaphylactic shock.

   a) **Maintain an open airway;** insert an endotracheal tube or perform a tracheostomy if necessary.

   b) Determine the CVP and **expand intravascular volume** rapidly, keeping the CVP below 150 mm.

   c) **Epinephrine,** aqueous, 0.3–0.5 ml, should be given subcutaneously and the injection site massaged; 0.1–0.2 ml may be given every 5–15 minutes thereafter if necessary.

    d) Aminophylline, 500 mg IV, and hydrocortisone, 100 mg IV, are effective for bronchospasm.

    e) Antihistamines are of little proved value but may block further histamine binding to target tissues.

II.   **ACUTE ADRENAL CRISIS** may be precipitated by numerous factors, including infection, surgical stress, and cessation of medication by the patient with Addison's disease or the patient who has some other illness for which he has been receiving therapeutic doses of corticosteroids.

    A. Prevention   Patients who have primary or secondary adrenal insufficiency or who have been receiving steroids for other reasons should increase their maintenance dosage of cortisone by 25–50 mg daily during acute illnesses not necessitating hospitalization. If patients with adrenal insufficiency require elective surgery, 100 mg cortisone acetate should be given IM 24 hours prior to operation and on the morning of operation; 100 mg hydrocortisone succinate or phosphate should be infused IV during surgery. Postoperatively, steroids may be tapered over 3–5 days to the usual maintenance dosage if there are no complications. If an emergency operation is required, 100 mg cortisone acetate should be given IM and 100–200 mg hydrocortisone infused IV before and during the procedure.

    B. Treatment   Objectives of therapy include correction of hypotension, fluid and electrolyte imbalance, hypoglycemia, and hypothermia, and control of underlying infection, if present. The therapeutic problems will vary, depending on precipitating factors and previous therapy, but substantial steroid dosages are indicated for all patients.

    1. Glucocorticoids

      a) 100 mg hydrocortisone succinate or phosphate are injected IV.

      b) 100 mg hydrocortisone are diluted in 1000 ml of 5% D/S and infused at a rate of approximately 250 ml per hour.

      c) 50–100 mg cortisone acetate are given IM.

      d) Generally, no more than 200 mg hydrocortisone are required during the first 12 hours of therapy unless the patient is very ill and in profound shock.

      e) Cortisone dosage after the first 24 hours of therapy is determined by the severity of the initial clinical manifestations and by the patient's response. Most patients will have responded dramatically, and cortisone can be administered orally in decreasing dosage over the ensuing 2–3 days until maintenance levels are reached.

    2. Mineralocorticoids   Generally these agents are not required; hydrocortisone in large dosage produces adequate salt retention. If mineralocorticoids are administered in addition to significant amounts of sodium, pulmonary edema may develop. However, for patients who are critically ill and severely hyponatremic, desoxycorticosterone acetate 5–10 mg IM, or 9-alpha-fluorohydrocortisone (Florinef) 0.2–0.4 mg orally may be given initially.

    3. Fluids and electrolytes   Requirements are determined by the clinical state and electrolyte abnormalities. Determination of serum Na^+, K^+, Cl^-, HCO_3^-, and BUN should be made as soon as the patient is seen. Administration of 2000–3000 ml 5% D/S IV during the first 24 hours will usually correct the salt and water depletion. However, significant dehydration or hyponatremia may not occur in patients who develop acute adrenal insufficiency following sudden cessation of therapeutic doses of corticosteroid drugs; in this situation large amounts of fluid are not required.

4. Other measures

   a) Hypotension usually responds to administration of saline and hydrocortisone, but if severe peripheral circulatory collapse is present, vasopressors may be necessary.

   b) Hypothermia and hyperthermia should be treated with routine measures.

   c) Unnecessary procedures and examinations should be delayed until the patient's condition has improved.

   d) Appropriate cultures should be obtained and administration of broad-spectrum antibiotics started routinely in most patients who suddenly develop acute adrenal crisis without apparent precipitating cause. In such cases infection is commonly responsible, and signs of infection may not be apparent because of dehydration and hypothermia.

   e) Hypokalemia and overhydration should be avoided.

III.   THE COMATOSE PATIENT   Disturbances of response to environment related to intracranial or systemic illness present a clinical picture ranging from slight confusion to deep coma. Because the cause of illness is often obscure, these patients present the ultimate in diagnostic and therapeutic difficulty. Certain therapeutic considerations take precedence over all diagnostic procedures when the patient is first seen. They are establishment of an airway and establishment of a secure route of administering intravenous fluids and medications by means of an 18-gauge needle or large intravenous catheter. Simultaneously, a search must be made for inapparent blood loss and for evidence of inadequate cerebral perfusion. Patients first seen in coma are often unattended persons whose illness has been neglected or persons who have attempted suicide. Because the history in such cases either is not immediately obtainable or may be unreliable, diagnosis must proceed despite lack of some useful information. Prompt diagnosis can greatly influence prognosis. Although intoxication with alcohol or sedatives is probably the most common cause of coma, the most frequently overlooked cause is hypoglycemia (obtain blood sugar!); it responds to the administration of 100 ml of 50% glucose by IV push. Parenteral use of CNS stimulants (Ritalin, Coramine) is contraindicated because of cardiac side effects and the danger of poststimulation rebound. The management of prolonged coma is discussed below.

A. Blood pressure must be maintained at levels adequate for cerebral perfusion. A usual minimum value is 80 mm Hg systolic; there may be exceptions.

B. Pulmonary ventilation should be assured as follows:

1. Search for dentures or intraoral foreign body.

2. Tape a short, hard-rubber or plastic oropharyngeal airway in the mouth to prevent the tongue from obstructing air flow. If the airway is too short it will not work and if too long it will produce coughing and laryngeal spasm by supraglottic irritation.

3. Control of secretions is obtained by:

   a) Frequently suctioning the nasopharynx with clean, lubricated catheters at moderate suction pressures (7–10 cm Hg).

   b) Positioning the patient on his side with face turned slightly toward the mattress and partially extending the neck; intermittent use of the Trendelenburg position may also be useful.

4. Hypoxia and cyanosis respond to oxygen supplementation. When the above measures are insufficient to control secretions, the cough reflex is absent, or prolonged mechanical respiratory assistance is required, a cuffed endotracheal tube may be inserted, to be followed within 36 hours by tracheostomy if coma persists (see Chapter 8).

C. Cutaneous pressure sores are avoided by turning the patient every 1–2 hours, keeping the bedding clean, dry, and wrinkle-free, and by padding the bony prominences. Alternating-pressure mattresses are helpful in preventing bedsores but do not replace fastidious nursing care.

D. Nutrition and hydration are often conveniently maintained by tube feeding if reflux and aspiration can be prevented (see Chapter 1).

E. Incontinence of stool and urine is the rule, necessitating prompt frequent changes of bed linen. Condom catheters may be used in male patients either intermittently or with appropriate safeguards against penile maceration. When an indwelling catheter is necessary, the use of a three-way catheter with continuous irrigation is recommended (see Chapter 9). Clamping the catheter for short periods of time helps maintain bladder tone.

F. Diarrhea is a common sequela of tube feeding but may also result from fecal impaction.

G. Corneal abrasion or opacification can be prevented by taping the eyelids shut or by using methylcellulose eyedrops.

H. Restlessness or delirium may occur transiently during the recovery period and attempts to modify such activity may only prolong it. Extreme restlessness or delirium of several hours' duration, in the absence of other signs of recovery, should be treated with a sedative appropriate to the underlying disease (barbiturate or phenothiazine). Seizures are treated with anticonvulsants.

I. Cerebral edema with attendant increased intracranial pressure may accompany various forms of central nervous system insult, including trauma, encephalitis, neoplasm, hypertensive crisis, and other cerebrovascular diseases. When increased intracranial pressure is observed in association with altered states of consciousness, some degree of cerebral edema may be presumed to be present. Deepening of the unconscious state or the development of brain-stem compression as indicated by changes in vital signs or cranial-nerve changes represents a neurologic emergency. When the cause of the increased pressure is unknown, arteriographic search for a focal organic lesion may be necessary immediately. In the interim, further progression can often be slowed and the process reversed and sometimes prevented by use of one or several agents to reduce cerebral edema.

The following therapeutic regimen is designed to alleviate and reduce irreversible brain damage while appropriate diagnostic and therapeutic procedures are being carried out. However, such a regimen in no way takes the place of definitive therapy.

1. **Dexamethasone (Decadron)** 10 mg may be injected by IV push. Maintenance doses of 4–6 mg IM q6h are used. Steroids offer the advantage of simplicity of medical management without risk of creating severe electrolyte disturbances. However, in cerebral edema steroids become effective only after 5–6 hours, and maximum effect is achieved only after 24 hours. Although any steroid preparation in equivalent dosage is effective, dexamethasone is preferred because of minimal salt retention.

2. **Twenty percent mannitol** solutions are given rapidly to relieve acute swelling that is life-threatening. A dose of 1.5 gm/kg body weight is given rapidly over a period of 30 minutes to 1 hour, depending on cardiac status. It is important to administer mannitol using a blood infusion apparatus with a filter to prevent entrance of undissolved crystals into the circulation. Before administration, an indwelling urinary catheter must be in place. Urinary output must be checked every hour and flow of more than 50 ml per hour maintained. Vital signs must be checked several times each hour and blood electrolytes several times daily. The above dose of mannitol may be repeated every 12 hours but usually is replaced by steroid therapy after 48 hours.

IV. **CEREBROVASCULAR ACCIDENTS**   Vascular accidents (thrombosis, hemorrhage) may be mimicked by other conditions (e.g., primary or metastatic brain tumor, encephalitis, and metabolic disorders such as hepatic coma, hypoglycemia, drug intoxication, etc.). Appropriate diagnostic measures should be carried out because a definitive diagnosis may not be immediately apparent. The ultimate prognosis cannot always be predicted during the first few days following an acute vascular accident.

A. **Supportive therapy** of stroke patients is most important. As many as three-fourths of cerebrovascular hemiplegics can achieve independent ambulation, self-care, and continence of bladder and bowel. In addition to general measures listed in the treatment of coma, certain special precautions and procedures should be instituted.

1. Large doses of barbiturates and narcotics should not be given. Certain patients may be inordinately sensitive to their effects; administration of these drugs may preclude careful serial evaluation of the neurologic status.

2. Muscle contractures should be prevented by using a small pillow in the axilla of a paretic arm and by splinting the wrist and fingers in neutral position with a gauze roll placed in the palm. Prevention of external rotation at the hip, knee flexion contracture,

and fixed foot drop by appropriate use of footboards and sandbags will greatly facilitate reambulation.

3. Elastic stockings or elastic wrapping up to the knee lessens the likelihood of phlebothrombosis and pulmonary embolism.

4. As soon as the patient regains consciousness, regular full-range-of-motion passive exercises should begin for all paretic limbs.

5. Intravenous fluid therapy via paretic limbs should be avoided whenever possible. The lower extremities should never be used for this purpose.

B. Hemorrhage Twelve percent of cerebrovascular accidents are due to intracerebral or subarachnoid hemorrhage. The patient should be put to bed; excessive movement and jarring should be avoided. If headache is severe, narcotics (despite their side effects) may be required; sedation in the form of chlordiazepoxide (Librium) may be given if agitation is a significant problem. Cerebral hemorrhage with hypertension is a critical therapeutic problem. In many patients, hypertension relates to brain-stem dysfunction from rapidly expanding intracerebral hemorrhage; therapy is supportive and directed against cerebral edema which surrounds the hematoma. In cases in which the hematoma develops more slowly and is not related to an extensive deficit in the dominant hemisphere, surgical evacuation may be helpful. Antihypertensive medication should be administered gradually regardless of the level of blood pressure.

Therapy of hemorrhage from rupture of arterial aneurysm or from bleeding arteriovenous anomalies has improved rapidly through advances in surgical technique. Survival and recovery is aided by immediate diagnostic arteriographic examination to allow for appropriate planning of the type and time of surgical intervention. It must be noted that some patients with aneurysms may have marked spasm of intracranial arteries at the time of aneurysm rupture. Angiography is contraindicated in these patients because of the possibility of worsening spasm by the procedure (with possible production of infarction distal to the site of spasm) and because spasm may prevent angiographic visualization of the affected vessel.

C. Embolus About 3% of vascular episodes result from emboli. Cerebral embolization, usually from thrombi in auricular appendages or mural thrombi in the heart, is prevented or decreased in frequency by anticoagulation. It is best to wait 5 days after the acute episode before beginning Coumadin anticoagulation to reduce chances of hemorrhage into the infarcted area. (The use of anticoagulants is discussed in Chapter 4.) Anticoagulation is contraindicated in patients with embolic infarction related to bacterial endocarditis.

D. Thrombosis of a major cerebral vessel accounts for 85% of cerebrovascular accidents.

1. **Ischemic attacks** due to disease of the basilar and carotid arteries present as recurrent, totally resolving deficits lasting less than 4 hours and usually less than 20 minutes. Nonarteriosclerotic causes include polycythemia, anemia, hypertension, cerebrovascular syphilis, cerebral lupus erythematosus, polyarteritis, and migraine. Each of these entities should be treated primarily. Among the arteriosclerotic group, anticoagulation is indicated for selected reliable patients amenable to careful follow-up. In most of these

patients, ischemic attacks will be less frequent or totally elimi-nated, and mortality will be lower, in spite of the added risk of hemorrhagic complications of therapy. In cases in which attacks are recent or increasing in frequency therapy may be initiated with heparin and Coumadin simultaneously. Heparin is discon-tinued after reaching "therapeutic" prothrombin times and Cou-madin is continued indefinitely. Anticoagulation should always be preceded by a lumbar puncture to help exclude hemorrhage or neoplasms. Since 20% of patients with intracerebral bleeding do not have bloody or xanthochromic spinal fluid initially, the administration of anticoagulants is always a calculated risk.

2. **Stroke in evolution** occurs when submaximal neurologic deficit de-velops progressively over a period of 12 to 24 hours. Most clinicians now feel that emergency anticoagulant therapy has little value in changing the outcome in such cases. Others still feel that clinical progression may be significantly reduced by anticoagulant therapy. Heparin and Coumadin therapy are usually begun simultaneously, and immediately, with only the latter maintained beyond the acute period. Coumadin may be continued for 6 months or lifelong. Appropriate diagnostic precautions and consideration of patient reliability must also be applied here. Use of low- and intermediate-molecular-weight dextran solutions in patients with incomplete lesions has been proposed, but their usefulness still remains to be verified.

3. **Completed occlusions** of cerebral, carotid, or vertebral arteries and submaximal deficits progressing to conclusion in less than 12 hours do not respond to anticoagulation. Because of the increased mortality from cerebral hemorrhage, anticoagulation is of no value in such cases.

    An unconfirmed report indicates that hyperbaric oxygen (at 2 atmospheres) benefits patients with cerebrovascular occlusive disease. However, nasal oxygen supplementation is incapable of increasing delivery of oxygen to the brain and is unnecessary except in patients suffering hypoxia from other cause (pulmonary, cardiac, etc.). Vasodilators such as carbon dioxide, papaverine, nicotinamide, histamine, procaine, cyclandelate (Cyclospasmol), isoxsuprine (Vasodilan), and stellate ganglion block have little or no effect on cerebral blood flow in infarcted areas of the brain. However, cerebral blood flow is markedly decreased by a fall in blood pressure, and efforts should be directed toward maintenance of an adequate systemic circulation.

V.   **STATUS EPILEPTICUS** Recurrent major convulsions without interim return of consciousness constitute a threat to life or may result in perma-nent central nervous system injury. Two major seizures without interval return of consciousness is status epilepticus.

A. **Supportive treatment**

1. An adequate orophryangeal airway or padded tongue blade is used in conjunction with oxygen supplementation via a short catheter taped to the airway. If such arrangement proves unsatisfactory, an endotracheal tube is inserted.

2. A reliable route of intravenous administration of medication is established and kept open with intravenous fluids.

3. Secretions are cleared by suctioning.

B. Drug therapy   The outline of therapy below is designed to avoid respiratory depression and long periods of disturbed consciousness.

   1. Intravenous diazepam (Valium) has advantages over more classical agents. It is especially effective in status related to old or slowly progressive cerebral lesions and may be effective in acute lesions as well. Efficacy will be evident after two 10-mg IV injections given 10 minutes apart at a slow rate—5 mg (1 ml) per minute. If seizure activity has not stopped within 10 minutes, other agents must be employed.

      Recurrence of seizures may require a repetition of the above-outlined regimen of therapy in as little as 1–2 hours after the initial administration. When administered repeatedly in a short period, the drug bears little advantage over other anticonvulsants because of cumulative sedative and some respiratory depressant effects.

      Continuous focal motor seizure activity without loss of consciousness and seizure activity with only momentary interictal intervals may respond well to an intravenous drip of 50–100 mg Valium in 1 L isotonic saline administered over 24 hours.

      When IV administration is not clinically feasible, the drug may be given IM at the same doses. Although the anticonvulsant effect of intramuscular diazepam is minimally delayed when compared to the IV route, the rate of absorption from injection sites is somewhat erratic and unpredictable.

      Oral diazepam or long-term use of parenteral diazepam has no place in the routine therapy of epilepsy.

   2. Barbiturates   Amobarbital (Amytal) or sodium phenobarbital (Luminal) may be given slowly (to avoid apnea). There is some evidence that apnea occurs more readily in patients previously treated with diazepam, and great caution should be exercised in administration of barbiturates to such patients.

      a) Phenobarbital 300 mg diluted in 12 ml of sterile saline (25 mg/ml) is given slowly (1 ml/minute) to a minimum dose of 150 mg or with additional increments until seizures stop. After an interval of 20 minutes the uncontrolled patient may be given an additional 120–180 mg in the same dilution at the same rate.

      b) Amobarbital 500 mg is diluted in 20 ml of sterile saline (25 mg/ml) and injected IV at the rate of 1 ml per minute to a minimum dose of 250 mg or with additional increments until seizures stop. In patients still uncontrolled another 250 mg of amobarbital may be given in the same way.

   3. Diphenylhydantoin (Dilantin)   Administered intravenously diphenylhydantoin has immediate anticonvulsant effect and can be used alone or in combination with other drugs, since it has little sedative or respiratory depressant effect. Many clinicians recommend its use before initiating barbiturate therapy. When it is administered properly there is little danger of significant side effects such as ataxia. The usual dose is 4 mg/kg body weight. In the adult an initial dose of 250 mg is given intravenously at a rate of 25 mg (0.5 ml) per minute. Cardiac arrest has been reported attendant to intravenous diphenylhydantoin therapy, but such reactions are thought to be due to excessive rates of administration or use of incompletely dissolved material. At room temperature 10 minutes must be allowed for the diphenylhydantoin to dissolve, but the period may be shortened by immersing the vial with diluent added in warm water. If necessary, the initial dose may be given intramuscularly. Subcutaneous administration should be avoided because of the highly alkaline nature of the solution. The initial dose is followed by 100–125 mg IM every 8–12 hours; oral therapy is instituted as early as possible. Objective results of diphenylhydantoin should be evident within 20 minutes; if it is unsuccessful, other drugs should then be used.

4. **Mannitol** When status is of long duration prior to therapy, the assumption can be made that significant cerebral edema is present and is contributing to the patient's persistent unconscious state. Unless there is evidence of heart failure, the patient should receive 20% mannitol in a dose of 1.5 gm/kg body weight over a period of 1–2 hours. (See page 356 for additional details.)

5. **Anesthesia** When seizures cannot be controlled by the above drugs within a period of two hours, general anesthesia (ether or thiopental) may be administered by an anesthesiologist.

6. **Paraldehyde** is an infrequently used agent in treatment of status epilepticus. Its main use currently is as an oil-retention enema in a dose of 0.2 ml/kg body weight.

VI. ACUTE PULMONARY EMBOLISM

A. **Oxygen** should be given by nasal catheter. If marked tachypnea, apprehension, or pleuritic pain associated with pulmonary infarction is present, meperidine 75–125 mg should be given IM. It is probably better to avoid morphine because of its bronchoconstrictor effects. Stool softeners to prevent straining are indicated.

B. **Cardiac arrhythmias,** which occur in more than 10% of cases, should be treated appropriately. If shock occurs, fluids and vasopressors should be given. Intravenous fluids should be monitored by central-venous-pressure (CVP) measurements; the CVP should be maintained below 150 mm saline to prevent pulmonary edema.

C. **Anticoagulation therapy** should be initiated with heparin administered IV as described in the section on anticoagulants in Chapter 4. A coumarin drug should be given orally, but heparin administration probably should be continued for 7–10 days to assure adequate anticoagulation. Anticoagulant administration should be continued for at least 6 weeks after the acute episode unless a chronic disease such as congestive heart failure which predisposes to venous thrombosis is present; under this circumstance long-term anticoagulation therapy should be considered. Thrombolytic drugs are still experimental agents undergoing extensive clinical investigation and are not available for general use, but may well be agents of choice in the future.

D. **Surgical embolectomy** is feasible in those rare instances of massive embolism to the main pulmonary artery or its major branches which is proved by pulmonary angiography.

E. **Inferior vena cava plication or ligation** is indicated in those patients who continue to have pulmonary emboli while adequately anticoagulated, those patients who experience septic pulmonary emboli usually from infected pelvic veins, and in those patients in whom anticoagulation is definitely contraindicated.

F. If thrombophlebitis is present, the usual local measures should be carried out.

VII. HEATSTROKE

A. The elevated body temperature should be reduced immediately. Clothing should be removed and the patient sprinkled with cold water or wrapped in a wet sheet; cooling will be promoted if an electric fan is aimed to blow directly on the patient. If temperature elevation is very marked, the patient should be placed in a tub of water to which ice is slowly added. The trunk and extremities should be massaged and the ice bath continued until the rectal temperature (checked every 10 minutes) falls to 102–103°F. The patient should then be removed from the bath because body temperature continues to fall another 3–4 degrees as a rule. If the rectal temperature falls below normal, the patient should be warmed cautiously with blankets. Reduction in temperature also may be promoted by the administration of a phenothiazine—e.g., prochlorperazine (Compazine) 10–15 mg IM—but significant hypotension may occur.

B. If shock occurs, central venous pressure should be measured and fluids should be given intravenously (often there is contraction of the extracellular fluid volume). Care must be taken not to administer fluids at too rapid a rate, in order to avoid precipitating pulmonary edema (which may occur spontaneously as well). Because hypernatremia is common, fluids should be hyponatremic (equal parts 5% D/W and isotonic saline). Vasopressor agents are contraindicated initially because their vasoconstrictor action interferes with heat loss; as temperature is reduced they may be given, if required.

C. Appropriate supportive care should be given. Convulsions may occur; the usual therapeutic measures should be carried out. Acute tubular necrosis may be a complication of heatstroke, and urine output should be measured frequently. Rarely, fibrinolysis, afibrinogenemia, and bleeding may occur. When one of these is suspected, fibrinogen levels should be determined and appropriate therapy given, if necessary.

D. During the period of convalescence, activity should be restricted for 10–14 days and exposure to sunlight avoided.

VIII. POISONING

A. Medicolegal responsibilities Preserve and transfer to proper authorities any objects that may have been found at the scene—e.g., bottles that might have contained poison or medicines, spoons, drinking glasses, etc. Adequate specimens of vomitus, stomach washings, etc., should be saved, if possible, for further analysis. Careful notes of observation and treatment should be made; these may be of value to the toxicologist and to the physician should he be called to testify in court. Do not sign death certificates of patients who have died under suspicious circumstances; if a patient dies from a suspected homicidal or suicidal poisoning, the physician must report the death to the coroner and the police.

B. Removal of poison from the body

1. Gastric intubation and lavage

a) Use the largest tube available; a regular stomach pump is preferred. Take the usual precautions to make sure the tube is not in the trachea; this may be difficult in the comatose patient. If in doubt, place the fill end of the tube in a glass of water; continuous bubbling on expiration implies the tube is in the trachea.

b) Keep the patient on his side and his head hanging over the edge of the bed. Lavage with isotonic saline with an antidote if one is available. Only small amounts of fluid should be used at one time to prevent the passing of poison into the small intestine. Lavage until the returns are clear. Leave 1.0 gm of activated charcoal in the stomach when lavage is completed. Pinch the tube slightly when withdrawing it.

c) The following are contraindications to gastric lavage: ingestion of strong corrosive agents (alkali and acids), ingestion of strychnine, ingestion of petroleum distillates, and coma.

2. Emesis is usually a very effective way of emptying stomach, but fluids (1–2 glasses) should be in the stomach or the stomach will not empty readily. Contraindications to inducing emesis are the same as those indicated above for gastric lavage. The following are effective emetics:

a) **Syrup of ipecac:** 10–15 ml to be repeated in 15–30 minutes if emesis does not occur.

b) **Apomorphine:** 0.03 mg/lb subcutaneously followed by levallorphan (Lorfan), 0.01 mg/lb, to terminate both the emetic and narcotic effects of apomorphine.

C. The usual supportive measures for respiratory depression, shock, etc., have been described in other sections. Excretion of poisons eliminated by the kidney may be speeded by administration of large amounts of fluid. Hemodialysis is of value in certain situations.

D. Special measures and antidotes   The number of potential poisons is so great that no physician or textbook can detail all pertinent current data. Many large cities have poison control centers manned day and night to answer emergency telephone calls from the public and from physicians. They maintain up-to-date information about the composition of most household and industrial substances that are potential poisons and the appropriate therapy to be given. A few comments about certain types of poisoning follow; this section is not meant to be comprehensive.

1. Acute salicylate poisoning   Early symptoms include vomiting, tinnitus, hyperpnea, fever, lethargy, and confusion. In severe poisoning, respiratory failure, convulsions, and coma may occur. The acid-base disturbances that may develop are influenced by salicylate dosage, duration of poisoning, and age of the patient. Hyperpnea, an early manifestation (due to CNS stimulation), causes respiratory alkalosis; later a severe metabolic acidosis (the precise mechanism of which is not known) may occur. As a rule, older children and adults usually have a respiratory alkalosis; infants, young children, and patients with severe salicylate poisoning may have a metabolic acidosis. Marked hypokalemia is often associated with the respiratory alkalosis.

Other complications that may occur include transient hyperglycemia and glycosuria; severe hypoglycemia; bleeding disorders, usually due to hypoprothrombinemia but occasionally caused by thrombocytopenia or other coagulation defects; cerebral or pulmonary edema; and, rarely, renal failure.

a) Treatment in adults is outlined below.

i) Obtain a blood pH to define the acid-base status. Clinical observations are of little value in determining acid-base status because the same signs and symptoms may occur whether the patient is alkalotic or acidotic, and in each instance the CO_2 combining power or CO_2 content will be low. The pH of the urine when less than 7.0 is usually of no value in reflecting the pH of extracellular fluid during the stage of respiratory alkalosis, since an acid pH may occur in respiratory alkalosis associated with marked potassium deficiency.

ii) Determine blood sugar, electrolytes, BUN, prothrombin time, and salicylate concentration.

iii) Perform gastric lavage if the patient is seen within 4 hours of ingestion of aspirin.

iv) Give 50 mg of vitamin K_1 oxide intravenously.

v) Start administration of 5% D/W intravenously.

vi) If the blood pH is high the patient is in the state of respiratory alkalosis, and the therapeutic measures of importance are the administration of adequate amounts of fluid (e.g., 2–3 liters of 5% D/W and 1 liter of isotonic saline during the first 24 hours, depending on the state of hydration) and large amounts of potassium.

Hypokalemia invariably occurs during the stage of respiratory alkalosis (unless renal failure is present) and may play an important role in the genesis of clinical manifestations. Large amounts of potassium are required, often 200–400 mEq during the first 24 hours. Further dosage will depend on clinical response and changes in blood chemistries.

vii) If the blood pH is low, metabolic acidosis has occurred. The therapeutic measures of importance are the administration of adequate amounts of fluid and alkali. The arterial pH, which serves as a guide to therapy, must be determined frequently because dramatic changes may occur rapidly, unaccompanied by any obvious change in physical examination or urinary pH.

Sodium bicarbonate should be given if the arterial pH is less than 7.2; 3–5 mEq/kg body weight may be given during the first four hours of treatment; 7.5% $NaHCO_3$ (45 mEq $HCO_3{-}$/50 ml) may be added to the fluids described in paragraph **vi.** Further amounts (150–250 mEq every 2–4 hours) may be given, depending on the clinical response and changes in arterial pH. Because of the large amounts of sodium and fluid administered, the patient should be watched carefully for signs of circulatory overload.

viii) Those patients not responding satisfactorily to the measures described above or those with limited cardiac reserve unable to tolerate the significant amounts of sodium required for alkalinization should be considered for extracorporeal hemodialysis (salicylates are not recovered efficiently with peritoneal dialysis).

b) Other measures: Sponging is indicated if hyperpyrexia is marked; short-acting barbiturates should be given if convulsions occur; calcium gluconate may be required if tetany occurs (rare, unless alkalinization has been excessive); artificial ventilation may be necessary if depression ensues.

2. **Acids** Lavage the stomach with large volumes of aluminum hydroxide gel, soapsuds, or milk of magnesia (10 ml/250 ml water). Alkalies are contraindicated in cases of oxalic acid (bleaching agent) poisoning; 10 ml of a 10% calcium gluconate solution may be given IV as often as necessary to combat the hypocalcemia associated with oxalic acid poisoning.

3. **Alkalies** Lavage the stomach with vinegar, 5 ml/250 ml water. A tracheostomy set should be readily available in case severe laryngeal edema occurs.

4. **Arsenic**

a) Irrigate the stomach with large volumes of warm water, then lavage with milk and raw egg white. Leave 50 ml 50% magnesium sulfate in the stomach.

b) In severe cases give dimercaprol (BAL) 3 mg/kg body weight IM immediately, and every 4 hours thereafter for 24–36 hours; dosage may be reduced subsequently. (For mild poisoning 50–75% of this amount may be given.) If severe reactions such as chills, fever, and hypotension accompany the administration of the drug, the dosage should be reduced.

5. **Barbiturates**

a) **General** Barbiturate intoxication is the most common cause of drug-induced coma and more than 75% of all suicidal deaths due to drugs result from barbiturates. The CNS depressant effect of the numerous barbiturate compounds is similar and varies from one compound to another in duration and rapidity of onset. The long-acting drugs are metabolized slowly and primarily depend on the kidney for elimination; the short- and intermediate-acting drugs are metabolized primarily by the liver and are much less dependent on the kidney for excretion. The potentially lethal dose for short-acting drugs is 3.0 gm; for long-acting drugs 6–9 gm corresponding to blood levels of 2 and 11–12 mg/100 ml, respectively. Blood levels are useful prognostically and in determining modes of therapy. Remember that psychiatric consultation is warranted in all suicide attempts.

b) **Supportive measures** are the most important. An adequate airway must be maintained (usually with cuffed endotracheal tube—tracheostomy if tube needed more than 48 hours); ventilation should be maintained with a mechanical respirator when necessary; intravenous saline should be given rapidly (monitored by CVP) and vasopressors considered if hypotension occurs.

c) **The stomach should be lavaged** if the patient is seen within 2–3 hours after drug ingestion. If the patient is comatose, a cuffed endotracheal tube should be inserted to minimize pulmonary aspiration. After gastric lavage is completed, the tube should be left in place to prevent gastric dilatation and regurgitation of gastric contents.

d) **Forced diuresis** enhances barbiturate excretion. The nonionized form of barbiturates readily permeates cell membranes, and the amount reabsorbed passively by the renal tubules is determined by the degree of ionic dissociation of the compound in the glomerular filtrate. Barbiturates are dissociated maximally when the pH of the tubular fluid is greater than the pK of the drug in question. The pK of phenobarbital is 7.2, and alkalinization of the urine significantly increases renal excretion by reducing the concentration of undissociated compound available for reabsorption. The pK of short-acting barbiturates is above the range of pH that can be achieved in the renal tubules; therefore, alkalinization is ineffective. With phenobarbital maximal renal clearance is achieved by a combination of forced diuresis and alkalinization; the renal clearance of short-acting barbiturates is roughly proportional to the increase in rate of urine flow.

As long as adequate urine flow is maintained (8–10 ml/min), the method of forced diuresis is relatively unimportant. A satisfactory program is to rotate the following solutions at a rate of 500 ml per hour: 500 ml of 5% D/W with 44 mEq of $NaHCO_3$, 500 ml of 5% D/W with 30 mEq KCl, 500 ml of normal saline. Additional quantities of bicarbonate may have to be given to keep the urine pH above 7.5. Urine flow may be enhanced initially by infusing 500 ml of 10% mannitol. Diuretics also enhance barbiturate excretion, may be used initially, and should be used if fluid retention occurs. Accurate records of fluids infused and urine output must be kept; bladder catheterization with closed urinary drainage is probably justified. Serum electrolytes, especially potassium, should be determined frequently, every 2 hours initially and every 6 hours thereafter. The rate of infusion of intravenous fluids should be monitored by the central venous pressure.

e) **Peritoneal dialysis** is indicated in the presence of severe renal impairment and in those patients whose cardiac status precludes vigorous fluid administration. Peritoneal dialysis is not more effective than forced diuresis in removing barbiturate from the body. Adding albumin to the dialysate will enhance barbiturate elimination, but the cost of albumin is frequently prohibitive.

f) **Hemodialysis** is an effective way of removing barbiturates, especially long-acting drugs, and is indicated in the following situations: shock, progressive clinical deterioration with more conservative therapy, ingestion of a potentially fatal dose, finding of potentially lethal blood levels, and in those patients with significant renal and cardiac disease in whom peritoneal dialysis is ineffective or contraindicated.

g) Other measures Analeptic agents provide little or no benefit worth the potential hazards associated with their use. Prophylactic antibiotics are not indicated; treat infections as they occur.

6. **Glutethimide (Doriden)** intoxication is serious, increasingly common, and is usually fatal when the dose is greater than 10 gm or the blood level greater than 3.0 mg/100 ml. Cyclic changes in central nervous system depression are frequently seen, and sudden apneic episodes with death occur. Supportive measures including gastric lavage, maintenance of a clear airway, rapid intravenous saline monitored by CVP, and vasopressors are most important. Peritoneal dialysis is not effective; hemodialysis is indicated when conservative supportive measures are failing, when potentially fatal doses have been taken, and when cardiac and renal disease preclude large volumes of intravenous saline. Catharsis and duodenal drainage have been advocated to interrupt the enterohepatic circulation, but these procedures have been difficult in comatose patients who frequently have adynamic ileus and who are susceptible to apneic episodes.

7. **Carbon monoxide** Remove the patient from the contaminated atmosphere, give 100% oxygen by face mask, and keep the patient at rest until oxygen-carrying capacity is normal.

8. **Cyanide**

   a) Give amyl nitrite inhalations immediately while preparing the following solutions.

   b) Give IV immediately:

   i) Sodium nitrite 0.3–0.5 gm. Methemoglobin is formed and combines with cyanide to form cyanmethemoglobin, which is nonionized and nontoxic.

   ii) Following the above, give sodium thiosulfate 50 ml of a 50% solution IV slowly (can be sterilized by boiling). This drug converts the cyanide ion, when released from cyanmethemoglobin, to thiocyanate.

   c) Methylene blue, though relatively ineffective, should be given if the above drugs are not available. Give 1 mg/kg body weight IV.

9. **Mercury**

   a) Give dimercaprol (BAL) promptly in a dosage of 5 mg/kg body weight initially, then 3 mg/kg in 3 hours.

   b) Lavage the stomach thoroughly with 5% sodium formaldehyde sulfoxylate solution; leave 250 ml in the stomach. If this solution is not available, lavage with water, and leave milk or raw egg white in the stomach.

   c) Observe carefully for the development of acute tubular necrosis. Stomatitis may be a serious problem; careful mouth care will be necessary.

10. **Methanol** Symptoms are often delayed 10–30 hours and are principally visual disturbances and acidosis. Gastric lavage with 3% solution of $NaHCO_3$ should be carried out immediately. Ethyl alcohol, which inhibits the metabolism of methyl alcohol, should be given in a dose of 60 ml initially followed by 9 ml each hour. The treatment of metabolic acidosis, which occurs characteristically, is described in Chapter 2.

11. **Phenol**

   a) Lavage should be done very cautiously with activated charcoal or milk immediately and then castor oil (which dissolves and retards absorption of phenol); alcohol and mineral oil are probably contraindicated.

   b) Acidosis, frequently profound, should be treated with intravenous $NaHCO_3$.

IX. **MYASTHENIA GRAVIS: MYASTHENIC AND CHOLINERGIC CRISES**

A. **General considerations** Myasthenia gravis is a motor end-plate disease that is manifested by rapid fatigue of voluntary muscles and delayed recovery following exercise. The diagnosis must be considered in patients with weakness and easy fatigue of voluntary muscle but without loss of muscle mass or disturbance of reflexes and sensation. Although initial presentations involving limb muscles are common, the most easily identified syndromes involve extraocular musculature with later involvement of swallowing, speech, and mastication. Among the 25,000 myasthenics in the United States, about 10% will develop ventilatory failure during the course of therapy and will require emergency medical management. These difficulties usually do not occur in a newly diagnosed patient. Therefore, many instances of myasthenic crisis can be distinguished from cholinergic crisis on the basis of accurate data concerning the patient's medication schedule, adherence to the schedule, and the clinical response to medication.

B. **Definitions**

1. **"Crisis"** in myasthenia gravis refers to respiratory failure requiring emergency assistance in maintaining an airway and mechanical respiratory assistance.

2. **Myasthenic crisis** is the failure of musculature resulting from inadequate anticholinesterase medication.

3. **Cholinergic crisis** results from overmedication with anticholinesterase drugs such as neostigmine (Prostigmin), pyridostigmine (Mestinon), and ambenonium (Mytelase). Characteristic symptoms include:

   a) Muscarinic: abdominal cramps, nausea, diarrhea, excessive salivation, anorexia, sweating, lacrimation, blurred vision, meiosis, and excessive bronchial secretion.

   b) Nicotinic: weakness, muscle fasciculations, slurred speech, dysphagia, and muscle cramps.

   Unfortunately, the skeletal muscle weakness of cholinergic crisis may precede the autonomic symptoms listed above.

C. Emergency care. The patient in obvious respiratory failure must have the airway cleared immediately and ventilation provided by a mechanical respirator. An endotracheal tube is used until the decision is made regarding tracheostomy. Care of the patient in these aspects is detailed in the section on Respiratory Failure (page 170). If the oral and tracheal secretions are profuse and watery, atropine sulfate 1.0 mg IV should be injected and repeated as necessary since overdosage with cholinergic·drugs is likely.

It is often wise to withhold all cholinergic drugs for a few days when the patient is on the respirator, even if the crisis is thought to be myasthenic and not cholinergic. By omitting the drugs one avoids cholinergic crisis, the stimulation of excessive tracheal secretions, the need for atropine, and the risk of diarrhea.

D. The Tensilon test is used by some in differentiation of myasthenic crisis from cholinergic crisis. The test is based upon objective muscular changes in response to intravenous administration of edrophonium (Tensilon). The clinical response is observed carefully and timed with serial observations of lid, eye, face, tongue, and extremity strength. The response to Tensilon is most evident 30 seconds to 2 minutes following injection. Tensilon 2 mg (0.2 ml) is given abruptly IV. The patient should be closely observed for evidence of improvement of myasthenic weakness or worsening symptoms of overdosage (cholinergic), indicated by increased weakness, facial or deltoid fasciculation, twitches or spasms of the lids. Tensilon is generally well tolerated except for a rare instance of cardiac arrhythmia. Unfortunately the response to Tensilon is often equivocal or variable from muscle to muscle.

E. Drug therapy. The use of drugs in myasthenic crisis is only of secondary importance and should not concern the attending physician until an adequate airway and adequate pulmonary ventilation have been assured. In a few days the judicious administration of drugs may be gradually instituted.

1. Myasthenic crisis

a) **Neostigmine (Prostigmin)** 1.0 mg IV is given and its effect assessed. Further doses of 1–2 mg IV or IM every 2 to 4 hours can be given. Be alert for overdosage effects.

b) Atropine sulfate 0.4 mg IV or IM will control muscarinic side effects of the neostigmine but should be used sparingly to avoid inspissation of bronchial secretions.

c) Diarrhea can be controlled with diphenoxylate (Lomotil) 2.5–5 mg two to four times daily by nasogastric tube.

d) **Drugs not to be given in myasthenic crisis** include barbiturates, ether, chloroform, and opiates. Quinine, quinidine, procaine amide, curare, muscle relaxants, corticosteroids, and ACTH also increase myasthenia. Although steroids may have a place as a secondary drug in refractory myasthenia, they are contraindicated in crisis. Some antibiotics (neomycin, polymyxin, colistin, kanamycin) should be avoided because of their neuromuscular toxicity. Penicillin, streptomycin, ampicillin, and tetracycline are well tolerated, even though streptomycin has caused neuromuscular block in experimental preparation.

2. Cholinergic crisis

    a) Atropine sulfate 1.0 mg IV should be injected immediately and repeated as necessary to alleviate distress from excessive secretions. Sustained cycloplegia and cutaneous flush should be used as signs of atropine overdosage.

    b) Diarrhea can be controlled as above (see paragraph **1.c.**).

    c) Although the use of pralidoxime (Protopam) has been advocated by some authorities to counteract nicotinic effects of anticholinesterase drugs, we see no need for its use in myasthenic patients.

X. **TETANUS**   In the event of injury that may be complicated by tetanus, immunization should be carried out. Patients who have been immunized in the recent past (as discussed below) may be given a booster dose of tetanus toxoid; those who have not been immunized, have massively contaminated or deep penetrating wounds, or are first seen later than 24 hours after the injury, may require tetanus antitoxin (TAT) in addition. A significant deterrent to use of TAT has been the high incidence of reactions following its administration, but the availability of human tetanus immune globulin makes the decision of whether or not to administer TAT prophylactically less difficult. Although it is expensive, its advantages are several: the likelihood of reactions such as anaphylaxis or serum sickness is remote; fewer units (compared to equine TAT) are given, and simultaneously administered toxoid may establish a higher degree of active immunity; blood antitoxin titers are more persistently and uniformly elevated than are those following administration of equine or bovine TAT (the half-life of human antitoxin is about 4 weeks, whereas that of animal antitoxin is about 10 days).

A. Prophylaxis

    1. Proper care of the wound   Thorough cleansing and debridement, with removal of devitalized tissue, are necessary to minimize conditions favorable to growth of anaerobic organisms.

    2. Penicillin and tetracycline, if started at the time of injury, may be as protective against tetanus as are ordinary doses of TAT, but that is controversial. Although these antibiotics control the growth of *Clostridium tetani*, thus eliminating the source of toxin, they will not offer protection against toxin already produced. They are indicated primarily for those patients who have large or multiple wounds or who have not been immunized .

    3. Immunization

        a) For previously immunized patients who have had full immunization with tetanus toxoid and a booster dose within 5–10 years, 0.5 ml fluid toxoid will be adequate therapy unless the patient is first seen 24–48 hours or longer after injury or the injuries carry a strong chance of resulting in tetanus (e.g., crush injuries, penetrating or puncture wounds, compound fractures, deep burns, and wounds containing devitalized tissue or foreign material). In these situations the patient should be given in addition 250–500 units human tetanus immune globulin or, if that is not available, 3000–5000 units equine TAT.

b) **For unimmunized patients,** active immunization with alum-precipitated toxoid should be started, and TAT administered if the wound is one that may be complicated by tetanus. As previously mentioned, administration of human tetanus immune globulin is preferable; the dose is 250–500 units IM. If equine TAT must be used, hypersensitivity to horse serum must first be excluded. Remind those patients in whom active immunization has been started to return at 4 weeks and at 4 months for the second and third injections of toxoid.

   i) A skin test is performed by injecting 0.1 ml of TAT diluted 1:10 into the forearm. A blood-pressure cuff should be in place on the upper arm, and a syringe of epinephrine (0.5 ml 1:1000 aqueous epinephrine) should be immediately available in case a reaction occurs.

   ii) If no reaction occurs within 15–30 minutes, 3000–5000 units TAT are given IM (but not in the extremity which received the toxoid). If the patient is first seen 24 hours or later after the injury, significantly larger doses (up to 20,000 units) may be given.

   iii) If reaction occurs, bovine TAT or human tetanus immune globulin must be given instead.

B. **Treatment** The mortality rate in tetanus is 30–50%. Prompt diagnosis and treatment are of the utmost importance. Muscle spasm must be prevented (by use of muscle relaxants and/or anesthesia), the source of toxin eliminated (by wound debridement and administration of antibiotics), and the toxin not yet fixed to the central nervous system neutralized (by administration of large doses of TAT). Careful nursing care and prevention of respiratory complications are important measures. An anesthesiologist should follow the patient closely in conjunction with the internist.

1. **Management of convulsions and spasms** Many drugs are available; those muscle relaxants and sedatives which are useful include parenteral methocarbamol (Robaxin), parenterally administered diazepam (Valium) or meprobamate, and barbiturates.

   a) **Meprobamate** abolishes seizures triggered by somatic stimuli (loud noises, lights, etc.) but does not cause central nervous system depression. The dosage is 400 mg IM every 3–4 hours (effects begin in 10–15 minutes and persist 3–4 hours). Seizures precipitated by visceral and proprioceptive stimuli are not well controlled, however, and phenothiazines (e.g., chlorpromazine 25–50 mg or prochlorperazine 5–10 mg IM every 3–4 hours) may be required in addition. If the meprobamate-phenothiazine combination is not effective, barbiturates (e.g., phenobarbital 100–200 mg IM every 3–4 hours) may be given also.

   b) **Methocarbamol** may be injected intravenously at a maximum rate of 3 ml/minute or diluted in 5% D/S and infused as rapidly as is necessary to control spasms. Generally, not more than 20–30 ml/day should be administered. The drug is contraindicated in patients with renal insufficiency.

   c) **Diazepam** 5–10 mg may be given intravenously every 4–6 hours.

d) **Barbiturates,** administered intravenously, may be used in place of, or in addition to, the previously mentioned agents. If used alone, thiopental 0.5–2.5 gm is diluted in 5% D/W to produce a 0.1–0.2% solution and infused over a 24-hour period.

2. Neutralization of toxin

a) Passive immunization should be accomplished by the intramuscular administration of human tetanus antitoxin 3000–6000 units. If equine TAT must be used the dose usually recommended is 100,000 units IV (half may be given IM), although recent studies suggest that a maximal dose of 10,000 units may be optimal.

b) Active immunization with toxoid should be started when feasible; tetanus does not confer immunity.

3. Other measures

a) Antibiotics—penicillin or tetracycline—should be given in large dosage.

b) Contaminated wounds should be debrided early unless the surgical procedures precipitate uncontrollable tetanic spasms. Antitoxin and antibiotics should be given before manipulation of the wound.

c) Tracheostomy should be performed early in all but very mild cases with infrequent seizures and cared for as described in Chapter 8.

d) Nutrition and electrolyte and fluid balance should be maintained with parenteral fluids; a feeding tube should not be inserted because of the danger of aspiration. Oral feedings may be started when all danger of tetanic seizures has passed.

Appendix I

Trade Names and Generic Names of Drugs

Because drugs are listed in the index by generic name, and because certain generic names may be unfamiliar, the following list contains the trade name (**boldface type**) and generic name of most drugs discussed in the Manual. The generic and trade names of *phenothiazines* may be found on page 17; of *digitalis preparations* on page 99; of *thiazides* on page 108; of *semisynthetic penicillins* on page 189; of *antacids* on page 237; and of *corticosteroids* on page 337.

Achromycin tetracycline
Aerosporin polymyxin B
Albamycin novobiocin
Aldactone-A spironolactone
Aldomet methyldopa
Alkeran melphalan
Amytal amobarbital
Ansolysen pentolinium
Anturane sulfinpyrazone
Apresoline hydralazine
AquaMEPHYTON phytonadione
Aralen chloroquine
Aramine metaraminol
Arfonad trimethaphan
Aristocort triamcinolone
Astrafer dextriferron
Atromid-S clofibrate
Aureomycin chlortetracycline
Aventyl nortriptyline
Azulfidine salicylazosulfapyridine

Benadryl diphenhydramine
Benemid probenecid
Butazolidin phenylbutazone

Calciferol vitamin D
Cardilate erithrityl tetranitrate
Cardioquin
  quinidine polygalacturonate
Cathomycin novobiocin

Cedilanid deslanoside
Chloromycetin chloramphenicol
Colace dioctyl sodium sulfosuccinate
Colcemid deacetylmethylcolchicine
Coly-Mycin colistin
Compazine prochlorperazine
Cordran fluranorenolone
Cosmegen dactinomycin
Coumadin warfarin
Cuemid cholestyramine
Cyclamycin triacetyloleandomycin
Cytomel triiodothyronine
  (liothyronine)
Cytoxan cyclophosphamide

Darbid isopropamide
Darvon propoxyphene
DBI phenformin
Decadron dexamethasone
Declomycin demethylchlortetracycline
Delatestryl testosterone enanthate
Deltalin vitamin D
Demecolcin deacetylmethylcolchicine
Demerol meperidine
Depo-Testosterone testosterone
  cypionate
Desferal deferoxamine
Diabinese chlorpropamide
Diamox acetazolamide
Dianabol methandrostenolone

Dibenzyline   phenoxybenzamine
Dicumarol   bishydroxycoumarin
Dilantin   diphenylhydantoin
Dilaudid   dihydromorphinone
Doriden   glutethimide
Dornavac   dornase
Doxinate
   dioctyl sodium sulfosuccinate
Dulcolax   bisacodyl
Durabolin   nandrolone
Dyazide   triamterene-thiazide
   combination
Dymelor   acetohexamide
Dyrenium   triamterene

Edecrin   ethacrynic acid
Elavil   amitriptyline
Elixophyllin   theophylline
Equanil   meprobamate
Erythrocin   erythromycin

Florinef   alpha fluorohydrocortisone
Fulvicin   griseofulvin
Fungizone   amphotericin B
Furacin   nitrofurazone
Furadantin   nitrofurantoin
Furoxone   furazolidone

Gantanol   sulfamethoxazole
Gantrisin   sulfisoxazole
Grifulvin   griseofulvin
Grisactin   griseofulvin

Halothane   fluothane
Harmonyl   deserpidine
Hyperstat   diazoxide
Hypertensin   angiotensin
Hytakerol   (A T 10; assayed as
   dihydrotachysterol)

Ilosone   erythromycin
Ilotycin   erythromycin
Imferon   iron-dextran
Imuran   azathioprine
Inderal   propranolol
Indocin   indomethacin
Inversine   mecamylamine
Ismelin   guanethidine
Isordil   isosorbide dinitrate
Isuprel   isoproterenol

Jectofer   iron-sorbitol-citric acid

Kantrex   kanamycin
Kaon   potassium gluconate
Kaopectate   pectin-kaolin

Kayexalate   polystyrene sodium
   sulfonate
Keflin   cephalothin
Kenalog   triamcinolone
K-Lyte   potassium bicarbonate
Konakion   phytonadione
Kynex   sulfamethoxypyridazine

Lanoxin   digoxin
Lasix   furosemide
Leritine   anileridine
Letter   levothyroxine
Leukeran   chlorambucil
Levophed   norepinephrine
Librium   chlordiazepoxide
Lincocin   lincomycin
Lomotil   diphenoxylate
Loridine   cephaloridine
Luminal   phenobarbital

Madribon   sulfadimethoxine
Mandelamine
   methenamine mandelate
Marplan   isocarboxazid
Mephyton   phytonadione
Mercuhydrin   meralluride
Mestinon   pyridostigmine
Metamucil   psyllium
Metopon   methyldihydromorphinone
Midicel   sulfamethoxypyridazine
Miltown   meprobamate
Moderil   rescinnamine
Modumate   arginine glutamate
Mono-Kay   phytonadione
Mucomyst   acetylcysteine
Mustargen   mechlorethamine
Myambutol   ethambutol
Mycostatin   nystatin
Myleran   busulfan
Myochrisine   gold sodium thiomalate
Mytelase   ambenonium

Nalline   nalorphine
Nardil   phenelzine
NegGram   nalidixic acid
Nembutal   pentobarbital
Neo-Synephrine   phenylephrine
Niamid   nialamide
Nilevar   norethandrolone
Norpramin   desipramine

Oncovin   vincristine
Orinase   tolbutamide

Panmycin   tetracycline
Panwarfin   warfin

Paregoric   camphorated tincture of opium
Parnate   tranylcypromine
Pentothal   thiopental
Peritrate   pentaerythritol tetranitrate
Persantine   dipyridamole
Pertofrane   desipramine
Phenergan   promethazine
Placidyl   ethchlorvynol
Plaquenil   hydroxychloroquine
Premarin   estrogenic substances, conjugated
Pro-Banthīne   propantheline
Pronestyl   procaine amide
Prostaphlin   oxacillin
Prostigmin   neostigmine
Protopam   pralidoxime
Purinethol   6-mercaptopurine
Pyribenzamine   tripelennamine

Quinaglute   quinidine gluconate

Regitine   phentolamine
Robaxin   methocarbamol
Robitussin   glyceryl guaiacolate

Seconal   secobarbital
Senokot   senna extract
Serpasil   reserpine
Singoserp   syrosingopine
Solganal   gold thioglucose
Solu-Cortef   hydrocortisone succinate
Sparine   promazine
Staphcillin   methicillin
Sulfasuxidine   succinylsulfathiazole
Sulfathalidine   phthalylsulfathiazole
Sumycin   tetracycline
Synalar   fluocinolone

Syntetrin   rolitetracycline
Synthroid   levothyroxine

Tacaryl   methdilazine
Talwin   pentazocine
Tandearil   oxyphenbutazone
Tao   triacetyloleandomycin
Tapazole   methimazole
Temaril   trimeprazine
Tempra   acetaminophen
Tensilon   edrophonium
Terramycin   oxytetracycline
Tetracyn   tetracycline
TetraMAX   tetracycline
Tetrex   tetracycline
Thiomerin   mercaptomerin
Thiotepa   triethylene thiophosphoramide
Thorazine   chlorpromazine
Tinactin   tolnaftate
Tofrānil   imipramine
Tolinase   tolazamide
Tylenol   acetaminophen

Urecholine   bethanechol

Valisone   betamethasone 17-valerate
Valium   diazepam
Vancocin   vancomycin
Varidase   streptokinase-streptodornase
Vasoxyl   methoxamine
Velban   vinblastine
Vioform   iodochlorhydroxyquin

Winstrol   stanozolol

Xylocaine   lidocaine

Zyloprim   allopurinol

Nomogram for Calculating the Body Surface Area of Adults*

---

*From Eugene F. DuBois, *Basal Metabolism in Health and Disease*. Philadelphia: Lea & Febiger, 1936. Copyright 1920 by W. M. Boothby and R. B. Sandiford.

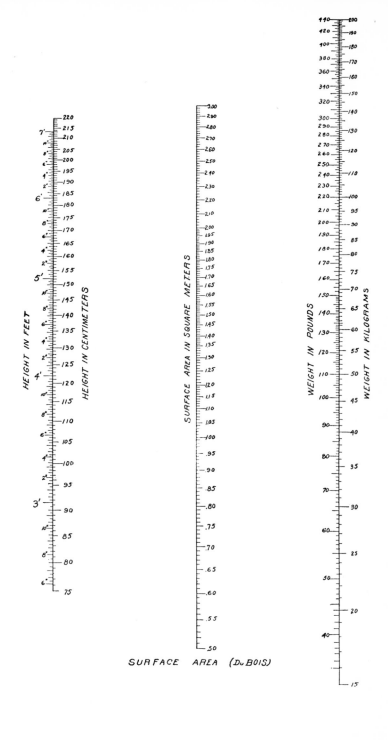

SURFACE   AREA   (DuBOIS)

Index

The index catalogs and cross-references the most important diseases, drugs, and subjects about which information may be sought quickly. All drugs are indexed by generic name; consult Appendix I for trade name–generic name equivalents. The primary reference dealing with preparations, dosage, actions, side effects, etc., of those drugs indexed under a number of headings is listed in **boldface** type.

Lawrence Block published his first novel in 1958 and has been chronicling the adventures of Keller since 1998. He has been designated a Grand Master by the Mystery Writers of America, and has received Lifetime Achievement awards from the Crime Writers' Association (UK), the Private Eye Writers of America, and the Short Mystery Fiction Society. He has won the Nero, Philip Marlowe, Societe 813 and Anthony awards, and is a multiple recipient of the Edgar, the Shamus and the Japanese Maltese Falcon awards. He and his wife, Lynne, are devout New Yorkers and relentless world travellers. To find out more visit his website at www.lawrenceblock.com

HIT ME

LAWRENCE BLOCK

An Orion paperback

First published in Great Britain in 2013
by Orion
This paperback edition published in 2013
by Orion Books,
an imprint of The Orion Publishing Group Ltd,
Orion House, 5 Upper St Martin's Lane,
London WC2H 9EA

An Hachette UK company

1 3 5 7 9 10 8 6 4 2

A CIP catalogue record for this book
is available from the British Library.

ISBN 978-1-4091-3517-3

Printed and bound by CPI Group (UK) Ltd,
Croydon CR0 4YY

The Orion Publishing Group's policy is to use papers
that are natural, renewable and recyclable products and
made from wood grown in sustainable forests. The logging
and manufacturing processes are expected to conform to
the environmental regulations of the country of origin.

www.orionbooks.co.uk

KELLER IN DALLAS

ONE

The young man, who would have looked owlish even without the round eyeglasses, unfolded a piece of paper and laid it on the counter in front of Keller. "The certificate of expertization for Obock J1," he said. "Signed by Bloch and Mueller."

He might have been a Red Sox fan invoking Ted Williams, and Keller could understand why. Herbert Bloch and Edwin Mueller were legendary philatelists, and their assertion that this particular stamp was indeed a genuine example of Obock's first postage due stamp, designated J1 in the Scott catalog, was enough to allay all doubt.

Keller examined the stamp, first with his unaided eye, then through the magnifier he took from his breast pocket. There was a photograph of the stamp on the certificate, and he studied that as well, with and without magnification. Bloch and

3

Mueller had sworn to its legitimacy in 1960, so the certificate was old enough to be collectible in and of itself.

Still, even experts were sometimes careless, and occasionally mistaken. And now and then someone switched in a ringer for an expertized stamp. So Keller reached for another tool, this one in the inside pocket of his jacket. It was a flat metal oblong, designed to enable the user to compute the number of perforations per inch on the top or side of a stamp. Obock J1 was imperforate, which rendered the question moot, but the perforation gauge doubled as a mini ruler, marked out in inches along one edge and millimeters along the other, and Keller used it to check the size of the stamp's overprint.

That overprint, hand stamped on a postage due stamp initially issued for the French Colonies as a whole, had the name of the place—Obock—in black capitals. On the original stamp, the overprint measured 12 1/2 millimeters by 3 3/4 millimeters. On the reprint, a copy of which reposed in Keller's own collection, each dimension of the overprint was half a millimeter smaller.

And so Keller measured the overprint on this stamp, and found himself in agreement with Mr. Bloch and Mr. Mueller. This was the straight goods, the genuine article. All he had to do to go home with it was outbid any other interested collectors. And he could do that, too, and without straining his budget or dipping into his capital.

But first he'd have to kill somebody.

The Dallas-based firm of Whistler & Welles conducted auctions of collectibles throughout the year. At various times they sold coins, books, autographs, and sports memorabilia, but the partners had started out as stamp dealers, and philatelic holdings remained the largest component of their business. Their annual Spring Equinox Sale, held each year in the Hotel Lombardy on the third weekend in March, was one Keller had wanted to attend for years. Something had always prevented him from attending. He'd marked up copies of their catalogs over the years, sent in unsuccessful mail bids on a few occasions, and one year had a hotel room reserved and a flight booked before something or other came up and forced him to cancel.

He'd lived in New York when Whistler & Welles put him on their mailing list. Nowadays he lived in New Orleans, and the name on their mailing list was one he'd borrowed from a local tombstone. He was Nicholas Edwards now, and that was the name on his passport, and on all the cards in his wallet. He lived in a big old house in the Lower Garden District, and he had a wife and a baby daughter, and he was a partner in a construction firm specializing in purchasing and rehabilitating distressed properties.

A year earlier, he'd looked with longing at the Whistler & Welles catalog. Dallas was a lot closer to New Orleans than to New York, but he and Donny Wallings were putting in twelve-hour days and seven-day weeks, just trying to keep up with everything they had going on.

But that was a year ago, before the collapse of the subprime mortgage market and everything that followed on its heels. Credit dried up, houses stopped selling, and they'd gone from more business than they could handle to no business to speak of.

So he could afford the time. A couple of days in Dallas? Sure, why not? He could even take his time and drive to Dallas and back.

And there were plenty of stamps on offer that he'd be eager to add to his collection, with Obock J1 at the very top of his wish list.

Now, though, he couldn't afford it.

* * *

The Lombardy, an independent, locally owned older hotel trying to survive in a world of modern chains, was starting to show its age. The carpet in Keller's room, while not yet threadbare, was due for replacement. A sofa in the lobby was worn on the arms, and the wood paneling in one of the elevators needed touching up. None of this bothered Keller, who found the hotel's faded glory somehow reassuring. What better venue for men of a certain age to compete for little pieces of paper that had done their duty carrying the mail long before any of them were born?

Whistler & Welles had booked a large conference room on the mezzanine for their three-day sale, which would begin promptly at nine Friday morning. New Orleans and Dallas were a little over five hundred miles apart, and Keller drove most of the way Wednesday, stopping for the night at a Red Roof Inn off a handy exit from the interstate. He checked into his room at the Lombardy a little after noon, and by one o'clock he was signing *Nicholas Edwards* on the bidder register and walking over to the long table where they were showing the auction lots.

By two thirty he'd had a look at all the lots that interested him, and had made cryptic notes in his auction catalog. Every sales lot was illustrated with a color photograph, so he didn't absolutely have to see them up close and personal, but sometimes you got something that way that you couldn't get from a photo in a catalog. Some stamps reached out to you while others put you off, and it probably didn't make any real sense, but the whole hobby was wacky enough to begin with. I mean, spending a fortune on little pieces of colored paper? Picking them up with tongs, putting them in plastic mounts, and securing them in albums? Why, for heaven's sake?

Keller had long since come to terms with the essential absurdity of the pastime, and didn't let it bother him. He was a stamp collector, he derived enormous satisfaction from the pursuit, and that was all he needed to know. If you thought about it, just about everything human beings did was pointless and ridiculous. Golf? Skiing? Sex?

Upstairs in his room, Keller reviewed the notes he'd made. There were stamps he'd initially considered and now decided to pass on, others he might buy if the price was right, and a few for which he'd be bidding competitively. And there was Obock J1. It was rare, it didn't come up that often, and this particular specimen was a nice one, with four full margins. Imperforate stamps had to be cut apart, and sometimes a careless clerk snipped off a bit of the stamp in the process. That didn't keep a letter from reaching its designated recipient, but it made the stamp considerably less desirable to a collector.

According to the Scott catalog, Obock J1 was worth $7500. In their catalog, Whistler & Welles had estimated the lot conservatively at $6500. The actual price, Keller knew, would depend on the bidders, those in the room and those participating by mail or phone, or via the Internet, and the hammer price wouldn't tell the whole story; to that you'd have to add a 15 percent bidder's premium and whatever sales tax the state of Texas saw fit to pile on. Keller, who wanted the stamp more than ever now that he'd had a look at it, figured he might have to bid $12,000 to get it, and the check he'd write out would be uncomfortably close to $15,000.

Would he go that high?

Well, that's why they had auctions, and why bidders showed up in person. You sat in your chair, and you'd decided in advance just how high you'd go and when you'd drop out, and then they got to the lot you were waiting for and you discovered how you really felt. Maybe you did exactly what you planned on doing, but maybe not. Maybe you found out your enthusiasm wasn't as great as you'd thought, and wound up dropping out of the bidding early on. Or maybe you found yourself hanging in far beyond your predetermined limit, spending considerably more than your maximum.

No way to guess how it would be this time. It was Thursday, and tomorrow's morning and afternoon sessions would both be devoted to U.S. issues, and thus of no interest to Keller. He wouldn't need to be in the auction room until Saturday morning, and the French Colonial issues, including Obock J1, wouldn't come up until early Saturday afternoon.

He went downstairs, walked outside. It was cool, but not unpleasantly so. Football weather, you'd call it, if the calendar didn't insist that it was March. Cool, crisp—a perfect October day.

He walked a couple of blocks to another hotel, where there was a queue of waiting cabs. He went to the first one in line, settled into the backseat, and told the driver to take him to the airport.

TWO

He'd been working on his stamps when the phone rang. He was alone in the house, Julia had left to pick up Jenny at day care, and he very nearly let the machine answer it because calls were almost invariably for Julia. But there was always a chance it was Donny, so he went and picked it up half a ring ahead of the machine, and it turned out to be Dot.

Not that she bothered to identify herself. Without preamble she said, "Remember that cell phone you had?" And she broke the connection before he could respond.

He remembered the phone, an untraceable prepaid one, and even remembered where he'd left it, in his sock drawer. The battery had long since run down, and while it was charging Julia and Jenny came home, so it was a good half hour before he was back in his den with the phone.

For years he'd lived in New York, a few blocks from the United Nations, and Dot had lived north of the city in White

Plains, in a big old house with a wraparound porch. That house was gone now, burned to the ground, and the same wind that had blown him to New Orleans had picked up Dot and deposited her in Sedona, Arizona. Her name was Wilma Corder now, even as his was Nicholas Edwards, and she had a new life of her own. Back in the day she had arranged the contract killings he had performed, but that was then and this was now.

Even so, he closed the door before he made the call.

"I'll just plunge right in," she said. "I'm back in business."

"And the business is—"

"Holding its own. Not booming, but a long way from flatlining, which seems to be what everybody else's business is doing."

"What I meant—"

"I know what you meant. You want to know what business I'm in, but do you have to ask? Same old."

"Oh."

"You're surprised? You're not the only one. See, there's this thing I joined, Athena International."

"It sounds like an insurance company."

"It does? It's what they call a service club, like Rotary or Kiwanis. Except it's exclusively for women."

"Can't women join Rotary?"

"Of course, because it would be sexist to keep them out. But men can't join Athena."

"That doesn't seem fair."

"Keller, if it bothers you, you can put on a dress and a wig and I'll drag you along to a meeting. If you're still awake at the end of it I'll buy you a pair of high heels."

"But you enjoy it."

"The hell I do. I must have been brain-dead when I joined.

We do things like pick up trash once a month around Bell Rock, and I approve of that, since I've got a view of the damned thing from my bedroom window, and it looks better without the beer bottles and gum wrappers. I'm not crazy about walking around in the hot sun hunting for other people's garbage, but I go once in a while. And we raise money to give some deserving girl a scholarship to college, and if I'm not out there running a table at the bake sale, or God forbid baking something, at least I'll write out a check. But I mostly pass on the monthly meetings. I've never been a meeting person. Endless talking, and then the damn song."

"What song?"

"The Athenian song, and no, I'm not about to sing it for you. But that's how we close the meeting. We all stand in a circle and cross our arms over our chests and clasp hands and sing this Mickey Mouse song."

"Minnie Mouse," he suggested.

"I stand corrected. The thing is, most of the members have careers of one sort or another, and we don't just pick up garbage. We network, which means we take in each other's laundry."

"Huh?"

"Beth's a travel agent, Alison's a real-estate agent, Lindsay does Tupperware parties."

"So you've been buying Tupperware," he suggested. "And houses."

"No houses. But when I went to Hawaii for a week I let Beth make the booking," she said, "and one of our members is a lawyer, and when I need a lawyer she's the one I go to. And of course I bought the Tupperware. You go to the party, you buy the Tupperware."

"And drink the Kool-Aid. I'm sorry, go on."

"Anyway," she said, "there they all were with their careers, and there I was, with all the money I needed, and it couldn't keep me from feeling time was passing me by."

"That's what time does."

"I know. But I couldn't shake the feeling that I ought to be doing something. But what? Volunteer at a hospital? Help out at a soup kitchen?"

"Doesn't sound like you."

"So I picked up the phone," she said, "and made a few calls."

"How'd that go? I mean, officially, aren't you dead?"

"As a doornail," she agreed. "Shot in the head and burned up in a fire. You Google Dorothea Harbison and that's what you'll find out. But the people who would call me to arrange a booking, they never heard of Dorothea Harbison. A few of them knew me as Dot, but most of them didn't even have that much. I was a phone number, and a voice on the phone, and a mail drop where they sent payments. And that was as much as anybody needed to know."

"And how much did you know about them?"

"My customers? Next to nothing. But I did have a couple of phone numbers."

And one day she drove to Flagstaff and rented a private mailbox at a franchise operation on South Milton Road, a block from the Embassy Suites hotel. On her way home she picked up a prepaid and presumably untraceable phone, and over the next few days she made a couple of calls. "I wondered what happened to you," the first man said. "I tried your number, but it was disconnected."

"I got married," she told him, "and don't bother congratulating me, because it didn't work out."

"That was quick."

"For you, maybe. You weren't there. Long and short, I'm here for you when you need me. Let me give you the number."

She had other numbers, too, of men who'd done what Keller used to do. Not all of those numbers worked anymore, but she was able to reestablish a contact or two, and one fellow said he could really use the work. Then she sat back and waited for something to happen, not entirely sure she wanted her new phone to ring, but it did, and within the week.

"And here's something interesting, Keller. The call was from someone I hadn't called myself, someone I hadn't even worked with before. One of my old clients passed the word, and here was this guy calling me out of the blue, with a piece of work to be done in the great state of Georgia. So I called the guy who'd told me how he needed work, and he couldn't believe I was getting back to him so quick. And I sat back and got paid."

Like old times, Keller suggested, and she agreed. "I'm still me," she said. "I'm a rich lady, and I look better than I used to. I moved to Sedona and the pounds started to drop off right away. The place is crawling with energy vortexes, except I think the plural is vortices."

"What are they?"

"Beats me, Keller. I think it's something like an intersection, except the streets are imaginary. Anyway, some of the women I know are fat as pigs, and they've got the same vortices I do. I belong to a gym, can you believe it?"

"You told me."

"And I've got a personal trainer. Did I tell you that, too? His name is Scott, and I sometimes get the feeling he'd like to get a little more personal, but I'm probably wrong about that. It's not as though I turned into whistle bait, and what would he want with a woman old enough to use a term like that? Whistle bait, for God's sake."

"I guess people don't say that anymore."

"They don't whistle much, either. Look, this is a mistake, isn't it? I shouldn't have called."

"Well."

"For God's sake, you've got your life to live. You've got a beautiful wife and an amazing daughter and you're the rehab king of New Orleans real estate. So why don't you just wish me luck in my new venture and hang up, and I'll leave you alone."

THREE

Keller limited himself to monosyllables en route to the airport, and gave the driver a tip neither large nor small enough to be memorable. He walked through the door for departing flights, took an escalator one flight down, and a bubbly girl at the Hertz counter found his reservation right away. He showed her a driver's license and a credit card, both in the same name—one that was neither J. P. Keller nor Nicholas Edwards. They were good enough to get him the keys to a green Subaru hatchback, and in due course he was behind the wheel and on his way.

The house he was looking for was on Caruth Boulevard, in the University Park section. He'd located it online and printed out a map, and he found it now with no trouble, one of a whole block of upscale Spanish-style homes on substantial landscaped lots not far from the Southern Methodist campus. Sculpted stucco walls, a red tile roof, an attached three-car garage. You'd think a family could be very happy in a house like that, Keller thought, but in the present instance you'd be wrong, because the place was home to Charles and Portia Walmsley, and neither of them could be happy until the other was dead.

Keller slowed down as he passed the house, then circled the block for another look at it. Was anyone at home? As far as he could see, there was no way to tell. Charles Walmsley had moved out a few weeks earlier, and Portia shared the house with the Salvadoran housekeeper. Keller hadn't learned the housekeeper's name, or that of the man who was a frequent overnight guest of Mrs. Walmsley, but he'd been told that the man drove a Lexus SUV. Keller didn't see it in the driveway, but he couldn't be sure it wasn't in the garage.

"The man drives an SUV," Dot had said, "and he once played football for TCU. I know what an SUV is, but—"

"Texas Christian University," Keller supplied. "In Fort Worth."

"I thought that might be it. Do they have something to do with horny frogs?"

"Horned Frogs. That's their football team, the Horned Frogs. They're archrivals of SMU."

"That would be Southern Methodist."

"Right. They're the Mustangs."

"Frogs and Mustangs. How do you know all this crap, Keller? Don't tell me it's on a stamp. Never mind, it's not important. What's important is that something permanent happens to Mrs. Walmsley. And it would be good if something happened to the boyfriend, too."

"It would?"

"He'll pay a bonus."

"A bonus? What kind of a bonus?"

"Unspecified, which makes it tricky to know what to expect, let alone collect it. And he'll double the bonus if they nail the boyfriend for the wife's murder, but when you double an unspecified number, what have you got? Two times what?"

Keller drove past the Walmsley house a second time, and didn't learn anything new in the process. He consulted his map, figured out his route, and left the Subaru in a parking garage three blocks from the Lombardy.

In his room, he picked up the phone to call Julia, then remembered what hotels charge you for phone calls. Charles Walmsley was paying top dollar, bonus or no, but making a call from a hotel room was like burning the money in the street. He used his cell phone instead, first making sure that it was the iPhone Julia had given him for his birthday and not the prepaid one he used only for calls to Dot.

The hotel room was okay, he told her. And he'd had a good look at the stamps he was interested in, and that was always helpful. And she put Jenny on, and he cooed to his daughter and she babbled at him. He told her he loved her, and when Julia came back on the phone he told her the same.

Portia Walmsley didn't have any children. Her husband did, from a previous marriage, but they lived with their mother across the Red River in Oklahoma. So there wouldn't be any kids to worry about in the house on Caruth Boulevard.

As far as the Salvadoran maid was concerned, Dot had told him the client didn't care one way or the other. He wasn't paying a bonus for her, that was for sure. He'd pointed out that she was an illegal immigrant, and Keller wondered what that had to do with anything.

* * *

That first night, he hadn't called Dot back right away. First he and Julia had tucked Jenny in for the night—or for as much of it as the child would sleep through. Then the two of them sat over coffee in the kitchen, and he mentioned that Donny had called earlier, not because some work had come in but on the chance that he might want to go fishing.

"But you didn't want to go?"

He shook his head. "Neither did Donny, not really. He just wanted to pick up the phone."

"It's hard for him, isn't it?"

"He's not used to sitting around."

"Neither are you, these days. But I guess it must be like old times for you. You know, with lots of time off between jobs."

"Stamp collecting helped take up the slack."

"And I guess it still does," she said. "And that way there's no fish to clean."

He went upstairs and sat down with his stamps for a few minutes, then made the call. "So you're back in business," he said. "And you didn't call me, and then you did."

"And I guess it was a mistake," she said, "and I apologize. But how could I be in the business and not let you know about it? That didn't seem right."

"No."

"And it's not like you're a recovering alcoholic and I'm opening wine bottles in front of you. You're a grown-up. If you're not interested you'll tell me so and that's the end of it. Keller? You still there?"

"I'm here."

"So you are," she said. "And yet you haven't told me you're not interested."

One of his stamp albums was open on the table in front of him, and he looked at a page of Italian stamps overprinted for use in the Aegean Islands. There were a few stamps missing, and while they weren't at all expensive they'd proved difficult to find.

"Keller?"

"Business dried up," he said. "There's no financing. We can't buy houses and we can't sell them, and nobody's hiring us to repair them, either, because there's no money around."

"Well, I'm not surprised. It's the same everywhere. Still, you've got enough money to see you through, haven't you?"

"We're all right," he said. "But I've gotten used to living on what I earn, and now I'm dipping into capital. I'm not about to run through it, there's no danger of that, but still…"

"I know what you mean. Keller, I've got something if you want it. I had a guy lined up for it and I just learned he's in the hospital, he flipped his car and they had to yank him out of there with the Jaws of Death."

"Isn't it the Jaws of Life?"

"Whatever. His own jaw is about the only part of him that didn't get broken. I guess he'll live, and he may even walk again, but there's no way he can get it all together by the end of the month and spare my client the agony of divorce."

"And the heartbreak of community property."

"Something like that. It has to happen before the first of April, and either I find somebody who can take care of it or I have to send back the money. You probably remember how much I like doing that."

"Vividly."

"Once I have it in hand," she said, "I think of it as my money, and I hate like the devil to part with it. So what do you think? Can you get away for a few days in the next couple of weeks?"

"My calendar's wide open," he said. "All I've got is a stamp auction I was thinking about going to. That's the weekend after next, if I go at all."

"Where is it?"

"Dallas."

There was a thoughtful silence. "Keller," she said at length, "call me crazy, but I see the hand of Providence at work here."

FOUR

The Lombardy had a buffet breakfast they were proud of, and in the morning Keller went down to give it a try. The problem with buffets, he'd found, was that you wanted to get your money's worth and wound up eating too much. He resolved not to do that, and helped himself to a moderate amount of bacon and eggs and a toasted bran muffin. When he was through he sipped his coffee and thought about the other items he'd noticed, and how good they'd looked. He sighed and went back for more.

And took another plate, as the sign advised him to. "I don't get it," he said to a fellow diner, a heavyset man with an over-size mustache. "Why does the state of Texas forbid me to pile new food onto an old plate?"

"Health regulation, isn't it?"

"I guess, but why? I mean, what am I going to do, pass germs to myself?"

"Good point."

"And this way they've got an extra plate to wash."

"Even more," the man said, "if you make enough return trips, and that smoked salmon is worth a try, believe me. They feed you a hell of a breakfast here at the Venetia. But maybe there's another reason for fresh plates. Maybe it's like putting new wine in old bottles."

"Well, that's something else I've wondered about," Keller said. "I know it's a metaphor, but what are you supposed to do with old bottles? Just throw them in a landfill?"

He went back to his table and ate everything on his plate, but didn't even consider going back for thirds. Instead he let the waitress pour him more coffee, signed his check, and carried the coffee over to the table where the mustachioed gentleman was working on his smoked salmon.

Keller put a hand on an unoccupied chair, and the man nodded, and Keller sat down. "You're here for the auction," he said.

"I have that look, do I?"

He shook his head. "The hotel," he said. "You called it the Venetia."

"I did? Well, that's a giveaway, isn't it? A very philatelic slip of the tongue. Or should that be slip of the tongs?"

Because he collected stamps, Keller knew that in the mid-nineteenth century Lombardy-Venetia had been a kingdom in the north of Italy forming part of the Austrian Empire. Starting in 1850, Austria produced stamps for Lombardy-Venetia, essentially identical to regular Austrian issues but denominated in centesimi and lire and, after 1858, in soldi and florins. Then in 1859 Lombardy was annexed to Sardinia, and seven years later Venetia became a part of the kingdom of Italy.

"But for philately," the fellow said, "I might never have heard of Lombardy or Venetia, let alone know to link the two of them with a hyphen."

"I haven't done much with Lombardy-Venetia," Keller admitted. "All those reprints, and so much counterfeiting. It's confusing, so I always find it easier to buy something else."

"Your Lombardy-Venetia's probably well ahead of mine, considering that I don't own a single stamp from the benighted place. Nothing but U.S. for me, I'm afraid."

"And that's the one thing I don't collect," Keller said. "I'm worldwide, to 1940."

"That way there's always something for you to buy. Which is a blessing or a curse, depending how you look at it. I don't even collect all of my own country. I did, but then I sold everything after 1900, and then I narrowed that down to the 1869 issue. I don't know if you know the stamps..."

Keller knew them well enough to hold up his end of the conversation. By the time they left the table they were Nicholas and Michael, sharing the comfortable camaraderie of fellow hobbyists who wouldn't be competing with one another in the auction room. In fact they wouldn't even be occupying the room at the same time, with U.S. on the block today and the rest of the world waiting its turn.

"Stamps in the morning, covers in the afternoon," Michael said. "There's a block of Scott 119, the fifteen-cent type two, that I wouldn't mind having. And this afternoon, well, this wouldn't mean much to a nonspecialist, but..."

Keller heard him out, wished him luck.

"Ah, but what's luck, Nick? I'm too old to chase 'em nowadays, but when I used to go out looking to pick up a woman, I'd tell myself maybe I'd get lucky. But you reach a point where getting lucky means going home alone. You know, you ought to drop by when the 1869 lots come up. Share in the drama without having a stake in the outcome. All the excitement and none of the risk — like watching a murder mystery on television."

Keller slipped into the auction room a half hour after the start of the morning session. The first several dozen lots were nothing too exciting, job lots and accumulations, and then the first of the Postmasters' Provisionals came up and the proceedings got more interesting. Sort of like watching a mystery on television, come to think of it.

He stayed longer than he'd planned, waiting for the large block of number 119 to be offered, and watched as his new friend hung in gamely while bidding climbed to four times the estimated value. Then Keller's friend dropped out, and the block was knocked down to a telephone bidder.

Not quite like a murder mystery on television, because it didn't end the way you wanted it to.

Keller slipped out of the auction room, left the hotel, and picked up his rental car. He'd brought his map along, but never took it out of his breast pocket. He had no trouble remembering the route to the house on Caruth Boulevard.

He drove past the house, taking a quick look at it, and all he really managed to establish was that it was still there. He couldn't stake the place out and watch the comings and goings, not in this neighborhood, where a man lurking in a parked car would be reported to the police in no time at all. Nor could he park a few blocks away and approach on foot, because if there was a single pedestrian over the age of six anywhere in the area, he'd managed to keep out of Keller's field of vision.

The right way, he thought, was to take a week or two, but the hell with that. This wasn't some well-guarded mafioso in a walled castle, with a moat full of bent-nosed alligators. This was a woman who had no idea just how much her husband wanted to be rid of her, and no reason to fear a stranger at her door.

Keller went back to a strip mall he'd passed earlier, with a Walgreens at one end and an Office Depot at the other. Park near one and walk to the other? No, he told himself. Why bother? Nobody was going to look at his license plate, and what difference did it make if they did?

He parked in front of the Office Depot and was in and out of it in ten minutes, paying cash for the clipboard and the pad of yellow paper. Duct tape? No, not necessary. He was going to buy a pen, then remembered that he already had one of his own.

What else? A box cutter, a letter opener, something sharp and pointed? No. He had his hands, and there would be knives in the kitchen if he felt the need.

He drove back to the Walmsley house and parked in the driveway, where anyone walking by could see his car and take note of the license plate. Fat chance, he thought, and walked up to the door and rang the bell.

Nothing.

Maid's day off, he thought. Getting lucky, he told himself, was when you rang a doorbell and nobody answered. That was even better than going home alone, and—

Footsteps, approaching the door. He waited for it to open, and when it didn't he poked the bell again, and this time the door opened immediately, and he found himself looking at his own reflection in the mirror that faced the door. Just for an instant, albeit a disconcerting one; then he lowered his eyes and looked down at the Salvadoran maid.

"Ah, good morning," he said. "Mrs. Walmsley?"

"No," the maid said, in Spanish or English, it was impossible to tell. "Her no *aquí*," she said, in a combination of the two.

"And Mr. Walmsley?"

"Him not *vive aquí*."

A shake of the head, good enough in either language.

"Is anyone else at home?"

Another head shake. The simple thing to do, Keller realized, was kill the woman, stuff her in a closet—or a laundry hamper, or a big hatbox. She was innocent, but then so was Portia Walmsley, for all he knew.

But Jesus, she was so tiny.

The client, he recalled, didn't care one way or the other about the woman. He wasn't paying a bonus for some illegal immigrant, and—

Bingo.

He brandished the clipboard, gave her a look at it. He hadn't thought to write anything on the top sheet of paper, but it didn't matter.

"INS," he said.

Her face remained expressionless, but eloquently so.

"Green card," he said.

"*No hablo inglés.*"

"*Carta verde,*" Keller said, straining his command of the language to the limit. "*¿Tienes un carta verde?*"

Una, he thought. Not *un,* for God's sake. *Una.* An INS man would know that, right? Jesus, you couldn't live in New York without knowing that much, let alone Texas, and—

Un, una, what difference could it possibly make? Her shoulders slumped, and she managed somehow to become even smaller. Keller felt horrible.

"I will be back," he said. "I'll go away now to have my lunch, and when I come back you can show me your green card. Your *carta verde, comprenez-vous?*"

Comprenez-vous? That was French, for God's sake, yet another language he was unable to speak. But it was clear that she *comprenezed* just fine.

"You come back?"

"In an hour," he said, and turned away, unable to bear the sight of her expressionless face.

He drove to the strip mall, parking this time near the Walgreens, and tossed the clipboard into a trash bin alongside the entrance. He wasn't hungry and he couldn't think of anything to buy, so he returned to his car and sat behind the wheel. Nothing to read, nothing to do, really, but let time pass. He fiddled with the radio, but couldn't figure out how to get it to play without running the engine. There'd be a way to do it, there always was, but every car maker felt compelled to work out its own way of doing things, and when you rented cars you could never figure out how to adjust the seats or play the radio or work the air-conditioning or dim the lights, and when you went to signal a left turn you generally wound up switching on the windshield wipers. The steering was always more or less the same, and so were the brakes, and it was a good thing or everybody would crash into everybody else.

They'd have newspapers in the drugstore. Magazines, maybe even paperback books.

No, the hell with it.

He gave her an hour and a half, then returned to the Walmsley house and parked once again in the driveway. He walked up to the door and rang the bell, and wondered if he might have been a shade precipitous in ditching the clipboard, because what if she opened the door with Portia Walmsley on her left and some slick immigration lawyer on her right? *Hang on,* he'd say. *Be right back, soon as I get my clipboard—*

No one came to the door. He rang the bell again, and listened carefully, and heard no footsteps. The car, the rented Subaru, had now become a problem, and he wished he'd left it at the strip mall and approached on foot. But that was a long way to walk in a neighborhood where everybody drove.

He couldn't leave the thing in the driveway. There was probably room for it in the three-car garage, since the estranged husband wouldn't have left on foot, but Portia Walmsley would almost certainly notice his car when she parked her own beside it, and—

He backed out of the driveway, drove fifty yards down the street, parked, and walked back. Rang the bell, listened for footsteps, knocked, listened again. He tried the doorknob, because you never know, but it was locked.

No problem.

FIVE

Keller had never been a thief, let alone a burglar. In his youth he'd been one of several young men who'd hung around the Old Man's place in Yonkers. The Old Man was Giuseppe Ragone, dear to the hearts of tabloid journalists, who wrote about him as Joey Rags. Keller had never called him that, or anything like it. In direct conversation, if he called the man anything it was Sir. To others, he'd refer to him as Mr. R. In his own mind, though, his boss was the Old Man.

And Keller liked hanging around. The Old Man would give him errands to run, packages to pick up and deliver, messages to pass along. Eventually he sent Keller along when disciplinary actions were called for, and something he saw led him to devise assignments that, in retrospect, Keller was able to recognize as little tests. Keller, unaware he was being tested, passed with flying colors. What the Old Man managed to establish was that Keller didn't flinch when called upon to pull the trigger. The Old Man had suspected as much, that was why he'd devised the tests, but it was all news to Keller.

So Keller went from being an errand boy to taking people out, and at first the people he took out were men who had somehow managed to get on the Old Man's hit list, and then the Old Man realized what a fine, dependable asset he had, and began renting Keller out to interested parties. Not many people knew Keller's name, the Old Man saw to that, but an increasing number of people knew he was out there somewhere, at the beck and call of Joey Rags, and that he did good work. So from that point on that was the only kind of work he was called upon to perform. There were no more packages or messages to deliver, no more errands to run.

A more conventional apprenticeship would have seen Keller grow into a jack-of-all-criminal-trades, with a working knowledge of various felonious enterprises. But Keller, forced to improvise, had picked up what he needed to know. Without ever becoming a disciplined student of the martial arts, he'd read books and rented videos, taken the odd class here and there, and was as proficient as he had to be with the usual run of weapons, and with his bare hands. Similarly, he'd become reasonably good at breaking and entering, and it didn't take him long to get into the Walmsley house.

It was the sort of house that would have a burglar alarm installed, and there was a decal to that effect, along with metallic tape on the ground-floor windows. But the alarm had not been engaged when the maid opened the door to him, and he didn't believe for a moment she'd have taken the time to set it before fleeing a house she'd never be likely to see again. If the Walmsleys had ever taken the trouble to teach her how to set it in the first place.

No alarm, then. The front door was locked, probably because it locked of its own accord when you pulled it shut. Keller could have forced it but didn't, nor did he force the door leading to the garage. He went around to the rear of the house, took one of the windows off its track, and let himself in.

The maid wouldn't be coming back. The house was a large one, and Keller went through it room by room, and it was easy to tell the maid's room, because it was the smallest room in the house, tucked in under the back stairs and alongside the kitchen. There was a wooden crucifix hanging from a nail on one wall, and there was a week-old copy of *El Diario,* and that was pretty much all there was aside from the bed and dresser. She'd thrown everything else in a suitcase and now she was gone, and she wouldn't be coming back.

The crucifix, he decided, had been a parting gift from her mother in El Salvador. That was the name of the country, while the capital city was San Salvador, but she probably came from somewhere else. Cutuco, he decided. Puerto Cutuco was the only other city he knew in El Salvador, and he knew it because one of the stamps of the 1935 series pictured the wharf at Cutuco. Another stamp in the same series showed a volcano, and he knew its name, but couldn't remember it.

As if it mattered. Her mother in Cutuco had given her the crucifix, he continued thinking, telling her to keep it with her forever and it would always protect her, and she'd dutifully mounted it on the wall, and in her haste she'd forgotten it. Terrified of the faceless Immigration and Naturalization Service (except it wasn't so faceless now, it had Keller's face on it), she'd abandoned the one thing she owned that tied her to her home and family. She wouldn't come back for it, she didn't dare, but its loss would always bother her, and—

Jesus, get over it, he told himself. She could let go of the crucifix a lot easier than he could relinquish the fantasy he was spinning, complete with a hometown from a stamp in his collection.

It bothered him, though. That he'd scared her the way he did. Still, what else was he supposed to do? He couldn't snap her neck just because she was in the way. She was tiny, she'd have to stand on a box to be five feet tall. It would be like killing a little kid, and that was something Keller had never done. Once or twice someone had offered a contract on a child, and he and Dot had been entirely in accord on the subject. You had to draw a line, and that was where you had to draw it.

But that was a matter of age, not size. The woman—and he found himself wishing he knew her name, now that he'd played such a role in her life—was certainly over twenty-one. Old enough to vote, old enough to drink…and old enough to be killed? Was he being politically incorrect by giving her a pass on the basis of her height? Was he being…well, he wasn't sure the word existed, but was he being a sizeist? A heightist? Was he altitudinally prejudiced?

What he was being, he told himself, was severely neurotic, and that was the occasional consequence of breaking into an empty house with nothing to do but wait for someone to appear. He'd done this sort of thing before, but that was in an earlier life. Now he had a wife and a daughter, now he lived in a big old house in New Orleans and had a business repairing and renovating other people's houses, and the new life suited him, and what was he doing here, anyway?

He looked at his watch, and every ten minutes or so he looked at it again.

Keller had read somewhere that all of man's difficulties stemmed from his inability to sit alone in a room. The line stayed with him, and a while ago he'd Googled his way to its source. Someone named Pascal had made the observation, Blaise Pascal, and it turned out he'd said a lot of other interesting things as well, but all but the first one had slipped Keller's mind. He thought of it now as he forced himself to sit alone in the maid's room, waiting for Portia Walmsley to come home.

And pictured the woman. When he was living in New York, he'd have taken the train to White Plains, where Dot would have given him the woman's photograph, which someone would have sent to her by FedEx, in the same package with the first installment of his fee. Instead, he'd booted up his computer, clicked on Google Images, typed in "Portia Walmsley," and clicked again, whereupon Google served up a banquet of pictures of the oh-so-social Mrs. Walmsley, sometimes alone, sometimes with others, but all of them showing a big-haired full-figured blonde with what Keller had once heard called a Pepsodent smile. Or was it an Ipana smile? Keller couldn't remember, and decided he didn't care.

Sitting alone in a room, with only one's own mind and an abandoned crucifix for company, wasn't the most fun Keller had ever had in his life. There was nothing in the room he could read, and nothing to look at but suffering Jesus, and that was the last place Keller wanted to aim his eyes.

Which, no matter where he pointed them, he was finding it increasingly difficult to keep open. They kept closing of their own accord. He kicked off his shoes and stretched out on the bed, just for comfort, not because he intended to sleep, and—

And the next thing he knew he was in an auction room, with one lot after another hammered down before he could get his hand in the air to bid. And a man and a woman were sitting on either side of him, talking furiously in a language he couldn't understand, and making it impossible for him to focus on the auction. And—

"Where is that damn girl? For what I pay her you'd think she could do what she's supposed to. *Margarita!*"

"Maybe she's in her room."

"At this hour?"

His eyes snapped open. A man and a woman, but now they were speaking English, and he could hear them on the stairs. He sprang from the bed, crossed to the door, worked the bolt. No sooner had it slid home than they had reached the door, and the woman was calling the maid's name—Margarita, evidently—at the top of her brassy voice.

"Give it up," the man said. "Ain't nobody home."

A hand took hold of the doorknob, turned, pushed. The bolt held.

"She's in there. The lazy bitch is sleeping."

"Oh, come on, Portsie." Portsie? "Couldn't nobody sleep through the racket you're making."

"Then why's the door locked?"

"Maybe she don't want you rummaging through her underwear."

"As if," Portia said, and rattled the doorknob. "This is something new, locking the door. I don't think you *can* lock it, except from inside. You slide a bolt and it goes through a little loop, but how can you do that from outside?"

"Maybe she's in there with a boyfriend."

"My God, maybe she is. Margarita! God damn you, open the fucking door or I'll call the fucking INS on you." There was a pause, and then Keller heard them moving around, and some heavy breathing.

"Hey," the woman said. "And what do you think you're doing, sport?"

"Rummaging through your underwear, Portsie."

"It's distracting me."

"That's the general idea."

"If she's in there fucking some pint-sized *cholo*—"

"She's not. She was in there, all by herself, and she locked the door."

"So where is she now?"

"Out."

"Out? How'd she get out?"

"Through the keyhole."

"You're terrible, baby."

"C'mon," he said. "I need a drink, and so do you. And that's not all we need."

And Keller stood there while their footsteps receded.

Once he'd had time to think about it, Keller realized he'd missed an opportunity. There they were, the target and the bonus, all ready to walk right into the room where he was waiting for them. And what had he done? He'd locked the door, as if he were not a hired assassin but the timid little chambermaid who'd been the room's rightful if unlawful occupant.

He was half asleep, and unprepared, and that's why he'd been so quick to lock the door. Alert and prepared, he'd have flung it open and yanked them inside, and in no time at all he'd have been around the block and out of the neighborhood, and they'd be working their way toward room temperature.

Now, because he hadn't been clever enough to let them burst in on him, he'd have to do the bursting.

SIX

It wasn't hard to find them. From the hallway outside Margarita's room, he could hear them — laughing, grunting, sounding for all the world like a pair of drunken lovers. He made his way to the door of the master bedroom, which they had not troubled to close, and there they were, doing the dirty deed. One glance established as much for Keller, and he quickly averted his eyes.

The woman was Portia Walmsley; Keller had glimpsed more than enough of her to match her with her pictures. Not that he'd been in much doubt, with her companion calling her Portsie. And the man looked vaguely familiar as well, though Keller couldn't think why. Had he seen him in the auction room? Jesus, was the sonofabitch a stamp collector?

He could take another look, but he didn't really want to. Keller had never regarded lovemaking as a spectator sport. When he was in high school a classmate had brought some dirty pictures to class, and Keller had looked at them, and found them erotic enough. But he wasn't in high school anymore.

Even without watching them he could tell they were pretty well wrapped up in each other, and unlikely to offer much resistance if he went in there and did what he was supposed to do. He rehearsed it in his mind, visualized himself moving purposefully into the room, taking the lover out of the play with a judo chop to the side of the neck, grabbing the woman and breaking her neck, then doing the same for the immobilized man. It would all be over before they knew it, almost before *he* knew it.

Go on, he thought. *Don't just stand there. You know what you're supposed to do. So why aren't you doing it?*

Maybe there was a better way.

If he just went in there and got the job done, he'd have earned his fee—plus a bonus for the boyfriend. But he'd also be leaving the kind of mess that would make headlines, and the cops would be all over their client. It was Walmsley's responsibility to provide himself with an alibi, and he'd probably come up with a good one, but would he have the sense to lawyer up right away and keep his mouth shut? Or would he fall apart when it became clear that he was the sole suspect?

Not Keller's worry. Walmsley could hang himself by talking, but he didn't know enough to hang anybody else.

Still, what if Keller left the Dallas cops a case they could close as soon as they opened it? He could see a way to do it, and earn a double bonus in the process.

It would take time, though. So he went back to Margarita's room to wait.

Was it the same crucifix? He could swear it was larger than he remembered.

He left the door open. He didn't really want to hear the two of them—though that wasn't nearly as bad as seeing them. But he wanted to know when they fell silent.

And, while he waited, he ran an amended scenario through his mind. He liked it, he thought it would work, but there was still one question he couldn't answer.

Could he do it?

For a couple of years now he'd been leading a very different life, and it struck him as possible that he'd become a different person in the process. He had a wife, he had a daughter, he had a house, he had a business. He might cross the street against the light, and he and Donny managed to keep their cash receipts a secret from the tax man, but all in all he was a law-abiding individual, a reasonably solid citizen. He'd always had a penchant for civic responsibility; he'd served on a jury when called, and volunteered at Ground Zero in the aftermath of 9/11. But all along he'd had this dark side, this other life, and he'd left that part of himself behind when he settled in New Orleans.

So maybe that was what had led him to throw the bolt and lock himself in the maid's room. And maybe he wasn't waiting now for a better opportunity. Maybe he was stalling, and waiting for a chance to pull the plug on the whole operation.

He mulled it over, running various possibilities through his mind. And then it struck him that he couldn't hear them anymore, and in fact hadn't heard them for a while now.

How long? Could they have put their clothes on and gone out? If so, he decided, then he was going to say the hell with it. He'd climb out the window and drive away, and leave Portia Walmsley to work out for herself what had happened to her maid and her window, one having jumped the track and the other having disappeared altogether. But she'd get to stay alive, at least until her husband hired somebody else, and she'd never know what a close call she'd had.

Scratch that, he told himself. Because there she was in the bedroom, lying on her back with her mouth open, snoring away in a very unappealing fashion. And, lying beside her and snoring twice as loud, was the oaf she'd picked to be her boyfriend. He still looked familiar, and Keller figured out why. It was the mustache, identical in shape to that of Michael, his companion at breakfast.

Keller found his way to the kitchen, and came back with a knife.

SEVEN

"Oh, it was a lazy day," he said. "I got to talking with a U.S. collector over breakfast, and wound up hanging out in the auction room to see how he did when his lots came up. I meant to call earlier so I could talk to Jenny before her bedtime, but I guess it's too late now."

His first call, when he got back to his hotel room, was on his other cell phone, the one he used only for calls to Dot. When there was no answer he put that phone away, got out the other one, and called Julia, and when he heard her voice he felt a great sense of relief.

After the phone call, after she'd told him about her day and he'd made up a day for himself, he tried to figure out what that sense of relief was all about. He hadn't been aware of any anxiety until the sound of her voice dispelled it.

It took him a few minutes to sort it out, but what he decided was that he'd been afraid his whole new life was gone, that he'd somehow thrown it away in the Spanish-style house on Caruth Boulevard. Then he'd heard her voice and been reassured.

Now, though, he wasn't sure how he felt.

He tried Dot again, watched a half hour of television, tried Dot one more time, and tried to decide if he felt like getting something to eat. He hadn't eaten since breakfast, so he ought to be hungry, but he didn't have much of an appetite. He checked the room-service menu and decided he could eat a sandwich, but when the waiter brought it he knew it was a mistake. There was coffee, and he drank that, but he left the sandwich untouched.

Years ago he'd learned how to clear his mind after a job. Very deliberately he let himself picture the master bedroom on Caruth Boulevard as he had last seen it. Portia Walmsley lay on her back, stabbed through the heart. Beside her was her unnamed lover, comatose with drink, his fingers clenched around the hilt of the murder weapon. It was the sort of image you'd want to blink away, especially if you'd had something to do with it, but Keller fixed it in his mind and brought it into focus, saw it in full color and sharp relief.

And then, as he'd learned to do, he willed the image to grow smaller and less distinct. He shrank it, as if viewing it through the wrong end of a telescope, and he washed out the bright colors, dimming the image to black and white, then fading it to gray. The details blurred, the faces became unrecognizable, and as the image disappeared, the incident itself lost its emotional charge. It had happened, there was no getting around it, but it was as if it had happened years and years ago, and to somebody else.

* * *

Keller, in line for the breakfast buffet, knew he was going to get his money's worth. He'd put the room-service tray outside his door without taking the first bite of the sandwich, and went to bed uncertain if he'd be able to sleep on an empty stomach. The next thing he knew it was morning, and one of the first things that came to mind was an expression his mother had used now and then: *My stomach thinks my throat's been cut*. Keller was shaving when the line came to him, which might have given him a turn, but he used a twin-blade safety razor, hardly something you'd use to cut a throat, your own or anybody else's.

He piled his plate high and looked around for an empty table, and there was his friend of yesterday morning, mustachioed Michael, wielding a fork with one hand and beckoning to Keller with the other. Keller, glad for the company, went over and joined him.

"Saw you yesterday morning," Michael said. "If I remember correctly, you were in the room when that big block got away from me."

"Quite a price it brought."

"Way more than my maximum, so I wisely sat back and let it go. And guess what?"

"You've been kicking yourself ever since."

"Around the block and back again. Oh, I know I was right to let it go, but when am I gonna get a shot at a piece like that again? Not until they auction off the collection of the sonofabitch who bought it, and by then it'll probably go for three times what it brought yesterday. Nick, I've bought some things I shouldn't have over the years, and I've paid too much for some of them, but that sort of thing never bothers me for more than a minute or two. It's the ones that get away that drive you crazy."

Obock J1, Keller thought.

He worked on his breakfast while Michael told him about the afternoon session, where he'd made up for the loss of the block by picking up all the covers he'd had his eye on, most of them at good prices. "But I wanted that block," he told Keller, "and I still want it. How about yourself? What are you looking to buy today?"

Keller had a seat in the auction room and was studying his catalog when he realized he'd forgotten to call Dot. He hadn't called Julia, either, to wish her a good morning. Should he duck out and make the calls? He thought about it, and then they started the sale and called the first lot, and he decided to stay where he was.

By the time they got to France and French Colonies, Keller had bid on ten lots and acquired six of them, letting the others go when the bidding climbed out of his range. As Michael had observed, a general collector always has plenty of things to buy, and Keller spent a few dollars and added a few stamps to his collection, issues from Albania and the Dominican Republic and Eastern Rumelia and Ecuador, none of them bringing more than a few hundred dollars. Then they got to the French section, where Keller's collection was strongest and where the lots he needed were higher in price, and harder to find. He sat calmly in his chair, but he felt anticipation and excitement coursing through him like an electric current.

The Obock stamp was valued at $7500 in Keller's Scott catalog, while his Yvert et Tellier specialized catalog of France and its colonies listed the stamp at €12,000, or almost double the price in Scott.

Both Scott and Y&T mentioned the reprint, Scott pegging it at $200, Y&T at €350. Keller couldn't remember what he'd paid, but thought it was around $150. Now he'd have the chance to bid on the original, and had a feeling it was going to bring a high price.

Back in New Orleans, before Dot's phone call, Keller had already had his eye on the stamp. At the time he'd decided the stamp was worth $10,000 to him, but wasn't sure he could rationalize spending that much money. Now, with his business on Caruth Boulevard successfully concluded, the money was there to be spent. He picked up a couple of lots—an early stamp from Diego-Suárez, an inverted overprint from Martinique—and when Obock J1 came up, he was ready.

Moments later, the stamp was his.

There were other lots that he'd marked in his catalog, but he was no longer interested in bidding on them. He felt as though he'd just fought a prizefight, or run a marathon, and all he'd done was raise a forefinger and keep it raised until he was the only bidder left.

The hammer price was $16,500, and he'd have to pay a 15 percent bidder's premium on top of that, plus whatever sales tax the state of Texas felt it deserved. Close to $20,000 for a homely little square of paper, but it was his to have and to hold, his to protect in a black-backed plastic mount, his to place in his album alongside the $200 reprint to which it looked essentially identical.

In the elevator he felt a twinge of buyer's remorse, but by the time he was in his room it had dissipated, leaving him with a warm glow of accomplishment. He'd had to hang in there, had to keep his finger in the air while other bidders in the room gave up and dropped out, then had to hold on until the phone bidder finally gave up and let go. It was a rare stamp, and other people wanted it, but the whole point of an auction was to see who wanted something the most, and this time around it was Keller.

He called Julia from his room. "I got the stamp I wanted, and it's a beauty. But I had to spend more than I expected, so I'm going to skip the afternoon session and hit the road early. I'll break the trip somewhere, and I should be home some time tomorrow afternoon."

She told him the latest cute thing Jenny had said, and a little gossip about the young couple who'd moved into the old Beaulieu house, and when the conversation ended he switched phones and called Dot, and this time she answered.

"I tried you yesterday," he said, "and then I was going to call first thing this morning but it slipped my mind, and I was all caught up in the drama of a stamp auction."

"With all the pulse-pounding excitement thereof."

"What I wanted to tell you," he said, "is it's all taken care of, and it couldn't have gone better."

"Is that so."

"Double bonus," he said.

"Oh?"

They were using a pair of untraceable phones, but even so he felt it best to be cryptic. "The primary is down," he said, "and the secondary objective is fully implicated."

"Do tell."

He frowned. "Is something wrong?"

"From a dollars-and-cents standpoint," she said, "I'd have to say there is. There's not going to be a bonus, let alone a double bonus."

"But—"

"As a matter of fact, we can forget about the second half of the basic fee. You know, the portion due upon completion of the assignment?"

"But the assignment was completed."

"I'll say."

"Dot, what's the matter?"

"You got up this morning, had a cup of coffee—right so far?"

"I had breakfast," he said, mystified. "And then I went to the auction room."

"Read the paper while you ate your breakfast?"

"No. I joined this fellow and we got to talking."

"About stamps, I'll bet. Good breakfast?"

"Yes, as a matter of fact, but——"

"And then you went to the auction room."

"Right."

"And bought some stamps, I suppose."

"Well, yes. But——"

"The Dallas morning newspaper," she said, "is called the *Dallas Morning News,* and don't ask me how they came up with a name like that. You can't beat Texans for imagination. Go buy the paper, Keller. You'll find what you're looking for right there on the front page."

EIGHT

He picked up the lots he'd won, paid for them, and packed them along with his other belongings in his small suitcase. He checked out of the Lombardy and drove off with his suitcase next to him on the front seat. Traffic was light, and he didn't have any trouble finding his way to the interstate. He headed for New Orleans, and found a country music station, but turned it off after half an hour.

He broke the trip at the same Red Roof Inn, used the same credit card. In his room he wondered if that was a good idea. But the trip was a matter of record, and one he had never attempted to conceal. Portions of it, of course, were off the record—the car rental, the visit to Caruth Boulevard—but he had no reason to hide the fact that he'd been to Dallas, and had the stamps to prove it.

He ate next door at a Bob's Big Boy, and it seemed to him that half the men in the room had mustaches. Like his philatelic friend Michael, and like the man whose fingers he'd curled around the hilt of Portia Walmsley's kitchen knife.

They'd found him like that, Keller had learned on page one of the *Dallas Morning News*. Still in a drunken stupor, still holding the knife, and still sprawled out next to the dead body of a woman.

Reading the paper, Keller had learned why the sonofabitch looked familiar. Keller had seen him before, and not in the auction room, or around the Lombardy. He hadn't seen the man himself, not really. He'd seen the guy's picture—online, in some of the photos that popped up when he asked Google Images for a peek at Portia. And it was entirely natural that he be photographed at her side. After all, he was her husband.

Charles Walmsley. The client.

A reconciliation, Dot had explained. Charles Walmsley had gone over to his wife's house, perhaps in the hope of getting one last look at her before he got to see her in her coffin. And evidently the old magic was still there, and, well, one thing led to another. And somewhere along the way he remembered that he'd better call off the hit.

So he made a phone call and figured that was that. A single phone call had put the operation in motion, so wouldn't a second phone call nip it in the bud?

Absolutely. But the person Walmsley called had to make a call of his own, and the person *he* called had to call Dot, and the new directive took its time working its way through the system. By the time Dot got the word, it was already too late.

Back home, Keller held his daughter high in the air. "Tummy!" she demanded, and he put his lips to her stomach and blew, making an indelicate sound. Jenny laughed with delight and insisted he do it again.

It was good to be home.

Later that evening, Keller went upstairs and settled in with his stamps. After he'd mounted Obock J1, he called Julia in and showed it to her, and she admired it extravagantly.

"It's like when somebody shows you their new baby," Keller said. "You have to say it's beautiful, because what else are you going to say?"

"All babies are beautiful."

"And all stamps, I suppose. That's the original on the right and the reprint next to it. They look the same, don't they?"

"I bet their mother could tell the difference," she said.

Two days later, Keller bought a new phone and called Dot. "Take down this number," he said, and read it off to her. She read it back and asked what was wrong with the old number. "It's no good anymore," he said, "because I smashed the phone and threw the pieces down a storm drain."

"I smashed a pay phone once," she said, "when it flat-out refused to give me my dime back. What did this phone do to piss you off?"

"I figured it would be safer to get a new phone."

"And I figure you're probably right. You okay, Keller? Last time we talked you were a little shaky."

"I'm all right."

"Because you didn't do anything wrong."

"Our client fell in love with his wife all over again," he said, "and I killed her and framed him for it. If I'd known what was going on, you can bet I'd have handled it differently."

"Keller, if you'd known, you wouldn't have handled it at all. You'd have bought some stamps and come home."

"Well, that's true," he allowed. "Obviously. But I still wish I hadn't made the phone call."

"To me?"

"To the cops, after I got out of there. I wanted to make sure they showed up before he could come to his senses and head for the hills."

"Hills would be hard to find," she said, "in that part of the country. Look, don't worry about it. You had no way of knowing he was the client, or that he'd canceled the contract. One way to look at it, he's a lucky man."

"Lucky?"

"You wanted the double bonus, right? That's why you left him with the knife in his hand."

"So?"

"So otherwise you'd have killed them both. This way at least he's alive."

"What a lucky guy."

"Well, yes and no. See, he's consumed with guilt."

"Because he didn't call it off soon enough?"

"Because he got drunk and killed his wife. He doesn't actually remember doing it, but then he can't remember much of anything after the third drink, and what's a man supposed to think when he comes out of a blackout with a knife in his hand and a dead woman next to him? He figures he must have done it, and he'll plead guilty, and that's the end of it."

"And now he's got to live with the guilt."

"Keller," she said, "everybody's got to live with something."

KELLER'S
HOMECOMING

NINE

Keller, his suitcase unpacked, found himself curiously reluctant to leave his hotel room. He turned on the TV, channel surfed without finding anything that held his attention, threw himself down on the bed, picked himself up, test-drove every chair in the room, and finally told himself to get over it. He wasn't sure what it was that he had to get over, but he wasn't going to find it sitting in his room. Or lying down, or pacing the floor.

One explanation occurred to him in the elevator. Keller, who'd lived all his life in and around New York, had never had occasion to stay at a New York hotel before. Why would he? For years he'd had a wonderfully comfortable apartment on First Avenue in the 40s, and unless he was out of town, or had been invited to spend the night in the bed of some congenial female companion, that was where he slept.

Nowadays the only female companion in his life, congenial

or otherwise, was his wife, Julia, and he lived in her house in New Orleans's Garden District. His name in New Orleans—and, for that matter, everywhere he went—was Edwards, Nicholas Edwards. He was a partner in a construction business, doing post-Katrina residential rehabilitation, and his partner called him Nick, as did the men they worked with. Julia called him Nicholas, except in intimate moments, when she sometimes called him Keller.

But she didn't do that so often anymore. Oh, the intimate moments were no less frequent, but she was apt to call him Nicholas then. And, he thought, why not? That was his name. Nicholas Edwards. That's what it said on his driver's license, issued to him by the state of Louisiana, and on his passport, issued to him by the United States of America. And that was the name on every credit card and piece of ID in his wallet, so how could you say that wasn't who he was? And why shouldn't his wife call him by his rightful name?

His daughter, Jenny, called him Daddy.

He realized that he missed them both, Jenny and Julia, and it struck him that this was ridiculous. They'd driven him to the airport that morning, so it had been only a matter of hours since he'd seen them, and he went longer than that without seeing them on any busy workday. Of course there'd been fewer busy workdays lately, the economy being what it was, and that in fact had a little to do with this visit to New York, but even so…

How you do go on, he told himself. And, shaking his head, walked through the lobby and out onto the street.

His hotel, the Savoyard, stood at the corner of Sixth Avenue and West 53rd Street. He took a moment to get his bearings, then headed uptown. There was a Starbucks two blocks from his hotel, and he waited at the counter while a young woman with a snake coiled around her upper arm—well, the inked representation of a snake, not an actual living reptile—made sure the barista understood exactly what she did and didn't want in her latte. Keller couldn't imagine caring quite that much about the composition of a cup of coffee, but neither could he imagine getting tattooed, so he let it go. When it was finally his turn, he asked for a small black coffee.

"That would be a 'Tall,'" said the barista, herself sporting a tattoo and a few piercings. She drew the coffee without waiting for his reply, which was just as well, because Keller didn't have one. The tables were all taken, but there was a high counter where you could stand while your coffee cooled. He did, and when it was cool enough to drink he drank it, and when he was done he left.

By then he'd come up with another explanation for his disinclination to leave his hotel room. He wasn't used to being in a hotel in New York, and consequently he wasn't quite prepared for what they cost. This one, decent enough but hardly palatial, was charging him close to $500 for no more space than they gave you in a Days Inn.

Spend that much on a room, you wanted to get your money's worth. If you never left the room, it would only be costing you $40 an hour. If, on the other hand, you used it solely to sleep and shower...

At 56th Street he crossed to the west side of the avenue, and at 57th Street he turned to his left and walked about a third of a block, stopping to look into the window of a shop that sold watches and earrings. Once Keller had heard one woman tell another on QVC that you couldn't have too many earrings, a statement that he had found every bit as baffling as the snake tattoo.

Keller wasn't really interested in looking at earrings, and it wasn't long before he'd turned to gaze instead across 57th Street. Number 119 West 57th Street was directly across the street, and Keller stayed where he was and tried to pay attention to the people entering and leaving the office building. People came and went, and Keller didn't see anyone who looked familiar to him, but 57th was one of the wide crosstown streets, so he wasn't getting a really good look at the faces of those who were coming and going.

It wasn't the hotel room, he realized. The price of it, the novelty of being in a New York hotel. He hadn't wanted to leave the room because he was afraid to be out in public in New York.

Where there were people who used to know him as Keller, and who knew, too, that one fine day in Des Moines, that very Keller had assassinated a popular, charismatic midwestern governor with presidential aspirations.

TEN

Except he didn't. It was a frame, he was the fall guy, and it cost him his comfortable New York life and the name under which he'd lived it. When all was said and done he didn't have any regrets, because the life he now led in New Orleans was worlds better than what he'd left behind. But that hadn't been the plan of the man who set him up.

That plan had called for Keller to be arrested, or, better yet, killed outright, and it had taken all Keller's resource-fulness to keep it from turning out that way. The man who'd done the planning was dead now, thanks to Keller, and so was the man who'd helped him, and that was as far as Keller saw any need to carry it. Someone somewhere had pulled the trigger and gunned down the governor, but Keller figured that faceless fellow was probably dead him-self, murdered by the man who'd hired him, a loose end carefully tied off. And if not, well, the best of luck to him. He'd just been a man doing a job, and that was something Keller could relate to.

And Keller? He had a new name and a new life. So what was he doing back in New York?

He walked back to the corner of Sixth and 57th, waited for the light to change, then crossed the street and walked to the entrance of 119 West 57th. This was a building he'd entered a dozen or more times over the years, and always for the same purpose. There had been a firm called Stampazine on the second floor, and every couple of months they held a Saturday auction, and there was always some interesting and affordable material up for grabs. Keller would sit in a wooden chair with a catalog in one hand and a pen in the other, and every now and then he would raise a forefinger, and sometimes he'd wind up the high bidder. At six or six thirty he'd pick up his lots, pay cash for them, and go home happy.

Stampazine was gone now. Had they closed before or after he'd left New York? He couldn't remember.

He recognized the uniformed lobby attendant. "Peachpit," he said, and the man nodded in recognition—not of Keller but of Keller's purpose. "Seven," he said, and Keller went over and waited for the elevator.

Peachpit Auction Galleries was a cut or two above Stampazine. Keller had never visited them during his New York years, but after he was settled in New Orleans an ad in *Linn's Stamp News* sent him to the Peachpit website. He bid on a couple of lots—unsuccessfully; someone else outbid him—but, having registered, he began to receive their catalogs several times a year. They were magnificently printed, with a color photograph of every lot, and he always found an abundance of choice material.

There was a way to bid online in real time, during the actual floor auction, and he'd planned on doing so but always seemed to be at work during their midweek auctions. Then a few months ago he'd had the day off—he and Donny had the whole week off, actually, although they'd have preferred it otherwise. And he remembered the Peachpit sale, and logged on and went through what you had to go through to bid, and he found the whole process impossibly nerve-racking. An auction was anxiety-ridden anyway, but when you showed up in person you could at least see what was going on, and know that the guy with the gavel could see you in return. Online, well, he supposed a person could get the hang of it, but he hadn't, and wasn't inclined to try again.

Then, a couple of weeks ago, Julia and Jenny walked into his upstairs office—Daddy's Stamp Room—to find him shaking his head over the new Peachpit catalog. Julia asked what was the matter.

"Oh, this," he said, tapping the catalog. "There are some lots I'd like to buy."

"So?"

"Well, the sale's in New York."

"Oh," she said.

"Daddy 'tamps," said Jenny.

"Yes, Daddy's stamps," Keller said, and picked up his daughter and set her on his lap. "See?" he said, pointing at a picture in the catalog, a German Colonial issue from Kiauchau showing the kaiser's yacht, *Hohenzollern*. "Kiauchau," he told Jenny, "was an area of two hundred square miles in southeast China. The Germans grabbed it in 1897, and then made arrangements to lease it from China. I don't imagine the Chinese had a lot of choice in the matter. Isn't that a pretty stamp?"

"Pity 'tamp," Jenny said, and there the matter lay.

Until the phone rang two days later. It was Dot, calling from Sedona, and the first thing she did was apologize for calling at all.

"I told myself I'd just call to see how you're doing," she said, "and to find out the latest cute thing Jenny said, but you know something, Keller? I'm too damn old to start fooling myself."

Dot still called him Keller. And that figured, because that's who she was calling to talk to. Not Nick Edwards, who fixed houses, but Keller. Who, in a manner of speaking, fixed people.

"The last thing I should be doing," she went on, "is calling you. There's two reasons why this is a mistake. First of all, you're not in the business anymore. I dragged you back in once, that business in Dallas, and it wasn't your fault that it didn't go off perfectly. But it wasn't what you really wanted, and we both agreed it was what the British call a one-off."

"What does that mean?"

"One time only, I think. What's the difference what it means? You went to Dallas, you came back from Dallas, end of story."

But if it was the end of the story, what was this? A sequel?

"That's one reason," she said. "There's another."

"Oh?"

"Three words," she said. "New. York. City."

"Oh."

"What am I even thinking, Keller, calling you when I've got a job in your old hometown? I didn't throw New York jobs your way when you lived there, *because* you lived there."

"I worked a couple of New York assignments."

"Just a couple, and they weren't exactly what you'd call problem-free. But at least you could walk around the city without wearing a mask. Now it's the one place in the world where it's not safe for you to be you, where even a waitress in a coffee shop can take a second look at you and reach for a telephone, and here I am calling you with a New York assignment, and that's as far as this is going, because I'm hanging up."

"Wait a minute," Keller said.

The receptionist at Peachpit told him to have a seat, and he leafed through an old auction catalog while he waited. Then a stoop-shouldered man with his sleeves rolled up and his tie loosened came to show him inside and seat him in a stackable white plastic chair at a long table. He had already prepared a slip of paper with the numbers of the lots he wanted to inspect, and he looked them over carefully when they were brought to him.

The stamps were tucked into individual two-inch-square pockets of a chemically inert plastic, each plastic pocket stapled to its own sheet of paper bearing the lot number, estimated value, and opening bid. Keller had brought a pair of tongs, and could have taken out a stamp for closer inspection, but there was no need, and the tongs remained in his breast pocket. Given that the catalog had already shown him clear color photos of all of these stamps, it probably wasn't necessary that he look at them in the first place. But he'd learned that actually looking at a stamp, up close and personal, helped him decide just how much he really wanted to own it.

He'd requested a dozen lots, all of them stamps he needed, all of them stamps he genuinely wanted—and he didn't want them any less now that he was getting a look at them. But he wasn't going to buy them all, and this would help him decide which ones to buy if they went cheap, and which ones deserved a firmer commitment. And, finally, which ones he'd go all out to get, hanging on like grim death, and—

"Hello, there! Haven't seen you in a while, have I?"

Keller froze in his white plastic chair.

"She loves watching you work with your stamps," Julia said. "'Daddy 'tamps,' she says. She has a little trouble with the *s-t* combination."

"I suppose philately is out of the question."

"For now. But before you know it she'll be the only kid in her class who knows where Obock is."

"Just now I was telling her about Kiauchau."

"I know. But see, I know how to pronounce Obock."

He was silent for a moment. Then he said, "There's something we have to talk about."

ELEVEN

They sat at the kitchen table with cups of coffee and he said, "I've been keeping something from you, and I can't do that. Ever since we found each other I've been able to say whatever's been on my mind, and now I can't, and I don't like the way it feels."

"You met someone in Dallas."

He looked at her.

"A woman," she said.

"Oh, God," he said. "It's not what you think."

"It's not?"

If he had to kill this man, how would he do it? He was close to sixty, and he looked soft and pudgy, so you couldn't call him a hard target. The closest thing Keller had to a weapon was the pair of stamp tongs in his breast pocket, but he'd made do often enough with nothing but his bare hands, and—

"I guess you don't recognize me," the fellow was saying. "Been a few years, and it's safe to say I put on a few pounds. It's a rare year when I don't. And the last time we saw each other the two of us were on a lower floor."

Keller looked at him.

"Or am I wrong? Stampazine? I never missed their auctions, and I'd swear I saw you there a few times. I don't know if we ever talked, and if I ever heard your name I've long since forgotten it, but I'm pretty good with faces. Faces and watermarks, they both tend to stick in my mind." He stuck out a hand. "Irv," he said. "Irv Feldspar."

"Nicholas Edwards."

"A damn shame Stampazine's gone," Feldspar said. "Bert Taub's health was bad for years, and finally he closed up shop, and then the word got around that he missed the business and wanted to get back into it, and the next thing we knew he was dead."

"A hell of a thing," Keller said, figuring something along those lines was expected of him.

"Plenty of other auctions in this city," Feldspar said, "but you could just show up at Stampazine and there'd be plenty of low-priced material to bid on. No fancy catalogs, no Internet or phone bidders. I don't think you and I ever bumped heads, did we? I'm strictly U.S. myself."

"Everything but U.S.," Keller said. "Worldwide to 1940."

"So I was never bidding against you, so why would you remember me?"

"I didn't come all that often," Keller said. "I live out of town, so—"

"What, Jersey? Connecticut?"

"New Orleans, so—"

"You didn't come in special for Bert's auctions."

"Hardly. I just showed up when I happened to be in town."

"On business? What kind of business are you in, if I may ask?"

Keller, letting a trace of the South find its way into his speech, explained that he was retired, and then answered the inevitable Katrina questions, until he cleared his throat and said he really wanted to focus on the lots he was examining. And Irv Feldspar apologized, said his wife told him he never knew when he was boring people, and that she was convinced he was suffering from Ass-Backward syndrome.

Keller nodded, concentrated on the stamps.

Julia said, "I knew there was something. Something's been different ever since you got back from Dallas, and I couldn't say what it was, so I had to think it was another woman. And you're a man, for heaven's sake, and you were on the other side of the state line, and things happen. I know that. And I could stand that, if that's what it was, and if what happened in Dallas stayed in Dallas. If it was going to be an ongoing thing, if she was important to you, well, maybe I could stand that and maybe I couldn't."

"That wasn't it."

"No, it wasn't, was it?" She reached to lay her hand on top of his. "What a relief. My husband wasn't fooling around with another woman. He was killing her."

"I don't know what to say."

"Do you remember the night we met?"

"Of course."

"You saved my life. I was taking a shortcut through the park, and I was about to be raped and killed, and you saved me."

"I don't know what got into me."

"You saved me," she said, "and you killed that man right in front of me. With your bare hands. You grabbed him and broke his neck."

"Well."

"That was how we met. When Jenny's old enough to want to know how Mommy and Daddy met and fell in love, we may have to give her an edited version. But that's not for a while yet. How was it? In Dallas? I know it went smoothly enough, and I think it's pure poetry that the man you framed wound up confessing."

"Well, he thinks he did it."

"And in a sense he did, because if he hadn't made that first phone call you would never have left the hotel."

"I probably wouldn't even have gone. I'd have sent in a few mail bids and let it go at that."

"So he got what was coming to him, and it doesn't sound as though either of them was a terribly nice person."

"You wouldn't want to have them to the house for dinner."

"I didn't think so. But what I wanted to know was how was it for you? How did it feel? You hadn't done anything like this in a long time."

"A couple of years."

"And your life is different from what it was, so maybe you're different, too."

"I thought of that."

"And?"

He thought it over for a moment. "It felt the same as always," he said. "I had a job to do and I had to figure out how."

"And then you had to do it."

"That's right."

"And you felt the satisfaction of having solved a problem."

"Uh-huh."

"At which point you could buy that stamp without dipping into capital."

"We only collected the first payment," he said, "but even so it more than covered the cost of the stamps I bought."

"Well, that's a plus, isn't it? And you didn't have any trouble living with what you'd done?"

"I had trouble living with the secret."

"Not being able to mention it to me, you mean."

"That's right."

She nodded. "Having to keep a secret. That must have been difficult. There are things I don't bother to tell you, but nothing I *couldn't* tell you, if I wanted to. How do you feel now?"

"Better."

"I can tell that. Your whole energy is different. Do you want to know how I feel?"

"Yes."

"Relieved, obviously. But also a little troubled, because now I seem to be the one with a secret."

"Oh?"

"Shall I tell you my secret? See, the danger is that you might think less of me if you knew." Before he could respond, she heaved a theatrical sigh. "Oh, I can't keep secrets. When you told me what happened in Dallas? What you did?"

"Yes?"

"It got me hot."

"Oh?"

"Is that weird? Of course it is, it's deeply weird. Here's something I'm positive I never told you. It got me hot when you killed the rapist in the park. What it mostly did was it made me feel all safe and secure and protected, but it also got me hot. I'm hot right now and I don't know what to do about it."

"If we put our heads together," he said, "maybe we can come up with something."

Back in his room at the Savoyard, Keller figured it out. Asperger's syndrome—that's what Feldspar had, or what his wife said he had.

Though Ass-Backward syndrome wasn't a bad fit.

"If I'd known what it would lead to," he said, "I'd have told you right away."

"But you didn't."

"No. I was afraid, I guess. That it would ruin things between us."

"So you didn't say anything."

"No."

"And then you did."

"Right."

She didn't say anything, but he felt besieged by her thoughts, bombarded with them. He said, "I figured I was done with it, I'd never do it again, so why bother mentioning it? I could just keep my mouth shut and seal off the episode and let it fade out into the past."

"Like the faces you picture in your mind."

"Something like that, yes."

"I guess you got another phone call."

"This afternoon."

"I noticed something was different," she said, "when Jenny and I got home from Advanced Sandbox. How's Dot these days?"

"She's good." He cleared his throat. "I reminded her what I'd told her right after Dallas. That I didn't want to do this sort of thing anymore."

"But she called you anyway."

"Well," he said, "it's complicated."

TWELVE

Keller, who'd found it hard to leave his hotel room earlier, now found it impossible to spend any time in it. He showered, got dressed, turned the TV on and then off again, and went out.

In New Orleans, Keller drove his pickup truck for business and Julia's car on other occasions. If he walked north for a couple of blocks, he could hop on the St. Charles Avenue streetcar. And there was a fair network of buses, and it was never hard to get a cab.

For all the choices available to him, Keller did a lot of walking. New Orleans was one of a relatively small number of pedestrian-friendly American cities. Not only could you get around on foot and find interesting things to look at while you did so, but New Orleanians—total strangers—would actually greet you in passing with a smile and a kind word. The ones who didn't might well draw a gun and hold you up, post-

Katrina street crime being a definite problem, but among the law-abiding citizenry you were apt to encounter a high level of politeness and genuine warmth. "Lovely morning, innit?" "Just grand! And how are y'all keeping this fine day?"

New York was at least as much of a city for walkers, to the point where Keller couldn't understand why some people lived in the city and still felt compelled to own cars. The sidewalks might not be as quaintly friendly as those of New Orleans—there was, after all, good reason for the popularity of the line "Can you tell me how to get to the Empire State Building or should I just go fuck myself?"—but nevertheless it was a walker's city, and Keller didn't have to think about it. He left his hotel and started walking.

After his shower, he'd checked in the mirror to see if he needed a shave. He'd decided he could wait until morning, and looked a moment longer at the face Irv Feldspar had been able to recognize. It had changed some since Feldspar (or anyone else in New York) had last had a look at it. Back then his hair had been dark brown, almost black, and it had grown further down on his forehead. When he surfaced in New Orleans, with his face in newspapers and on TV, not to mention on post office walls, he wore a cap all the time, and tried to figure out how to dye his hair gray.

Julia had dyed his hair for him, not gray but a sort of tan shade she called mouse brown. And she had cut his hair short, and had given him a receding hairline. He'd had to shave the stubble where the hairline grew back, but he didn't have to do that anymore, as Time had worked its own barbering tricks on him. Julia still touched up the dye job periodically, but the dark roots she'd had to lighten were now evolving into gray roots she needed to color.

And yet for all that transformation, worked by Julia and by

the years, a guy Keller didn't recall at all had placed him immediately. Of course he'd seen him in context, he knew him from one stamp auction and recognized him at another, so if they'd run into each other on a subway platform, say, Feldspar might not have given him a second glance.

If he had, Keller could have thrown him in front of a train.

"You may have read about the case," Dot said. "Or caught it on the evening news. Political corruption in northern New Jersey."

"I'm shocked," Keller said.

"I know. It's almost impossible to believe. Elected public officials taking bribes, laundering money, selling kidneys—"

"Selling kidneys?"

"So I understand, though who'd want to buy a politician's kidney is a question I'd be hard put to answer. You must have seen something in the paper or on TV."

"In New Orleans," he told her, "we don't pay much mind to political corruption in faraway places."

"Y'all like to eat your own cooking?"

"There you go," he said.

"A lot of people got arrested, Keller, and a couple of them went so far as to resign, but most of them are out on bail and still collecting their municipal paychecks. But it looks as though they'll all have to step down sooner or later, and the abbot will probably have to give up his position, and—"

"The abbot?"

"Well, I don't see how he can go on heading the monastery."

"There's an abbot heading a monastery?"

"Keller, that's what they do. Not all of them can be partners with Lou Costello." She paused, and he realized too late that she'd been waiting for him to laugh. When he didn't, she said, "I don't know how any of this works. I guess he can go on being a monk, unless he gets defrocked. And as for the other monks, well, I guess they'll go on doing what they do. What do they do, anyway?"

"Pray," Keller guessed. "Bake bread. Make cordials."

"Cordials?"

"Bénédictine? Chartreuse?"

"Monks make those? I thought that was Seagram's."

"Monks started it. Maybe they sold the business. I think basically they pray, and maybe work in the garden."

"The garden-variety monks work in the garden," she suggested. "The laundry-variety monks keep themselves occupied with money and kidneys. See, the abbot was in cahoots with all the politicians."

"Felonious monks," Keller said. "Dot? You don't think that was funny?"

"I chuckled a little," she said, "the first time I heard it."

"I just made it up."

"You and every newscaster in the country."

"Oh."

"Long story short," she said, "here's the long and the short of it. The abbot's the guy who knows where all the kidneys are buried. If he talks, nobody walks. Keller? You beginning to get a sense of what your role's going to be?"

To Keller, the word *monastery* called up an image of a walled medieval building, set off somewhere in a secluded rural location, its design combining elements of a Romanesque cathedral and a fortified castle. There'd be those narrow windows, to shoot arrows out of, and there'd be places to sit on the battlements, whatever exactly battlements were, while you poured boiling oil on people. And there'd be a dungeon, and there'd be little individual cells where the little individual monks slept. And there'd be grains of rice, to kneel on during prayer.

And singing, there'd be lots of singing. Gregorian chants, mostly, but maybe some sea chanteys, too, because Keller tended to mix up chants and chanteys in his mind. He knew the difference, but he mixed them up anyhow.

You wouldn't look for a monastery on a quiet residential block in the East 30s. You wouldn't expect to find a monastic order housed in a five-story limestone-front row house in Murray Hill.

Yet there it was.

It stood on the downtown side of East 36th Street between Park and Madison, flanked on either side by similar structures. A small brass plaque identified one of them as the Embassy of the Republic of Chad, while the other looked to be what all of these houses had once been—an elegant private residence. Between them, the building whose plaque read simply THESSALONIAN HOUSE looked no more monastic than either of its neighbors.

Dot had referred to Paul Vincent O'Herlihy, abbot of the Thessalonians, as a fine figure of a man, giving the words a touch of stage-Irish lilt. Keller knew why when he checked him out via Google Images. The abbot was tall and broad-shouldered, heavily built but not fat, with a leonine head and a full mane of white hair. He had one of those open faces that tend to inspire trust, often unwarranted, and Keller could see right away how, if this man were to become a monk, he might very well wind up as the man in charge. With the same looks and bearing, he could as readily have become some city's commissioner of police, or chairman of the board of a Wall Street firm, or an insurance company CEO. Or, back when Tammany Hall ran New York, he might have been mayor.

Likes his food, Keller had thought, noting O'Herlihy's bulk, the fit of his jacket, and in his head he heard the voice of a middle-aged Irishwoman: *"Ah, but doesn't he carry it well?"* Likes a drink, Keller added, taking note of the florid complexion, the network of broken blood vessels in the cheeks and nose. *"Ah, shure, and don't they call that a strong man's weakness?"*

He was in there now, this fine figure of a man. He'd been there when a crew of federal agents came to the door and rang the bell. (If there was one; Keller noted a great brass door knocker mounted in the middle of the door, and perhaps that had been what the Feds used to make their presence known.)

Keller liked the idea of them using the knocker. When they rounded up drug dealers, they generally used a battering ram and knocked the door down. That was how they did it on TV, anyway, and it was impressively dramatic. But when they had to pay a call on a man of God, they didn't even need to disturb the tranquillity with a doorbell's chime. A discreet knock would serve.

So they'd knocked, Keller decided. And he knew that the visit had been no surprise to Father O'Herlihy, that he'd been forewarned by a phone call and was accordingly forearmed, with his attorney at his side when the door opened.

Had they cuffed him for the ride downtown? It was usually mandatory, but maybe they'd spared him that indignity. Keller couldn't remember seeing news photos of a priest in handcuffs, and it was the kind of image that tended to stay with you.

Keller walked to the end of the block, crossed the street, and looked back at where he'd been. Having posted bond,

Father O'Herlihy was now free to go where he pleased, but Keller was willing to bet he was under self-imposed house arrest, living the cloistered life in Thessalonian House. He'd be comfortable there, and those walls would keep him safe from reporters and photographers and other intrusive types.

And, of course, from Keller.

Suppose he just walked up and thumped away with the brass door knocker? Somebody would open the door. And who was to say it wouldn't be the man himself?

Keller, who was ordinarily inclined to take his time, had been in a hurry once in Albuquerque. And so he'd gone straight to the home of the designated victim, walked from his rented car to the front door, and rang the bell. The door was opened by the man in the photo they'd sent Keller, who'd promptly killed him and left. The girl at the Hertz counter said, "So soon? Is there something wrong with it?" He said something about a change in plans, and flew back to New York.

Keller couldn't believe the duty of opening the front door would fall to the abbot, not even in more ordinary circumstances. So Keller would have to deal with whoever came to the door, and then there'd probably be other people to deal with before he got to O'Herlihy.

He turned his back on the monastery and started walking.

Keller had lived for years in an Art Deco apartment building on First Avenue in the 40s. He had rented the apartment, then bought it when the building went co-op. Since then it had appreciated enormously in value, although he supposed it must have dropped some in the current recession.

Not that it mattered, because he was pretty sure he didn't

own it anymore. How could he? He hadn't paid the maintenance since his world turned upside down and left him running for his life. It had probably taken the co-op board a while to figure out how to proceed, but they'd have long since worked it out, and someone else would be living there now.

It was, he thought, stupid to walk over there, stupid to show his face in his old neighborhood. But he couldn't seem to help himself, and while his mind wandered here and there— thinking about O'Herlihy, thinking about stamps, thinking about Julia and Jenny—his feet insisted on carrying him to the block he used to live on, and planted him in a doorway directly across the street.

There was a light on in his window.

He felt very strange. Years and years ago, he'd had occasion to walk down the suburban street where he'd lived as a boy. By then it had been ages since he and his mother lived there, and he'd never had an urge to go back, and that unplanned visit hadn't had much impact. Someone had painted it another color, he'd noted, but the old basketball backboard was still mounted on the garage. It seemed to him that the shrubbery looked different, though he couldn't have said just how.

And he'd turned away and never given the place another thought.

Now, though, it was somehow different. He hadn't moved out of this apartment. He was just there, and then one day he wasn't. He'd sneaked back in the dead of night, slipped the doorman a few bucks to look the other way, and went upstairs to retrieve his stamp collection. Only he was too late for that...

And so he'd gone off, never to return. Until now, when he was suddenly back in New York. He wasn't Keller anymore, and he didn't live here anymore, and just what did he think he was doing here, anyway?

He walked halfway across the street until he could get a look at the doorman. The fellow was wearing the uniform they all wore, maroon with gold piping, but as far as Keller could make out there was nothing else familiar about him. It had been a couple of years, and a certain amount of staff turnover was to be expected. And if Keller didn't recognize the guy, why should the guy recognize Keller?

He probably wouldn't. That didn't necessarily mean Keller could get past him, but it seemed likely Keller could at the very least get close to him, close enough to get his hands on him. And there was the package room, right off the lobby. He could put the guy in the package room and they wouldn't find him until morning.

And then all he'd have to do was go upstairs, and give the doorbell a poke—no knocker on his door, not unless the new tenant had added one. *"Hi, I'm your neighbor from downstairs, I don't mean to disturb you but I've got water coming through my bathroom ceiling—"*

Then the door would open, and there'd be a man or a woman standing there—or a man *and* a woman, or two men, or two women, it hardly mattered. And he didn't have a weapon, but he had his hands, and that was all he'd need.

He drew back into the shadows, flattened himself against the brick wall of the building behind him. Across the street, the doorman stepped out onto the street for a quick cigarette break. He still didn't look familiar to Keller, who found himself wondering why he'd been contemplating snapping the guy's neck and sticking him in the package room.

Just so he could go upstairs and kill some stranger for no good reason at all.

The impulse—or fantasy, or whatever you might want to call it—was gone now. Go home, he told himself sternly.

He stepped over to the curb, held up a hand for a cab. One came along, its dome light lit, and headed his way, whereupon Keller shook his head and waved him off. Keller wasn't able to see the expression on the driver's face, but he could imagine it.

He started walking.

He walked all the way back to his hotel, and he took his time getting there. On the way, he stopped for a slice of pizza and ate it standing at the counter, drank a cup of coffee at the diner that had been his regular breakfast place. He bought a newspaper at a deli, dropped it unread into the next trash can he came to.

And wondered throughout just what he was doing.

He wasn't entirely certain whether or not he recognized anybody. There were faces that looked familiar, but the waitress at the diner wasn't the one who'd served him all those breakfasts. She'd have finished her shift hours ago.

There'd been changes in the neighborhood. He saw a bank that hadn't been there before, and a chain drugstore. What was missing? It seemed to him that a Chinese restaurant was gone, and a dry cleaner, and what happened to the shoe-repair guy? Or was he over on the next block?

He was exhausted by the time he got back to his hotel. He took a shower, drank a bottle of water from the minibar. And went to bed.

THIRTEEN

Keller's first thought was to have breakfast in the hotel. They had a huge buffet, but they charged $35 for it, and he couldn't see starting the day with $35 worth of food in his stomach. He went across the street to an imitation French bistro, where an Asian girl with her hair in pigtails brought him a croque madame, which was essentially a grilled ham-and-cheese sandwich with a fried egg on top. He had orange juice, and a side of home fries, and finished up with a two-cup pot of filtered coffee, and the check came to $31.25, plus tip.

But it was money well spent, he decided, because his attitude was better after breakfast. A good night's sleep had rid him of most of last night's mood, and the meal had finished the job.

And, speaking of jobs, it was time he got to work on his.

Abbot O'Herlihy, Paul Vincent O'Herlihy, was tucked away in the Thessalonian residence in Murray Hill. There were, as far as Keller could make out, only two ways to carry out his assignment. He could get the man to leave the building, or he could contrive to get himself inside it.

The first way was better, he decided, if he could find a way to manage it. The second way had two parts to it, getting in and getting out, and both of them could present problems. Not that getting O'Herlihy out of his refuge was a piece of cake, but there ought to be a way to manage it.

It was Tuesday morning, and, according to his watch, not quite a quarter to ten. The Peachpit auction would take the form of morning and afternoon sessions Wednesday and Thursday. All of Wednesday was given over to general foreign, with British Commonwealth in the morning and the rest of the world in the afternoon. Thursday morning was a specialized offering of U.S. issues, and the final session on Thursday afternoon was devoted to a remarkable collection of German offices and colonies, including that stamp from Kiauchau he'd pointed out to his daughter.

So he had all of Tuesday, and Wednesday night and Thursday morning. And he could miss one or both of the Wednesday sessions if he had to, but he really wanted to be in the room Thursday afternoon when they sold the German collection.

And Thursday night he wanted to be on his way to New Orleans. The last flight out was JetBlue's, at 8:59, and with luck he'd be on it.

He walked all the way to Thessalonian House, and it looked no different than it had the previous afternoon. The brass knocker was just as inviting, the heavy door just as forbidding. He looked over at it from the uptown side of the street, and barely slowed as he passed on by.

He didn't see a pay phone at the corner of 36th and Park,

and walked another block to Lexington. No pay phones there, either, and he walked a block uptown before he found one, and it didn't work. He had a prepaid cell phone in his pocket, which he'd bought at the New Orleans airport, and he'd hoped he could use it to call Julia, but it looked as though he was only going to be able to get one call out of it.

Well, too bad.

He punched in 911, spoke briefly, and disconnected. Then he walked over to the curb and slipped the inoffensive phone down a storm drain.

He retraced his steps slowly, south to 36th Street, west toward Thessalonian House. He was halfway to Park Avenue when he heard the first siren, but maintained his measured pace. By the time he reached the scene, three city vehicles had already arrived, two NYPD squad cars and an FDNY hook and ladder.

Not surprisingly, a crowd was gathering, with a couple of uniformed cops moving spectators to the uptown side of the street, and firefighters setting up barricades to block the sidewalk on either side of the monastery.

Keller picked out one of the cops and asked him what was going on. The man didn't answer, but a fellow spectator chimed in. "Guy broke in, shot two nuns, and he's holding the rest of 'em hostage."

The doors opened, and the monastery began to empty out, the sidewalk filling up with men, some of them in robes, some in business suits. The man who'd just spoken said he might have been wrong about the nuns, and a woman said you didn't have nuns in a monastery, and another man said, "What meat can a priest eat on Friday? None. Get it?"

Keller was the first to spot the bomb squad truck, but he let somebody else point it out. It looked like one of the Brink's ar-

mored cars used to transport large amounts of cash, but it said
BOMB SQUAD on the side, in letters large enough to command
attention. "Oh, it must be a bomb," someone said, and everyone immediately moved one step in from the street.

So did Keller, even though he couldn't imagine what protection an additional foot of distance from a blast could possibly afford. And in any event he knew there was no bomb,
having called in the threat himself.

Another cop, younger and larger than the first, was standing off to the side. He was smoking a cigarette, and Keller got
the impression that doing so was against department regulations, and that the man didn't give a damn.

Keller moved closer to him, but not too close, and asked if
the building across the street was the Thessalonian monastery.

The cop bristled. "And if it is?"

"I just wondered," Keller said. "A fellow I went to school
with, a good friend, actually, he was going to join the Thessalonians."

"Oh, yeah?"

"He thought very highly of them," Keller said. "But you
know, you lose track of people. I don't know whether he
joined up or not. Say, isn't that—"

"Father O'Herlihy," the cop said. "He hasn't got enough on
his plate, he needs a bomb threat on top of everything else."

The man in question looked to Keller as though very little
stayed for very long on any plate of his. He had a full face and
an extra chin, and looked massive even though his robe hid his
figure. His was a plain brown robe, but somehow it seemed
less plain and even less brown than those worn by the other
monks. He was quite clearly in command, and while Keller
couldn't make out what he was saying he could see how the
rest rearranged themselves according to his orders.

"And here comes *Eyewitness News,*" the cop said sourly. "Fuckin' media won't leave the man alone. Jersey's got a certain level of corruption, and it don't matter whether you're the Church or some local businessman, you gotta go along to get along. But maybe you see it different."

"No, I'm with you," Keller said.

"But as soon as a man of God's involved, and especially if he just happens to be a *Catholic* man of God, then it's all over the goddamn papers. These days, beating up on the Church is everybody's favorite sport. Not too many years ago this woulda got swept back under the rug, where it belongs."

"Absolutely," Keller said.

"What did the man do, for Christ's sake? I didn't hear no scandals about altar boys. All right, somebody goes and sells a kidney, that's gonna draw attention. I'll grant you that. But is it any reason to sling mud at a man who does as much good in the world as Father O'Herlihy?"

Keller was ready to express agreement, when someone off to the side said, "Hey, look, a dog!" And indeed a uniformed bomb squad officer was fastening a leash to the collar of a sprightly beagle.

"Jesus," somebody said. "Don't tell me the monks are selling drugs on top of everything else."

"It's a bomb-sniffing dog, you moron," someone else said.

"It's cute, whatever it is," a woman said.

"We had one just like that when I was a kid," a man said. "Dumber than dirt. Couldn't find food in his dish."

The dog disappeared into the building, and the conversation looked for other topics. The abbot continued to move among his corps of monks, patting this one on the back, touching this one on the shoulder, looking like an officer rallying the troops.

"Hey, O'Herlihy," someone called out. "I hear you're running a special on kidneys this week!"

The crowd had been buzzing with casual conversation, and it stopped dead, as if someone had unplugged it. Keller sensed his fellow spectators gathering themselves, brought up short by the combination of shock and a sense of opportunity. The speaker had clearly crossed the line, and they were deciding whether to disapprove or join in. It would depend, he figured, on whether they came up with things too clever to suppress.

But the abbot made the decision for them. He broke off his conversation, spun around to his left, and stalked up to the curb. He drew himself up to his full height and silenced the crowd with a stare.

Then he spoke. "Disperse," he said. "All of ye. Have ye nothing better to do? Go about your proper business, or return to your homes. There's no need for ye here."

And damned if they didn't do exactly that, and Keller with them.

FOURTEEN

I t was pretty impressive," he told Dot. "He just assumed command."

"I guess he must be used to it. Comes with the job, wouldn't you say?"

"I suppose so, but I got the feeling he's been like that all his life. I can picture him as a ten-year-old in the schoolyard, settling disputes in kickball games."

"I always wanted to play kickball," Dot said, "but at my school it was boys only. I'll bet it's different now."

He'd bought another prepaid phone, with a chip good for one hundred minutes or one call to 911, whichever came first. His first call was to Julia; he told her how it felt to be in New York, and how the auction was shaping up, and she filled him in on Jenny's day, and passed on some gossip about a couple two doors down the street. He hadn't told her anything specific about his assignment, and didn't talk about it now.

To Dot he said, "I'm not sure I accomplished anything with that call I made."

"Oh, I don't know, Keller. You got a look at him, didn't you?"

"It's not as though I hadn't seen enough pictures of him."

"But seeing him in person's a little different. You got a sense of the person."

"I guess."

"And you established for certain that he's in residence there. You'd assumed as much, but now you know it for a fact."

"I suppose you're right."

"You don't sound convinced, Keller. What's the matter?"

"The phone."

"Why'd you toss it? I know they log 911 calls, but I thought your phone's untraceable."

"They can't tie it to me," he said, "but they can tell what numbers I call with that phone. Then all they have to do is walk back the cat."

"To Sedona," she said, "and to New Orleans. No, you wouldn't want them to do that. So what's the problem? You bought a disposable phone and then you disposed of it."

"I paid seventy bucks for that phone," he said, "and I made one useless call with it, and now it's floating in the New York sewer system."

"I doubt it's floating, Keller. It probably sank like a stone."

"Well."

"And landed on the bottom," she said, "unless an alligator ate it. Remember Tick-Tock the alligator? In *Peter Pan*?"

"Wasn't that a crocodile?"

"Keller, I know there's a difference between alligators and crocodiles, but is it one we have to care about? Tick-Tock swallowed a clock once, and that's why you could always hear him coming."

"Probably how he got his name, too."

"Odds are. You know, I always wondered how come it didn't run down. You figure it was like a self-winding watch? Just swimming around was enough to keep it going?"

"Dot—"

"So here's your phone," she said, "and this alligator swallows it, and now what happens if somebody calls you?"

How did he get into conversations like this? "Nobody has the number," he said.

"Is that a fact?"

"Besides, I turned the phone off after I made the call. So it wouldn't ring."

"That was wise of you, Keller. Because all you need is an alligator in the sewer with a phone ringing inside his belly."

"And anyway it's a myth. There aren't really any alligators in the New York sewers."

She sighed heavily. "Keller," she said, "you know what you are? A genuine killjoy. You got any inside information about Santa Claus, kindly keep it to yourself. And I wouldn't worry too much about the seventy dollars. It's not gonna keep you from buying any stamps, is it?"

"No."

"Well, there you go. How's New York?"

"It's okay."

"You comfortable there?"

"Pretty much. At first I was worried someone would recognize me, but nobody did, so I stopped worrying."

"I guess so, if you actually started a conversation with a cop."

"Until this moment," he said, "it never occurred to me that I was doing anything risky."

"Maybe you weren't, Keller. The world has a short memory, and I have to say that's just as well. Look, you'll figure out a way to get the job done. You always do."

Keller had Thai food for lunch. You could get perfectly decent Thai food, and almost everything else, in New Orleans, but there was a Thai restaurant two blocks from his old apartment that he remembered fondly. He walked over there, and the hostess put him at a table for two on the left wall, about halfway between the front door and the kitchen.

He was studying the menu when the waitress brought him a glass of Thai iced tea before he could ask for it. How did she know that was what he wanted? He reached for it, and she said, "Papaya salad? Shrimp pad thai, very spicy?"

Was the young woman psychic? No, of course not. She remembered him.

And so had the hostess. Because, he realized, this was the table where he'd always sat years ago, and the meal was the one he'd almost invariably ordered.

Now what? He'd always paid cash, so they wouldn't know his name. Still, they would certainly have seen his photograph, in the papers or on the TV news. But would it have registered out of context?

More to the point, what should he do now? Get up and make a run for it? Or, more discreetly, invent a pretext: "Uh-oh, forgot my wallet, I'll be back in a minute." And they'd never see him again.

But wouldn't that create suspicion where it might well not already exist? And once he'd done that, they'd have reason to wonder what was the matter, and at that point one of them might link this old customer of theirs to a photo dimly recalled, and they could call 911 and it wouldn't even cost them a $70 phone.

On the other hand, he'd be gone by then.

But the authorities, who'd had years to get used to the idea that Keller the Assassin had been liquidated by his employers, would have reason to believe he wasn't dead after all. And there'd be a manhunt, and attention from the media, and what would happen to his life in New Orleans?

The papaya salad came. If he wanted to allay suspicion, he thought, then he ought to act like a man with nothing to hide. So he picked up his fork and dug in.

It was just as he remembered it.

So was the pad thai—the rice noodles nicely slippery on the tongue, the shrimp tender and flavorful, the whole thing fiercely hot. He'd lost his appetite when he realized he'd been recognized, but it returned in full measure once he started eating, and he cleaned both his plates. He might have ordered dessert, there was a baked coconut rice pudding he used to like, but he decided not to push it.

He scribbled in the air, and the hostess brought the check, took his money, and brought his change. He left a tip designed to be generous without being memorable, and on the way out the hostess said, "Long time we don't see you."

"I moved away."

"Ah, that's what I say! Somebody say maybe you don't like us no more, but I say he move. Where you now, Upper West Side?"

"Montana."

"Oh, so far! What city?"

The first thought that came to him was Cheyenne, but that was in Wyoming. "Billings," he said, pretty sure it was in Montana.

"My brother's in Helena," she told him. "Big problem getting people there to try Thai food. So he put sushi on the menu. Sushi very big in Helena."

"In Billings, too."

"They come for sushi," she said, "and then maybe they try something else. Smart guy, my brother. Almost went broke, thought of sushi, and now he's making lots of money."

"That's great."

"You get to Helena, you try Thai Pagoda. Nice place." She frowned. "Cheap rent, too. Not like here. You come back when you in New York, okay?"

"I will."

"You looking good," she said. "Lost some weight!"

"A couple of pounds."

"Almost didn't recognize. Then it comes to me. Table seven! Thai iced tea! Papaya salad! Shrimp pad thai!"

"That's me, all right."

"Very spicy! Make sure very spicy!"

Keller, back in his hotel room, sat in front of the television set watching NY1, the twenty-four-hour local news channel. It was pointless, he knew; if somebody at Thai Garden did make the connection and felt compelled to rat him out to the law, the media wouldn't be reporting it for at least a couple of hours. But he sat there for a half hour anyway, and learned more than he needed to know about the sports and weather, along with ongoing coverage of the bomb scare at Thessalonian House. Once again he got to hear the abbot thunder at the crowd, bidding them to disperse, and even spotted himself in the act of dispersal.

That gave him a turn, but he realized that no one could have identified him on the basis of what he'd just seen. He was part of a crowd shot, seen from a distance, and he had his back to the camera. If he hadn't known he was there, he doubted he'd have recognized himself.

There was, of course, no bomb to be found. The beagle's name turned out to be Ajax, which struck Keller as a pretty decent name for a dog, bomb-sniffing or otherwise. There was a brief interview with Ajax's handler, a light-side-of-the-news piece that Keller found reasonably interesting, and then the announcer's voice turned serious as she talked about the criminal nature of bomb threats, and the need to respond to each of them, and the high cost involved.

"Every call reporting a bomb is logged, and every caller identified," she said. "If you make a false report, it's just a question of time before the long arm of the law reaches out and takes hold of you."

Well, maybe not, Keller thought. Not unless the long arm of the law could reach all the way down into the sewers, and yank his phone out of the alligator's belly.

In the hotel's business center, Keller logged on to the Peachpit site and checked the current status of the lots he was interested in. With one or two exceptions, the opening bids were un-changed. He noted the changes in his catalog and was ready to return to his room when he thought of something.

Google. Who could imagine life without Google?

He was on the computer for fifteen minutes more, and made a few more notes. Then he pulled down the History menu and deleted that day's searches, his and everybody else's.

Then back to his room.

FIFTEEN

I'd like to talk to Abbot O'Herlihy," Keller said. His voice, he noticed, was pitched higher than usual. He hadn't planned on it. It just came out that way.

"That would be Abbot Paul," said the monk who'd answered the phone. "And I'm afraid he's not taking any calls."

"I think it would be a good idea for him to take this one," Keller said, and he could only hope he'd said it ominously.

There was a thoughtful silence. Then, "Perhaps you could tell me the nature of your business with the abbot."

"It was almost thirty years ago," Keller said, "and he wasn't Abbot Paul then. He was Father O'Herlihy, with a parish in Cold Spring Harbor. And I was little Timmy Hannan, just ten years old, and, and—"

"I'm putting you on hold," the monk said, and Keller heard a click, and then spent a full five minutes listening to recorded Gregorian chants.

Keller was just beginning to get into the music when it cut out in the middle of a phrase, and the voice that took over was very different from that of the mild-mannered chap who'd answered the phone. He placed it at once, the timbre, the authority, the slight but unmistakable touch of brogue.

"Who is this?"

"Someone you knew in Cold Spring Harbor."

"Tell me your name." Not *What's your name?* but *Tell me your name.* This man, when he prayed, probably gave orders to God.

"Timothy Michael Hannan, Father, but you called me Timmy."

"Did I? And when was this, by God?"

"Almost thirty years ago. You did...bad things."

"Bad things."

"And I forgot! I blocked it all out, and last week I saw you on television, and I heard your voice, and—"

"And it all came back to ye, did it?"

Remarkable how the son of a bitch managed to put you on the defensive. Keller, in his high-voiced role as little Timmy Hannan, damn near cowered.

He drew a quick breath and said, "Father, they want me to go to the media, to the district attorney, to the diocesan office, but first I wanted—"

"Wanted what?"

"To meet with you. If I could just have a few private minutes with you this afternoon, or perhaps this evening—"

"Private minutes."

"Because, I don't know, maybe it's a false memory. God knows I want it to be. If we could just meet in person, in private—"

"Tomorrow."

"Uh, I was hoping we could find some time today."

"Tomorrow morning," the abbot said, "a car will call for me at nine forty-five to take me to the New York Athletic Club. Do ye know where that is?"

"I can find it."

"No doubt ye can. I am a member, and I will arrange for ye to be admitted as my guest. Spell your name for me."

"T-I-M—"

"Your last name, ye idiot."

Keller wasn't sure how to spell it, Hannan or Hannon, but he figured he was all right either way. He spelled it with two *a*'s.

"You'll arrive at ten fifteen, no sooner and no later. They'll give ye a pass and a locker key, and tell ye how to find the steam room. Strip to the skin, put your clothes in a locker, fasten the key around your wrist, and help yourself to a towel. I'll be taking the steam before my massage. You'll come join me, and we'll have our 'private time.'"

Keller wasn't sure how to reply to that. While he was working it out, the phone clicked in his ear.

Hell.

Wednesday morning's session at Peachpit would feature Great Britain and the British Commonwealth, and there were several lots that Keller was hoping to bid on. The starting time was ten o'clock, and he'd just agreed to show up at the New York Athletic Club at ten fifteen.

Or had he? It seemed to him that he, in the persona of little Timmy Hannan, hadn't been provided with much opportunity to agree or disagree. He'd been issued his instructions, and it seemed to be a given that he would follow them to the letter. And to the number, which was precisely fifteen minutes after the Peachpit crew began selling British stamps.

It was impossible to predict the pace of an auction; the more competitive the bidding, the longer it took to get through the lots. But no matter how you figured it, Keller couldn't keep his date with the abbot without missing the first half of the session, and the tyranny of alphabetical order placed British East Africa very much in that time span.

British East Africa was what philatelists designated a dead country. The first time Keller heard that term he visualized an arid wasteland, with the skulls of cattle scattered here and there, and noxious vapors rising from the occasional water source. In due course he learned that the term merely indicated that a particular stamp-issuing entity was no longer operating under that name.

Keller's collection had a cutoff date of 1940. He'd stretched that out to include British Commonwealth issues through 1952, the end of George VI's reign constituting a natural stopping point. And lately he seemed to be stretching his limits for other countries as well, to accommodate World War II issues. All in all, though, his collection held no end of dead countries, and the list kept growing. Even Czechoslovakia had become a dead country, once it divvied itself up into the separate Czech and Slovak Republics.

British East Africa had its philatelic birth in 1890, when the British East Africa Company overprinted three Indian stamps for use in the territory under its administration. The next eight years saw the appearance of just over a hundred British East Africa stamps, some of them created specifically for the colony, others overprinted on stamps of India or Zanzibar. Then British East Africa was incorporated as the East Africa and Uganda Protectorate, which was subsequently folded into the Kenya Colony, which gave way to what collectors knew as K.U.T., for Kenya Uganda and Tanganyika, which Keller always thought of as an African version of the Atchison, Topeka, and Santa Fe.

Dead countries, all of them.

Commencing in 1890, British East Africa issued seventeen stamps with the design of a crowned sun, ostensibly symbolizing light and liberty. The following year, a shortage of certain denominations led the postal authorities to surcharge others, changing their denominations either by hand stamp or by pen and ink and creating eight collectible stamps in the process. One of these, listed in the Scott catalog as number 33, consisted of a two-anna vermilion stamp surcharged half an anna in manuscript, and marked as well with the initials A.B., for Archibald Brown.

Keller had no idea who Archibald Brown might be, and didn't much care, but he wanted the stamp. It was unused, with only a trace of original gum, and the centering was not absolutely perfect, but the color was bright and unfaded, and an accompanying Sergio Sismondo certificate proclaimed it genuine and free of flaws.

Scott valued the stamp at $6000, and Peachpit's presale estimate was $3500. A mail or Internet bidder had submitted an opening bid of $2750, and no one had topped it when Keller had last checked. But there was no telling what would happen when it went under the hammer.

How much did he want it? How high would he go for it? Well, that was one of the things you found out when you sat in an auction room. You might have a top figure in mind, but when the time came you might find out you didn't really want it all that much. Or you might go much higher than you'd planned.

Could he get there in time? No, not a chance. British East Africa 33 was lot number 77, and would surely be sold in the first hour of the auction. At ten fifteen he'd show up at the NYAC, and by the time he was actually inside the steam room it would be ten thirty, and he couldn't envision a scenario that left Paul Vincent O'Herlihy dead and Keller dressed and in Peachpit's auction room by eleven o'clock.

Get real, he told himself. It's only a hobby.

It was only a hobby, and the stamp was only a stamp, but that didn't mean he could get it out of his head. He had dinner at a deli that was famous for giving you more food than you could eat, and it lived up to its reputation. The waiter was surprised, and seemed slightly offended, when Keller didn't want to take home the leftover half of his enormous sandwich. "That's a whole meal you're throwing away," the man told him. "Didn't your mother ever tell you they're starving in Africa?"

And there he was, back in the blighted landscape of British East Africa, with its long-horned cattle skulls and poisoned water holes. And now, thanks to this helpful son of a bitch, the picture included little black children, their stomachs bloated with kwashiorkor, flies buzzing around their mournful eyes. It was a hard image to get rid of, and the only solution was to resume thinking about the stamp.

And he went on thinking about the stamp for the rest of the evening, except when he forced himself to think about what he would do in the steam room. He could guess why O'Herlihy had chosen it as the venue for their meeting, as it combined convenience with security. He was going there anyway for his massage appointment, so there'd be no unexplained absence from the monastery. And how could Timmy Hannan, with only a towel to cover himself, wear a wire into a steam room?

Keller hadn't planned on wearing a wire, as a recording of the proceedings was the last thing he wanted. But it would be nice to have a weapon.

A gun, say. Keller wasn't that crazy about guns. They were noisy, unless you used a suppressor. They left nitrate particles on your hand, unless you wore gloves. Sometimes they jammed, and sometimes they misfired. And, unless you got fairly close to your target, there was always the chance that you would miss. If you were close enough to rule out a miss, well, you were probably close enough to get the job done without a gun.

Still, O'Herlihy was an awfully large man. Sheer bulk was part of what made him so imposing. It might be mostly fat, but simply carrying all that weight around could make a man strong, couldn't it? So there was a certain appeal in being a couple of steps away from him, maybe even three or four steps, and pointing a gun at him, and finding out if he could stop the bullets by sheer force of will.

Well, forget that. They wouldn't make you go through a metal detector to get into the New York Athletic Club, but there'd be other people in the locker room, and possibly in the steam room as well, and even if he took a second towel and wrapped the gun in it—no, never mind, he couldn't go in there with a gun.

Not that he had a gun, or knew offhand where to get hold of one.

Then what? A knife? Anything large enough to do the job would be a problem to conceal.

He walked around, letting his mind play with the problem. He remembered a television program he'd seen ages ago, in which the murder weapon was an icicle. A nice touch, he'd thought at the time. It was a locked-room murder, if he remembered correctly; the murderer and the victim were found in the room, the victim stabbed to death, and no murder weapon to be found. Because it melted.

Did they solve it? Find water droplets in the wound and put two and two together? Or did the killer get away with it? He couldn't remember, and didn't see that it mattered. Nor did he see where he was going to find an icicle at this time of year, let alone carry it into a steam room.

Maybe the best he could hope for from tomorrow's meeting was to lay the groundwork for another meeting at a more promising venue. And then what? Set up something for Thursday afternoon and miss his shot at the German Colonials?

He spent twenty minutes in a chain drugstore. Then he headed back to his room at the Savoyard and went to bed.

SIXTEEN

It was a quarter after seven when Keller opened his eyes, and he was grateful for the opportunity to get up and start the day. He'd set the bedside alarm clock for eight and backed it up with an eight fifteen wake-up call, and he shut off the first and canceled the second and got under the shower, hoping the spray would sluice away the residue of the dream.

He'd dreamed about the stamp, of course, and managed to incorporate the old naked-in-public-places dream that he'd had in one form or another for most of his life. It had pretty much stopped since he wound up in New Orleans, but here it was again, with him sitting in Peachpit's auction room and suddenly realizing that he was wearing a T-shirt and nothing else.

And all night long he kept realizing it was a dream, and turning over and going back to sleep, and slipping right back into the dream all over again, trying to find a way to make it

LAWRENCE BLOCK

come out right. He missed out on the lot he wanted to buy, and he made mistakes and bought other things that he didn't want or need, and throughout it all he was hoping nobody would notice that he didn't have any pants on.

Only a dream, he thought. Only a dream, only a hobby, only a stamp.

Hell.

Downstairs, he visited the business center and checked the stamp's current price. It was unchanged, still $2750. Keller had decided the most he was willing to pay was $4500, and he registered on the site and entered the bid. He waited a minute or two and refreshed the page, and saw that the opening bid had now increased to $3000. That meant he was the high bidder, and someone else would have to raise it another $1750 to top his maximum.

Was it time to meet O'Herlihy? No, not even close. He had plenty of time for breakfast, but he'd just committed himself to pay $4500 for a stamp, and it would cost him more than that by the time he was done. The auction gallery tacked on a buyer's premium of 20 percent, and there was New York sales tax on top of that, so a lot he bought for $4500 would cost him something over $5800, which wasn't that much less than its $6000 Scott valuation.

Shelling out $35 for breakfast never seemed like a great idea to Keller, but it was even less attractive after the bid he'd just made. So he passed on both the hotel's buffet and the ersatz bistro and found a vendor's cart on one of the side streets. He got a croissant and a cup of coffee, which was as much as he wanted, and the bright-eyed immigrant, no doubt from a dead country, gave him change back from his $5 bill.

The croissant was fine, and so was the coffee, and they had

pedestrianized Times Square since he moved away, so he was able to pull a little chair up to a little table and have his breakfast in — well, not peace and quiet, not exactly, but it was pleasant all the same.

When he was done he glanced at his watch. There was time, he saw, but he'd have to hurry.

He walked quickly back to his hotel. The business center had four people in it, but it had five computers, and Keller was grateful for that.

The New York Athletic Club was on the corner of Seventh Avenue and Central Park South, not far from the Savoyard and even closer to the Peachpit offices on 57th Street. Parked out in front, next to a convenient fire hydrant, stood a black limousine, its chauffeur chatting away on a no-hands cell phone. And waiting, Keller suspected, to drive the abbot back to the monastery.

Keller had put on a suit and tie, thinking the place might have a dress code, and realized the absurdity of it when a couple of overage preppies passed him wearing workout clothes. Still, the suit might make a decent impression on the desk attendant, who looked up at his approach. "Hannan," Keller told him. "I'm Father Paul O'Herlihy's guest."

"You have some ID?"

To sit in a steam bath? Keller had a full set of ID, but nothing that proclaimed him to be Timothy Hannan.

He patted his pockets. "No idea I'd need it," he said. "I don't like to leave my wallet in a locker."

The clerk, whose totem animal was clearly the weasel, explained that all guests had to show identification. "I'm afraid I can't make an exception," he said.

Oh, I'll bet you can, Keller thought. "Fine," he said, and

turned toward the door. "I'll just tell the abbot that the fellow behind the desk took his job a little too seriously."

He took three steps, but before he could take a fourth the weasel must have imagined the conversation he'd wind up having with Father O'Herlihy. In view of the abbot's prominence, he suggested, and because Mr. Hannan hadn't been informed of standard procedures, well, perhaps these were special circumstances. And here's a locker key, and to get to the locker room, all you do is...

Well, Keller thought, now for the hard part.

In the locker room, one flight below ground level, two men in their fifties were discussing a proposed corporate merger while they got back into their business attire. "These things always take too long," one of them said. "But then everything's like that these days. I'm with my girlfriend the other day and I realize I can't wait for it to be over. I didn't want the pleasure, I wanted the memory of the pleasure."

The other nodded. "Some days," he said, "all I want is to move everything in my life from the in-box to the out-box."

Keller picked up a towel and found the right locker. He stripped and loaded his clothes into it. There was a wooden hanger for his jacket, another for his shirt. Before he took off his pants, he drew his homemade weapon from his pocket. He'd bought a few yards of picture-hanging wire at the drugstore the night before, and in his room he'd bent it back and forth until he'd equipped himself with a piece two feet long. He'd fashioned a loop at either end and wound up with what ought to be a perfectly serviceable garrote, which he now wound around his left wrist.

It looked like a bracelet, an arts and crafts project from some facility for the developmentally challenged, but when

Keller slipped his hand through the locker key's elastic band, it pretty much blended in. And he could have it off his wrist and his hands in its loops in a matter of seconds. He'd spent half an hour last night trying, and if practice hadn't made him perfect, it had at least made his movements swift and sure.

He secured the towel around his middle and headed for the steam room.

And walked into a fog bank. One thing he somehow hadn't taken into account was the presence of steam, though it now seemed to him an obvious component of a steam room, like water in a swimming pool. The steam was hot, and right there in his face, and he couldn't really see anything, just colorless shapes looming in the colorless mist.

While he couldn't see much, that didn't mean he was himself invisible. He learned as much when a voice he recognized said, "Hannan? Over here."

He blinked, moved toward the voice. Either the steam was clearing or his eyes were getting used to it, because he could see a little better now. There were seven men—well, he could only assume they were men—seated on ledges on three of the room's sides. The abbot of the Thessalonians was all by himself at the extreme right of the far wall.

"Sit beside me, Hannan. No, get closer, but not so close that your leg is touching mine. Ye might fancy that but I would not."

Keller so arranged himself that there was a good six-inch gap between his leg and O'Herlihy's. He'd have preferred to be on the man's other side, so that his wire-wrapped wrist would be shielded from view, but there was a wall on that side.

"Now remove the towel."

Oh, Jesus, Keller thought.

"So that I may assure myself you're not wearing a wire, lad. I've no interest in any part of your wretched self that's beneath the towel."

But he was in fact wearing a wire, Keller thought, and then realized the man was talking about a recording device, not something Keller hoped to loop around his thick neck. Keller lifted the towel, and the man looked at him and looked away so quickly that Keller found himself feeling somehow inadequate.

"Now we can talk, Hannan. If we keep our voices at this level these other men won't hear us. The steam's an insulator. And it will probably keep ye from recording this, should ye be equipped with some new device I'm unable to detect."

"I'm not."

"Ah, well, I'm sure I can take ye at your word."

The sarcasm was razor-sharp, and came wrapped in the rank odor of yesterday's alcohol draining from the man's pores. That, Keller guessed, was the point of the steam bath; it drew out yesterday's poison and made room for today's.

And room would be needed, because O'Herlihy's breath carried a slightly different scent, one of alcohol not yet processed by that bulky body. So he'd had a drink to start the day. Some sort of whiskey, by the smell of it.

Ah, well. A strong man's weakness.

"Now I'll talk," O'Herlihy said, in a cloud of whiskey breath. "And ye'll listen. If ye'd called six months ago with the same sorry tale I'd have told ye to feck off. And hung up on ye, and taken no calls from ye afterward. Do ye know why?"

Keller shook his head.

"Because I'm not queer," he said, "and there's women who'd swear to it. There's a woman who was a housekeeper of mine, in Cold Spring Harbor and other parishes, and I'd still see her after I went with the Thessalonians. Not as often, as I was older and felt the heat less, and she's along in years herself, but still has her charms. But they'd be wasted on ye, wouldn't they? You're a gay boy yourself, are ye not?"

"No, I—"

"Of course ye are, and fixing to blame myself for your sorry state. Six months ago the press'd pay no mind to ye. They'd have heard rumors of this woman of mine, and one or two others who needn't concern you, and they'd dismiss your dirty talk out of hand. But now I'm in the public eye, and if nothing else they'd have to refute your bloody words, and she'd get dragged into it, and I won't have that. Do ye follow me, lad?"

"Father, I must have made a mistake."

"Indeed ye did, thinking to squeeze money out of myself."

"No," Keller said. "No, I honestly thought—Father, I have these memories, but they can't be true, can they?"

There was a pause. The door to the steam room opened. A man left, and two others entered.

"There might be something in those memories," O'Herlihy said grudgingly. "There was another priest in the same parish, as thin as I was stout, and as dark as I was fair. Father Peter Mullane was his name, and he had a weakness for boys, and—"

"Father Peter," Keller said, glad for a straw to grasp at.

"You recall him, lad?"

"I'd forgotten him completely, but as soon as you said his name I could picture him. Very slender, and dark-haired, and—God, I can see his face now!"

"Well, ye needn't start searching for him. The poor man's twenty years dead. And didn't he take his own life? Whatever grief he caused ye, he's paying for it many times over. Burning in hell for all of eternity, if ye believe the shite we taught ye."

Scotch, Keller thought, getting the strongest whiff yet of the man's breath. He said, "Father, I don't know what to say. I made a terrible mistake."

"Ye did, but at least spare me the burden of hearing your confession." A sigh. "Well, they'll get my testimony, the bastards, and there'll be some misfortunate men in New Jersey, but it can't be helped." He snorted, and then seemed to remember there was someone sitting beside him. "And that's nothing to ye, is it? Ye can go now, and we needn't set eyes on one another again."

Keller glanced at his wrist, where the garrote reposed, ready to be uncoiled and put to work. In a hot steamy room full of witnesses, against a man twice his size who'd yank it out of his hands and lash him with it.

Right.

SEVENTEEN

I felt like a worm," he told Dot. "I'm not sure, but I think he had me groveling."

"That's not how I picture you, Keller. Did you go to Catholic school?"

"No. I was in a Boy Scout troop that met in the parish hall of a Catholic church, but the scoutmaster wasn't a member of the clergy."

"So he just wore one of those silly little soldier suits."

"It was a Boy Scout uniform," he said, "and it never looked silly to me. Though I guess it might nowadays. You know, I don't think it was the religious aspect that got to me. He just plain assumed command of the situation."

"I guess he's used to it."

"Yesterday I thought maybe the robe had something to do with it, but this time all he had was a towel draped over his lap. Dot, the guy was sweating out yesterday's Scotch and he already had a good start on today's. His nose is red and his face is full of broken blood vessels. It's a shame the client can't wait for cirrhosis to take him off the board."

"We don't get paid for cirrhosis," she said, "and the client can't wait, not if he's made up his mind to testify. But I have to say I don't know how the hell you're gonna get to him. There's no way he'll take another meeting with you, is there?"

"No, I had my chance. If I'd just gone ahead and given it my best shot—"

"You'd be dead," she said, "or in jail. Say you brought it off. Then what? Dash out of the steam room with half a dozen witnesses in hot pursuit, pause to unlock your locker and put on your suit and tie your tie—"

"I wouldn't have bothered with the tie."

"Well, I hadn't realized that, Keller. That'd make all the difference, all right. Get dressed, rush past everybody, ring for the elevator—"

"I'd have taken the stairs. But I get the message, Dot. I know you're right. I just feel there should have been something I could do."

"The question," she said, "is what can you do now, and I have the feeling the answer is nothing. Say he keeps the same schedule every day as far as the steam room and massage are concerned. He walks what, ten or a dozen steps from his door to the limo? And if he's not escorted, at a minimum he's got the limo driver standing there holding the door."

"It wouldn't work."

"No, of course not. And what are your chances of getting inside the residence?"

"None, as far as I can see."

"Well, Keller, what does that leave?" She didn't wait for an answer. "Look," she said, "except for the money, what do we care if some of New Jersey's finest get a small fraction of what's coming to them? I'll give back the money. That's easy enough."

"You hate to give back money."

"I do," she said, "because once I have it in hand I think of it as my money, and giving it back is like spending it, and what am I getting for it? Well, in this case what we're both getting is piece of mind, and you could say we're paying for it with somebody else's money."

"Don't give it back just yet," he said. "Maybe I'll come up with something."

When he got out of the New York Athletic Club, Keller had had a fleeting thought of rushing to the auction gallery. But that was ridiculous; it was after eleven, and the most spirited bidding since the sale of the Ferrary collection couldn't have delayed the sale of British East Africa number 33. Besides, he'd already put in a high bid, which he'd second-guessed himself into raising after downing his croissant and coffee.

He'd rushed back to the hotel computer and upped his own bid from $4500 to $6000, and the instant he'd done so he began to have regrets. If he got the stamp for that bid, tax and buyer's premium would boost it to something like $7700, and that was far more than the stamp was worth to him.

Well, it was done. Before, he'd worried that he would miss out on the stamp, and now he was worried that he'd get it, and it was hard to say which was worse. It would work out however it worked out, and in the meantime he'd pushed it out of his mind and gone to his rendezvous with the Thessalonian abbot.

For all the good that did him.

Afterward, flushed from the steam bath and the ignominy

of it all, he returned to the Savoyard. He walked right past the business center and went to his room, and after he'd spoken with Dot he walked right past the business center again and continued four blocks uptown. He was a full half hour early for the afternoon session, and one of the assistants was happy to check on lot 77.

"Went for eighty-five hundred," the woman reported. "All of British Africa was going way over estimate. All the best stuff, that is. Well, that's the beauty of auctions. You never know."

"Like life itself," Keller said.

"Well, in my life," she said, "sometimes you know. But auctions, all it takes is two bidders who both really want the same lot. And this is just a stamp. With postal history, where every cover is essentially unique, well, there's no predicting. One piece will go for ten or twenty times estimate and another won't bring a single bid. You really never know."

She steered him to a refreshment table, where Keller joined a couple of other bidders who were drinking coffee and chipping away at a platter of sandwiches. Keller helped himself, and listened while one man told another how he'd been unable to interest his son in stamps, but his grandson was shaping up as an ardent young philatelist.

"Right now he likes first-day covers," the man said, "which is fine at his age, but I take him to shows, and he'll sit and go through boxes of covers, and you can see his imagination growing."

"So it skips a generation," his friend said.

"Exactly. Well, not to say what I shouldn't, but better he should take after his grandfather than his father in certain respects."

"And we'll leave it at that," the friend said, "before *I* say what I shouldn't."

The men walked off, laughing. Keller finished his sandwich and took his coffee into the auction room. He took a seat, paged through a catalog, and tried to get in the mood.

Without much success. The auction began at its appointed hour, and Keller couldn't get lot 77 out of his head. He was at once relieved not to have to pay the $6000 plus extras that his bid had committed him to, and disappointed to have missed out on the stamp. On the one hand he was a fool to have bid as much as he did; on the other, the high bidder had evidently seen something in the stamp that Keller had not, and maybe he knew something; maybe Keller should have been in there all the way.

He had, he realized, a severe case of the woulda-coulda-shouldas, and recognizing the syndrome wasn't enough to make it go away. Here he was, in a comfortable chair with a whole afternoon of worldwide stamps up for sale, and he couldn't concentrate on what was going on now because he was trying to rewrite what had already taken place hours ago.

The first lot he'd circled was a 1919 set of Albanian overprints, with a catalog value just under $500 and an estimate of $350. Keller had looked at the stamps, and figured he'd go $375, maybe $400. The bidding opened at $200, and there were no bids from the live online participants, no phone bids reported by either of the women manning the phones. Keller was one of a mere dozen bidders physically present in the room, and none of his companions showed any interest in the Albanian set.

Nor did Keller. He sat there as if mummified while the set was sold to the book bidder for $200.

Wonderful. That gave him something new to regret.

After an Egyptian lot got away from him, knocked down to an Internet bidder for less than he'd been prepared to pay,

Keller knew what he had to do. There was an exercise he'd developed to keep his work from exacting a psychic toll, and if it worked with dead people, why shouldn't it work with a stamp from a dead country?

First, he found the photo of lot 77 in his catalog and stared intently at it. Then he closed his eyes and held the image in his mind—the vivid color, the details of the design, the hand-stamped overprint, the handwritten initials. He brought the image in close, so that it was larger than its actual size.

And then he turned it over to the Photoshop of his mind. He let the colors go dim, the vermilion washing out, the black overprint fading to gray. He pushed the stamp away, letting it recede in the distance, growing smaller and smaller in his mind's eye. It became a distant colorless blur, and grew smaller and smaller until it vanished altogether.

By the time the lots from France and the French Colonies came up, he was back in the game.

EIGHTEEN

Back at his hotel room, Keller found another reason to be glad he'd missed the British East Africa stamp. The way things stood, it looked as though he wasn't going to be able to carry out his assignment. Dot would have to refund the advance payment, and he wouldn't be getting paid.

With nothing coming in, he'd have to pay attention to his expenses. He still had substantial funds in an offshore bank, but he'd been dipping into them just to cover ongoing household expenses, ever since the economic downturn flattened the business of rehabbing houses and flipping them. He could still afford to buy stamps, but he could spend more freely out of profits than out of capital.

He put away the stamps he'd just purchased, including a high value from Gabon that had eluded him for years. He was happy to have them, but maybe it was just as well he'd missed out on the stamps from Albania and Egypt.

Maybe he should skip tomorrow's afternoon session, with all of that outstanding German Colonial material. Maybe he should move up his departure. He could probably still get a seat on tonight's 8:59 flight to New Orleans. He wouldn't save anything on the hotel bill, it was hours past checkout time, but he'd be home a day earlier, and that had to be worth something.

Call Dot, tell her there was nothing for it but to give back the money.

Hell. Maybe he should have one last look at the monastery.

It looked as impregnable as ever.

Oh, he could get a foot in the door. All he had to do was bang away with the knocker, and some creature in a plain brown robe would open it. But it wouldn't be O'Herlihy, because when you were the abbot, you didn't have the job of opening up for visitors. Instead you kept busy telling everybody else what to do, or stayed in your room, sucking on the Scotch bottle.

Or did monks have cells? They seemed to in books, but then they weren't cloistered in Murray Hill town houses, not in the novels he'd read. O'Herlihy, he somehow knew, would have a large and well-appointed bedchamber all to himself, unless he managed to smuggle in one of those women he'd been bragging about.

Would that bedchamber front on the street? Could the man be standing at his window now, looking out at the passing scene? Looking out, perhaps, at the man he knew as Timothy Hannan?

Keller, on the north side of the street, drew back into the shadows.

If you knew which room was his, and if it did indeed look out on 36th Street, then what?

A bomb? Not a huge one to demolish the whole building, but something more along the lines of a hand grenade. Lob it through the window in the wee small hours of the morning, by which time O'Herlihy would have taken in enough Scotch to render him unconscious. Boom! The man would never know what hit him.

Of course you'd have to know which window belonged to his room. And you'd also have to know where to get your hands on a grenade.

Hmm. If he could just find another way into the building. A back door, say. So that he could contrive to be inside when all but a skeleton crew of monks had retired for the night, and their abbot along with them. Then, gliding down the corridors like a ninja, he could find O'Herlihy's room with the man passed out and snoring, his intimidation factor severely diminished. Keller, who could bring any weapon he wanted, might as easily dispatch his quarry with his bare hands.

He turned to his right, counting his steps as he walked to Madison Avenue, where he turned left and walked a block south. At 35th Street he turned left again, and counted his steps again, stopping when he reached the number he'd tallied earlier. Now, unless he'd screwed up somehow, the building in front of him was one that backed up on Thessalonian House.

And a handsome building it was, four stories tall, with a limestone facade and Greek Revival pillars. Like Thessalonian House, it had surely started life as a private home, and was just as surely something else now. There was a brass plaque alongside the door, but Keller couldn't make out what it said, and—

"Edward!"

The voice was familiar, even if the name was not. Keller

117

turned, and there was Irv Feldspar, the man who'd recognized him from years ago at Stampazine. He was wearing a tweed jacket and a checked shirt and a big smile, and he hurried along the sidewalk to where Keller was standing.

"Edward Nicholas," he said, panting from the effort. "Knew you right away. Never thought you'd be a member, living where you do. New Mexico, didn't you say?"

"New Orleans."

"Well, I was close. But of course we've got plenty of out-of-town members. We just don't get to see them so often. You're here for the presentation?"

"I was just walking down the street," Keller said. "And I'm afraid I'm not a member of anything, Mr. Feldspar."

"Please, make it Irv. And do you prefer Ed or Edward?"

"Well, I—"

"Or Eddie, even, for all I know."

"Actually," he said, "my name's Nicholas Edwards, so—"

"Well, I was close. Nick? Nicholas?"

"Either one, Irv."

"So you're not a member of the Connoisseurs? Your feet just brought you here? Well, I have to say you've got smart feet. We meet the first and third Wednesday of the month, drinks and hors d'oeuvres for an hour, then a one-hour presentation, and we're out by half past seven. Tonight we've got a visiting speaker from Milwaukee, an expert on the philately of the Civil War. Come on."

Feldspar had taken him by the arm and was urging him toward the door. Keller said again that he wasn't a member, but that didn't seem to matter. "You're my guest," he said. "You'll have a drink, you'll have something to eat, and you'll see some great philatelic material and listen to a terrific talk. And you'll meet some wonderful fellows. Franklin Roosevelt was a member of this club, FDR himself. Come on, Nick, you don't want to miss this."

"It was pretty interesting," he told Julia. "The place is the next thing to a mansion, and it belongs to the club. Someone gave it to them a hundred years ago, and there's no mortgage, and because they're nonprofit there are no taxes to pay. And they can afford to put out a spread of food and drinks before every meeting, and it's all free."

"And the people were nice?"

"Very pleasant fellows. And a couple of women, too. Irv kept introducing me to people, and he got a couple of names wrong, but they know him well enough to be used to him."

"Ass-Backward syndrome," she said. "How was the presentation?"

"That's what I wanted to tell you about. It was Civil War philately, which of course means the USA—"

"And the CSA, buster."

"Well, yeah. But it's an area I don't collect, so that made the material on display less interesting to me than it might have been otherwise. But the talk was fascinating, and I learned some things I never knew. Do you know what happened in 1861?"

"Well, I guess I do," she said. "Y'all started a damn war for no good reason."

"Besides that," he said. "See, someone in Washington realized that all those U.S. post offices in the southern states had large stocks of U.S. stamps on hand."

"So? They couldn't mail letters with them. They were a separate nation by then, even if nobody in Washington was willing to acknowledge it."

"Sometimes," he said, "you're more southern than usual.

This fellow in Washington was worried that those stamps constituted a danger to the Union. Confederate agents could smuggle them across the border and sell them at a discount to unscrupulous parties. On the one hand that would raise funds that could be used to aid the secessionist cause, and at the same time it could undermine the integrity of the United States mails."

"Would that work?"

"I don't see how. We're talking about stamps, for God's sake. But in order to nip such a scheme in the bud, the Post Office recalled all the current stamps and rushed a whole new series of stamps into production, with no end of complications that would only interest a stamp collector, and at a cost that had to be ten times what those mythical southern smugglers could have netted for their stamps."

"Yankees," she said. "Was it a southern boy who gave the presentation?"

"As a matter of fact he was from Milwaukee."

"Maybe his granddaddy moved north," she said, "though why he'd want to do that is beyond me. I'm just having fun, you know, when I get like this."

"I know."

"It sounds as though you had a good time. Are the dues very high?"

"Two hundred dollars a year."

"That's hardly anything. What, four dollars a week?"

"It's even less for out-of-town members. He offered to sponsor me."

"Who, Mr. Asperger?"

"Feldspar. I'd need references, but there are enough dealers I've done business with. And I'm a member of the American Philatelic Society."

"I think you should join."

"Well, I'll think about it. Who knows when I'll be back in New York?"

"But you feel okay there?"

"Pretty much." She hadn't asked about the job that had brought him there, nor had he volunteered anything. "But I'll be glad to get home."

"Me, too. Tomorrow night, you said? I'll pick you up at the airport."

"It'll be way past Jenny's bedtime. Anyway, I left the pickup in long-term parking."

"So what's there for me to do?"

"You could leave a light on."

"I could. And there'll be a fresh pot of coffee waiting for you. They don't make it with chicory up there, do they?"

"They don't."

"In that case," she said, "I guess you'll be glad to get home."

NINETEEN

The parlor floor of the Connoisseurs, half a flight up from street level, was given over to the club's offices, along with their extensive philatelic library. The meeting was held on the second floor, with food and drinks arrayed on a table in a room at the front of the building; a room for displays and lectures was at the rear. Keller made himself a light Dewar's and soda and helped himself to cheese and crackers and salted nuts while Feldspar introduced him to various members, all of whom seemed more than happy to have him in their midst.

"A general worldwide collector," said one man, whose name Keller recognized from articles in *Linn's*. "The wonderful thing about it is that there's always something to buy. And that's also the horrible thing about it—there's always something to buy."

Keller figured he'd remember that one. But he missed a lot

at first because his mind was largely occupied with figuring out how the club could provide access to Thessalonian House. There was a stairway leading to the upper floors, although a velvet rope indicated it was off-limits. Still, if he found a way to conceal himself in a men's room when the meeting broke up, the velvet rope would hardly stop him from ascending to the top floor, and from there he ought to be able to get onto the roof.

And then what? If all of these buildings were tenements, they might have been built right up against one another, enabling an adventurous fellow to spring from one roof to another. But that only worked if the buildings in question were the same height, and it seemed to him that the monastery was taller by a story. And both structures were on a block in Murray Hill that had never been given over to tenements, and the gap between this building and O'Herlihy's was almost certainly one that not even Nijinsky could span.

And if he somehow found himself on the monastery's roof? Then what?

No, forget the roof. The club surely had access to the rear courtyard, from the basement if not from the parlor floor, so that's where he could direct his efforts, if indeed he could hide out while everybody else went home. The club's rear exit would be locked, but fire laws assured that they could be opened from within. And there'd be a rear door for the monastery, and if he could work out a way to open it, why then he'd be in the basement of the monastery, surrounded by cellar-dwelling monks wondering who he was and what in hell he was doing there.

That was as far as he got before the formal meeting began. Then the guest speaker began talking and showing his PowerPoint presentation, and Keller had the good fortune to get caught up in it and, at least for the time being, forget all about Father Paul Vincent O'Herlihy and the impregnable fortress that kept the man out of harm's way.

Thursday morning, Keller woke up early. During his shower he realized that he felt good, and wondered why. He decided that somehow, during the night, he'd resigned himself to the failure of his assignment, and would be glad simply to be getting home.

He found the same food cart as yesterday, ordered the same breakfast of croissant and coffee, and told himself he'd just saved another $30. And yesterday, by God, he'd fed himself all day for the couple of dollars breakfast cost him. The coffee and sandwiches at Peachpit had been a satisfactory lunch, and he'd skipped supper after having enjoyed the food and drink at the Connoisseurs. And now, while he enjoyed feeding his trim body a light breakfast, the plump and stately P. V. O'Herlihy would already be pouring the first of today's whiskey down his throat while he prepared to sweat out yesterday's, and—

Wait a minute.

He dropped the remains of his croissant in the trash, followed it with his unfinished coffee. No time to waste. Things to do, people to see.

Alphabet City had already changed substantially when Keller was last there, its nasty tenements getting rehabbed left and right for young monied tenants. Now it was even harder to recall what a foul pit it had once been.

But he was comforted to see it was still a place to cop, if you could use your eyes and knew how to comport yourself. Keller, on East 5th Street between Avenues C and D, watched business being done, and got into character. He picked out the right man to approach and braced him.

"Got that," the fellow said. "Say you want a set of works, too? You sure 'bout that? Nobody shoots this shit, man. These downs, they ain't like lady or smack. You shoot up, you gone get abscesses."

"It's for a friend," Keller told him.

"The very best," the man said reverently. "It's not a single malt, mind you. Some of the special-batch single malts can get up there in price, but what we have here is a blend of several malt whiskeys, aged for an astonishing sixty years."

"And you say it's five hundred dollars?"

"A towering sum for a bottle of Scotch," the man admitted. He was wearing the vest and trousers of a three-piece gray suit, with a fresh white shirt and what Keller had to think was the tie of a good regiment. His hair was styled and his mustache trimmed, and he looked just right for his role behind the counter of a Madison Avenue purveyor of fine wines and spirits.

"The price," he continued, "is ten times that of any number of truly excellent Scotches. But to keep it in perspective, we've any number of bottles of wine for which we'd have to get three or four times as much, and some that are quite stratospheric in price. A Latour of the right vintage, a Lafite Rothschild—and to open such a bottle is to finish it. An hour or two and you've emptied it, whereas a liter of whiskey can be best enjoyed a dram at a time, over months or even years. And every time your man has his sip, he's reminded of the generosity of the giver."

"It certainly looks expensive," Keller said.

"At the very least, the packaging is equal to the contents.

Notice the bottle is sealed with lead over its twist-to-open cork stopper. Notice the wooden casket that holds the bottle, brass-bound and equipped with its own tiny brass key. It looks not only expensive but special. One glance and the recipient cannot fail to be aware of the high esteem in which you hold him."

"Well, that's important," Keller said, and drew out his wallet.

What was called for, Keller thought, was a Bunsen burner. And if he were back in his high school chemistry lab, he'd have the use of one. But he was in his room at the Savoyard, and had to make do with a candle.

He'd opened all fifteen of the purple-and-yellow capsules, and their contents pretty much filled the steel serving spoon. He'd bought it, and the little votive candle as well, at a housewares store. The spoon had been paired with a serving fork, which he'd discarded on the way back to the hotel. The candle came in a little glass container, and the Hebrew lettering on its paper label suggested it was some sort of Jewish memorial light.

He added a few drops of tap water to the grains of powder, then held the spoon in the candle's flame. A Bunsen burner couldn't have served him any better; the powder liquefied, and he was able to draw up almost all of it into the hypodermic syringe.

Now the bottle. Remove the lead seal? No, he'd never get it back just right. Easier to go right through the seal and the cork beneath it. Would it reach? Yes, easily, and he depressed the plunger all the way.

After he'd rinsed out both spoon and syringe, he had a look at the bottle. There was a visible pinhole in the lead seal. He could probably let it go, but could he fix it?

The lead extended almost two inches down the neck of the bottle. Keller helped himself to a small piece of the lowest portion, used the spoon and the candle to melt it, and used the softened lead to patch the top of the seal. The pinhole was gone.

He placed the bottle in its handsome wooden container, fastened the little lock. Reached for the wrapping paper.

TWENTY

Dear Father O'Herlihy,

First I must apologize for my intrusion into your life. I should never have bothered you, especially at a difficult time. Although my memory seemed real to me, you helped me to see that it was false, and I find myself wondering how many others have been unjustly smeared as a result of such false memories.

But I must thank you for removing the veil. I now understand what really happened, and that is the first step toward recovery. I feel much better already.

So I hope you will accept this gift as a token of apology and gratitude. I hope it brings you closure equal to mine.

Yours in Christ,
Timothy Michael Hannan

Keller looked over what he'd written out on a sheet of hotel stationery. He added a set of quotation marks around *memory* in the third sentence, and frowned at the last line. Closure? Oh, it was cute enough, but was cute what was wanted here? He crossed it out, and considered other last lines, and rejected them all. Was anything needed after *gratitude*? Not really.

On the front of the card he'd bought it said THANK YOU!, the words surrounded by unidentifiable flowers, and inside he copied his amended draft, using handwriting quite different from his own. The letters were small and carefully formed, and he felt they made a nice match with the voice and manner he'd given young Hannan.

Near the end, he hesitated. *Yours in Christ.* Was that too much?

Oh, the hell with it. He left it in.

Keller, carrying a shopping bag and wearing a brand-new short-sleeved shirt with a button-down collar, let the Savoyard's doorman flag a cab for him. In the cab he put on the plain dark blue tie he'd tucked in the bag, checking the rearview mirror to get the knot right.

Still in the bag, along with the gift-wrapped bottle of Scotch, was a billed cap the same medium blue as the shirt. The clerk who'd sold it to him had called it a Greek fisherman's cap, but to Keller it looked like something a messenger might wear.

The cab dropped him at the corner of 36th and Madison, and once it had driven off he put the cap on his head, tucked the package under his arm, and dropped the empty shopping bag in a trash basket. Then he walked straight to Thessalonian House, where he finally got the chance to use the brass knocker. It was satisfying, and enough time passed so that he was about to do it again, when the door opened to reveal a plump little monk in a nut-brown robe.

"Express rush delivery," said Keller, in Timothy Hannan's voice. "For Abbot Paul O'Herlihy. You'll make sure he gets it right away, won't you?"

Two blocks from the monastery, Keller ditched the Greek fisherman's cap and caught another cab back to his hotel. He took a quick shower, put on a clean shirt, finished packing, and went downstairs to check out. He shook off the doorman and walked, arriving at the Peachpit offices in plenty of time for a pre-session sandwich and coffee.

Before things got underway, he went to the men's room and locked himself in a stall, where he had a chance to count the cash in his money belt. He had a little over $12,000, and it was okay with him if he spent every cent of it.

Keller got to JFK hours before his flight. He remembered, finally, to buy a plush rabbit for Jenny, who collected stuffed animals as ardently as he collected stamps. He checked his bag, the rabbit snugly stowed inside it, and picked up his boarding pass, then found a bar with a TV tuned to local news. He ordered a Diet Coke, and of course the third news item reported a new link between sugar-free soft drinks and cancer. The barmaid evidently heard the item herself, and glanced at Keller even as he was looking her way.

Neither of them had to speak a word. She scooped up his glass, dumped its contents, rinsed it, and looked inquiringly at him. He pointed to a bottle of beer, which she uncapped and placed before him, along with the glass. He reached for his wallet, but she shook her head and walked off to serve somebody else.

The beer lasted Keller for most of an hour. He was waiting for a particular news item, not really expecting to hear it, but disappointed all the same.

Waiting was always the hardest part.

Around seven thirty he realized that a sandwich and the better part of a croissant didn't amount to a full day's rations. He moved from the bar to a nearby table, where he ordered a Caesar salad with grilled shrimp and a second beer. The salad wasn't bad. Neither was the beer, but half of it was plenty.

He could see and hear the bar's TV from where he was sitting, so he got another go-round with the sports and weather and various fires and traffic wrecks. And nothing much else.

Just as they were about to call his flight for boarding, he took out his cell phone and called Dot. "I'm heading home," he said.

"Well, I can't say I'm surprised. I don't know why I sent you in the first place. I'll send back the money."

"No, don't do that," he said.

"No?"

"Not just yet," he said. "Wait three days and see what happens."

"Three days?"

"Maybe four."

"Four days. I could do that. I mean, they don't know you're on your way home, do they?"

He ended the call, stopped in the men's room. Was the phone compromised? Even if it wasn't, what did he need with it now? He took it apart, snapped the chip in half, and did other things to render the thing inoperative. He dropped the different components in different trash receptacles and went to board his plane.

*　*　*

"She's going to love this," Julia said, brandishing the rabbit. "Not only is it wonderfully soft and squishy, it's from her daddy. Why don't you go put it in her bed and she'll find it when she wakes up?"

Was there anything more beautiful than Jenny sleeping? He tucked in the rabbit at her side and returned to the kitchen, where he looked at his wife and found an answer to his question.

"I'm a rotten husband," he said. "I didn't bring you anything."

"You came back in one piece," she said. "That's good enough. Did you bring a story to get me all excited?"

"Not quite yet."

That puzzled her, but she let it go. "Not a problem," she said. "Tonight you won't need a story. You know what they say about absence? Well, it's not just the heart that grows fonder."

"Now, here's a stamp I'm happy to have," Keller said, lifting Gabon number 48 with his stamp tongs. "If you just take a quick look, you'd think it was the same as this one here. Denomination's the same, five francs, colors are the same, and you've got the same picture. That's a woman of the Fang tribe, and isn't she pretty?"

"Pity," Jenny agreed.

"When I was a little boy, I had some of these stamps. Well, ones just like them. The low values. You see this stamp? It shows a warrior, also of the Fang tribe, and he's a man, and very fierce. But I saw the fancy headdress and always thought he was a woman. Funny, huh?"

"Funny."

"Now what makes this stamp different," Keller said, even as he slipped the stamp into the mount he'd cut for it, "is the inscription. It says 'Congo Français,' and the other one says 'Afrique Equatoriale,' so it belongs to the first of the two sets. It goes in the last blank space on the page, one I've been looking to fill for years now. There. Doesn't it look nice?"

"Nice 'tamp."

"Gabon was a French colony in West Africa," he told her. "It issued stamps until 1934, when it was merged into French Equatorial Africa. Now of course it's an independent country, but Daddy's collection only goes to 1940, so his Gabon stamps stop in 1933."

"Maybe Daddy'll take us to Gabon someday," Julia said. "You know what we ought to get? A globe, so you could show her where all the countries are. I can see how you thought the warrior was a woman. Though you might have noticed that he's holding a couple of spears."

"A fierce woman," he said. "A globe's a good idea. That's probably what I should have bought instead of the stuffed rabbit."

"Well, globe or no globe, don't try to take the rabbit away from her. She'll tear your arm off."

"Rabbit," Jenny said.

"A bunny rabbit," Keller agreed. "One of your better words, isn't it? Now, these stamps are interesting. They aren't very pretty, but there's a great story that goes with them. See, they're from German East Africa, which was a German colony before the First World War."

"Like Koochoo, which Daddy told you about, except even your mommy can tell where this one's located."

"Kiauchau."

"Gesundheit. I was close, wasn't I?"

"You were," Keller said. "But listen to this, will you? During the war, the post office in German East Africa couldn't get stamps from the fatherland, so they had these printed by the evangelical mission in Wuga—"

"Wuga," Jenny echoed.

"See, sweetie? Now Daddy's talking your language."

"—but before they were needed, new stamps did arrive from Germany. Then, with British troops advancing, the postal authorities buried all of the Wuga stamps—"

"Wuga. Wuga."

"—to keep the Brits from capturing them. Stamps! Why would they care if the enemy captured the stamps? They were overrunning the whole colony, for God's sake."

"Who thought that up, the same genius who ran your Yankee post office during the War of the Northern Aggression?"

"You'd almost think so," he said. "After the war, before the colony was taken away from Germany and parceled out to Britain and Belgium, the Germans dug up the stamps. Most of them were so damaged from being buried that they had to be destroyed, and the rest weren't exactly pristine, but they took them home and auctioned them off."

"And you've got a whole sheet of them."

"Of the seven and a half heller, yes. It's the least expensive of the three denominations, but an actual unbroken sheet— well, let's just say I wasn't the only person who wanted it."

No one actually present in the room had fought him for it, but there was competition online, and a phone bidder who just wouldn't quit. But here he was, trimming a large sheet of plastic mounting material to fit, and preparing a blank album page to receive it.

The sheet was fragile, and he handled it with great delicacy.

He'd have done so anyway, but having shelled out a small fortune for it made him especially careful with it.

Would he get the money back? He'd put on CNN at breakfast, behavior uncharacteristic enough to get a raised eyebrow
from Julia, if not a question. He'd been hoping for a particular
news item from New York, the same one he'd hoped for at the
airport bar.

No luck. And there were so many things that could go
wrong, the most likely of which being that O'Herlihy would
decide to save this magnificent bottle for a special occasion, or
even attempt to curry favor by passing it on to a bishop. Keller
had an awful vision of the brass-bound casket ascending up
the hierarchy, until it wound up carrying off the Holy Father
himself.

Things to think about while affixing an extraordinary pane
of stamps to an album page. And while Jenny was standing
patiently at his side, waiting for him to tell her more about
what he was doing. So he told her how the Belgian portion
of German East Africa had been known as Ruanda-Urundi,
but when it became independent it split into two countries,
Rwanda and Burundi.

"Wanda," Jenny said. "Rundi."

TWENTY-ONE

I t's Dot."
   He looked up. It was remarkable how stamps took him into another dimension. He hadn't been aware that Julia had left the room, hadn't heard the phone ring, hadn't heard her return, and here she was, handing him the phone.

"Well, congratulations," Dot said. "Your horse came in and paid a good price."

"Oh?"

"There's an online news feed that keeps you up to the minute," she said, "and the story's breaking right now. Respected religious leader, blah blah blah, extreme stress, blah blah blah, expected to provide invaluable testimony, blah blah blah."

"Sounds as though it's mostly blah blah blah."

"Well, isn't that always the way, Keller? Everything is mostly blah blah blah. What it boils down to, evidently the poor fellow got this special bottle of whiskey and it was so good he drank more than his usual amount."

"His usual amount," Keller said, "was enough to float a battleship."

"Oh, this is interesting. Preliminary examination suggests that the alcoholic intake was exacerbated by barbiturates. The man washed down sleeping pills with booze, and that's never a good idea, is it?"

"No."

"Death by misadventure," she said. "Now I have to wonder how you got him to take the pills. And if I had to guess, I'd say you dissolved them in the whiskey. Which would be good."

"Why?"

"Because once the lab works its magic on the leftover booze, they'll know what really happened. And that'll keep the client from whining that he doesn't want to pay us for something that happened all by itself. Not that I'd let him get away with that, but who needs the hassle?"

"Not us."

"You betcha. So I don't have to give the money back, and they have to send us some more. You happy?"

"Very."

"And New York was all right?"

"New York was fine."

"And I'll bet you brought home some stamps. Well, you must want to go play with them, so I'll let you go now. Now put Jenny on the phone so Aunt Dot can give her a big kiss."

"See?" Keller said. "I told you it wasn't exciting."

"It was a problem," Julia said, "and a complicated one, and you tried different things, and in the end you found the solution. How could that fail to be exciting?"

"Well…"

"Oh, because there was no action? No slam-bang adventure? The life of the mind is exciting enough, at least for those of us who have one."

It was evening, and Jenny had gone to bed, clutching her new rabbit. Julia and Keller were at the kitchen table, drinking coffee with chicory.

"I wasn't sure it would work," he said.

"But you came home anyway."

"Well, if it didn't work, what was I going to do about it? I didn't have anything else to try." He thought for a moment. "Besides, I was ready to come home. I had you and Jenny to come home to."

"Otherwise you'd have stayed there."

"Probably. But there wouldn't have been any real point to it."

"More coffee?"

"No, I'm good. Does it bother you that he was a priest?"

"No, why should it?"

"Well, it's your church."

"Only in the most tenuous way. I'm the child of lapsed Catholics. I was baptized, that was their sole concession to their own upbringing, but it was pretty much the extent of my own involvement with the Church."

"I never asked you if you wanted Jenny baptized."

"Don't you think I'd have said something? Do you even know what baptism is for?"

"Isn't it to make you a Catholic?"

"No, darling, guilt is what makes you a Catholic. What baptism does is rid you of original sin. Do you suppose our daughter is greatly weighed down by the burden of original sin?"

"I don't even know how you could go about finding an original sin these days."

"I suppose selling somebody else's kidney might qualify. And no, what do I care about some fat drunken priest whose greatest boast was that all his sins were strictly heterosexual? You want to know what's exciting?"

"What?"

"That you can tell me all this. That we can sit here drinking coffee —"

"Damn good coffee, too."

"—and either of us can tell the other anything about anything, and how many people have anything like that? God, though, I have to say I'm glad you're home."

"Me, too," Keller said.

KELLER AT SEA

TWENTY-TWO

Whan Julia and Jenny got home from day care, Keller was sitting in the kitchen with a cup of coffee and a magazine, *The American Stamp Dealer & Collector*. He'd picked it up after he got off the phone, but couldn't keep his mind on what he was reading. It was restless, darting all over the place. So he was more than happy to set it aside and ask his daughter what she'd learned in school that morning.

It wasn't a school, and the harried woman who ran it didn't try to teach her charges much; she was happy if she managed to keep them from hitting each other and screaming their little heads off. But Jenny, Julia had reported, called it school, and took the whole enterprise very seriously. As far as she was concerned, she went there to learn stuff, and it seemed to piss her off that they weren't teaching her to read.

So Julia had picked up a book on phonics, and Jenny was learning to sound words out. You couldn't always understand what she was saying, because there were words she couldn't yet get her tongue around, but damned if she wasn't reading.

She had her lunch and went in for her nap, and Keller asked Julia if she'd like to go on a cruise.

"A cruise," she said. "You mean like on a ship? Yes, of course that's what you mean. A cruise. You know, that sounds heavenly. When were you thinking? In the winter?"

"Actually," he said, "it would be sooner than that."

"Late fall?"

"A lot sooner."

"Oh. Can you get away?"

"There's no work," he said. "Getting away has never been less of a problem. Donny called me this morning, very apologetic. He's hired on with a contractor based over in Slidell. Says the pay's not much but he's sick of sitting in front of the TV while he runs through his savings. At least he'll have something to do and some money coming in."

"That part's good. But he must feel awful."

Donny Wallings had given Keller a job when he'd first moved in with Julia, and almost before Keller knew it he'd found himself a partner in an enterprise that bought distressed homes, patched them up, and flipped them. That worked well in the early post-Katrina days, but then the economy cratered and there was no money to be had for home renovation loans, no money to finance home sales. And, just like that, no business.

"He was concerned about us," Keller said. "But I told him we were okay."

"Are we? I mean I know we are, but can we afford to pick up and go on a cruise? You know, if we can it's actually the perfect kind of vacation. I bet Jenny'd love it, too. There are plenty of cruises out of New Orleans, and you can literally walk from here to the cruise port. Unless our ship uses the Poland Avenue terminal, and that's what, a ten-minute ride?"

"We'd be leaving from Fort Lauderdale," he said.

"In Florida?" She looked at him. "You've got a particular cruise in mind. Did somebody call this morning? Besides Donny?"

He'd just got off the phone with Donny when it rang again. He picked it up, and Dot said, "Keller, I can't help thinking you need a vacation. But before I go any further, there's something I have to ask you. Do you get seasick?"

"Seasick?"

"You know, rushing to the rail, tossing your cookies, feeding the fish? Seasick, Keller. What happens to you on the high seas?"

"I don't know," he said.

"You've never been on a boat? And the Staten Island Ferry doesn't count."

"I've been on the Gulf," he said. "I don't know if that counts. A friend of Julia's, well, he and his wife are actually friends of both of us by now—"

"Do I really need to know that part, Keller?"

"Probably not. I've been out a few times. Fishing, but I have to admit I never caught anything."

"But you didn't get seasick? Have they got waves there?"

"It's the Gulf of Mexico," he said, "so yes, there are waves, but they don't toss you around all that much. One time it was a little choppy, but I hardly noticed it."

"So you're a good sailor, Keller. And the cruise ships have stabilizers, and you can always take Dramamine, so I'm sure you'll do fine. Keller? Where'd you go?"

"I'm right here, waiting for you to tell me what you're talking about."

"Oh," she said, "I thought it was perfectly obvious. You're going on a cruise."

* * *

"Saturday," Julia said. "Monday, Tuesday, Wednesday, Thursday, Friday, Saturday. Why are you looking at me like that?"

"If you were Jenny," he said, "I'd congratulate you for getting your days right."

"My point is there's not much time."

"I know."

"I suppose we'd have to fly over there on Friday."

"The ship doesn't sail until late afternoon. We could get a flight Saturday morning and be there in plenty of time."

"It sails from Fort Lauderdale and returns to Fort Lauderdale. So you're back where you started. There's a pointlessness about it that's curiously appealing."

"There is?"

"Yet at the same time," she said, "it won't be entirely pointless, will it? You'll be working."

"That's right, and I can see where that might be a dealbreaker right there. There's something I'll have to do."

"Something you'll have to do. Some passenger for whom the cruise will have a surprise ending. Do they still bury people at sea?"

"I don't think so."

"There's probably an ecological argument against it, though I couldn't think why. People are biodegradable, aren't they?" She stepped behind him, put her hands on his shoulders, and began to knead the muscles. "You're all tense," she announced. "This feel good?"

"Very."

"I know what you do," she said, "and I don't entirely know how I feel about it, but I don't seem to mind. I honestly don't."

"I know."

"But I'm not there when it happens, am I? And in a sense I wouldn't be this time either, in that I wouldn't be in the room when—when what? When push came to shove?"

"When it goes down," he suggested.

"That works. I wouldn't be in the room, or I suppose you call it a cabin. Or is it a stateroom? Is there a difference between a cabin and a stateroom?"

"I have no idea."

"Does Dot know you're thinking about taking me along?"

"She suggested it."

"You're kidding."

"She apologized for the fact that it wasn't that long since New York, and I said I didn't really feel like being separated from you again so soon. 'It's a nice big cabin,' she said. 'Plenty of room for two.' And she went on to say I'd be a lot less conspicuous if I had a companion."

"That actually makes sense."

"I guess."

"'Look at that handsome gentleman all by himself. I wonder what his story might be.' But with me along you're far less interesting. I want to come."

"To make me less interesting?"

"Partly that. Partly because I've never been on a cruise. Partly because I don't feel like being home in New Orleans while you're island-hopping. And partly because it scares me."

"Then why—"

"'Do the thing you're afraid of.' I read that somewhere. Don't ask me where."

"I won't."

"But as for taking Jenny—"

"No."

"Even if I were deranged enough to think it was a good idea, we don't have time to get her a passport. She'd need one, wouldn't she?"

"It doesn't matter, because neither of us is nuts enough to take her. But yes, she'd have to have a passport."

"These days you just about need one to cross a state line. Well, this way she'll have her own vacation." She went to the phone, dialed a number she didn't have to look up. She said, "Claudia? Julia Edwards. Darlin', Nicholas told me how Donny's hired on with a crew, and I just want to say I was glad to hear it. Not that he had to but that he was able to, you know? And I know Nicholas already told Donny that we're fine here, but I wanted to say so myself, to you…"

Keller knew where the conversation was headed, but didn't feel the need to listen to it. He reached for his magazine and got lost in an article about a recently discovered cache of letters to and from a young Mississippian in Pemberton's army who'd been killed during Grant's siege of Vicksburg. He surfaced in time to hear Julia say she had a real big favor to ask, and Claudia should feel completely comfortable saying no. Then he went back to a letter filled with the youth's big plans for after the war was over. The letter was dated March 7, 1863, at which time its author had all of three months to live.

"…can't thank you enough," he heard, which wouldn't stop her from trying. Phone calls in New Orleans seemed to go on longer than in most places, especially if there was a woman on either end of the line. He tuned out again, and stayed lost in the magazine until Julia returned to the table.

"We're all set," she announced. "Claudia can't think of anything she and Donny'd rather have than Jenny's company for a week, not to mention her kids'll be over the moon about it. They place her somewhere between a baby sister and a house pet. And she loves going over there, so she'll just have a slightly longer visit than usual."

He got to his feet. "I'd better book our flight," he said.

"You've got the easy part, mister. I have to figure out what to pack."

TWENTY-THREE

Cruise ships out of Fort Lauderdale docked at Port Ever-glades, a six-mile cab ride from the airport. Keller paid the driver, who wished them both *buen viaje,* which was close enough to bon voyage for Keller to figure it out.

If packing for Julia had been a trial, she'd nevertheless managed to narrow down her choices to fit in a single medium-size suitcase. Keller's bag was smaller, and he carried his and wheeled hers through the cruise terminal and down the walkway to where their ship was receiving passengers.

Their ship, the *Carefree Nights,* looked large to Keller, but not after he'd seen the leviathans berthed on either side of her. Their cabin was on the second of five passenger decks, and once they were in it Keller excused himself and made his way back to the terminal.

He'd had an eye out for a man in a Hawaiian shirt and a New York Yankees baseball cap, and the guy had evidently had his eye out for Keller, too, because they'd exchanged nods and glances the first time through. Keller found him now, and, though it struck him as unnecessary, went through the prescribed ritual.

"Mr. Gallagher?"

"Absolutely," the man said. "Mr. Shean?"

"Positively."

"That fuckin' Dot," said the man, whose name was no more Gallagher than Keller's was Shean. "I swear the woman watches too much TV. Like we're not gonna be able to find each other." He took off his cap, set it on the floor under his seat. "There's some who look good in hats and some who don't, and we know which kind I am. And this fuckin' shirt." He glanced at the shirt Keller was wearing. "That one's her idea, too, right?"

The polo shirt, with narrow red horizontal stripes on a navy field, was one of Keller's favorites. He couldn't think of a response, and that turned out to be response enough.

"Actually," Gallagher said, "it's an okay shirt. Here, have a seat. I wish I could tell you to enjoy the boat ride, that it's all taken care of. Though how anybody could enjoy a boat ride's beyond me altogether."

"I guess it's not your thing."

"Let me put it this way, Shean. I take lots of showers. You know why?"

Keller could guess—guilt, a need to expunge the recent past. But that wasn't it.

"Because I don't even like bathtubs is why. They show *The Poseidon Adventure* on TV, I change the channel. The remote's on the fritz, I'll walk across the room to do it."

Keller, who couldn't help thinking of the man as Gallagher, felt that showed real commitment.

"What I like," Gallagher said, "is the long shot. I'm not talking gambling here, Shean. I'm talking riflery. I grew up in L.A., I never touched a gun my whole life, and I went in the service and they took me out to the rifle range, and I couldn't miss. Qualified as expert rifleman first time out, and the next thing I know I'm in sniper school. Join the army, learn a trade."

It would have been different, Keller thought, if he'd joined the navy.

"So I get a call. The subject's holed up in a house in Hallandale. That's a little ways south of here. Takes some doing, but I find a spot where I can set up. Minute he walks out the door, he's mine."

"But he never leaves the house."

"Oh, Dot told you? Maybe he leaves and maybe he don't, I couldn't tell you, because all I ever see is this black Lexus with tinted glass all around. Fuckin' car comes and goes, in and out of the attached garage. Is he ever inside it? Maybe yes, maybe no. When he's home, does he ever stand in front of the nice big picture window? Again, maybe yes, maybe no, because it's got curtains and they're never open. Two weeks I'm sitting on that house, and I never get a glimpse of the son of a bitch, let alone get to draw a bead on him. So let me ask you, Shean. What would you do?"

"I don't know. Maybe try to get into the house."

Gallagher shook his head. "What I didn't mention," he said, "is they got guards posted. There's a car just sits across the street twenty-four seven, three shifts, two men to a shift. UPS shows up, somebody pops out of the car, braces the driver, takes the package, and walks it up to the door. The newsboy knows the drill; he don't even throw the paper onto the porch, he brings it straight to the car and lets them deliver it for him. Nobody gets close to the house, let alone into it."

Keller thought of Thessalonian House, the phoned-in bomb threat, the meeting in the steam room. "You'd have to draw him out," he said.

"How?" Keller didn't have the answer, and Gallagher said, "Yeah, well, there you go. Then I get the word, they're so fuckin' proud of themselves, on account of they got him booked on a cruise, and there's a cabin just waiting for me. Yeah, right. So that's where you come in."

"He gets seasick," Dot had said. "Who knew? And even if I had known, nobody asked me. The client went ahead on his own and hooked him with a free cruise."

"How?"

"'Dear Mr. Dimwit, you've won a free all-expenses-paid cruise of the West Indies on the Good Ship Lollipop.'"

"And he fell for it?"

"Keller, how many times have the cops mailed out announcements to all the mopes with outstanding wants and warrants? 'You just won a free flat-panel plasma TV! Show up such and such a place, such and such a time, to claim your prize!' These are wanted criminals, Keller, and you'd think if they wanted a television set they'd go out and steal one, but year after year the cops throw a party like this, and year after year morons show up for it."

"Even so."

"I know, I know. Maybe he was going stir-crazy, cooped up and guarded around the clock. Maybe he just wanted to assert himself. 'Yes, I need your protection, but I still get to live my life.' And who knows if he'll actually wind up getting on the ship? He could come to his senses by Saturday, but let's hope he doesn't. Because he's a lot softer target on open water. As long as you're not stuck in your cabin, puking your guts out."

"No way I'm getting on a boat," Gallagher said. "Sitting here is as close as I want to get, and we're on a concrete floor on dry land, and I swear I can just about feel the motion. So I thought, okay, I got a couple of days, maybe I'll get a shot. Yeah, right. You know what I wanted to do? The garage door rolls up, the black Lexus comes out, and what I wanted to do was empty a clip into the fucking thing."

"That might work," Keller allowed.

"If he's in the vehicle, and if it's not reinforced and bulletproof six ways and backwards, and if I get lucky. Shean, getting lucky's not what I'm about. What I'm about is the subject's in the crosshairs and a single well-placed shot puts him forever in the past tense."

Keller thought that last phrase was a nice one. He had a feeling Gallagher must have heard it somewhere before making it his own.

"So I got no real complaints," Gallagher said, "on account of I get to keep the advance. It would have been nice to close the deal, but I got paid and I get to go home now, and that's not so bad. I thought they might get sloppy today, but the Lexus pulled out of the garage same as always, and I kept my finger off the trigger. I jumped in my ride and got here before they did, and if you were already here I'd a pointed him out to you, but I didn't see anybody fitting your description, and nobody approached me looking for Mr. Gallagher."

"I came straight from the airport."

"I found this seat," Gallagher said, "on account of the good view it gave me, and twenty minutes goes by, and thirty, and forty, and where is he? Did he get past me? Well, you're not here, so there's nobody to point him out to, but if I don't see him get on maybe he changed his mind, in which case my job's not done. You follow me?"

"Sure."

"Then he shows, and he's got this babe with him." Gallagher cupped his hands and held them in front of his chest. "Va-va-voom, right? Maybe she's old enough to vote, but not by much. Maybe Latina, maybe not, and what's the difference what she is? The woman is a total fox." He sighed. "Son of a bitch's got thirty-five, maybe forty years on her. Was she in the house all along? I never saw her, but I never saw him, neither, or anybody else but the guys sitting in the car across the street. My guess is that's where the forty minutes went, driving somewhere to pick her up, and she's still got packing to do, and makeup to freshen and all those things women find to do with time." He shook his head. "I'm talking too much. Sorry. I been sitting on my ass for two weeks, staring at nothing and doing less, and the only talking I've done's been to the weather guy on TV. 'Oh, yeah? Call that a perfect day, asshole? It's too fuckin' hot.'"

"Well," Keller said.

"Right. Here's the photo they sent me. He lost the beard since it was taken, and in my opinion he shoulda kept it, but otherwise he looks about the same. Don't ask me what name he's using."

"They booked his cabin under his own name," Keller said.

"Carmody, huh?"

"Michael Carmody. I'll check the passenger manifest. Anyway, he's got one of the premium cabins on the Sun Deck, and there are only four of them, so he won't be hard to find."

"Please," Gallagher said, holding a hand to his stomach.

"Stop it with the nautical terms, okay? I had lunch just three hours ago."

"Sorry."

"I been sitting here all along," Gallagher said. "And I been keeping one eye on the entrance and exit over there, and they haven't come back."

"Him and his girlfriend?"

"Why would they come back? If they weren't fixing to take their boat ride they wouldn't've come here in the first place. No, I'm talking about the muscle."

"Muscle."

"Security, bodyguards, whatever you want to call 'em. The two guys in suits who walked him and her through the door and up to where they look at your tickets and make sure you're getting on the right boat."

"He had escorts."

"Yeah, that's as good a word as any, though it's got a couple different meanings. I had an escort the other night, called a number in the phone book. Two hundred and fifty bucks and she had one eye on her watch the whole time. Nice tits, I got to admit. That's worth something, right?"

"Sure. Uh, his escorts—"

"Frick and Frack. I figure they're just seeing him to his room, checking out the basic situation. But they don't come back. No way anybody suckered them into thinking they won a cruise, so how do you figure that?"

Keller checked his watch. The escorts still had an hour before the scheduled departure time, but if they were still on the ship this late, they were probably there for the duration. The target's minders, unable to dissuade him from the cruise, had simply booked a cabin for a pair of their own men. If a private citizen like Dot had been able to get Keller on the ship, why couldn't the other side, with the full force of the law working for them, do as much themselves?

He asked Gallagher how he'd know them.

"You watch football? One's built like a tight end, the other's more of a running back. That give you a picture?"

"Sort of."

"Just look for two guys in suits. Not gonna get many of those on a fuckin' cruise, are you? And I know what you're gonna say."

"Oh?"

"'Suppose they change their clothes?' Which, granted, they might. So look for two guys who look like they're wearing casual clothes for the first time in twenty years. Hey, you'll spot 'em, Shean. They'll stick out like a couple of thumbs."

TWENTY-FOUR

A little after six, while Keller and Julia were in the Club Lounge for the Bon Voyage cocktail party, the *Carefree Nights* set sail for the Bahamas. Members of the dining room staff passed trays of drinks, and Keller picked off a pair of margaritas. He barely touched his, and offered it to Julia when she'd finished her own, but one was all she wanted.

She fell into conversation with an older woman who turned out to be from Mobile, and the two of them got caught up in a spirited game of Who Do You Know? That left Keller and the woman's husband to talk about sports or the stock market, say, but the fellow wasn't much of a talker, and the set of his face and the way he walked suggested that he might be recovering from a stroke. He seemed content to listen to the two women, or not listen, and that was fine with Keller, who was too busy scanning the room to pay much attention to anything else.

He didn't see Michael Anthony Carmody, whose photo was now in Keller's back pocket. Nor did he see any men in suits, or indeed anyone built like a football player, whether a tight end or a running back. Aside from the ship's staff, most of the people in the room looked as though they'd had their AARP cards long enough to forget where they'd put them. Carmody wouldn't stand out in their company, but his entourage would.

"Like thumbs," he said, not realizing he'd spoken out loud until Julia and her new friend shot him a glance. "Nothing," he said. "Just thinking out loud."

"Well, I'm not planning on thinking for the next seven nights," said the woman from Mobile. "Out loud or otherwise. I do enough of that back home. All I plan on doing is drinking and eating and laying out in the sun."

"And shopping," her husband said, proving he could speak after all.

"Well, maybe a little bit of that," she said. "Just to stay in practice."

After the lifeboat drill, Keller found his way to where they posted the names and cabin assignments. There was no Carmody listed, and Keller wasn't surprised. He figured it wouldn't be the trickiest thing in the world to get yourself listed under an alias, as long as you carried legitimate ID. Wasn't that what celebrities did? And didn't the people trying to keep Carmody alive have more than enough clout for that?

He went all the way through the list, and all four Sun Deck cabins were occupied, and none of the names meant anything to him.

There was an elevator—with the median age of this crowd, there would really have to be—but Keller took the stairs to the Sun Deck. There was a pool, which surprised him; he somehow hadn't imagined that you'd carry a pool of your own out into the middle of the ocean. Lounge chairs ranged around the pool, and there was what looked to be a health club, with a couple of treadmills and a Universal machine. And, toward the rear of the ship, he saw a little block of staterooms.

The stern, he thought. That was what they called the back end of the ship, and the front was the bow. And port and starboard were left and right.

Keller, wondering why you needed a whole new vocabulary the minute you left shore, felt the ship's motion. He hadn't really paid any attention to it until now. It didn't bother him, not as much as the new names for left and right and front and back and up and down. *Topside,* he thought. *Below.* Jesus.

He wasn't seasick, not at all, but all the same he found himself feeling a common bond with Gallagher.

At dinner, they shared a table with three other couples, and Keller didn't find out much about any of them. The conversation was mostly of other ships and past cruises, and that left him and Julia without much to contribute. It also made their company hugely useful to the others, who were able to tell them which ships they should avoid, which ones they were sure to love, and no end of other tips that demanded little more from Keller than a thoughtful nod, or the observation that he'd certainly have to keep that in mind.

Keller didn't see Carmody anywhere, or anybody who looked young enough to be his daughter, or to move Gallagher to cup his hands and say whatever it was he'd said. Va-va-voom?

Of course Carmody, like any of *Carefree Night*'s passengers, had the option of dining in his stateroom. And if his companion was indeed of the va-va-voom sort, and if this was a maiden voyage for the two of them, well, it stood to reason that the man might be reluctant to leave his cabin, at least for the first day or two. And there was also the chance that—

"Oh, my," Julia murmured.

Keller looked up, and saw where she was looking, and noted that half the people in the dining room were looking in the same direction.

Va-va-voom!

"I didn't know it would be like this," Julia said.

"What? The ship? Our cabin?"

They were back in their cabin now, and free at last to talk about the strawberry blonde knockout who'd stopped all dining room conversation in its tracks.

She shook her head. "Seeing him ahead of time. Oh, come on. That was him, wasn't it? The man playing Mr. December to her Miss May? Except that sweet young thing's barely made it into April. Is statutory rape legal in international waters?"

"I don't think anybody's going to arrest him."

"Still, he's got to be your assignment. Did you get a look at the two hoods keeping the charming couple company? A nice little table for four, and they all came in together and left together. I'm sure those two were carrying guns."

"The two younger men, you mean."

She gave him a look. "Just tell me I'm not spinning an elaborate story out of thin air. It's him, isn't it?"

"I wasn't going to say anything."

"No, and I wasn't going to try to coax it out of you, because I wasn't sure I wanted to know. Although it might be worse, having to be careful not to get too friendly with any of the women because one of their husbands might be the very man my husband was here to—do I want a euphemism? To nullify, to take off the board, what?"

"There's just the two of us here," he pointed out.

"You're right. To kill. Although I'm not sure you're going to have to kill anybody. She'll do it for you."

"Because she's young?"

"Darling, did you look at her? And don't tell me you didn't, because every man on the ship did, even the gay waiter. Her youth is just part of it. The woman oozes sex. It drips from her. Didn't you notice?"

"Well—"

"Of course you did, and why shouldn't you? Right now you'd love to be in bed with her, and don't deny it, because so would everybody else, and once again I'm including the gay waiter. Girls don't do a thing for me, darling, and even so *I'd* like to be in bed with her."

"Really?"

"I wouldn't literally *want* to, but I picture her with that pouty mouth and that hot body and those get-lost-in-here eyes and my mouth waters. Doesn't yours?"

She didn't wait for an answer. "But she's not here," she went on, "so neither one of us is going to get her tonight. But we're here in this lovely stateroom, and the two beds have an aisle between them, but I don't see why we'll need more than one bed anyway, at least for the next hour or so. There's a little movement to the ship, I think they call it a swell, and I can see where it might actually add something to the proceedings, can't you? And speaking of swells, what have we here? Hmm?"

A little later she said, "I got carried away there. I wonder how thick these walls are. Do you suppose people could hear me?"

"Only the ones in the Western Hemisphere."

"Was I really that loud?"

"You were a perfect southern gentlewoman."

"That sweet young thing got things started, but then she disappeared and it was just us, and wasn't it lovely? I was wondering. Do you figure she's a prostitute? Or just a talented amateur?"

"Probably somewhere in between, would be my guess. She's his girlfriend for the duration of the cruise, and when we dock in Fort Lauderdale there'll be a present for her."

"And by a present you mean—"

"Cash, I would think."

"But they wouldn't have set a price ahead of time."

"No, because it wouldn't be a price. It would be a week of sun and sea for her, with a present at the end of it. But she'd expect the present, and he'd know it was expected."

"How big a present?"

"No way to know. I would think it would have to be at least a thousand, and that seems a little low. Say two, three thousand."

"And it could be more."

"It could, but I wouldn't think it would be a whole lot more than that. Say five thousand tops—*if* he's rich, and if he likes to throw it around. What?"

"I didn't say anything."

"No, but you were about to."

"Well," she said. "The present comes at the end of the trip, right?"

"So?"

"So I was just thinking," she said, "that if all goes well from our point of view, she's essentially getting screwed, isn't she?"

TWENTY-FIVE

Keller woke up when the ship cut its engines. It was six thirty, and he figured that was Nassau he could see through the window. Or were you supposed to call it a porthole? It was large and square, not small and round, so that argued for window. And it was on the ship's starboard side—Keller had figured that out earlier. Could you call it a porthole if it was on the starboard side?

Julia was sleeping soundly. He showered and dressed and went to the dining room, where they were serving a buffet breakfast, with a happy chef on hand to make you whatever sort of omelet you wanted.

Keller wasn't sure he wanted that much human contact. He sat by himself at a table for two, nodded at the waiter's offer of orange juice, nodded a second time for coffee. He picked out a plateful of items from the buffet, and was agreeing to a second cup of coffee when Carmody's pair of bodyguards showed up.

It took him a moment to recognize them, because they'd finally embraced casual dress. At dinner their suits had given way to blue blazers and Dockers, and this morning they'd come all the way down to floral-patterned short-sleeve shirts. Something in their stance suggested they didn't feel entirely happy with their attire, but Keller wondered if maybe he was imagining that part.

He'd been giving the two some thought. Last night, before he drifted off, he'd wondered what he was going to do about them; this morning, in the shower, he'd had them on his mind.

Because, no question, they were a complication. They'd make it more difficult to get to Carmody, or even to do reconnaissance toward that end. But he had a week, and Carmody had already shown that he wasn't going to spend every minute in his stateroom, so Keller figured the opportunity would arise before the ship was back in Port Everglades.

So he could probably arrange some sort of accident. But with these two around, would it pass as an accident? Not likely. If they couldn't keep their charge safe, the least they could do was straighten things out after the fact. They'd turn the ship upside down looking for Carmody's killer, and if the net they cast didn't scoop up Keller, it still wouldn't make his life simpler, or the remainder of the cruise more comfortable.

Keller got to his feet, set his napkin beside his plate. "I'll be back," he told a passing waiter. "Don't clear the table."

Julia opened her eyes when he let himself into their stateroom. "Forgot something," he said. "Go back to sleep." He rummaged in his bag, found what he was looking for, and hurried back to the dining room.

His table was as he'd left it, and the waiter had refilled his coffee cup. More important, Carmody's minders were still at their table. They were in fact built like football players, though a little small for the pros. College, Keller decided, and not the NCAA top tier but one level below it. Appalachian State, University of Delaware—something like that.

What Keller hoped was that they'd have football-player appetites. They were both at the table now, with plates of food in front of them. Keller's best chance would have been right after they ordered their coffee and headed for the buffet, but he'd needed to get to the cabin first.

Packing for the cruise, Keller had made do with a small bag, but had managed to find room for more than his clothes. He knew he wouldn't have access to chain drugstores or neighborhood hardware stores or ghetto entrepreneurs, not aboard ship, so he'd brought along what he thought he might need. His toilet kit included some special pills and powders, besides the usual aspirin, and an improvised garrote, of the sort he'd made and discarded in New York, was wound into a coil and tucked into the toe of a spare shoe.

And he'd packed the HandyMan traveler's tool kit that had belonged to Julia's father. It was a sort of industrial-strength Swiss army knife, with a few implements Keller doubted he'd need. There was a little chrome-plated hammer, handy if he needed to check somebody's patellar reflex, and a pair of needle-nose pliers, and a belt punch. But there was also a knife blade long enough to be useful.

He sipped his coffee and set about watching the two men without being obvious about it. A waiter approached, filled their coffee cups. The running back took a sip, put his cup down, and got to his feet. He picked up his plate, and evidently the tight end reminded him that you were supposed to use a clean plate each time, because he returned his plate to the table and headed for the buffet.

A waiter appeared immediately and whisked away the abandoned plate. The tight end stayed seated and had a sip of coffee.

Come on, Keller urged him silently. *The bacon's crisp, the sausages are tangy. What the hell, let the guy make you an omelet.*

For a moment Keller thought his message had gotten through, because the man's hands fastened on the arms of his chair as if to brace himself for the hard work of standing up. But no, the son of a bitch stayed where he was, and all he did with his hands was reach for his coffee.

The running back took his time and came back with a plate piled high with enough food for both of them, and evidently the tight end thought it looked pretty good, because even as his friend was brandishing his fork, he was moving his hands again to the arms of his chair. And this time he followed through and got to his feet, plate in hand, and it was the running back's turn to remind him about the fresh plate requirement, and the tight end gave a laugh and put his plate back on the table.

Well, maybe they weren't terribly bright. Keller found that a hopeful sign.

But, bright or not, it seemed as though one of them was always going to be at the table. And if he waited any longer they'd leave the table together, and he wouldn't get another shot until breakfast the next day, if then—tomorrow morning might as easily find them at a table for four, with Carmody and his sexpot.

Keller took the little vial of pills from his pocket, uncapped the lid, shook two white tablets into his palm. Anyone watching would have seen him pop them into his mouth and chase them with a sip of water, but in fact the pills remained in his hand.

The ship had drawn up at the dock, and at nine its passengers would be able to disembark and spend the morning in Nassau. Keller's plan would work better, he knew, if they were in open waters with a lively sea under them. That would add verisimilitude, but at the same time it would add a degree of difficulty to his own moves.

Still, this was his chance, and he took it.

He got to his feet, walked down the aisle toward the table where the running back was plying his fork with enthusiasm. The deck was perfectly firm underfoot, no surprise given that the *Carefree Nights* lay at anchor, but Keller managed to teeter a bit as he walked, as if he might have equilibrium problems even on dry land.

He made sure not to overdo it, aiming for a diagnosis of *unsteady on his pins,* but when he reached their table he contrived to lose his balance big-time, lurching into the running back's chair and grabbing onto the man's shoulder for support.

While the fellow reacted, Keller reached with his left hand and dropped one of the pills in the man's coffee.

"Jesus! You all right, fellow? Here, let me give you a hand."

"Sorry, sorry. I was fine when the ship was rocking and rolling and now I can't—oops!"

And one more hearty lurch, this time into the now-standing running back, who had to work to keep his own balance now that Keller had assumed the role of loose cannon. But somehow both men stayed on their feet, even as somehow the second pill found its way into the other coffee cup.

Apologies from Keller, assurances from the running back. And then Keller was on his way back, passing his own table, and giving here a lurch and there a lurch, until he had made his stumbling way out of the dining room altogether.

*   *   *

As far as Keller could make out, everybody in Nassau had just disembarked from one of the cruise ships that thronged the docks. He figured there had to be other people around, but that they had the good sense to stay away from the harbor.

"Who buys all these T-shirts?" Julia wondered. "'Grandma and Grampa went to Nassau and all I got was this lousy shirt.' How stunningly original. Is there a tourist attraction on God's earth where they don't sell that shirt?"

"Auschwitz," Keller suggested.

"Were you ever here before?"

"Nassau? No. Were you?"

"Once," she said. "A man brought me here for a dirty weekend. I never heard the term before, and I gather it's English."

"He was English?"

"Welsh. His wife was English."

"Oh."

"Are you jealous?"

"It was before we met, wasn't it?"

"Oh, years ago."

"Then no," he said. "I'm not jealous."

Something in a shop window caught her eye, and they talked about that for a few minutes, while Keller glanced around to see if the two football types were around. He'd kept an eye out earlier, but hadn't seen either of them leave the ship, with or without Carmody and the girl.

Then Julia broke a silence to say, "It never happened."

"What never happened?"

"The married Englishman."

"Welsh," he said. "The wife was English."

"What difference does it make? I just told you it never happened. Neither of those two people ever existed, and I've never been to Nassau before."

"Oh."

"You really weren't jealous, were you?"

"Would you be happier if I said I was?"

"No, silly. I just didn't know if you would be or not, and I wanted to find out. Because you're a strange and unpredictable creature, Nicholas Edwards."

"I'm strange? You're the one who just dreamed up an adulterous affair with an English twit."

"Welsh," she said. "The wife was English."

They were heading back to the ship when they heard the siren. It was loud, and of a type familiar to Keller from films set in Europe—a long high note followed by a long note an octave lower, a sort of *ooh-gah-ooh-gah* effect. An ambulance roared past them, and it looked boxy and old-fashioned, but was unmistakably an ambulance.

Julia wondered if it was on its way to their ship. Keller hoped so.

They had lunch on the ship, and shared a table with two women, both of them retired schoolteachers from Crawfordsville, Indiana, along with a stockbroker and his wife who had retired to Florida from North or South Dakota, Keller wasn't sure which. The ambulance and its mission gave the six of them something to talk about.

"Now, I don't believe I met either of the two men," one of the schoolteachers said. "If I've got the names right, one was a Mr. Westin and the other was a Mr. Smith."

"Should have been Smith and Wesson," the stockbroker

170

said. "Way I heard it, after they took them off to the hospital, the cabin attendants packed up their bags, and they found a small arsenal there. A couple of guns, anyway, and ammunition to fit them."

"My goodness. On a cruise?"

"Oh, men and their guns," the second teacher said. She was taller and bulkier than her companion, and built not unlike a tight end herself, or maybe a linebacker. "I understand there are men who feel naked without their guns. But here we are having lunch, and not knowing what they ate that made them so ill."

"Nothing they ate," the broker said. "It was evidently an allergic reaction to some sort of drug. Analeptic shock, I think they call it."

"Anaphylactic," the first teacher said.

"Guns and drugs," the broker's wife said. "And it makes you wonder, doesn't it? Two men, traveling together, and sharing a cabin."

Her husband asked her what that was supposed to mean. She said it was just something to take into account.

In their own cabin, Julia said, "I'm still trying to figure it out. Was she suggesting they're gay? And what would that have to do with them both getting sick at the same time?"

Keller shrugged. "Beats me. AIDS, maybe?"

"I suppose. 'Two men sharing a cabin.' I don't know if you saw the look she got when she said that, but the schoolmarms didn't appreciate the implication. Given that they're two *women* sharing a cabin."

"And they're annoyed because they're lesbians?"

"Or they're not lesbians, and that's why they're annoyed. At the implication."

"The world's a complicated place," Keller said.

TWENTY-SIX

The lounge chair Keller selected gave him a good view of the block of four staterooms, one of which housed Carmody and his strawberry blonde. He sat down, put his legs up, and set about the business of anointing himself with suntan lotion. It boasted a high SPF number, and he found himself wondering if there was any point to the whole process. Wouldn't it be simpler to skip the lotion and stay in your cabin? Wouldn't you come out about the same?

Earlier, Keller had checked the listings, and found that Mr. Aldredge Smith and Mr. John Westin had occupied a cabin one flight below. That was unfortunate, because if their removal to a hospital in Nassau had left a Sun Deck stateroom vacant, Keller might have used it as a base of operations.

Keller hadn't thought to pack a bathing suit, but the shipboard shop had been happy to sell him one. It was black, and not too skimpily cut, but he still felt conspicuous in it, though less so than if he'd stretched out on the lounge chair in long pants and a shirt. And the sun felt good, and the ship had set sail shortly after lunch for Virgin Gorda, wherever that was, and Keller found its motion soothing. All he had to do was lie there and relax and keep his eyes open.

The third requirement turned out to be impossible. *Your eyes are closed,* he realized at one point, and told himself he'd have to do something about it, but by then it was too late. His mind had found a corridor to explore, and he drifted right off...

And came to abruptly. There was no sudden noise, and no one jostled his lounge chair or walked past it to block the sun. He wondered later if it might simply have been an unconscious awareness of her presence that did it, because when he opened his eyes there she was, not ten yards away from him, Ms. Va-va-voom herself, sitting sidesaddle on a lounge chair of her own, and applying coconut-scented suntan oil to those portions of her anatomy not covered by the scarlet bikini.

Which was to say almost all of her.

She took her time oiling her golden-brown skin, and it seemed to Keller that she was caressing herself as much as she was protecting it from the sun. He didn't want to stare at her, but seemed incapable of averting his eyes, and the next thing he knew she was looking right back at him.

He looked away, but it was as if he could see her no matter where his eyes were turned. He looked her way again, and she was still gazing at him, with an expression on her face that was not quite a smile, although it was definitely headed in that direction.

Then she turned her eyes from him, and swung her legs up onto the lounge chair, and worked the controls to lower the back into a horizontal position. She was still sitting up, and

Keller watched as she put her hands behind her back, uncoupled the bikini top, and removed it altogether.

She couldn't have exposed her breasts to him for more than a couple of seconds, but they were longer seconds than most. Then she was lying facedown on the lounge chair.

Had anyone else seen what Keller had seen? He looked around and saw no one who gave any evidence of having witnessed the performance. Had it been for his benefit? Or had he merely chanced to be present when a free-spirited creature displayed her charms without thinking twice about it?

Her head was turned to one side, resting on her arm, and facing toward Keller. Her eyes were closed. And she was smiling.

Go back to his cabin? Go to the bar for a drink, or the lounge for a cup of coffee? Find his way to the library and pick out something to read?

Or wait for her to give up on the sun and return to her cabin, so that he could see which one it was?

Keller closed his eyes to give the matter some thought, and once again the combination of sun and waves carried him off. He didn't doze for long, but when he opened his eyes he saw that the girl had changed position. She was lying on her back now, and was once again wearing the bikini top.

And she was no longer alone. On the lounge chair just beyond hers, wearing knee-length Bermuda shorts and a loose-fitting shirt with a palm tree on it, sat Carmody himself. His feet were bare—a pair of pink flip-flops rested at the foot of his chair—and from the knees down the man was fish-belly white, while from the knees up he was pretty much invisible, with the shirt and the shorts and his sunglasses and his pink cotton sun hat covering up most of him.

The contrast between the two of them, dramatic enough in

the dining room, was far greater beneath the sun. Earlier he'd looked old enough to be her father, or perhaps her father's older brother; now you'd be more apt to cast him as her dead grandfather.

She was lying down. Carmody's chair was in what the airlines call the full upright position, and he sat there looking like a man waiting for his number to be called. Then, after a few moments, he reached out and rested a hand on his companion's shoulder. Keller thought that was a tender gesture until the hand moved lower and slipped inside a cup of the bikini halter.

Keller looked away, willing the old goat to keep his hands to himself, and when he looked their way again it was as if his wish had been Carmody's command. Both the man's hands were now resting on the arms of his own lounge chair.

Well, that was better. On the other hand, a little more touchy-feely and they might get up and return to their cabin, and Keller could note its number. And he wished that would happen sooner rather than later, as there was a limit to how much sun he could handle.

But how much sun could Carmody take? Not too much on those pale white legs, so...

Hell. Keller watched as Carmody picked up his towel and draped it carefully over his feet and lower legs. Taking the sun without taking the sun, he thought. Wonderful.

Time to give up and get out of the sun himself? Wait, Carmody was saying something.

"Carina? You don't want to get too much sun, honey."

"Feels so good," she replied, so softly that Keller could barely make out the words.

"I can think of something else that'll feel good. Time to go inside, Carina."

"Give me a few more minutes, Mickey. You go. I'll be there by the time you're out of the shower."

"You and the sun," Carmody said.

"Makes me warm. You like me warm, don't you, Mickey?"

The man answered by leaning over to cop another feel, and Carina contrived to show her appreciation by squirming a little on the lounge chair. Then Carmody slipped his feet into his flip-flops, told her not to be too long, and stood up.

Keller gave him a head start. He got to his feet, and out of the corner of his eye he thought he saw Carina glancing at him. He didn't turn to check, but took off in Carmody's wake.

He followed the man around the pool and over to the four cabins. Carmody led him to one of two on the far side, so if he'd stayed where he was he'd only have been able to halve the possibilities from four to two, but now he was half a dozen steps behind the man by the time he'd used his key card to let himself into number 501.

The door closed, and Keller moved in front of it. His immediate mission had been one of reconnaissance, and it had paid off, but did he have to stop there? If he knocked, Carmody would open the door. And once he did, he was there to be taken.

Keller's swimsuit had a pocket, but all it held was his own key card. No garrote, no HandyMan, no pills or powders. All he had were his two hands, but if he needed more than that to cope with Michael Carmody he was in the wrong business.

He looked in both directions, and there was nobody around. How soon would the girl come back? Could he dispatch Carmody in time to be out of the room before she made her appearance?

If not, well, that would be bad luck all around, especially for her. Keller preferred to avoid that sort of situation, but sometimes you couldn't, and he had learned to do what had to be done.

He knocked on the door, listened for footsteps.

And didn't hear any. No, of course not, the son of a bitch was taking his shower. He wouldn't be able to hear Keller knocking, or if he did he wouldn't feel the need to cut short his shower to go see who it was.

Knock again? He was about to, but now there was someone in view, a maid pushing a service cart. And when she passed there would be somebody else, and sooner or later the girl would show up, and Keller would have to wait for a better time.

Maybe it was time to check out the library, see if he could find something to read. First, though, he'd get his own shower.

Mickey, he thought. Mickey and Carina. Well, the afternoon hadn't been a total loss. He now knew which cabin they occupied. And, though he couldn't see what good it did him, he knew what they called each other.

TWENTY-SEVEN

Julia had made a new friend during the afternoon, and worked things out so that the two couples could share a table for four at dinner. They were Atlantans, though both had grown up in the Midwest. The husband, Roy, said he had the perfect job. He worked for an insurance company, but he didn't sell anything, or weasel out of paying claims, or sit at a desk and crunch numbers. Instead he flew around the country and met with groups of insurance agents, explaining why they should push his company's policies instead of the competition's.

"I buy the pizza, I buy the doughnuts, I've always got the latest jokes, and whenever I show up everybody's glad to see me. I swear it never feels like I'm working."

"He works very hard," said his wife, who was called Myrt, which Keller figured had to be short for Myrtle. "On and off planes all the time."

"The planes are fine," Roy said. "It's the blankety-blank airports. But don't get me started."

Nobody did, and the subject shifted to the two men who'd left the ship, and whom everybody had taken to calling Smith and Wesson, and who were assumed to be very dangerous men. Mafia torpedoes, the consensus seemed to be, no doubt dispatched to kill one of the passengers, or even a crew member.

"It could be anyone," Myrt said darkly. "The captain looks perfectly decent, but he could have gambling debts."

"Are we playing Pick the Victim?" her husband wondered. "My candidate's Foxy Grandpa. Oh, you know who I mean. The dirty old man with the hot redhead."

"Gambling debts, Roy?"

"Hell, who needs a motive? I'd kill him myself if I thought it'd get me a shot at her."

"Oh, Roy," Myrt said, and swatted him with her napkin. "Am I gonna have to keep you on a leash?"

"Arf arf," Roy said.

"I swear, men are terrible creatures. Still, I have to say this is more interesting than our last cruise."

"You had a good time."

"Well, I did, but the conversation! Perforations, inverted underprints—"

"Overprints," Roy said.

"Like it matters? Roy," she announced, "took me on a cruise for stamp collectors. Can you imagine? Every time we landed and the wives went shopping, all of the men rushed to the nearest post office."

Roy said it wasn't quite like that, and Myrt said it was close enough, and Roy said only thirty-some passengers were stamp collectors, it was just a small portion of the whole, and Myrt said yes, but those were the people they had to sit with every night at dinner, and finally Keller was able to get a word in edgewise.

"You're a collector," he said.

"Guilty as charged, but I never would have brought it up, because there's nothing less interesting than someone else's hobby."

Was that true? Keller didn't think so, and had found most people to be at their best when talking about their hobby or pastime. But what he said was, "Well, I wouldn't be bored. I'm a philatelist myself."

"I guess you just might be, if you can pronounce it correctly. Myrt still has trouble after all these years. What do you collect, Nick?"

Keller told him, and Roy nodded respectfully. "Classic general worldwide," he said. "Got to admire that. Myself, well, nothing quite that ambitious, but I've got a batch of collections going. My main interest is stamps of Turkey, and don't ask me why. No Turkish ancestors, no connection of any sort, and I've never been to the country and don't expect I'll ever get there. I just like the stamps, for some reason."

It made perfect sense to Keller.

"And of course along with Turkey I collect a batch of dead countries connected to Turkey, like Hatay and Latakia."

"And Eastern Rumelia," Keller offered.

"You bet. And, let's see, besides Turkey I have one topical collection. I collect fish."

"That's fish on stamps," Myrt said, as if otherwise Julia might think Roy had a collection of actual fishes.

"Now, I like fish," Roy said, "though I wouldn't want it served to me every night. And when I was a kid I had an aquarium and I used to like watching the fish, until they all died and I emptied the fish tank and gave it to my mother to grow ferns in. And I've been fishing, but only a couple of times in my life, and I don't care if I never waste time again in that particular fashion. But I do like stamps with fish on them. I just like the way they look, all the different species."

That made sense to Keller, too.

Keller, stretched out on his bunk, turned at the sound of Julia's key card in the lock. She entered, holding the plastic rectangle aloft like a Plains Indian brandishing a scalp.

"That's the key to 501?"

She shook her head. "It's a spare key to our cabin. I just let myself in with it."

"Oh."

"Silly me, locking myself out. In a minute I'll take the key back." She tapped it with her thumbnail. "There's no way she'll give me a key to Carmody's cabin. You need to show ID and sign for it. But I saw where she keeps the keys, and how they're sorted. Now if somebody could get her to come away from the desk for a minute or two, someone else could slip away with the key to 501."

"Last time I passed the desk," Keller said, "there were two girls behind it. They looked enough alike to be Xerox copies, but there were two of them."

"Two to a shift," Julia agreed. "Two on duty from eight in the morning till four in the afternoon, and two others from four to midnight."

"And only one after midnight?"

"Pilar is so glad she does not have the graveyard shift this week. She had it last week, and you get so lonely."

"You got friendly with her."

"It never hurts to be friendly," she said. "She's from the Philippines."

"I think they all are."

"Uh-huh. All the dining room and housekeeping staff, and the ones on the desk. The cruise director and his staff are American, except for the ones who aren't. And the crew's a mini United Nations, with a lot of Eastern Europeans. The chef is Swiss. Pilar doesn't like the Ukrainians."

"Why not?"

"She says they're not nice. I was thinking if we waited until one o'clock, and then you found a way to lure the attendant out from behind the desk, all I'd need is a couple of minutes to get the key to their cabin."

"Maybe you should do the luring."

"No," she said, "because I saw where the keys are. You can play helpless confused man in need of help. Besides, if anybody happens to see me behind the desk, it'll be less unsettling than if they were to see you."

"Because you look more like a Filipina?"

"Because I'm a girl, silly. Women are less threatening. How could you not know that?"

He didn't say anything, and she asked him if something was bothering him.

"I'm just wondering," he said, "if this is really something you want to do."

"The key will help, won't it?"

"It might. It certainly wouldn't hurt."

"Well," she said, "I want to help."

He made one change to Julia's plan, delaying the starting time an hour to give the girl on the desk a little more time to appreciate the loneliness of her situation. At a couple of minutes past two, Keller approached the desk, where the attendant met him with a big smile.

"I was wondering if you could help me," he said. "The only thing is, I don't know if it's okay for you to leave the desk."

"It's not rush hour here," she said. "How can I help?"

There was a notice on the board he couldn't understand, he said, and he led her down a corridor to where notices were posted, and pointed to one he'd scouted out earlier. Its message, some drivel about evacuation in the event of fire or shipwreck, was pretty clear, but she was evidently willing to believe he was somewhere in the early stages of cognitive decline, and worried about drowning, and so she explained it all very clearly and carefully.

Keller asked if there were many shipboard fires, and after she'd reassured him on that score he raised the subject of piracy. That was pretty much limited to the Indian Ocean, she said, and the only real pirates in the Caribbean these days were running gift shops. He laughed at that, and found a joke to tell her in return, and she was polite enough to pretend it was funny.

She went back to her post and Keller returned to his cabin, where Julia showed him a key card. "What did I tell you?" she said. "Nothing to it."

In the morning they left the ship with Roy and Myrt, whose last names turned out to be Huysendahl. The wives had shopping to do, and Roy suggested a visit to the post office. "You won't find anything," Roy said. "Not if your collection's got a 1940 cutoff date. And I probably won't find anything, either."

"Not much from Turkey," Keller said.

"Doesn't seem likely, does it? But they might have some fish stamps. It's a popular topic, and easier to justify for a Caribbean island than some landlocked African dictatorship that gets three drops of rain every two years."

The post office had a special philatelic window, and a display showing just what stamps were still available for purchase. There was a very attractive set of stamps showing brilliantly colored reef fish, along with a six-stamp souvenir sheet; they'd just come out, and Roy picked up four sets, sheets included. "One for me and the others for some guys I know'll want them. Cheaper at the post office than from a new-issues dealer."

Back on the ship, Julia showed off a blouse she'd bought. "I don't know that I'll ever wear it," she said, "but it was cheap, and Myrt bought one, so I picked it up in the interest of female bonding. Did you find any stamps to buy?"

He showed her the two souvenir sheets he'd bought, one with fish, another showing the various islands that comprised the British Virgins. "They're souvenir sheets," he said, "so I bought them for a souvenir."

"And in the interest of male bonding?"

"I suppose. He's a nice fellow."

"Myrt thinks the four of us should make *dîner à quatre* a regular thing. Could you stand sharing a table with them every night? Just the four of us?"

"Saves trying to find things to say to new people."

"That was my thought. The British Virgins. You know what a British virgin is? A ten-year-old girl who can run faster than her brothers. Actually, that's an old joke about Cajuns. But I'm not sure it really works to adapt it. The British don't have that reputation."

"Quite the reverse," he said. "'Dead? Sacre bleu, Monsieur, I thought she was English!'"

"Oh, I heard that joke years and years ago," she said. "And it's still awful."

TWENTY-EIGHT

At dinner that night, Keller waited until he'd finished his main course, a nice piece of fish that had been swimming not too many hours ago. If it had been on a stamp, he thought, Roy would have snatched it away from him.

He put his fork down, patted his pockets, said, "Hell," and got to his feet. "Something I forgot," he said. "I'm not interested in dessert, so please go ahead without me. I'll join y'all for coffee if I get done in time."

The elevator might have been faster, but he didn't even think of it until he'd already climbed the first flight and started on the second. He was breathing hard when he reached the Sun Deck, but caught his breath by the time he was slipping the key card into the door of the Carmody stateroom. The lock turned and he was inside.

The maids serviced everybody's cabin during dinner, turning down beds, turning on lights, drawing curtains, and leaving a square of foil-wrapped chocolate on the pillow. The Sun Deck staterooms were essentially two-room suites, and Keller moved around the place looking at things and wondering what he was doing here. It put him in position for an ambush, but that would only work if Carmody turned up alone. And he might: he had a lot of years on his bladder and prostate, and could well feel the need for a quick pee before catching up with the lovely Carina in the lounge, where tonight's scheduled entertainment included a comedian and a torch singer.

But there was at least as good a chance that they'd return together, and then what did Keller do? He'd have the advantage of surprise, and he was a skilled professional up against two amateurs, one an out-of-shape older man and the other a woman. He was confident in his ability to take out both of them, and could probably do so before either one made enough noise to attract attention. And if they did get out a cry, so what? She'd sound as though she was feigning passion, while he'd come off as a self-styled Tarzan, pounding his chest and yowling in triumph.

If he was alone, that was how he'd want to do it. The girl was collateral damage. It was safer and easier to do two for the price of one, and while Carina was a good example of what Mother Nature could do when inspired, she was unlikely to find a cure for cancer or bring about a lasting peace in the Middle East. She'd assumed a certain risk when she agreed to share a cabin with a man like Carmody, and if her luck was bad, well, that was just bad luck. Killing her would bother Keller for a while, but he knew how to deal with that sort of thing, and he'd get over it.

That's if he was alone. But he wasn't, he had Julia along, and it was hard to know how Julia would take one death, let alone two. She knew that his assignments occasionally included women—Dot had more than once called him an equal-opportunity killer—but this was a woman she'd seen up close, and that made it different.

Well, maybe both he and Carina would be lucky this time, and Carmody would come back all by himself. But then what? Carina would return sooner or later and find the body, and just how much of a flap that raised would depend on whether or not he could make it look like natural causes. If he couldn't, there'd be cops on board the next time they made port, and he could probably handle the questioning until he had a chance to get off the ship and disappear, but once again, dammit, he wasn't alone, he had Julia along.

He paced the floor—the Sun Deck cabins provided ample room for pacing—and his mind kept working, trying to find a way, and then he stopped pacing and stopped thinking and froze in his tracks.

There was a key in the lock. So soon? How could they be done with dinner already?

He braced himself. Let it be Carmody, he thought, and the door flew open.

It was Carina.

His hands were out in front of him, ready to stifle her cries of alarm. But there were no cries, nor did she seem at all alarmed.

"Thank God!" she said.

Huh?

"The way you look at me," she said, moving closer to him, kicking the door shut. "And I know you saw the looks I gave you in return. But you have not approached me, and I saw you leave the dining room, and I thought maybe he's going to my cabin, and I made some excuse, and—"

She really was quite beautiful.

"But there's no time," she said. "Not now, he'll be here any minute. Oh, I want to be alone with you! What shall we do?"

"Uh..."

"Later tonight," she said. "One o'clock. No, one thirty, he'll definitely be asleep by then. I'll meet you on Deck Two out on the afterdeck."

"Uh, port or starboard?"

"All the way at the back," she said. "Behind the library. At the rail, at one thirty. Can you be there? Oh, I hope you can. Oh, God, there's no time, but kiss me. You have to kiss me."

And she pressed her mouth to his.

"I don't get it," he told Julia. "I wonder what she wants."

"Your fair white body, if I had to guess."

"Not unless she thinks I'm a Hollywood casting director," he said. "And it's just as well I'm not, because she wouldn't get the part. She's not that good an actress."

"It was an act?"

"'Oh, I want to be alone with you! What shall we do?' Yes, I'd say it was an act."

"I don't know," she said. "I frequently want to be alone with you. *What shall we do?* I ask myself that all the time."

"You usually come up with something."

"I asked myself just before you got back, and what I came up with was that we should call Donny and Claudia's. It's early, they'll be up, and with any luck so will Jenny."

Everyone was still awake at the Wallings house, and everybody talked to everybody else, until Donny Wallings took the phone and said, "This is costing y'all a fortune, and y'all are having fun and so's Jenny, so I'm gonna say good-bye now."

They ended the call, and Julia said, "She's having a wonderful time."

"That's great."

"She'll probably want to stay there forever. With her new family, that she now likes ever so much better than her old one."

"Maybe we can rent out her room."

"Go ahead, make fun of a mother's tears. Did you enjoy it? Was it hot?"

"Was what hot?"

"Kissing her. It must have been, that woman's one of the chief causes of global warming."

"It was just...I don't know. Dumb."

"Dumb?"

"I knew it had to be an act, and that she had an agenda. And even if it wasn't, I didn't want to be there."

"Poor baby. Was she at least a good kisser? Did she use her tongue?"

"Julia—"

"And press her tits against you? I'm sorry. I'm embarrassing you, aren't I?"

"I don't know. Yeah, sort of."

"If she doesn't want your body—"

"She doesn't. It was an act, pure and simple."

"Pure? Simple?"

"Well—"

"What do you suppose she wants?"

"I'll find out in a couple of hours."

"Well, I guess you will. One thirty, did you say?" She started to say something more, than stopped herself.

"What?"

"No, it's nothing. Well. What I was going to say was we could fool around a little first, to take some of the pressure off, but you're not in the mood, are you?"

"Not really, no."

"I'm as bad as she is, trying to make this about sex, and it's not about that, is it? And I at least should know better. Have you got something to read? I'll let you alone."

When Keller left their cabin, it was a little after one and most of the ship's passengers had retired for the night. There were still some holdouts in the bars and lounges, making up in volume what they'd lost in number, and a few passengers hung around on deck, looking out at the stars or thinking deep thoughts at the rail.

He got to the spot designated for their rendezvous a good ten minutes ahead of schedule, and found a vantage point nearby where he could observe Carina's approach and assure himself that she didn't have anyone trailing her. He'd changed to dark clothing, and found a dark spot to lurk, and evidently succeeded in rendering himself invisible; a couple passed within a few feet of him, pausing to kiss with surprising passion, and then walked on, never aware that he was almost close enough to reach out and touch them.

One thirty came and went. Keller stayed where he was, half hoping she'd stand him up. But then, seven minutes late by his watch, she hurried by without seeing him, positioned herself at the rail, and looked around in what looked like genuine concern.

"Right here," Keller said softly, and came out where she could see him.

"Oh, thank God. I thought that you weren't coming, or that you came and left when I was not here. I had to wait until he was sleeping. But come here, come kiss me."

She moved toward him, stopped when he held up a hand. "No kisses," he said. "You've got an agenda, and I want to know what it is."

"Agenda?"

"Tell me what you want."

"The same thing you want," she said. "I saw you looking at me."

"Lots of men were looking at you."

"Yes, and women, too. But there was something about the way you looked at me." She frowned, the original act shelved for now. "You don't want to fuck me?"

"You're a very attractive young woman," he said, "but I'm married, and no, I don't want to have sex with you."

She said something in a language he didn't recognize, frowned again, then looked up to meet his eyes as recognition dawned in hers. "Then what were you doing in my cabin?"

His hands were at his sides, and he raised them to waist level. There was no one around, and all he had to do was break her neck and fling her overboard. If she managed to cry out first, it might pass for a scream she'd uttered on the way down.

"Maybe we want the same thing," she said.

Oh? "Tell me what you want."

"What do I want?" She said the foreign word again. "What do you think I want? I want you to kill my husband."

TWENTY-NINE

Julia had been awake at one o'clock, reading what she'd called a novel of magnolias and miscegenation, but she was sleeping soundly when he let himself into the cabin. He didn't think he'd be able to sleep himself, but a hot shower took some of the tension out of him, and he went right out.

In the morning he told her what happened. "Apparently they're married," he said. "That's why it took as long as it did for them to get to the ship Saturday afternoon. They went through a quickie wedding ceremony first."

"Why? To make the cruise line happy?"

He shook his head. "Not the cruise line. The Witness Protection Program. After he testifies, they'll set him up in some little town somewhere out west, but the only way she can be part of the deal is if she's his wife. And I guess he didn't think the local talent in East Frogskin would be up to his standards, so he bit the bullet and proposed."

"How romantic. But why did she go along? And why change her mind and want him dead?"

"Two questions with one answer."

"Money?"

He nodded. "He's got a lot of money, or at least she thinks he does. And she's living the life we figured, going on dates and getting presents, and the life's not that great and neither are the presents, and these are her peak years."

"She's got a lot of her youth left."

"But she can see what's coming. And here's this rich guy who wants to marry her."

"But that means living in, what did you call it? East Frogskin? And that's more than she signed on for?"

"Actually," he said, "I think it's exactly what she signed on for, but that was before she had a chance to think it through."

"And now she wants to tear up the contract. Can't she divorce him? Get an annulment? Oh, but she wants the money."

"She also would like him to be dead."

"Oh, it's personal?"

"He takes a lot of Viagra," he said, "and he has certain preferences in bed that she doesn't care for."

"Like what?"

"She didn't get specific."

"What a tease. I bet I can guess, and I'd like to sit her down and explain that once you get used to it it's actually quite enjoyable. Are you blushing?"

"No. It's not just what he likes to do, it's apparently that now that they're married she finds everything about him objectionable."

"And if he dies she's a rich widow."

"She was pitching one of the minders, the shorter of the two."

"The running back."

"Right. I guess he didn't push her away when she made her move."

"I guess he didn't have a wife along."

"I don't know if he was stringing her along, or if she'd even made her pitch about how they could be together forever if only something happened to her husband. I can't think he'd have actually followed through with it. But when he and the tight end went off in the ambulance, her whole plan fell apart."

"And that's when she started giving you the eye."

"Along with a peek at what she had under her bikini top."

"And she thought it worked, because there you were waiting for her in her cabin. And when she found out she was wrong, she just went and made another plan. Except it's the same plan, isn't it? But with a different prize instead of her body. What's she offering? It would almost have to be money."

"An unspecified amount, payable after the estate's settled."

"Lord, who wouldn't rush to commit murder for terms like that?"

"She's given up the idea that I'm blinded by lust, but she evidently still thinks I'm pretty stupid. I agreed, and the first thing I explained was that we couldn't see each other again. No more secret meetings, no kisses, no long looks. And I told her what we'd do for now was nothing at all, not until the last night of the cruise."

"So that we'll be off the ship by the time they find him."

"And so will everybody else. She'll be unable to rouse him, and they'll haul him off to a Fort Lauderdale hospital and pronounce him dead, and once the estate clears probate I'll get my very generous payment from an extremely grateful widow."

"So what's the next step?"

"Breakfast," he said. "I'm starving."

"I mean—"

"I know what you mean. There's no next step until the night before we dock in Fort Lauderdale. All you and I have to do between now and then is enjoy the cruise."

"My God," she said. "What a concept."

"And another little collection I've got," Roy said, "is mourning covers. You probably know what those are."

"With the black bands?"

"That's right. They've been around about as long as stamps, since sometime in the mid-nineteenth century. Stationers made up envelopes with the black bands printed on 'em, and that's what you bought for notes of condolence. They got a lot of use, mostly in Europe and America, and then right around 1940 the whole custom pretty much died out. Which is ironic, considering how people were dying faster than ever once the war started."

"Interesting thing to collect," Keller said.

"Morbid, you mean? That's what Myrt says, but it's no more about death than my other collections are about Turkey and fish."

"I meant interesting because of the variety. Different stamps, different dates, different countries."

"And sometimes the letter's still in the envelope," Roy said, "and like as not it barely mentions the deceased. Just a nice newsy letter, who's getting married, who just had a baby, who got a new job. And oh, by the way, I'm sorry for your loss. Now that's interesting, don't you think?"

"Very."

"Well, different times. Now what would they send, text

messages? 'Heard N8 dead. Bummer. R U OK?'" He sighed. "The covers, I must have close to two hundred of 'em. They're not high priority, but when I see one that's a little different, or that I like, well, I pick it up. But I've got to figure out what to do with the damn things. I've got a Scott Specialized album for my Turkish, and I print out my own pages for the fish, but all I've managed to do so far with my mourning covers is heave 'em in a box. Sometimes I haul 'em out and look at 'em, and then I just toss 'em right back in the box."

And did Keller collect any postal history, or just stamps? As a matter of fact, Keller said, he'd begun picking up covers mailed in Martinique, if they were interesting and attractive and reasonably priced. Martinique wasn't exactly a specialty, but he had all of the country's stamps through 1940, and had begun acquiring minor varieties, and somebody gave him a cover once, and—

"Say no more, Nick. I can see the same thing happening with Turkey, when I run out of stamps to buy. Ah, here come the ladies. I wonder what they found to buy this time."

The cruise was an unalloyed pleasure once he was free of the need to do anything. The Huysendahls continued to provide good company, and the shore visits weren't limited to shopping for the wives and postal expeditions for him and Roy. Twice they signed up for shore excursions, and got to see some wildlife and swim beneath a waterfall, or at least look at it.

As he'd noted the first night, one of the chief activities of people on a cruise seemed to be talking about other cruises they'd taken, and Keller, who'd never thought much about cruises, began to see what a world of possibilities they presented.

A smaller ship would be nice. *Carefree Nights* was comfortable and luxurious enough, but cruising on it was like being a guest in a huge floating hotel. In one port, they'd been berthed next to an actual sailing ship, carrying just over a hundred passengers. It had engines, so they could make good time when they had to and never worry about getting becalmed, but the ship was really beautiful with its sails flying, or whatever it was that they did.

A more interesting itinerary would be a plus, too. Cruising the Baltic, cruising the South Pacific—there were some genuinely exotic routes available to cruise ships, going places he'd like to see.

Places he'd like to take Jenny. She was sure to love life aboard ship, and there were plenty of activities for kids if he and Julia wanted some private time.

Plenty to think about. And he'd much rather keep his mind busy with that sort of thing than with their final hours aboard the *Carefree Nights*. Which didn't promise to be all that carefree.

THIRTY

The fish on the dinner menu that last night was marlin, lightly grilled and served with a brown butter sauce. The two women ordered it, as did Roy. Keller asked for the filet mignon, medium rare.

"Well, that's a switch," Roy said. "This must be the first time I've seen you have anything but fish. I was beginning to wonder if you shouldn't be the one collecting fish stamps."

When you ordered fish, the waiter took away your ordinary table knife and gave you an oddly shaped fish knife. No one ever seemed to use it, and Keller figured any piece of fish he couldn't cut with the side of his fork was one he didn't much want to eat.

When you ordered steak, they brought you a steak knife.

At one thirty, Keller scanned the Sun Deck. All was quiet, and he couldn't see anyone around. At dinner they'd requested that all bags be placed out in the corridor by three a.m., so that crew members could collect them prior to departure, and the occupants of all four Sun Deck cabins had already complied.

Keller positioned himself in front of the door to stateroom 501. Several pieces of luggage were on the deck to his right. There was music playing within the cabin, barely audible through the heavy door, and the DO NOT DISTURB sign was suspended from the knob.

He had the key in his pocket, the one Julia had picked up for him, but he left it there and knocked. Carina opened it at once, wearing a pale yellow nightgown to which he supposed the word *diaphanous* might apply. He got a whiff of her perfume and a sense of her body heat as she reached to embrace him, then stopped herself when she realized that wasn't in the script anymore.

Instead she made do with stating the obvious: "You're here."

He was, and so was Carmody, stretched out on the bed on his back, naked to the world but for a pair of boxer shorts and an arresting amount of body hair. The man's mouth was hanging open and he was breathing slowly and heavily through it. The music Keller had heard through the door was still low in volume. Soft jazz, and Keller recognized the song but couldn't put a name to it.

"I put the powder in his nightcap," she said. "He drank it."

No kidding, Keller thought.

"He wanted to fuck me," she said, "but he passed out instead. You know where I can get some more of that powder?"

Keller had obtained it by crushing two capsules, collecting the powder in a folded-up slip of paper. As arranged, he'd met Carina that afternoon and passed it to her, along with instructions for its use. If he'd given it to her earlier she might have rushed things, and he hadn't wanted that.

"Out like a light," she said. "Look at him, hairy like an ape. You know what I almost did?"

"What?"

"Put a pillow over his face. I thought, what if he wakes up? But he wouldn't wake up. He's dead to the world, and a few minutes with a pillow over his face and he'd stay that way forever. Save you the trouble, huh?"

Satin Doll, Duke Ellington and his orchestra. That's what was playing.

He said, "It's good you restrained yourself."

"Why? I would have paid you all the same. You're the one gave me the magic powder."

"You want it to look like death by natural causes."

"So? He stops breathing, his heart stops beating, he's dead. What's more natural than that?"

"He'd have these pinpoint hemorrhages in his eyeballs."

"So his eyes bleed, what do I care? What's it gonna hurt him if he's dead?"

"They'd see the hemorrhages," he said patiently, "and they'd know immediately that he'd been smothered."

"Oh, fuck," she said. "Like *CSI*?"

"Something like that. And who do you think they just might suspect of smothering him?"

"Fuck. Good I didn't do it."

"I'd say."

"So," she said. "How you gonna make it look natural?"

He moved quickly to the side of the bed, drew the steak knife from his pocket, and sank it between two of Michael Carmody's ribs and into his heart. The body shook with a brief tremor, the hands raised up an inch or so from the bed, and then all was still.

"Holy fuck!"

"Well," Keller said.

"You just killed him. Just like that."

"You're a rich widow. That's what you wanted, isn't it?"

"But you stabbed him! The knife's right there sticking out of him!"

"Good point," Keller said, and removed the knife. There was hardly any blood on it.

"But won't they see the wound? How's that gonna look like natural causes?"

"Now, that's a good question," he said, and reached for her.

THIRTY-ONE

The ship docked in Port Everglades before breakfast, and at nine o'clock passengers were allowed to disembark. Keller collected their bags in the cruise terminal, and a cab had them at the airport three hours before their flight home.

They found a place to have coffee, and Julia said, "You didn't say, and I didn't ask, but I'll ask now. It's done, isn't it?"

"It's done."

"I want to hear, but I don't want to hear now. Okay?"

"Sure."

"I miss Jenny. I miss her like crazy. I've been sort of holding that off to one side, how much I miss her, but now we're on dry land and we'll be home in a couple of hours and it's okay to let myself feel it. I miss her something fierce."

"So do I."

"They were nice, weren't they? Roy and Myrt."

"Very."

"And there was a lot to him besides the stamps. That opened the door, but he's an interesting person in other respects, don't you think?"

"Definitely."

"I wouldn't mind seeing them again. I wonder if we ever will."

"We have their email."

"And they have ours, but did you see all the people exchanging email addresses last night? How many of them do you think will ever get in touch?"

"We could make a point of it," he said. "Maybe go on a cruise with them again sometime."

"With Jenny, though."

"Absolutely."

"And with no—"

"Work connected to it. Again, absolutely."

"That might be fun. Okay, I think I'll read the paper now. There won't be anything in the paper, will there? No, of course there won't, it's far too soon. Honey? We'll talk later."

"Okay."

"When I'm ready."

"Right."

Keller always liked the New Orleans airport, not least of all because it was named for Louis Armstrong. He didn't know who O'Hare was, but doubted he ever amounted to much as a horn player. Neither did JFK or LaGuardia. Orange County had named an airport after John Wayne, and that was pretty good, and there was Bob Hope Airport in Burbank, but Keller figured New Orleans had them all topped.

They drove straight from the airport to the Wallings house. Donny wasn't home from work yet, but Claudia and the kids were there, and something unwound in Keller the second he saw his daughter, something he hadn't even known was coiled tight. He picked her up and nodded happily as she told him a million things, some of which he could even understand.

Claudia poured coffee and put out a plate of cookies, and Julia unzipped her bag and played Lady Bountiful, passing out presents for everybody. Claudia got a blouse, which she professed to love, and for Donny Julia'd picked out a Hawaiian-style sport shirt with a desert island motif.

"I don't know if he'll ever wear it," she said.

Claudia said, "Are you kidding? He'll love it, and you know it's something he'd never pick out and buy for himself. The hard part'll be getting that man to take it off."

The kids got what they got, and seemed content. And, as soon as they decently could, they packed up Jenny and headed for home.

He'd found a spare moment to call Dot from the Fort Lauderdale airport, reporting success in an ambiguous sentence or two, ringing off after she'd expressed congratulations. Now he busied himself with the week's worth of mail. There was a new list from one of his favorite dealers, ten pages of Portugal and Colonies, and while it was hardly a priority, he'd been a week away from his stamps and couldn't resist.

He was circling an 1899 set of four Lourenço Marques overprints when Julia came into the room. He looked up and saw her face.

"I found the story online," she said.

"And?"

"It was simple and straightforward. An American couple, Mr. and Mrs. Michael Carmody, were found in their cabin, the victims of a double homicide. He'd been stabbed once, she'd been stabbed multiple times. The cabin was ransacked, and the apparent motive was robbery. The killer left behind an extra key card for the cabin, and one seems to have gone missing from the desk."

Keller nodded. That was the connection they were supposed to make.

"The murder weapon was also left behind. It was a steak knife, suggesting that a member of the kitchen or dining room staff might have been responsible."

"I can see how they might think that."

"Yes." She was sitting down now. Her hands were loosely clasped on the table in front of her, and she was looking down at them. "I knew you had to do it that way. Not the knife, I didn't even think about how, but I knew you were going to kill them both."

"I didn't really have much choice."

"No."

"The minute she walked in on me in their cabin, it was pretty much settled. When I met her out on deck in the middle of the night—"

"Two a.m., wasn't it?"

"Something like that. When she said what she wanted, I thought about doing her right then and there. Put her down fast and fling her overboard."

"And take care of him later?"

"If I could figure out a way. What I decided was the best thing to do was wait until the last night."

"And do them both."

"Yes."

She thought about this. "If you did what she thought you were going to do, made his death look like a heart attack— could you have done that?"

"I could have tried. But a good medical examiner wouldn't

be fooled. And the guy was going to be a star witness, and his two bodyguards had gone down the first day out of port."

"One of them died."

"I didn't know that."

"It was in the article. And the other one's still in the hospital in Nassau. Just a coincidence, as far as the early story is concerned, just a sign that this was a hard-luck cruise, because they don't know there's a connection between those two men and the Carmodys."

"They will."

"If he died and she didn't, they'd question her."

"Right."

"And she'd fall apart."

"Within a couple of hours, would be my guess."

"Even if it passed for a heart attack—but it wouldn't, would it?"

"If it was a genuine bona fide heart attack," he said, "and she's the just-married younger wife, who's pretty much of a semipro hooker, they'd still grill her six ways and backwards."

"Yes, of course they would. And she'd give you up in a New York minute, so there's no question, you had to do them both. Multiple stab wounds?"

"The first one killed her," he said. "The others were for show."

"So at least it was fast. For whatever that's worth." She looked up. "Oh, what am I going on about? She was trash to the bone, she was trying to get her husband killed, so why should her dying bother me? 'Cause she was a woman? Like that makes a difference? Please."

He didn't say anything.

"They were both horrible people, and the two bodyguards

were a pair of thugs, and what do I care about any of them? You know what it is?"

"You were there."

"That's exactly right. I was there. If I stayed home and you flew off somewhere and came back and told me the story, I wouldn't be able to wait to get you in bed. Now all I am is slightly sick to my stomach. And I wasn't just there, darling. I was a participant. I got you the card key."

"That's true."

"Doesn't that make me an accessory? Of course it does. I don't mean legally, I don't care about that. I mean the way I feel. Is there something I can do? So I don't feel like this?"

"Take a shower."

"Seriously?"

"Seriously."

She went off to do so, and he returned to his price list, but had trouble staying focused. He was still sitting there when she came back wearing a robe with her hair wrapped up in a white towel.

She said, "I couldn't see what good a shower would do, but I have to say I feel a little better. Isn't there something you do afterward to get over it?"

He'd performed the exercise the previous evening, before he fell asleep, and he talked her through it now: picturing the victim, concentrating hard on the image, and then turning it over to the Photoshop of the mind: shrinking it, fading it, pushing it off into the distance, until it was an undefined gray dot that ultimately vanished altogether.

"It's hard to do," she said.

"It gets easier with practice."

"I suppose it must. I'll work with it. And I may take more

showers than usual over the next week or so. But I don't want to have to do this again."

"No."

"I'm not sorry I was there. This is something you do, and I'm fine that you do it, and I even like it a lot more than I don't. And I should know what it's like, what it feels like. I didn't, and now I do."

"But once is enough."

"Once is plenty. Oh, a price list. 'Portugal and Colonies.' Are you finding stamps that you need?"

"A few."

"That's good," she said. "What and where is Lourenço Marques?"

"It's part of Mozambique."

"Well, I know where that is. And they have their own stamps?"

"Not since 1920."

"I guess nothing lasts forever. You know what I'm going to do now? Besides making the mental picture shrink and turn gray? I'm going to email Myrt Huysendahl to make sure we don't lose touch. Do you think Jenny would like a small-ship cruise of the Turkish Riviera?"

"You know, I'll bet that's what she was saying earlier."

"Must have been. I think you and I would like it, and Roy could see where his stamps come from. I'm going to be fine, you know."

"I know," he said.

KELLER'S
SIDELINE

THIRTY-TWO

I'll tell you what's annoying," Dot said. "I was in Denver myself this past weekend."

"What's the matter with Denver?"

"Nothing," she said, "aside from the fact that I had a perfectly nice room for two nights at the Brown Palace, and I didn't get to sleep in it."

"Insomnia?"

"I never have insomnia, Keller. Nothing keeps me awake. That's one of the benefits of leading a blameless life. I slept fine, but not in my room. And don't ask."

"I won't."

"I had a dirty weekend. Flew up to Denver and slept with a strange man."

"Oh."

"That's it? 'Oh?' That's all you've got to say on the subject?"

"You said not to ask."

"It's an expression, Keller. If I really didn't want you to ask I wouldn't have brought it up in the first place."

"Oh."

"You're just insisting on hearing it all, aren't you? All right. I met this man on JDate. You know what that is?"

"I've heard of it," he said. "It's an online dating site. But isn't it for Jewish people?"

"So?"

"I never knew you were Jewish."

"Look at it this way, Keller," she said. "I'm a lot closer to being Jewish than Stuart Lichtblau is to being sixty-two."

"Oh."

"He's a widower," she said, "and I gather he was sixty-one when his wife died, but that must have been fifteen years ago. He spent a few months mourning her and a few more searching for a replacement, and then he discovered he liked being single, and ever since he's been spending his golden years screwing his brains out."

He couldn't say *Oh* again, but what else was there to say? He asked her if she'd had a good time.

"Yes," she said, "and no. He's retired, he had a chain of record stores that he sold back when people still bought records, and he's got this town house in a gated community in Aurora. His bed's the size of a tennis court, and I bet he spends more on Viagra than you spend on stamps. I have to say he taught me some new tricks, though I can't say my life's fuller for having learned them. And I had good food to eat and pricey wine to drink, and he treated me like a lady, and you know what? I couldn't wait to go home."

He thought about it. Then he said, "What's annoying?"

"Annoying?"

"You said what's annoying is you were in Denver this past weekend, but…"

"Right, right. I could have done it while I was there. Except of course for the fact that it's your line of work, not mine. But, you know, call it irony. I made a trip to Denver, and now you have to make a trip to Denver. Assuming you feel like taking the job."

"You have a job for me."

"Well, of course," she said. "Why else would I be calling? Just to tell you I got laid by a foxy old Jewish guy?"

He dialed the number, and when the woman answered he said, "Mrs. Soderling? This is Nicholas Edwards in New Orleans. We spoke last week."

"Yes, Mr. Edwards."

"I hope you still have the stamps."

"Why, of course I do. And I hope you're still interested. I believe I was to expect you sometime the middle of next month."

"I was wondering if we could move it up," he said. "I'm going to be making a trip to your part of the country early next week, and I hoped to come see you as early as this Friday, if that's convenient."

He listened for a few minutes, made notes, exchanged pleasantries. He found Julia in the kitchen, stirring something that smelled wonderful. "Friday's fine," he told her. "Her husband's collection is still intact, and she's happy I'm still interested."

"And she's in Denver?"

"Cheyenne. Well, outside of it. She gave me directions, and anyway I'm sure the rental car'll have GPS."

"So you'll fly to Denver and drive up to Cheyenne."

He shook his head. "I'll fly to Cheyenne," he said, "although I'll probably have to change planes in Denver. I'll drive from Cheyenne to Denver, and then I'll drive back to Cheyenne, and I'll fly home from there."

"Even though you'll once again have to change planes in Denver."

"Right."

"Because if anybody asks, you flew out to Cheyenne to buy a stamp collection and flew straight home afterward. Denver? You were only in Denver to change planes."

"That's the idea."

"Is the collection worth the trip?"

"I won't know until I see it," he said, "but I was going to take the chance anyway."

"Before you heard from Dot."

He nodded. "The husband collected for years," he said. "He subscribed to a couple of publications, and he was a life member of the American Philatelic Society, and he was sitting on the sofa reading the latest issue of *Linn's* when he had a heart attack and died."

"I suppose that's not a bad way to go."

"She watched it happen. That part couldn't have been much fun. Anyway, by the time the body was in the ground she started getting letters. 'So sorry at your hour of grief, but we'll make sure you get the best price for your husband's stamps.'"

"Vultures," she said.

"When the first letter came she was pleased, because she figured she'd deal with these people and be done with it. But when all the other letters flooded in she began worrying that she'd make a mistake and deal with the wrong person. They were all in such a rush to send a buyer to her home that she got a little suspicious."

"So she picked someone she hadn't heard from at all."

"Me," he agreed. "Remember Mrs. Ricks?"

"Was that the one near Audubon Park?"

"That's her."

"This woman in Cheyenne is a friend of Mrs. Ricks?"

"No, never met her."

"But she's from New Orleans?"

"Never even visited."

"Then—"

"You know that kids' game, Telephone? Where a message passes all around the room, and gets garbled along the way?"

"I played it as a child," she said. "But as I remember, it never worked out the way it was supposed to. The message didn't get garbled. It just made its way around the room."

"Well," he said, "the same thing happened with Mrs. Ricks's message, which was that there was a young man in New Orleans who bought stamps, and you could trust him all the way."

"I remember now," Julia said. "You bought her stamps, and then they turned out to be worth more than you thought. And you handed her an extra check out of the blue."

"Well, it just seemed like the right thing to do," he said. "It never occurred to me she'd run around telling everybody."

"I know they're very valuable," Edith Ricks had said.

She perched on the edge of a ladder-back chair and fixed her clear blue eyes on Keller. On the coffee table between them were three stacks of albums designed to hold sheets of mint postage stamps.

There was coffee as well, in two bone china cups, and shortbread cookies on a matching plate. The coffee was strong, and flavored with chicory, and he was fairly sure she'd baked the cookies herself.

"When my husband was a young boy," she said, "his father realized that there was a foolproof way to invest. You didn't have to pay a commission to a broker, and your money was safe, because it was guaranteed by the government."

Keller had seen this coming. "He bought stamps at the post office," he said.

"Exactly! He bought full sheets, and put them in these folders with this special paper to keep them in perfect condition—"

Glassine interleaving, Keller thought.

"—and he tucked them away for safekeeping. And for quite a few years he continued his regular visits to the post office. Then he got out of the habit, but now and then he'd show me some of the stamps. They go all the way back to 1948, when his father first got started."

That figured, Keller thought. It was in the years right after the Second World War that the whole country discovered the can't-lose investment potential of mint U.S. postage stamps.

"And now he's gone," she said.

"I'm sorry."

"It's been almost five years since he passed," she said. "And, you know, I've thought about the stamps. If we'd had children, I wouldn't even consider selling them now. I'd pass them on."

"That would be ideal," Keller said.

"But I lost one baby, and then I could never have another. I have a niece and nephews, but we're not close. And I don't really *need* the money, but I'm not *doing* anything with the stamps, and who knows what would become of them if anything happened to me?"

A clock chimed. They were in the parlor of a substantial three-story house on Hurst Street, just east of Audubon Park.

Keller could have had a look at one of the albums, but felt he ought to wait for an invitation. Besides, he was in no hurry. He knew what he would find, and what the ensuing conversation would be like.

"I know there are people who deal in postage stamps," she said, "and I did look in the Yellow Pages once, but that's as far as I went. Because it's very difficult to know whom to trust."

"Your husband never did any business with stamp dealers?"

"Oh, no. He and his father dealt only with the post office. So I really didn't know how to avoid being cheated, and then I was talking to a friend, and she mentioned that someone had told her that the young man who married the Roussard girl had an interest in buying old stamp collections, and..."

She'd gone to school with Julia's mother, who had herself died many years ago, but that was enough of a connection to suggest that he was the sort of person she could admit to her house, and entertain with coffee and cookies. He'd be well-mannered and soft-spoken, and wouldn't try to cheat her out of her inheritance.

Nor would he. But he was going to have to break her heart.

THIRTY-THREE

The stamp business was Julia's idea.

He'd come home from a day on a construction crew, his muscles sore from ten hours of installing Sheetrock, his head throbbing from ten hours of salsa music pouring out of one crew member's boom box. He'd been paid in cash at the day's end, and he put three twenties and a five on the kitchen table and stood there for a moment staring at his earnings.

"Let me draw you a bath," Julia said. "You must be exhausted."

The bath helped. He returned to the kitchen, where the four bills were still on the table, along with a welcome cup of coffee. "I must be out of shape," he told Julia. "Used to be Donny and I'd work dawn to dusk and I'd feel fine at the end of it. Tired after a long day, but not like I'd just had a beating."

"You're not used to it."

"No," he said, and thought for a moment. "And it's different. We had a business, we were working to accomplish something. Now all I'm working for is six fifty an hour."

"Which you don't really need in the first place."

"Donny got the guy to take me on. I didn't really know how to turn it down. Donny's doing me a favor, I can't throw it back in his face."

"There ought to be a way," she said. "You don't want to keep on doing this. Or do you?"

"I suppose my body would get used to it before too long. But what's the point? We don't need the money."

"No."

"And even if my body gets used to it, I'm not sure my head will. They're mostly Hispanic, which is fine, except that the opportunity for conversation is limited. But the music they like, and the volume they play it at—"

"I can imagine."

"What am I going to tell Donny? 'Thanks all the same, but I've got a ton of money in an offshore account.'"

"No."

"'And now and then I get a phone call and...' Well, obviously I can't tell him that part, either."

They talked about it, and the following afternoon Julia followed Jenny into the den while he was working with his stamps. She stood there silent while he was cutting a mount. When he looked up she said, "I was thinking."

"Oh?"

"You need a business."

"I do?"

"Something," she said. "So that there's something that you do, so it'll make sense to Donny that you don't need to swing a hammer."

"That'd be nice," he allowed. "And it's not just Donny. There must be a lot of people who wonder just what it is I do."

"Not so much in this town. New Orleans is full of people who don't seem to do much of anything. But it wouldn't hurt if you had some visible source of income."

"I've had that thought myself," he said. "But there's nothing I know all that much about."

"You know a lot about stamps, don't you?"

"So I could go into the business?" He thought about it, frowned. "The dealers I know," he said, "work all the time. And they're constantly making little sales and filling orders and doing all this detail work. I don't think I'd be good at it. I enjoy buying stamps, but if you're going to make a business out of it, the part you have to enjoy is selling them."

"If the buying part's what you like, couldn't you make a business out of that?"

He extended a hand, indicating first the album on the desk in front of him, then the double row of albums in the bookcase. "I'm already doing that part," he said, "and it keeps me busy, but it's hard to call it a business."

"Did you ever meet my friend Celia Cutrone? She was a year behind me at Ursuline. Skinny little creature then, but she filled out. Yes, you did meet her, she was at Donny and Claudia's cookout."

"If you say so."

"She brought her big old dog, and the two of you were talking about dogs."

He remembered now, an owlish woman with a wonderfully well-behaved Great Pyrenees, and he'd found himself remembering Nelson, the Australian cattle dog he'd had for a while, until the dog walker walked off with him.

"We didn't talk about stamps," he said. "Did we?"

"Probably not. She's not a stamp collector."

"Oh."

"She's in the antiques business, but she doesn't have a shop or list things on eBay. She's what they call a picker."

He'd heard the term. A picker went around and scooped up items at garage sales and junk shops and wholesaled them to retailers.

"I could do that," he said. "I guess the way to get started is run standing ads in all the neighborhood papers. The ones they give away."

"Shoppers, they call them. And you wouldn't want to forget Craigslist."

"Craigslist is free, isn't it? Running ads in it, I mean. And ads in the shoppers can't cost the earth."

"And then there'd be word of mouth," she said. "'You know those old stamps Henry had all those years? Well, the nicest young man came over and paid me decent money for them.'"

"'The one who married the Roussard girl, and he's surprisingly polite for a Yankee.'"

"Word of mouth," she said, "New Orleans–style. You can run all the ads you want, but once you get them talking about you, you're in business."

He thought about it. Low start-up costs, nothing like opening a store. Even so...

"I don't know," he said.

"Whether you'd enjoy it?"

"Oh, I'd like it well enough. What I don't know is if there's any way to do it and come out ahead. I wouldn't want to cheat anybody, and I wouldn't get big prices from the dealers I sold to, and I could see myself putting in a lot of hours and barely breaking even."

"Hours doing what?"

"Well, driving around and looking at people's stamps," he said. "And then looking at them some more afterward, and figuring out just what I bought and what it's worth and who's the best buyer for it."

"And you might spend hours doing these things and make chump change for your troubles."

"Chump change," he said.

"Isn't that the expression?"

"It sounded funny," he said, "coming out of your mouth. But yes, that's the expression, and it's probably what I could expect to earn."

"So?"

He looked up at her, and got it.

"I don't have to make money," he said. "Do I?"

"No. We've got plenty of money. And every once in a while you get a call from Dot, and we get more money."

"All I need," he said, "is something that looks like a business. I need a sideline, but it doesn't have to be a profitable one. It could even lose money and that would be all right. In fact, we could declare a net profit whether we actually earned one or not. Pay a few dollars in taxes and keep everybody happy."

"You've got that quick Yankee mind," she said. "I do admire that in a man."

THIRTY-FOUR

Keller, in the parlor of the house on Hurst Street, spent as much time as he could leafing through the stack of mint sheet albums. The contents were what he'd anticipated, panes of commemorative stamps ranging from 1948 to sometime in the early 1960s, when James Houghton Ricks had stopped paying regular visits to the post office.

That was the collector's name, Keller had discovered, even as he'd learned that his hostess's name was Edith Vass Ricks, and that her husband was actually James Houghton Ricks, Jr., and was called Houghty to distinguish him from his father, although there was nothing remotely haughty about Houghty.

Mrs. Ricks spoke softly and expressively, and Keller found her words soothing without having to pay very much attention to them. All these stamps, he thought. All commemoratives, all three-centers for years, until the first-class rate went up to four cents.

"The condition's good," he said.

"They were placed in those books," she said, "and never touched."

That was no guarantee, Keller knew, not in the New Orleans climate. Mold and mildew could find their way into a sealed trunk, and even between the glassine interleaving of a mint sheet album.

"It must have seemed like such a good idea at the time," he said gently. He kept his eyes on the panes of stamps. "But there was something people didn't realize."

"Oh?"

"You can't sell stamps back to the post office," he said. "They're not like money. All you can do with them is mail letters."

He glanced at her, and she did not look happy, but neither did she appear to be taken entirely by surprise. He explained, not for the first time, how it worked. A stamp, while indeed issued by the government, was not currency. It represented the government's obligation to provide a service, and in that respect it never expired. The stamp you bought in 1948 was still valid as postage sixty-some years later.

"Of course there's inflation," he said. "Postal rates go up."

"Every year, it seems like."

It wasn't quite that often, but Keller agreed that it did seem that way. He pointed to a sheet of red stamps showing a young man's face with a flag on either side, one with only a scattering of stars, the other with considerably more.

"Francis Scott Key," he said. "The flag on the left flew over Fort McHenry during the War of 1812, and when it survived the bombardment, he's the one who wrote a song about it."

"'The Star-Spangled Banner,'" she said.

"It only had fifteen stars," he said, "because we only had fifteen states at the time. And this other flag has forty-eight, because Alaska and Hawaii weren't admitted to the union until 1959. I suppose that's another sort of inflation. But when this three-cent stamp came out it would carry a letter, and now it would take fifteen of them to do that job."

"That many?"

Well, fourteen, Keller thought, plus a two-cent stamp to make up the deficit. But her question didn't seem to require an answer.

"You'd cover both sides of the envelope," she said. "And all those stamps would add weight, and you'd wind up needing another stamp, wouldn't you?"

"You might."

She'd been to the post office, she told Keller, just to establish a baseline value for the stamps, and the postal clerk had told her essentially the same thing. But he'd been brusque with her, and she'd thought he might be shading the truth in order to keep the line moving. She'd taken it as an article of faith that, if all else failed, the post office would buy the stamps back from you.

But if that wasn't true, and she could see now that it wasn't, and if the stamps were too common for collectors to be interested in them, then what was she going to do with them?

"I don't mail ten letters a month," she said. "I pay bills, and I write a note if somebody dies or a baby's born, but you couldn't put fifteen stamps on one of those little envelopes, and how would it look if you did? If the post office won't take the stamps back, would they at least let me trade them in for the new ones?"

"I'm afraid not."

"You buy it, it's yours. No refunds and no exchanges. That's about it, then?"

"That's their policy."

"So these are worthless, then. Is that about the size of it? I can just put them out with the trash?"

Not quite, he told her. And he explained that there were brokers who sold stamps at a discount, somewhere around 90 percent of face value, to volume mailers looking to trim their costs. These brokers replenished their stock by buying holdings like that of Mrs. Ricks, paying 70 to 75 percent of face value for them. He'd be happy to give her contact information for one or two brokers and she could deal directly with them.

Or, if she wanted, he'd buy the stamps himself. He could only pay half their face value, but it would save her negotiating with the brokers, along with the nuisance of packing the stamps for shipment.

"And taking them to the post office," she said darkly. "And paying the postage!"

"Now, if there's anyone you know who might enjoy having the stamps," he said. "Church youth groups always welcome donations. Or a Boy Scout troop, or—"

But she was shaking her head. "Add them up," she said. "See what they come to, and what you can pay me. I just want them out of here."

The total face value of the lot ran to $1838, and he divided the sum in half and counted out nine $100 bills and added a twenty. She said she owed him a dollar, and insisted on paying it. As he was packing up what he'd bought and wondering if he'd come out ahead by the time he was done shipping it, she asked him if there was anything else he could use. She had books that she wouldn't mind selling, and some of them were pretty old. Did he have any interest in books?

Just stamps, he told her. If she happened to have any old envelopes with stamps on them, he'd be glad to take a look at them and let her know if they were something he could use.

She snapped her fingers, which was something you didn't see often. "In that trunk," she said. "You know, I've been meaning to get rid of that, but it's way up in the attic and I don't go there if I can help it. But there's a little stack of envelopes there. People in the family used to save letters, you know, and in Houghty's family as well, and some of them go all the way back to the war."

He knew which war she meant.

"A few times," she said, "I thought some of those stamps might be worth something, and what I ought to do was soak them off the envelopes, but—"

"No, never do that."

"Well, I guess I'm glad I never got around to it, from the tone of your voice! But isn't that what collectors do?"

"Not with old envelopes. No, you don't want to do anything of the sort. There are people who collect the whole envelope—covers, they call them—and they like them even better with the letters intact."

"That's what's in the attic. Envelopes with letters in them. And then there's some that don't even have any stamps on them, though how they got through the mail without them is beyond me. You probably won't want those, will you?"

"Maybe we should see what's up there," he said.

There were forty-one envelopes, and they fit quite comfortably in a box that had once held fifty Garcia y Vega cigars. "I don't think there are any outstanding rarities here," he told Mrs. Ricks, "but I can pay you twelve hundred dollars for these."

"That much for those old letters?"

"I'm pretty sure I'll come out okay at that figure," he told her. "And if I don't, well, I'll just add them to my own collection."

But he didn't collect U.S.—or Confederate, either, for that matter—and he knew just where to send the material he'd purchased. He'd met a fellow at an auction in Dallas, a dealer-collector hybrid from Montgomery who specialized in the postal history of the Confederacy, and when he got home he was able to put his hands on the man's business card.

He picked up the phone in his stamp room, dialed the number. "I've got a few pieces that might interest you," he said. "Can I send them for your offer?"

The offer came by return mail, in the form of a check for an even $15,000. There was a note along with it, allowing that one particular item alone might bring almost that much at auction. "But we'll never know," the fellow said, "because it's found a permanent home in my personal collection. You come up with any more goodies like this, you know where to send them."

He put the check in the bank, and added another a few days later, from the gentleman in Connecticut who bought and sold discounted postage; the mint stamps he'd paid $919 for had returned $1286. That was no more of a profit than he deserved, considering his time and shipping costs, but the $15,000 from the Alabaman, welcome though it was, left a sour taste in his mouth.

He spent a few days thinking about it, and then he made a phone call and showed up at the Hurst Street address with a check for $3500. "Those covers were better than I realized," he told Edith Ricks. "And it seems only fair that you should share in the profits."

She was astonished, and tried to get him to come in for another round of coffee and cookies, but he pleaded another appointment and went home. "It's not as though she needed the money," he told Julia, "but she was certainly happy to have it."

"That's the way it is with money," she said. "It's welcome wherever it goes. You didn't have to pay her extra."

"No."

"She'd never have known what you got for those covers."

"No, of course not."

"Conscience money."

"Is that what it was? It just seemed, oh, I don't know. Appropriate?"

"I'll tell you what it is, even though you didn't mean it that way. But that's how it'll turn out."

"What's that?"

"Bread upon the waters," she said. "You'll see."

And he did get a few nibbles over the next month or so, though none of them amounted to much. He told a woman in Metairie that her late husband's boyhood stamp collection, housed, as Keller's own had been, in a *Modern Postage Stamp Album,* would be best donated to charity—a church rummage sale, perhaps, to save the cost of shipping it to one of the stamp charities.

Another woman had a soldier's letters home, or in any event the envelopes they'd come in. The letters themselves had disappeared, and she had no idea who the sender might be, or the recipient, either; they'd turned up, carefully wrapped in oilcloth, when her husband had taken down a wall to enlarge their kitchen.

The letters, an even dozen of them, had been posted from Germany in the immediate aftermath of World War II, and bore stamps issued by the Allied Military Government. The stamps were common, but the covers were interesting, and Keller's offer of $20 for the lot was accepted.

It was also high, as he found out when he emailed a couple

of scans to an eBay dealer who did a lot with covers. The man's offer was $1.50 a cover, $2 less than Keller had paid for the material, and he'd have the trouble and expense of mailing them to upstate New York.

He mailed them off, took the loss. He could have kept them, but this way he'd recorded another transaction for his sideline.

Bread upon the waters, but nothing much to show for it, and when the calls stopped coming he more or less forgot about Edith Vass Ricks.

And then he heard from the woman in Cheyenne.

THIRTY-FIVE

Keller packed everything he needed in a wheeled case that was well within the airline's limits for a carry-on. He checked it anyway, because he didn't want some zealous security officer to confiscate his stamp tongs.

Which seemed unlikely, but Keller had known it to happen. A perfin and precancel collector he'd met at a show had told him about it, how the woman from Homeland Security had glared at his tongs as if they were an AK-47. "Look at this," she'd said, holding them aloft. "Five, six inches long! Made of steel! You could put somebody's eye out with these!"

"I extended my index finger," the man told Keller, "and I was just about to point out how easily I could use it to gouge her eye out, but something stopped me."

"Just as well, I'd say."

"Oh, I know. I'd be awaiting trial even as we speak. But can you imagine taking a man's tongs from him? That particular pair didn't even have pointed tips, I want you to know. Rounded, so you couldn't stab yourself by accident."

Or even on purpose, Keller thought, packing two pairs of tongs (one with rounded tips, the other with tips just made for stabbing) and two magnifiers and, of course, his catalog. He checked his bag straight through to Cheyenne, and boarded his flight to Denver with his laptop in a padded briefcase and his cash in a money belt around his waist.

The airport in Denver had a free wi-fi connection, so he logged on and checked his email. He'd been outbid in an eBay auction, and the email invited him to raise his bid and win the lot after all. But of course the other bidder had waited until the last minute to top him, so the auction was over by the time Keller received the invitation.

Not that he'd have bothered anyway. He always bid his maximum at the beginning, and if someone else was willing to outbid him, then that person wanted it more than he did. He'd explained as much to Julia once, and she'd told him his attitude was remarkably mature. He still hadn't decided whether she was being ironic.

He thought of killing time at a couple of favorite sites, but decided to save his battery instead. He logged off and carried his briefcase to the men's room, where he locked himself in a stall and took out the envelope Dot had sent. It held a pink ruled index card with one side blank and a name and address and phone number on the other.

He'd memorized that information earlier, and had considered destroying the index card afterward, but dismissed the notion as stupid. He'd also considered copying the data into a computer file, and decided that would be even stupider. For now the man whose name was on the card was alive and well, and that meant there was no risk in having the card in his possession. If something happened to the fellow, then something would happen to the card as well. You could get rid of an index card, you could burn it or shred it or chew it up and swallow it, but once it was on a computer it had eternal life.

The envelope also contained two small photographs, which Keller could only assume were of the same man. One was taken from the side, and showed him walking along a street, with a shoe repair shop behind him. The other was full-face, and had probably been taken at fairly close range and with a flash, because it had caught the subject blinking. If the subject had any strong features, neither photograph had managed to capture them. You couldn't use them to make an ID, just to rule out other fish that might turn up in the net.

Keller, who hadn't needed to use the toilet, flushed it anyway in the interests of verisimilitude. The rushing water proved a stimulus, and he used the toilet after all, and then flushed it again, which was rather more verisimilitude than the occasion would seem to require. Way more, he found upon exiting the stall, as he seemed to be the only person in the restroom.

He walked away, frowning.

His Cheyenne flight was on a regional carrier, and the plane was a small one, with minimal capacity for overhead luggage storage. Most of the passengers had to check their putative carry-ons at the gate, and Keller, who'd checked his all the way through, felt he was ahead of the game.

The pilot spent most of the hour apologizing for the rough air, which didn't seem all that rough to Keller. The landing was certainly smooth enough. He collected his bag, picked up the car Hertz had waiting for him. It was a perky little Toyota, slate blue in color, and it had a GPS system, but Keller didn't have an address to program into it, so he just followed the signs to the motel strip on West Lincolnway. Ten or a dozen of them huddled there, like cattle bracing against a storm, and he passed three for no particular reason before pulling into a La Quinta.

It seemed to him he'd stayed at a La Quinta not too long ago, but he couldn't remember where, or whether he'd liked it. He tried phrases in his mind: *Oh, La Quinta, that was the nice clean one. Oh, La Quinta, with the moldy carpet.* One seemed as likely as the other, and what difference did it make? If this one had a moldy carpet, or a flickering TV, or a bad smell, well, he'd go to the one next door.

The woman behind the desk had an easy manner that inspired confidence, and the room she gave him was perfectly acceptable. He unpacked, shifting his stamp tongs to his breast pocket.

His cell phone got a signal right away. His first call was to Julia, just to let her know he'd survived a couple of hours in the air. She didn't offer to put Jenny on, nor did he ask. He was working, and that part of his life could wait until the job was done.

He made a second call, to Denia Soderling, who immediately invited him to dinner. There was enough for two, she said, if he hadn't eaten. He said he was tired, which was true enough, and that it would be better to start fresh in the morning. He wrote down the directions she gave him, and they agreed that he'd show up around nine thirty or ten.

He ate across the street, at a family restaurant that proclaimed itself locally owned and operated. He had shrimp in a basket, which didn't strike him as all that local, and a small garden salad, and drank a glass of iced tea. The menu promised him unlimited refills on the iced tea, but one glass was plenty.

Back in his room, he took a shower and decided his shave could wait until morning. The TV had a satellite connection, and got what seemed to be an infinite number of channels. He put on CNN while he booted up his laptop and checked his email. No email of note, and no news he cared about. He turned everything off and went to bed.

Ten hours later he was eating breakfast down the street at Denny's. An hour and a half after that he was looking at stamps.

THIRTY-SIX

The first thing that struck Keller, when Denia Soderling showed him into her husband's den, was that no one could have designed a better room for a stamp collector. Walls paneled in knotty cedar, half a dozen rifles and shotguns in a glass-fronted cabinet, a pair of swords crossed on one wall, a matched pair of dueling pistols to their right. A picture window opened onto a rail-fenced paddock, where a pair of horses as well matched as the pistols stood enjoying the morning sun. And the window faced north, Keller saw, so the sun wouldn't come into the room and cause trouble.

One of a pair of glass-fronted bookcases held books unrelated to stamp collecting, most of them history, along with a dictionary of quotations and a few volumes of poetry. The other case contained the owner's philatelic library. There was a full set of the Scott catalogs, each volume two or three years old, and there were other catalogs as well, Michel and Yvert and Gibbons and more. And the shelves were filled with books and pamphlets on one stamp-related subject or another. The majority dealt with European nations and their colonies, but Keller spotted Michael Laurence's study of the ten-cent covers of 1869. He'd almost bought the book himself, even though he didn't collect U.S. issues and had no real interest in the subject. J. S. Soderling had evidently had the same impulse, and acted on it.

The second thing Keller realized, and he did so even as he was looking around and taking everything in, was that it shouldn't have been necessary for him to check his carry-on bag. Bringing his own tongs to a room like this had to be right up there with carrying coals to Newcastle.

He confirmed this when he opened the bookcases where the stamp albums were housed. One shelf held the tools of the well-equipped philatelist, and Soderling had equipped himself fully. There were magnifiers and watermark detectors and guillotine-style mount cutters and, not surprisingly, an even dozen pairs of tongs. There were tongs with pointed tips, with blunt tips, with spade-shaped tips, with rounded tips. There were tongs with angled tips, for getting at otherwise inaccessible stamps, and tongs with their arms angled in the middle, which no doubt made them particularly well suited for some special purpose, although Keller couldn't think what it might be.

And then there were the stamps. The albums stood up in rows—France and Colonies, Portugal and Colonies, Italy and Colonies, Germany and Colonies. Russia. Eastern Europe. No U.S. that he could see, and no British Empire, and no Latin America, either. No Asia or Africa, aside from the colonial issues. But all of continental Europe was there, from Iceland

and Denmark clear across to Russia and Turkey, and the albums filled two large bookcases. Most of them were from the Scott Specialized series, but there were leather-bound stock books as well, and blank albums.

"It's overwhelming," Denia Soderling said, and Keller was surprised to realize she was in the room with him. They'd entered it together, but he'd been so transported by the room and its contents that he'd lost track of her. But there she was, a tall and slender woman with just a touch of gray in her dark hair.

"It's quite a room," Keller said.

"Jeb loved it. If he wasn't at the desk working on his stamps he'd be in the leather chair with his feet up, reading about some battle in the Thirty Years' War. Or the Hundred Years' War, I'm afraid I can never keep them straight."

"One was longer."

"Once a war lasts thirty years," she said, "I can't see that another seventy would make much of a difference. I can't tell you how many times I've come into this room since Jeb passed. I can't keep from coming in, and I can't make myself stay for more than a few minutes. Do you know what I mean?"

He nodded.

"I tried to look at the stamps. And I thought he might have left a letter for me, telling me what to do with them. I couldn't find anything. And of course there were all those letters from all those dealers. Overwhelming, all of it."

"I can imagine."

"Now you're going to want to spend some time just looking, aren't you? And you don't need me watching over your shoulder, and frankly I'd just as soon not spend any more time in this room than I have to. In fact, I think I'll go out and ride for an hour. I try to ride every day. I think it's good for me, physically and emotionally, and I know it's good for the horses."

Keller voiced his agreement without being at all certain what he was agreeing with. Her words had washed over him without entirely registering. Something was evidently good for the horses, and it seemed safe to be in favor of it.

He carried the first volume of Portugal and Colonies to the desk and opened it.

At one point the door opened, although he never heard it. Then she was at his side, announcing that she'd brought him a cup of coffee. It was black, she said, but if he took cream or sugar —

He told her black was fine. She told him to let her know when he was ready for a lunch break, and he said he would.

She withdrew, leaving the coffee where he could reach it but far enough away so he'd be unlikely to knock it over. Well, she'd probably brought coffee to her husband in similar circumstances. She'd had plenty of time to work out just where to put the cup.

And coffee was just the ticket. He could use a cup of coffee, no question about it.

First, though —

By the time he reached for the coffee, it was cold.

"Are you sure you won't have another sandwich, Mr. Edwards?"

"No, I'm fine," he said.

She'd served him lunch at a glass-topped table on the back patio, where the view was the same as the one from the stamp room's window. The two horses were keeping each other company in the paddock. Both were chestnut geldings, and wonderfully gentle, she'd told him, and added that she'd been out for an hour on the one with the star on his forehead. And did he ride, by any chance?

He shook his head. "Stamps keep me busy," he said.

"They certainly kept Jeb busy," she said, "although he was always eager to spend plenty of time in the saddle." The double entendre was clearly unintentional, and she colored when she realized what she'd said. Keller, who'd been about to suggest she call him Nicholas, decided they'd be better off staying with Mr. Edwards and Mrs. Soderling for the time being.

He said, "About the stamps."

"Yes."

"Do you have any sense of what you'd like to get for them?"

"Well, as much as I can."

"Of course."

"I know Jeb put a good deal of money into his collections. His line of business was quite volatile, he had interests in oil and cattle and real estate, so we'd be rich one day and broke the next and rich again the day after. When there was plenty of money he'd buy stamps, and when his cash flow tightened up he'd bide his time."

"Did he keep records of what he spent?"

"I don't believe so. He got a lot of his income in the form of cash, so he preferred to pay for his stamps that way. Something to do with taxes, I suppose."

And the nonpayment thereof, Keller thought.

"He said stamps were an investment, that the better ones would go up in value. But he also said it wasn't like the stock market, that you couldn't expect to get close to retail when you sold. And there was one time when he talked about selling."

"Oh?"

"When the market crashed a few years ago. 'Maybe I'll sell

the stamps,' he said. 'That'd keep us going a while, anyway.' But I don't think he was serious, and nothing ever came of it. You asked me if I had any idea what they're worth. I don't, not really, but I would think it would come to six figures, wouldn't you?"

He took a moment before answering. Then he said, "I could make a phone call right now, and move some money into my checking account. And then I could write you a check for a quarter of a million dollars. I'd be running a certain risk, because there are rare stamps that haven't been authenticated by experts, and they might or might not turn out to be genuine. It's a chance I'm prepared to take. But I don't think it would be the best deal for you."

"Because it might be worth more."

"Possibly a great deal more," he said. "I only collect stamps up to 1940, and your husband's collections go all the way to the present. The modern material's out of my area of expertise. And in some of his collections, Russia in particular, there's a ton of specialized material, imperfs and errors and other varieties."

"He had no use for the Russians," she said, "but he liked their stamps."

"Well," he said. "The point is I can make you that offer, but I'd advise you to turn it down. If this were a much smaller collection I'd take it on consignment, giving you an advance and a share in whatever I received over a certain figure. But that's not really good, either."

There was still some iced tea in his glass, and he took a drink of it. "Here's what I'd propose," he said. "I'll act as your agent, and I'll call the three dealers most likely to be ideal purchasers of your husband's stamps. I'll make appointments for them each to send a representative within the next week.

Ideally we'll have them here on three consecutive days, and we'll get sealed bids from each of them, and the high bidder gets the collection."

"And they'll all be able to get someone here on the day you specify?"

"If any of them can't," he said, "I'll call the next name on the list."

"And you think one of them will pay significantly more than a quarter of a million dollars."

"Yes."

"As to how much more—"

"I'd be guessing."

"I understand. But that guess would be at least a half a million?"

"Probably more."

She thought for a moment. "And if their offers turn out to be lower than you expect—"

"That won't happen. But if it does, yes, I'll still pay you the quarter million."

"And you'll be here when they come?"

"To protect your interests. Yes."

"And what about your own interest, Mr. Edwards? You'll be stuck in Cheyenne for a week, and of course you'll be entitled to a portion of the price I receive, but do you have a figure in mind?"

THIRTY-SEVEN

Getting from Cheyenne to Denver was simple enough. You got on I-25 and drove south for a hundred miles, and if it took you more than an hour and a half you weren't keeping up with the light Saturday morning traffic. He held the Toyota steady at four or five miles over the posted speed limit, thus inviting neither the attention of a highway patrolman nor the scorn of his fellow motorists.

He'd programmed the GPS with the address from the pink index card, and its soothing ladylike voice didn't have much to say for most of the way on the interstate. She perked up as they got close to Denver, and guided him southwest on I-76 to where that highway ran into I-70. There he let her talk him through a complicated cloverleaf ("Prepare to keep to the left, followed by a keep to the left...") that left him heading south on Wadsworth Boulevard.

He went on doing as instructed, until he made a turn into

Otis Drive and she told him, not without a measure of self-satisfaction, "You have arrived."

He hadn't quite, though. Not yet, because the street number of the house to his right, conveniently painted on the curb, was 4101, and the number he'd punched into the GPS was 4132. That would put it halfway up the block and on the left-hand side.

Where there were a couple of cars parked, two of them with flashing lights mounted on their roofs. And where all those people were standing.

And where the house, on the other hand, was not.

"You hear about houses burning to the ground," he told Dot, "but I always thought it was a figure of speech, because they never do. They burn, all right, and the property winds up being a total loss, but you still have walls standing."

"But not this time?"

"Burned to the foundation," he said, "which extended maybe a foot and a half above the ground, but that's it. Don't ask me how it happened."

"Keller, who else am I gonna ask?"

He and Dot had cell phones that they used only to call each other, and even then only when it was important that no record of the call exist. He'd had that phone with him, but waited until he'd driven a mile or so from what used to be 4132 Otis Drive. He pulled into a strip mall and parked in front of a furniture store that had closed for the night, if not forever, and he called the one number the phone was programmed to call, and she picked up midway through the second ring.

And now he held the phone in his hand and stared at it.

"Keller? Where'd you go?"

"You thought I did it," he said.

"Well, sure. I gave you a name and an address."

"And a picture and a phone number."

"Let's just stick to the name and the address, okay? I gave them to you, and sometime last night the address ceased to exist and the name wound up in the hospital."

"And you assumed I was responsible."

"Put yourself in my place, Keller. What would you have thought?"

"But to burn down a whole house?"

"I know, it's like that essay everybody had to read in high school, burning down the house to roast the pig. I forget who wrote it."

"Charles Lamb."

"Now how would you happen to know that, Keller? Don't tell me, I'll bet he's on a stamp. Do you suppose there's an alternate universe where Charles Pigg wrote a famous essay about lamb chops?"

"Uh…"

"Never mind. I thought it was pretty heavy-handed for you, not your usual style. Collateral damage and all that. Though the collateral damage could have been a lot worse. Two kids, and thank God it was Friday."

"Friday?"

"No school on Saturday, so they were both away from the house on sleepovers. Keller, you're right there in Denver and I'm filling you in from what I skimmed off the Internet. Here's a radical idea. Why don't you pick up a newspaper and call me back when you're up to speed?"

He bought the *Denver Post* from a convenience store clerk who seemed anxious that Keller was about to hold her up, and relieved when he didn't. The story wasn't hard to find, and he read it through twice and called Dot.

"Severe injuries," he said. "But he's expected to live."

"For now," Dot said.

"He had fish tanks," he said. "Aquariums, except I guess the plural is aquaria."

"Thanks for pointing that out."

"All destroyed, of course. His wife was away when it happened."

"That'd be Joanne."

"Joanne Hudepohl, right. She's described as distraught."

"There's a surprise. Your house is gone, fish tanks and all, and your husband's in the hospital with tubes coming out of his toes. Wouldn't you be distraught?"

"I suppose."

"Unless she did it," Dot said. "That's what you're thinking, isn't it? And it's what I'd have been thinking myself if I hadn't pretty much taken it for granted that you were the one who did it. She was out chauffeuring the kids to their sleepovers, wasn't she?"

"She dropped off her son first," he said, "and when she delivered her daughter, the other mommy invited her in. And there were two other mommies on hand, as it was a four-girl sleepover."

"How old were the daughters?"

"I don't know," he said. "What difference does it make?"

"None," she said, "only it's beginning to sound like a movie they were showing on cable the other night. Except those girls were college age, and they should have been ashamed of themselves. What did the four mommies do, break out the gin bottle?"

"I think it was wine. At some point she called her husband,

and he told her to stay as long as she wanted because he was busy with his fish."

"I suppose he was pasting them in an album," she said, "like you and your stamps."

"She called home before she left," he said, "but when he didn't answer she assumed he was asleep. Then she drove home in time to watch the firemen at work. They'd taken him to the hospital by then."

"So her alibi's solid."

"It looks that way."

"Just good luck that she wasn't home herself when everything went pear-shaped."

"Pear-shaped?"

"I've been watching English mysteries on the BBC," she said. "And once in a while an expression creeps into my speech. She wasn't home, and neither were the kids. Just her husband."

"And the fish."

"Collateral damage," she said. "Innocent byswimmers. It's awfully damn convenient for her, isn't it?"

"It does look that way."

"Not that she did it, but that she had it done. I suppose the same possibility might occur to the cops."

"You'd think so."

"And they'll ask her a couple of questions, and she'll fall apart."

"Amateurs generally do."

"Is she our client, Dot?"

"I think she's got to be somebody's client," she said, "but I don't know if she's ours or not. The job came from a broker who got it from a cutout, and there are too many levels for anybody to get through. There's no way she can implicate us, in case that's what you were wondering."

"The question did come to mind."

"We're clear," she said, "and why shouldn't we be? You didn't do it."

"No."

"So what you can do now," she said, "is catch the next plane back to Julia and Jenny. If the Fish Whisperer recovers, I'll tell my guy that we're keeping the advance payment and washing our hands of the whole business."

"And if he dies?"

"Then I ask for the second payment. Why not? Who's gonna prove you didn't do it, or sub it out to somebody?"

"So there's nothing I have to do?"

"Like what? Put on a white coat and hang a stethoscope around your neck? And sneak past hospital security so you can punch the guy's ticket? He ceased to be our problem when his house went up in flames."

"I guess you're right."

"Of course I'm right. Go home, Keller."

"Well," he said, "I can't. Not for a while."

Back in his room at La Quinta, Keller took a long hot shower. When he was done drying off, he tossed his towel on the floor of the shower stall.

That's what the little card told you to do, but it was hard for Keller to get used to it. If you returned your towels to the rack, that meant you wanted to use them again. If you felt fresh towels might be a good idea, you were supposed to throw them on the floor. This would save water, the management explained, and fight global warming, so Keller figured it was the least he could do.

But he couldn't throw a towel on the floor without imagining the look on his mother's face.

He got into bed, letting his mind conjure up a conversation with his long-gone mother. They hadn't had many conversations during her lifetime, and Keller had since wondered if the woman might not have been suffering from some degree of mental illness or impairment, but on balance she'd certainly been a good mother to him, and there were times when he regretted the talks they hadn't had. So he had them now occasionally, when he waited for sleep to overtake him.

They began by talking about the towel, and why he'd thrown it on the floor. *Well, if that's what they want you to do,* she said, *that's a different story. But I didn't bring you up that way.*

And then they were talking about Denia Soderling and her husband's stamps. He'd be in Cheyenne for most of the week, he told his mother, because he'd booked appointments with three dealers who'd be sending buyers to the Soderling home on three successive days, starting Monday. That gave him all day tomorrow to go through the albums and pick out the stamps he wanted as his commission.

My stars, Johnny. You've gone clear across the country to spend a week in the middle of nowhere, and all you're getting for your trouble is some stamps?

He tried to explain, but his mother wasn't having any. *If I sent you to town to sell our cow,* she said, *I swear you'd come home with a handful of magic beans. You remember that story? You used to love that story, and I used to love telling it to you, but I never for a moment thought you'd take it as gospel.*

It had struck Denia Soderling as a perfectly reasonable solution, and it even seemed to make sense to Dot, although she'd have been just as happy to see him back home in Louisiana. But why couldn't his mother seem to grasp it? He marshaled his facts and restated his arguments, and the next thing he knew it was morning.

THIRTY-EIGHT

Denia Soderling must have heard him pull into the drive, because she met him at the front door with a cup of coffee. "I know you want to get right to work on the stamps," she told him.

He set himself up in the stamp room, with a pad and pencil close at hand, along with his tongs and a box of small glassine envelopes. And he'd brought his own Scott Classic catalog along; he used it not only as a price guide but as a checklist, circling the number of each new acquisition, so that it served as a full inventory of his collection.

The bookcase full of albums was daunting, but you had to start somewhere, and he began with Italy and Colonies. He opened it to the Italian Aegean Islands. But for stamp collecting, Keller figured he wouldn't know a thing about the Turco-Italian War of 1911–12, which ended with Italy in control of three provinces in Libya and thirteen islands in the

Aegean Sea. The largest island was Rhodes, which he figured most people had probably heard of, though they might have trouble finding it on a map. The others were Calchi, Calino, Caso, and Coo, Lero, Lisso, and Nisiro, Patmo and Piscopi, and Scarpanto, Simi, and Stampalia, and it had taken many hours at his desk to enable Keller to reel them off like that.

Turkey officially ceded the islands to Italy in 1924, under the Treaty of Lausanne, but as early as 1912 the Italians had begun overprinting stamps for use there, and each island had its own stamps. One island's stamps looked rather like another's, the overprints constituting the only difference, but Keller liked them, and some of the early issues, though priced at only a few dollars apiece, were virtually impossible to find.

They were well represented in Jeb Soderling's collection. Keller, tongs in hand, went to work, selecting a stamp, slipping it into a glassine envelope, noting its catalog number and price. Calchi 5, $3.25. Calino 4–5, $6.50. Caso, same numbers, same value, and Soderling also had the Caso Garibaldi issue, the only Garibaldi set Keller still needed. Caso 17–26, unused, lightly hinged: $170.

And so on.

There was a moment when he sensed Denia Soderling's presence in the room, but by the time he looked up she was gone, and a fresh cup of coffee had replaced the empty one. He was working his way through French Colonial issues by then, and got all the way to an early overprinted issue from Gabon, when she returned to ask if he'd like to break for lunch.

"In a few minutes," he said, without raising his eyes from the stamp. Then he forgot about her, and about lunch, and the next thing he knew the door had opened and closed again, just barely registering on his consciousness, and there was a tray at the far end of the desk holding a plate of sandwiches and a glass of iced tea.

He forced himself to take a break, ate the sandwiches, drank the iced tea. Away from the stamps, even for the short time he spent eating his lunch, his mind returned to the burned-out suburban home a hundred miles to the south. He'd caught a Denver newscast on the motel's TV before breakfast, read a morning paper while he ate his breakfast, and as far as he could make out the situation was essentially unchanged. Richard Hudepohl remained in critical condition, a fire department spokesman attributed the fire's rapid devastation to the use of "multiple accelerants strategically deployed," and Joanne Hudepohl, having released a statement through an attorney, seemed to have lawyered up.

No concern of his, Keller assured himself. It was impossible to keep from thinking about it, but there was nothing to do about it, and it vanished from his mind the moment he returned to the stamps.

It was hard to know when to stop. Jeb Soderling's collection had no end of stamps lacking in Keller's, but it wasn't his intention to go through it like locusts through a field of barley. He worked diligently, keeping a running tally as he went along.

At one point he looked over at the window and was surprised to note that day had apparently turned to night. He hadn't glanced at his watch, and didn't do so now. He told himself it was time he got out of there, but first there was one more album he ought to have a look at...

By the time he emerged from the stamp room, it was almost ten o'clock. He was pretty sure Denny's would be open, not that he felt much like eating.

But the dining room table was set for two, and before he knew it she had steered him to a chair and suggested he pour the wine. While he filled their glasses from the opened bottle of California Cabernet, she brought their dinner to the table—a tossed salad in a large wooden bowl, a pot of chili.

He'd been ready to apologize for his lack of appetite, but once he got a whiff of the chili he had nothing to apologize for. He polished off one bowl and let himself be talked into another.

"I know beer's the natural accompaniment to chili," she said, "but my husband preferred wine. He said a full-bodied red transported the dish from a West Texas juke joint to a three-star restaurant."

"It's great chili," Keller said.

"The secret's the cumin," she said, "except it's not much of a secret, because you can smell it, can't you? But there is a secret. Would you like to know what it is?"

"Sure."

"Coffee. Leftover coffee, although I suppose you could make a pot for the occasion if you didn't have any left over. You simmer the beans in it. You can't taste it, can you? I can't, not even if I know it's there. But it *is* there, and it makes all the difference."

Over coffee—in china cups, not in their chili—he told her that he'd finished selecting the stamps that would constitute his commission on the sale. He estimated the fair market value of what he'd picked out at around $50,000, though of course the book value was a good deal higher than that.

The stamps, he added, were in the shoe box she'd given him that morning. And the box would remain in the stamp room until it was time for him to take it back to New Orleans.

"Of course," she said. "It wouldn't be safe to leave it in your motel room."

Keller supposed that was true enough, although he hadn't even thought of that aspect of it. The stamps weren't his yet, and wouldn't be until the rest of the collection was sold.

"And that brings up another question," she said. "We'll have a stamp dealer here on each of the next three days, and I don't suppose they'll breeze in, flip through albums for half an hour, and breeze out again."

Keller agreed that it would take each dealer the better part of a day.

"And you'll be here while they are? Not that I wouldn't be safe, but—"

"Whenever somebody's looking at the stamps," he said, "I'll be in the room with him."

"Today's Sunday, so Monday Tuesday Wednesday, and then you'd fly back on Thursday."

He nodded. He'd booked his flight as soon as he'd confirmed the appointments with the three dealers.

"Well, isn't it a nuisance having to drive back and forth each day? Not to mention the waste of money? I'm sure the guest-room bed is at least as comfortable as you'd get in a motel room, and the coffee's better. I would think you'd get more rest without the traffic noise, too. You could stay here tonight, as late as it is, and tomorrow you could fetch your things and check out of your room. Doesn't that make sense?"

THIRTY-NINE

K eller, back at La Quinta, heard the phone ring once as he emerged from the shower. When it didn't ring a second time, he reached for a towel and dried off, then found his cell phone on the dresser. It was turned off, so he turned it on to find out who'd called. There weren't any calls, and even if there had been, how could he have heard the ring if the phone was turned off?

He picked up the room phone and rang the front desk, where a man who sounded as though he had better things to do informed him there had been no calls to his room. Keller hung up and worked on the puzzle for a moment before he remembered he had another phone, the one he used only for conversations with Dot.

But that phone often went unused for weeks on end, and he kept it turned off unless he was expecting a call or had one to make. Where was it, anyway?

He couldn't seem to find it, and decided that was ridiculous, because he knew it was here, in this small room. Hadn't he just heard it ring?

If it rang once, it could ring again, and couldn't he make that happen? All he had to do was use his other phone to call his own number.

But he couldn't do that, he realized when he had his regular phone in hand, his thumb poised over the numbers. Because, of course, he didn't know his own number, and had never added it to his speed dial. Why would he? He never had occasion to call it himself, or to give it out to others. Only Dot used it, and only for calls that had to be kept private.

So much for that shortcut. He had a phone he couldn't locate, and it was somewhere within earshot, but he couldn't make the damn thing ring. All he could do was keep looking for it, knowing it was there, drawing precious little joy from the knowledge, and wishing it would ring.

It rang.

And, of course, there it was on the desk, invisible beneath a complimentary copy of *Cheyenne This Week,* which he'd picked up and paged through and tossed aside earlier. Evidently he'd tossed it right on top of his phone, but it had landed in such a way that it looked to be lying flat, an illusion that the ringtone instantly dispelled.

"Hello," he said.

"Well, hello yourself," Dot said. "Are you all right? You sound as though you just ran up three flights of stairs."

"I'm fine."

"Whatever you say, Pablo."

Pablo?

"You're still there, right? Counting stamps?"

"I'm here, but I'm not counting anything."

"Not even your blessings? Well, whatever you do with stamps. I don't suppose you lick them, but then neither does anybody else these days, not since the Post Office switched from lick-and-stick to whatever they call the new ones."

"Self-adhesive."

"Catchy. When's the last time you actually licked a stamp, Pablo?"

He did so whenever he had a letter to mail, but Dot didn't need to hear about discount postage. "It's been a while," he said, "but why are you calling me Pablo?"

"To keep from calling you by name."

"Oh."

"It's reflexive," she said. "I have this habit of calling you by name, using your name the way other people use commas. Not your new name. The old one, the one that's one silly little vowel away from your occupation."

Huh?

"I guess there's nobody who calls you that anymore, is there?"

Julia did, sometimes. She'd known him before he'd picked the name Nicholas Edwards off a child's tombstone, and like everyone else she'd called him by his last name, Keller. She never slipped and called him Keller in front of other people, and he didn't think Jenny had ever heard the name spoken, but when they were making love, or when she was in the mood to make love, all at once he was Keller again.

But less so lately. Subtly, gradually, Nicholas was displacing Keller in the romance department, edging him out in the bedroom...

"Hence Pablo," Dot said. "If you hate it I can probably come up with something else. I just always liked the name."

"Pablo."

"You hate it, don't you?"

"It's fine. Is that why you called? To see if I liked being called Pablo?"

"No, I just wanted to check in. I guess you've been keeping busy with stamps."

"Pretty much."

"Well, it's not as though you missed anything. Richard Hudepohl's still got a pulse, and nobody knows who burned his house down with him in it."

"The wife hasn't talked?"

"She hasn't," Dot said, "and I have to say I don't blame her. I've been thinking about her."

"Oh?"

"I think she's our client."

"Isn't that what we said the other day?"

"Not exactly, because at the time I thought she'd set it all up. Took the kids, left the house, and made sure she stayed away until the deed was done."

"Makes sense."

"It does," she said, "except it doesn't. Pablo, she hasn't got a thing to wear."

"Huh?"

"What woman gets someone to burn down her house with all her clothes in it? That might seem like a good idea to Charles Lamb, but I bet Mrs. Lamb would see it differently. Mrs. Hudepohl, the good news is that your husband is dead. The bad news is your fifty pairs of shoes are history."

"She had fifty pairs of shoes?"

"If she did, Pablo, she doesn't anymore. And her husband's not even dead."

He thought about it. "All right," he said. "She hired us, but while I was taking my time, somebody else went ahead and did the job. Who?"

"Suppose we just call him the other guy."

"Okay. Who hired the other guy?"

"I don't know," she said. "I know the wife didn't, and she's pissed."

"Pissed."

"Royally. I got a call from somebody who got a call from somebody who got a call from her. I know, it sounds like a bad song. The way she sees it, whoever burned her house down has to be the stupidest, craziest, most amateurish moron in the business."

"Well," Keller said, "I have to say I agree with her on that one."

"It's a pretty good description of our friend the other guy, isn't it? I passed the word that it wasn't us, so either one of the sub-brokers made more than one phone call—"

"Or someone else had the same idea she did. Are we sure she didn't make arrangements with some joker she met in a bar, then call in a pro when she figured he wouldn't go through with it?"

Dot was silent.

"And he went through with it after all? Except burning down the house that way called for some expert knowledge, wouldn't you say? I certainly wouldn't have known how to do it."

"You wouldn't have done it in the first place."

"Well, there's that. Still, does it sound like the work of some tattooed joker that you'd find on the Internet and meet in a bar?"

"Or find in a bar," she said, "and meet on the Internet. I've got some calls in, Pablo, and I think I might make a few more.

On the one hand, what do we care? Nobody's asking us to give back the first payment, and there's no way to earn the balance, so for us the war is over. Even so…"

"It'd be good to know."

"It would," she agreed. "I'll be in touch. You're with the Stamp Widow tomorrow? Keep your phone handy."

FORTY

The first stamp buyer was due at ten thirty, so Keller had a quick breakfast at Denny's, read the Denver paper's coverage of the Hudepohl case, and got to the Soderling house a little before ten. He wanted to make sure the fellow didn't get there first.

The previous evening, when Mrs. Soderling proposed he stay the night and check out of his motel in the morning, he'd invented a reason why that wasn't a good idea, some work he needed to do that very night on his computer. This morning, after his shower and shave, he packed up everything and stowed his bag in the Toyota's trunk.

But he kept the room, and even left the DO NOT DISTURB sign on the knob so the maid wouldn't assume he'd left early. Just keeping his options open, he told himself.

"I was up early," he told Denia Soderling. "I'm afraid I've already had my breakfast."

261

"But I'll bet you can manage another cup of coffee," she said. And he agreed that he could.

They sat together at an outdoor table, and quite out of the blue she began talking about the Hudepohl case. Had he been following it? He said he hadn't, which eliminated the possibility that he might disclose something that hadn't made the papers, but led her to furnish a full account of everything that had.

"That poor woman," she said. "She's lucky to be alive."

"If she'd been home—"

"Exactly! And her children. They seem quite certain it's arson, but you have to wonder."

"I guess you do."

"He kept tropical fish, didn't he? I wonder if there might have been chemicals involved. Spontaneous combustion, you know."

She topped up his cup of coffee, and when she put the pot down her hand brushed his. It might have been accidental, he told himself. Just like the fire on Otis Drive.

The stamp buyer, whose name was either Griffin or Griffith, was a short and slender man who wore a red-and-black striped vest with a black pinstripe suit. He had a narrow face, a sharp nose and sharper chin, and a full head of lustrous auburn hair, so full and so lustrous Keller was reasonably certain it was a wig. He looked as though he ought to be dealing blackjack in a casino, or touting horses at a track, and he bolstered this image when he hung his suit jacket over the back of his chair. The more you saw of his vest, the more it held your attention.

Then, as he seated himself at Jeb Soderling's stamp table, he completed the picture with a green eyeshade. He'd turned down the offered coffee, shook off the suggestion of tea or water, and drew a pair of tongs from one vest pocket and a magnifier from another.

"Europe," he said.

His voice was soft, and if he'd been a stage actor he'd have been inaudible past the first row. Keller, sitting just across the table from him, had to work to hear him.

"From Iceland to Turkey," Keller said.

"Actually," the man said, "there's some question as to whether Iceland is in fact a part of Europe. There's a geological fault line that runs right through the country. One side's Europe, other's North America. Philatelically, of course, it's grouped with the Scandinavian countries. I don't remember your name."

"Edwards."

"Edwards. Are you planning on sitting here the whole time? Because once I begin I won't want to talk, and I won't want to be talked to, either. I assure you I'm perfectly comfortable sitting alone with the collection."

"I'll stay," Keller told him.

The man didn't say anything. Neither did Keller, and eventually the man let himself be outwaited. He drew a breath and let it out without quite sighing.

"There are approximately a third of a million Icelanders," he said, as softly as he said everything, "and they are all descended from five Viking men and four Irish women. If you're going to stay here, you might as well bring me some albums."

Keller got to his feet.

"Not Iceland," the man said, answering a question Keller had not been about to ask. "France. I'll begin with France."

* * *

When he left his motel that morning, he'd set his phone—the one reserved for calls to and from Dot, the one he was already thinking of as the Pablo phone—on vibrate. He'd never done that before, and when a call actually came in it took him a moment to realize what it was. A strange sensation, really, as if a large centipede were dancing around in his breast pocket.

He withdrew to a corner of the room, pushed the appropriate button, but didn't say anything. Neither did Dot at first, but then she said, "Pablo?"

"Yes," he said, very softly.

"There are people around," Dot said.

"Yes."

"Dangerous people? Or just ears that don't need to hear our conversation?"

"Ears."

"Well, don't put me on speakerphone, okay? I got past a few middlemen. You can forget the moron with the tattoos. Her father was a magazine distributor, dealt with some people who knew some people. Died some years ago, but a while back he introduced her to a guy, then told her he was the man if she needed some heavy lifting done. Long story short, she called the guy. Remember me? I'm Benny's little girl, di dah di dah di dah, and he told her who to call and what to say, and she did and she did. Pablo? Are you still there?"

"Yes."

"Thought I lost you. Did you get all that?"

"Yes."

"I'd love to know what you think about it, but it's hard to get much from a man who never says anything but *yes* and *ears*. But if the other guy wasn't somebody that she found, that opens things up."

"All," Keller said.

"It opens it all up?"

It was frustrating, having to talk like this. The little man with the eyeshade seemed entirely caught up in the task at hand, which had him paging through the Benelux countries. Had he even noticed that Keller was on the phone, and could he possibly be giving any attention to the conversation?

It seemed unlikely, as softly as Keller was talking, and as preoccupied as the man was with the stamps. But anyone who spoke so softly was apt to have acute hearing, Keller figured, and along with his sharp nose and chin the guy had ears like a bat, so how could you be sure?

"Pablo? Where'd you go?"

"Why?"

"Why does it open it up? That's obvious, isn't it? But that's not your question. Why, why, why. Why did she want him hit? Is that it?"

"Yes."

"Good question," she said. "I'll get back to you."

The little man's name turned out to be neither Griffin nor Griffith, but was in fact Griffey, E. J. Griffey. He had shown up at ten thirty on the dot, and was in the stamp room murmuring about Iceland well before eleven. When Denia came into the room around twelve thirty to suggest lunch, he said politely that he'd had a large breakfast and would prefer to work straight through. Then he returned to the album he was examining, and made a note in his little notebook.

Keller stayed in the stamp room and ate the sandwich she brought him. A little before two, Griffey stood up and said something Keller didn't quite catch. He asked him to repeat it, and it turned out to be "bathroom." Keller walked him to the door, pointed him to the room he wanted. Griffey left, and took his notebook with him.

When the door closed behind him, Keller whipped out his phone and called Dot. As soon as she answered he said, "The fire was supposed to kill them both. Maybe the whole family, but let's say the other guy knew about the Friday night sleepovers. What he didn't know was it was going to turn into Girls' Night Out. He thought he'd get Mr. and Mrs. H. Gave her plenty of time to get home, spread his accelerant, set a timer, took off."

"Right."

"You figured all that."

"Pretty much. She hired you, and somebody else hired the other guy. If you'd gotten there first, what do you suppose the other guy would have done?"

"What I'll do," he said. "Go home. Why should we care who did what and why, Dot?"

"We shouldn't."

"And yet we do," he said.

"So it appears. I've got an idea, I'll talk to you—"

"Later," he said, and rang off even as Griffey opened the door.

"A sealed bid," E. J. Griffey said, brandishing an envelope with his firm's name and address in its upper left corner. Collectors of commercial covers called that sort of printed return address a *corner card,* a term that had always struck Keller as curious, a bit of philatelic whimsy, an insistence on employing a vocabulary that was as esoteric as thieves' argot. Covers, corner cards...

"Now I have a suggestion," the little man was saying, his voice a little more forceful though still low in volume. He and Keller had joined Denia Soderling in the parlor, where the three glasses of red wine she'd poured remained untouched. "What I recommend is that you open this envelope now. You'll see a figure which I think will please you, and which I suspect is higher than any other bid you're likely to receive. But if you open the envelope now and accept the bid on the spot as a preemptive offer, thus enabling me to make immediate arrangements for packing and shipping, I'll raise my own bid by ten percent."

He expanded on the subject, countering their objections. The other bidders would be disappointed? Why, this sort of thing happened all the time. They'd get over it.

Keller took the envelope from him, weighed it in his hand as if to assess its contents. "I think we'll stay with the original plan," he said. "Three sealed bids, and we'll open them all at the same time, and the high bid gets the collection."

Griffey started to offer an objection, then took another direction. "Suit yourselves," he said. "I'm confident my bid will turn out to be the high one. When that comes to pass, just remember you could have had ten percent more."

"My turn to make a suggestion," Keller said, and noted with satisfaction the quick flash of surprise on Griffey's face. "Raise your own bid."

"I beg your pardon?"

"You've just established that you're willing to pay ten percent more than the sum you wrote down. That was a nice tactic, but now that it hasn't worked, do you want to risk losing the collection because you didn't submit your highest offer?"

Griffey stared at him for a long moment, and all that

showed on his face was the effort it took to keep it expressionless. Then he snatched the envelope out of Keller's hand and
marched into the stamp room with it.

He returned, envelope in hand. "My card's in here," he
announced, "along with my firm's bid. I think...well, never
mind what I think. I assume you'll open all the bids the day
after tomorrow. Please call right away to let us know that our
bid was high."

Or that it wasn't, Keller thought, as his hostess showed E. J.
Griffey to the door.

FORTY-ONE

K eller's room was on the second floor, just to the left of the staircase. Even as the sound of Griffey's rented car was dying in the distance, she'd said that he'd probably want to freshen up before dinner, and suggested he get his bag from the Toyota. Had he even mentioned that he'd packed and left the motel? Or had she just assumed it?

Either way, here he was in a guest room, with a large four-poster topped by a patchwork quilt. The design, squarely geometric, looked Amish to him, but he didn't know much about quilts. Nor, he supposed, did he know much about stamps, not in comparison to a fellow like E. J. Griffey, who could flip through a few dozen albums in a matter of hours and come up with a professional assessment of their value.

On the other hand, what did E. J. Griffey know about fashioning a length of picture-hanging wire into a garrote?

*   *   *

After a shower and a change of clothes, Keller got his regular cell phone from his suitcase and called Julia. The brief conversation was ordinary enough, but he felt oddly detached from it. Should he mention that he'd relocated to the Soderling home? It wasn't information she needed, he hadn't bothered to tell her the name of his motel in the first place, but even so…

He called Dot on the Pablo phone. No answer, and after the fourth ring a male voice, computer-generated, invited him to leave a message. He rang off.

"I didn't know what to do while the two of you were in the stamp room," she said. "I would have gone for a ride, but somehow I felt I ought to be here, although I can't think why. So I cooked."

She'd prepared coq au vin. The *coq,* she told him, had grown up a mile and a half away, where he and his flock mates ranged free and enjoyed an organic diet. The *vin* was the same Pommard they were drinking. Jeb had enjoyed establishing a wine cellar, and ordered cases from a wine merchant on New York's Madison Avenue.

She'd changed for dinner. She'd changed the blouse and slacks for a simple black dress that showed a hint of décolletage.

And she was wearing perfume. He caught the scent when she came around behind him to pour his coffee.

"That Mr. Griffey," she said. "There was something very forbidding about that little man. I'd have been at a loss, trying to deal with him on my own. But you handled him brilliantly. You could see it in his face, that he'd been outmaneuvered and didn't know how to respond. And he sat right down and raised his own bid."

"Or didn't," Keller said. "For all we know he came back with the same envelope and never opened it."

"Do you think that's what he did?"

He shook his head. "I nicked the original envelope with my thumbnail," he said, "and the envelope he came back with didn't have the nick."

"How on earth did you think to do that?"

"I don't know," he said, "and I'm not sure it made any difference, but he must have changed his bid, and he certainly wouldn't have lowered it. I wonder how much he raised it."

"What figure do you think he wrote down?"

"I couldn't even guess."

"More than a quarter of a million?"

He nodded.

"So you won't get to buy Jeb's stamps."

"I'm afraid not."

"Should we open the envelope? We could steam it open and reseal it. No one would ever know."

"We could cut it open," he said, "because no one but the two of us will ever see the bids anyway. And they're your stamps, so you get to decide, but I'd rather stick to the script."

"And open them all at once," she said. "Like kids on Christmas? So as not to spoil the surprise?"

He thought about it. "That might be some of it," he admitted, "but I have the sense that we're in a stronger position if we don't know. I can't explain why, but—"

"No one can read our minds," she said, "if there's nothing in them. It's fine with me, Nicholas. I'd rather go with your instincts than mine."

Nicholas.

A few sentences later, almost to make a point, he managed to use her name in conversation. Mrs. Soderling.

"Denia," she said at once. "You're my houseguest now, and my negotiating partner. You can't go on calling me Mrs. Soderling."

"Denia."

"It's an unusual name, I know, but it's better than the one given me at birth. Can you guess?"

He couldn't.

"Gardenia," she said. "Flower names are all right, but some are better than others. Rose and Iris, for instance, are less of a burden than Pansy or, I don't know, Forsythia?"

"I don't think I've ever known a Forsythia."

"Neither have I, but I did know a girl named Dahlia, and that wasn't too bad. My mother wore this overbearing scent called Jungle Gardenia, and evidently it had a profound visceral effect on my father, who bought it for her by the half gallon. And insisted on it for my name. I hated it, and as soon as I was old enough I had it changed legally."

"To Denia."

"Yes, which I like, except for the nuisance of having to explain its derivation. I have a complicated relationship with the scent. I can't imagine wearing it, and I find it slightly sickmaking, but at the same time it smells like Mommy, and that means warmth and comfort, doesn't it?"

"It sounds complicated."

"It might be," she said, "but how often do I encounter it? Not once a year, I wouldn't think. Generally speaking, I find things don't have to be all that complicated, Nicholas."

Oh?

"Some more wine? We really ought to finish the bottle."

He covered his glass. "I'm already having trouble keeping my eyes open. It was oddly exhausting, sitting across the table from Mr. E. J. Griffey."

"I can imagine."

"And there's a call I have to make before I turn in."

"To New Orleans?"

To Sedona, but she didn't need to know that. "I spoke to her earlier," he said, "but I like to check in before I call it a day."

"He was having an affair," Dot said. "Why won't you boys learn to keep it in your pants?"

Keller, sitting on the edge of the bed in the guest room, felt the rush of blood to his face.

"Pablo? You there?"

"I'm here."

"Can you talk?"

"I'm the one who called," he reminded her. "I'm in the client's house, but I'm alone."

"You're in the client's—oh, the stamp lady. Not the *client* client."

"Who doesn't have a house in the first place."

"Not anymore. Well, he was having an affair, he had a tootsie on the side, and he wanted a divorce. And he was talking about a custody fight, and bringing up a lot of dirt on her, because she'd had an affair of her own a few years ago, which she regretted and thought they'd gotten past, and now he threw it in her face, and she just wanted him dead, the son of a bitch, and she remembered the man her father introduced her to, and—well, the rest is pretty much the way we figured it."

"Jesus," he said. "You got all this from the broker? From one of the cutout men?"

"No, of course not. She wouldn't spew all of this to some guy, and if she did he'd never pass it on to me."

"Then—"

"She told me. But can we cut to the chase, Pablo? She wants to call it off."

"The client."

"Right."

"Wants to call off—"

"The contract. She wanted us to do something, remember? And now she's changed her mind."

"When did this happen?"

"In his hospital room, seeing him all helpless there with tubes coming out of him. Do you want to know exactly what passed through her mind?"

"Uh—"

"Okay, she's in his room, he's unconscious, nobody's around, and it occurs to her that she can finish the job and no one will be the wiser. Pinch a tube shut, pull one out, pour something in his IV—there's a dozen ways to do it, and she realizes she loves him and she wants him to pull through. I'll spare you the emotional part, that comes under the heading of girl talk, but the bottom line is she loves him again and just wants him to live and be hers."

"Dot—"

"You know, same reason you're Pablo, I ought to be somebody else. You're not as addicted to saying names as I am, but now and then it slips out. How's Hilda?"

"Hilda?"

"If you have to call me something, Pablo, well, Hilda'll do. No, come to think of it, it won't. It's too close to my official name these days. Make it Flora, okay?"

"If you say so. How did she get in touch with you?"

"She didn't, Pablo. I got in touch with her. How? I picked up the phone and called her."

"Who gave out her number?"

"Nobody, but how many Joanne Hudepohls are there? Her cell phone's listed, so I dialed it, and she answered on the first ring. You'd have thought she was waiting for my call."

"What phone did you—"

"Easy there, Pablo. A new phone, bought for cash and unregistered. Same as this one, but just for her. And I got her number via a Google search, and I used a computer in a Kinko's in Flagstaff. There won't be any trail, paper or electronic, and as soon as all of this is over the Joanne phone goes in a storm drain."

"Maybe you should ditch it now."

"I might need to talk to her some more."

He frowned. "Why, for God's sake?"

"Once she got that we didn't burn her house down—"

"She knew somebody else did. And she only made that one call to her father's buddy."

"Right."

"So she knows about the other guy, and that somebody else hired him." He thought for a moment. "The girlfriend?"

"Gotta be. Or the girlfriend's jealous husband."

"The girlfriend's married?"

"That I couldn't tell you. But the girlfriend has to be the connection."

"And the girlfriend, and thus the other guy, might not feel the game is over."

"Right. They might try again. She's hired people from a security agency to protect her husband in the hospital, and she'll keep them on after he's released."

"Assuming he pulls through," he said. "But why do we care?"

"Pablo, that sounds so cold. 'Why do we care?' A man's life

hangs in the balance, and his wife is in peril, and you ask a question like that."

"And if I wait long enough," he said, "maybe you'll answer it."

"Opportunity," she said. "I hear it knocking. Pablo, get some rest. I'll get back to you."

FORTY-TWO

He spent a restless night, got up early, and found coffee poured and breakfast ready when he got downstairs. She said she hoped he liked huevos rancheros, and told him the eggs were from the same organic poultry farm that had supplied last night's free-range cockerel.

"One-stop shopping," she said. "I'd call it a Mexican breakfast, but according to Jeb, a Mexican breakfast is a cigarette and a glass of water. Do you suppose that's an ethnic slur? I suppose I could ask Rosita."

"Rosita?"

"That's right, you haven't met her. She stays out of sight, and she's straightening your room even as we speak. More coffee?"

No perfume this morning, and no décolletage. There'd been something on offer during the dinner hour, and he'd found a way to let it go without giving offense, and he had every reason to feel relieved.

But was it relief that he felt? Not entirely. He'd dodged a bullet, but what he felt was the skimpy self-satisfaction of a dieter who'd passed up dessert.

Martin Rombaugh struck Keller as a man who'd never passed up a dessert in his life, and there was nothing skimpy about his self-satisfaction, or his satisfaction with life in general. He was a big man with a hearty laugh, and he showed up fifteen minutes early for his ten thirty appointment.

"Afraid I'd have trouble finding the place," he said, "and then I didn't. Your directions turned out to be foolproof. Marty Rombaugh, representing Colliard and Bowden, and Lou Colliard specifically asked me to convey his sympathies, Mrs. Soderling. He'd met your husband on several occasions, he'd valued him as a customer, and..."

There was more, but Keller tuned it out. Soon enough they were seated across from each other in the stamp room, but Rombaugh had said yes to coffee, and hadn't protested when a plate of cookies accompanied it. "Homemade," he announced, after a bite. "Have one?"

Once again, Keller passed up dessert.

The hours went more quickly in Rombaugh's company than in Griffey's. The big man paged through albums as rapidly, made notes as cryptically, but kept up a running conversation throughout. He'd been ten when he started collecting stamps, joined a local stamp club where he could trade off his duplicates, decided to specialize in U.S. and took a table at a stamp show to sell off his foreign, spent so much time at a downtown stamp shop that they gave him a job, and had explored many facets of the hobby and business ever since, all of which he was apparently eager to share with his new friend Nicholas.

It could have been tiring for Keller, but he realized early on that he wasn't required to comment. When he did, Rombaugh was happy to engage in the back-and-forth of dialogue, but when Keller remained silent, Rombaugh was just as content to keep up the conversation on his own.

Keller found most of it interesting, and even informative. And, when his attention flagged, he could safely let his mind go elsewhere.

When his phone vibrated, Keller excused himself and took the call in the far corner of the stamp room. Rombaugh closed one stamp album and reached for another, clearly wrapped up in his task.

Should he leave the room? Rombaugh wouldn't hear anything, he decided, and wouldn't know what he was listening to even if he did.

He said, "Yes?"

"There's someone in the room."

"Sort of."

"How can someone be sort of in the room? Never mind, you can't talk freely, and I don't need to know. You got a pencil handy?"

"A pen."

"That'll do. If there's anything you need to erase just cross it out. Meanwhile, write this down."

She read out an address and he dutifully jotted it down on the back of Martin Rombaugh's business card.

"The girlfriend," she went on. "Her name is Trish Heaney, which I suppose must be short for Patricia. The Trish part, I mean. I don't think the Heaney part is short for anything."

"Right."

"Though I suppose it could be short for Heaniapopoulos. You don't think that's funny, do you?"

"Right."

"The girlfriend's got a boyfriend. Not the one we know about, with the tubes coming out of him. This guy's more of an ex-boyfriend, the kind of old pal a gal might call on in a pinch. His name's Tyler Crowe. He's younger than Hudepohl, but prison ages a man, and you'll never guess what he did that got him three years in Cañon City."

He could guess, but didn't want to say the word.

"Arson. You see where this is going, Pablo?"

Like Griffey, Marty Rombaugh didn't want to interrupt his work for lunch. But neither did he care to miss a meal, and polished off the sandwiches Denia provided.

A little after three he pushed back his chair and heaved a sigh. "Stamps," he said. "Just little pieces of paper, but they're more than that, aren't they?"

"They are."

"You didn't know Soderling, did you?"

"No."

"Neither did I, but you can tell a lot about a man from his collection. This was an orderly and systematic gentleman, but there was a lot of romance there as well, a little dash, a certain flair. I can't tell you how I know that, but I do."

"I know what you mean."

"You're not from around here."

"My wife and I live in New Orleans."

He'd mentioned his wife to keep the man from jumping to a certain conclusion, and he saw the word register. "You're basically a friend of a friend," Rombaugh said, "advising the lady on the disposal of her husband's holdings."

"I buy and sell some," Keller said. "Someone recommended me, but when I saw the extent of the collection—"

"You figured deeper pockets were required. I suppose the lady will be compensating you for your trouble."

The sentence didn't have a question mark at its end, but invited a response. Keller didn't supply one.

"Who'd they send yesterday, if you don't mind my asking? I bet it was the Griff, wasn't it?"

"If you mean Mr. Griffey——"

"Yeah, the little guy. He and I spend our lives tagging each other all around the country. All those Russian locals, the zemstvo issues, they might as well be from Uranus for all he knows about them." He paused, frowned. "That's the planet Uranus, but when you just say it, well, it comes out off-color. I should have said Jupiter. It's less open to misinterpretation."

"Well," Keller said.

"He'd lowball you on the Russian stamps. Other hand, he'd go high on some of the Czech and Polish overprints, on account of there's forgeries there that he probably wouldn't spot. Including one or two that Kasimir Bileski signed off on."

"Really."

"Just for curiosity, what did the Griff offer you?"

"He gave us a sealed bid."

"So? Come on, don't tell me you didn't sneak a peek."

"We didn't."

"Playing it absolutely straight, eh? Well, cards on the table. This is a very sweet little collection, and not even all that little, and my own compensation is tied to what I bring in to my employers. So what can you and I do just between ourselves to make that happen?"

Keller thought it over. "There is one thing," he said at length.

"I'm all ears."

No, he thought. Griffey was all ears, and might have flown

if he'd been able to flap them. As for Rombaugh—well, never mind.

"Figure out the absolute maximum the collection is worth to you," he told the man. "The most you can pay and still make your employers happy."

"And?"

"And that's your bid," Keller said. "Write it down and seal the envelope. If it's higher than either of the others, you win."

The address Dot had furnished was on Arapahoe Street, in that part of downtown Denver known as LoDo. Keller wasn't clear on where the term came from, but if he had to guess he'd have opted for LOwer DOwntown, the same way New York's SoHo and NoHo were NOrth and SOuth of HOuston Street.

He programmed the GPS accordingly, and halfway to Denver he thought about Dot, and how she'd driven all the way to Flagstaff to use a rental computer to chase down Joanne Hudepohl's phone listing. Because if she used her own computer, there'd be an electronic trail you couldn't rub out.

Well, what about his GPS? He'd already punched in the address on Otis Drive, including the precise number of the house that had burned to the foundation. And now he'd added another address, the LoDo loft that was home to Trish Heaney, and it didn't have to go up in smoke to draw attention from the authorities. All the trouble he'd gone to, flying in and out of Cheyenne, and he'd be returning his Cheyenne rental car with a GPS showing just where he'd been in Denver.

He took the next exit off the interstate, found a place to park, thought the whole thing over. The simplest thing, he realized, was to take out the Pablo phone, call Dot, and tell her he wanted to scrap the whole thing. They had the first payment, and that was plenty. Then he could turn the car around and have a romantic dinner with Denia Soderling.

"I'm going to have to go to Denver this evening," he'd told Denia, after Marty Rombaugh had delivered his sealed envelope and taken his leave.

She'd offered to hold dinner, and he said he wasn't sure how long his business might take. "Here's a house key," she said. "In case you're very late. But I'll probably be up, and if you're back before ten we can dine together."

And if he went back now? The sun wasn't even down yet, and he'd have to explain how his urgent business engagement had wrapped itself up in no time at all. Various possibilities suggested themselves—a medical emergency, a canceled flight—and he told himself he was overthinking the situation.

He could delete the Arapahoe Street address, but wouldn't it still be recorded somewhere in the gadget's history? Probably, and he'd only saddle himself with the difficulty of finding Tricia Heaney's loft without the patient guidance of the nice GPS lady.

He started the car, got back on the road. "Recalculating route," the voice said, infinitely patient, and only the slightest bit judgmental. He beamed the invisible woman a silent apology for deviating from the script, and followed her instructions all the way to LoDo.

"You have arrived," she said, and there was the address he wanted, a squat six-story brick building with big industrial-type windows.

Keller was glad he wasn't contemplating arson. The building looked like a hard structure to burn down.

FORTY-THREE

Keller, returning to Arapahoe Street from where he'd parked the car, reminded himself that he didn't have to do anything. He was simply a private citizen, paying a call on a woman at her residence. If she wasn't home, or if she wouldn't let him in, or if the right opportunity failed to arise, he'd go back to Cheyenne and eat a good dinner.

And there was Trish Heaney's building, right where he'd left it, with a row of buttons next to the windowless red door. Helpful little cards marked each button, and he pressed the one that said HEANEY.

Waiting, he reminded himself that he'd committed himself to nothing. That he'd neither misrepresented himself nor broken any laws.

"Yes?"

Just a citizen, ringing a doorbell.

"Hello? Who is it?"

"Officer Griffey," he said. "Police."

There was a lengthy pause.

Well, he'd just broken a law. It shouldn't take too long to drive back to Cheyenne. He wouldn't even need the GPS, although it would probably be simpler to use it. The Soderling address was already programmed into the system, and the woman with the soothing and infinitely patient voice was waiting to guide him home, and get him there in plenty of time for dinner. And Denia was a good cook, no question about it, and—

The buzzer sounded. He pushed the door open and went on in.

The elevator was industrial, but it had been converted to self-service when the building turned residential. There'd been a 4 next to the bell marked HEANEY, so he pushed the appropriate button and rode to the fourth floor. The elevator door glided open, and there she was, holding a drink in one hand and a cigarette in the other.

While he hadn't formed a mental picture of her in advance, it would have been hard to improve on reality. Trish Heaney was no more than five foot four, but she made an impression. She wore wheat-colored jeans and a fuzzy pink sweater, both garments skintight. The jeans would have been tight on anyone who wasn't severely anorexic, but most women who could have squeezed themselves into the jeans would have found the sweater a loose fit.

And that might have been true of this woman, he thought, before some obliging nip-and-tuck artist had put her in competition with Dolly Parton. The result was impressive, he had to admit, but no more convincing than the vivid red hue of her upswept hair. She had a butterfly tattoo on her neck, and the Geico gecko inked onto the back of one hand, and enough piercings to put a metal detector on tilt, and God knows what else she had underneath the sweater and jeans.

"You're a cop," she said. "You don't look like a cop."

"You don't look like a kindergarten teacher."

"Who said I was—" She broke off, frowned, took a deep drag on her cigarette. "That supposed to be a joke? You want to show me some ID?"

"I could," he said.

Or, he thought, he could cut to the chase. One hand cupping her chin, one hand grabbing that mop of red hair. Be over before she knew it.

"So?"

"But once I do," he said, "this becomes official. You sure that's what you want?"

"I don't know what you're talking about."

"There's a guy in the hospital, touch and go whether he lives or dies. I won't mention his name, but you wouldn't be living here if he wasn't paying for it."

"This is my place," she said. "The deed's in my name. And I still don't know what you're talking about."

Was this working? Keller wasn't sure. The cigarette smoke was bothering him, and so was her perfume, an overpowering floral scent redolent with musk.

He said, "Sure you do, Trish. You were all set to get Richard Hudepohl away from his wife, and then you realized he'd be broke after the divorce. But suppose he didn't have to go through a divorce? Suppose something happened to his wife and kids?"

"Not the kids," she said, and put her hand to her mouth.

"Not the wife, either," Keller said, "because old Tyler burned the house down with the wrong person in it."

"She took his car," she said, "and all Tyler saw was the car, and the kids in the backseat. He couldn't see who was driving it. If you're wearing a wire, that's too fucking bad. You never did read me my rights."

"Or show you my ID," he reminded her. "Because this isn't official. Trish, there'd be nothing easier than hanging this on Tyler, and if he's in it then you're in it, and having your rights read to you isn't going to help you. But I'm the only person who made the connection, and why would I want to see you go to prison?"

She looked at him, breathed in, breathed out. Really a bad idea, that perfume she was wearing. He could see how it might work on a primitive level, but it was so blatant, and so unpleasant—

"What do you want?"

"Your boyfriend's professional services, Trish. I got property that's underwater."

She frowned. "How can it burn if it's underwater?"

"It's an expression," he said. "It means I owe more money on it than it's worth. The bank's set to foreclose on the mortgage, and when that happens, my investment goes up in smoke."

"Unless—"

"Unless the property goes up in smoke first. Call him, get him to come over here. You'll both make a few dollars, and I'll forget what I happen to know about you and a man named Hudepohl. And Trish? Have you got a gun in the house?"

"Why?"

That was as good as a yes. "Get it for me," he said.

FORTY-FOUR

Halfway to Cheyenne, he spotted a sign for a country-style chain restaurant and found it at the next exit. The menu ran heavily to quaint—*Grampa Gussie's Crispy Taters, hand-cut wif his own Bowie knife*—but the food was what you'd get pretty much anywhere. He ate half of a grilled cheese sandwich and drank a few sips of his iced tea and let it go at that.

He stopped at La Quinta and caught the late local news on the CBS affiliate in Denver. A jeweler on Colfax Avenue had been robbed, apparently by a gang who'd been making a habit of this sort of thing. And the weather was going to be more of the same, although it took the weather girl ten minutes to convey that information.

Nothing about anyone named Hudepohl, or Heaney, or Crowe.

*   *   *

At first he thought Denia had retired for the night. The ground-floor lights were mostly turned down, and he used the key she'd given him and softened his step once he was inside.

The dining room table was cleared, the room dark. He padded across the carpet toward the staircase when she spoke his name. He turned, and saw her in an armchair in the dimly lit parlor. She was wearing a robe, and her feet were bare.

"It won't be any trouble to warm something up for you," she said. "But I've a feeling you've eaten."

"The fellow I had to meet was hungry," he said, "so I kept him company."

"I didn't have any appetite," she said, "so I had a couple of drinks instead and wound up going to bed on an empty stomach. And then I couldn't sleep after all, and I still didn't have any appetite, and I was too restless to lie there and wait for sleep to come. Do you ever have nights like that?"

"Once in a while."

"This is a robe of Jeb's. That's his actual name, incidentally. J-E-B, it's not short for anything, though people assume it's short for Jebediah. I don't think I've ever known anyone named Jebediah. Have you?"

"I don't believe so."

"I'm a little drunk, Nicholas. Why don't you sit in that chair there? I want us to have a little conversation, if you don't mind. That's all I want, just a conversation, but I do want that. Is that all right?"

"Of course."

"It has his smell. The robe, I mean. I ought to give all his clothes to the Goodwill. What am I keeping them for? But I like to smell them. And there's a flannel shirt of his that

I like to sleep in sometimes. And sometimes I put on this robe."

He didn't have anything to say to that.

"Widows are easy. You must have heard that, Nicholas."

"Uh."

"Everybody knows it, too. I'm not sure it's true, but I do know that everyone believes it is, or wants it to be. I'm a reasonably attractive woman, Nicholas, but I'm hardly a movie star or a supermodel. And men who I swear never looked twice at me while Jeb was alive, men who were his friends, men who are married to friends of mine..."

She shook her head, raised her glass, sipped its contents. "Passes were made," she said. "What an odd way to put it. 'Passes were made.' Well, they were, verbal and physical. Made and deflected, with no embarrassment on either side. I was not tempted."

"No."

"But I get lonely, you know. And I miss intimacy. Physical intimacy."

"Well."

"This is whiskey," she said, brandishing her glass. "I usually have a glass or two of wine of an evening. Tonight I've been drinking whiskey because I wanted it to hit me, and it has. Can you tell I'm drunk?"

"No."

"I'm not slurring my words, am I?"

"No."

"Or speaking in too loud a voice, the way drunks do?"

"No."

"What happens in Vegas stays in Vegas. Of course you've heard that slogan."

"Yes."

"My husband and I subscribed to that philosophy. He had to do a certain amount of travel for his business, and if he had an opportunity for a dalliance, he was free to pursue it. When he was at home he was married, and faithful. When he was miles away, he was a free agent."

"I suppose a lot of couples have that sort of understanding."

"I would think so. I'm going upstairs now. I'm sure I'll be able to sleep. I'm glad we've had this little talk, aren't you, Nicholas?"

"Yes, I am."

"And tomorrow's our last day. I can't remember the name of the buyer we'll be seeing tomorrow."

"I believe it's a Mr. Mintz."

"As in pie? Shame on me. It's ridiculous to make jokes about a person's name, and the person will have heard all of them, time and time again. When he's gone we'll open the envelopes. And you'll be able to have dinner, won't you?"

"Yes, of course."

"Boeuf bourguignon, I think. With the little roasted potatoes, and a salad. Good night, Nicholas. No, I can get upstairs under my own power. It's just my tongue that's loosened, that's all. I'll see you at breakfast."

He had a shower. He'd felt the need for one ever since he left the Arapahoe Street loft. He toweled dry, brushed his teeth.

Too late to call Julia. He'd thought of calling her from La Quinta, decided not to, and now it was too late. Was it too late to call Dot? Probably not, but he didn't want to call Dot. It was possible she'd called him, or tried to. He'd turned his phone off earlier and had never turned it back on.

He got in bed, turned off the light. What happens in Cheyenne, he thought, stays in Cheyenne.

He didn't think he was going to be able to sleep, and thought about putting on a robe and going downstairs to drink whiskey. But he didn't have a robe, and didn't much care for whiskey, or for the whole sad business of sitting up late drinking it.

He owned a robe, a very nice maroon one with silver piping. It had belonged to Julia's father, who'd been an invalid during the short time Keller had known him. Mr. Roussard hadn't known quite what to make of Keller, though they got along well enough, and then the man's illness ran its course, more or less, and he was gone.

Keller had admired the robe once, and after her father's ashes had been scattered in the Gulf, Julia got the robe dry-cleaned and told him it was his now. He liked owning it, but he hardly ever wore it. It didn't smell of the old man, or of the sickroom, the dry cleaner had seen to that, but still it stayed unworn in Keller's closet. Robes, pajamas, slippers, they worked fine for some men, not so much for others, and Keller—

Dropped right off to sleep, thinking of robes and slippers.

FORTY-FIVE

The representative of Talleyrand Stamp & Coin arrived twenty minutes late. Keller, on the patio with a second cup of coffee, watched as the fellow parked his black Lincoln Navigator in the driveway and headed for the front door, briefcase in hand. Like his predecessors, he wore a conservative suit and a tie; in manner and body type he fell somewhere between the two.

"Pierce Naylor," he said, first to Keller, then a moment or two later to Denia Soderling. "Lew Mintz couldn't make it. As I understand it, I'm the third stamp buyer to cross this threshold in as many days. Ma'am, you must be sick to death of the whole tribe of us."

"It's been no hardship for me," she said. "Mr. Edwards has enabled me to stay very much in the background."

"You're fortunate," he said. "The less time you spend around stamp buyers, the better off you are. Well, it's my intention to make this as simple and easy for you as I possibly can, and profitable in the bargain. Unless I've been misinformed, you were visited in turn by E. J. Griffey and Martin Rombaugh, and I'd be surprised if either one of them got out of here in less than five or six hours."

Keller was preparing a reply, but Naylor didn't wait for one. "That's far more of your time than I intend to take," he said, "nor will I eat you out of house and home, as I'm sure Marty Rombaugh made every effort to do. One hour's all I'll need."

Oh?

In the stamp room, Keller indicated the chair that had served Griffey and Rombaugh in turn. Naylor stayed on his feet and walked over to the shelved stamp albums. "Spain," he announced, and carried an album to the table. Still standing, he opened it apparently at random, studied the stamps, flipped a few pages, closed the album, and returned it to the shelf. He spent a little more time with Sweden, and not much time at all with Turkey.

"All right," he said, after replacing the Turkish album where he'd found it. "Griffey and Rombaugh, with Griffey leading off. He'd have tried to make his offer preemptive, but that little ploy quite obviously didn't work. And Marty would have tried to add a little sweetener. He'd top Griffey's bid and slip you a little something for your troubles. But that couldn't have worked, either, because the stamps are still here, aren't they?"

Keller agreed that they were.

"How high did Griffey go? And was Marty able to top it?"

"We haven't opened the envelopes."

"You're kidding," Naylor said, and looked intently at him. "You're serious," he announced. "Well, that makes it interesting, doesn't it? Why don't we bring in Mrs. Soderling? I have a suggestion to make."

"You want us to open both envelopes," she said. "In front of you."

"That's right."

"And you'll guarantee to top the high bid by twenty percent. I believe that's what you said."

"It is."

"But you barely looked at the stamps. How can you know they're worth that much?"

"I know the Griff," Naylor said. "I know Marty Rombaugh. If they say the collection's worth X dollars, I know it's worth that and more."

"Twenty percent more," Keller said.

"That's right. I looked briefly at three albums, and that was enough to give me a sense of the quality and the degree of completeness. I'll take the word of my predecessors as to the actual value, and at the same time I'll trust them to have shaded their bid enough to leave ample room for profit. Enough room so that I can bid twenty percent higher and still come out ahead."

"Or back out," Keller said.

"I beg your pardon?"

"Suppose we open the envelopes," he said, "and one bid's three times as high as the other, so high that you wouldn't even want to match it, let alone top it by twenty percent. 'My employers would never go for that,' you'd say, and what could we do about it?"

"Not a damn thing," Naylor allowed. "But so what? You'd go ahead and sell the stamps to Griffey or Rombaugh, whoever's the higher, but that's what you'd do anyway, isn't it?"

There had to be a flaw in the argument, but Keller couldn't spot it. Denia questioned the fairness of it. Wouldn't they be giving Naylor an edge over the competition?

"I had that edge from the start," he said, "because I'm the last of the three players in the game. If I'd already come and gone, and one of the others got to go last, he'd be giving you a version of the same pitch. Ma'am, you want to be fair to yourself, and to do right by the man who gathered all these philatelic treasures together in the first place. Which is to say you want the highest price. And that's exactly what you'll get if you open those envelopes."

It was getting on for noon when they opened the envelopes. By ten minutes to four, the entire cargo compartment of the oversize SUV was filled to capacity, with one additional carton, its seat belt securely fastened, riding shotgun. There was another box on the floor containing a two-quart Thermos bottle and half a dozen sandwiches in individual self-sealing plastic bags.

"I'll drive straight through," Pierce Naylor said. "It's around nine hundred miles to St. Louis, all of it on interstates, and with the sandwiches and coffee I'll never have to leave the vehicle. Very thoughtful of you, Mrs. Soderling. I'll have FedEx get your Thermos back in good shape."

"It's a spare, Mr. Naylor, and the cap's chipped. Don't bother returning it."

"You're sure? Because it wouldn't be any trouble. Well, then. Mr. Edwards, Mrs. Soderling. A pleasure doing business with you."

They stood in silence and watched him drive off. He'd flown from St. Louis to Denver, where he'd reserved the Navigator, making sure he got the largest SUV any of the rental outlets had on offer. If he'd missed out on the collection, he'd have driven back to Denver and flown home. But he'd been successful, so he'd drive home, pay the car rental people a drop charge, waste his return air ticket, and his employers would count it all money well spent.

"It was remarkable how smoothly it went. He called the firm he works for, and someone there called a bank and arranged a wire transfer, and in no time at all Mrs. Soderling's bank confirmed that the money was in her account."

"I guess I knew you could do that," Julia said, "but it never would have occurred to me. And she's happy with the price?"

"Very much so."

"And your other business?"

"All taken care of. I'll be home tomorrow."

She put Jenny on, and he listened happily as she babbled away about a puppy. Was it too early to get her a dog? This was not the first time he'd asked himself this question, and the answer still seemed to be yes, that she wasn't old enough yet. Soon, though.

He rang off, switched phones, called Dot. "You won't believe this," she said, "but the damnedest thing happened on Arapahoe Street in downtown Denver. An ex-con not too long out of Cañon City looked up his old girlfriend and slapped her around enough to leave marks. So she got her gun and put three rounds in his chest, and then I guess she felt remorseful, because she turned the gun on herself."

"These things happen."

"One in the heart. I understand men go for head shots, the mouth or the temple, but a girl wants to look her best."

"So they say."

"And they found something, don't ask me what, that has

them looking at the dead guy for that house that burned down a few nights ago."

"Maybe there was something in his wallet with the address on it."

"Of the house that went up in smoke? That might do it. Whatever it is, my guess is it's enough for them to clear the case. Time for Pablo to head for home."

"Tomorrow," he said. "Uh, as far as us getting paid—"

"Won't be a problem."

"When the husband recovers—"

"That won't be a problem, either."

It took him a moment. "You're saying he—"

"Died, Pablo. *El esposo es muerto.* Or should it be *está?* I think *es,* because it's a permanent condition."

"I thought she hired security."

"She did, amigo, but all the king's horses can't keep a man's kidneys from quitting on him. Acute renal failure, and I gather the only surprise at the hospital was that he lasted as long as he did. And this way she got to forgive him and fall back in love with him and get revenge on the people responsible for his death, and she doesn't have to worry that he'll find some other tootsie and put her through it all over again. Which we both know he would have done sooner or later. I have to say she comes out of this in good shape, Pablo. The little lady got her money's worth."

FORTY-SIX

The boeuf bourguignon was tender and savory, the little potatoes crisp on the outside and soft in the center. The wine was a Burgundy, appropriately enough, full-bodied and hearty, but neither of them managed more than a glass of it.

They talked through the meal, but mostly about the philatelic transaction. Of the two bids they'd opened, E. J. Griffey's was the higher by a substantial margin, and that had surprised them both.

Over coffee, she said she wanted to pay him a bonus. The stamps he'd selected, he told her, were ample compensation for his time. He'd enjoyed the visit, and he'd learned a great deal from the three men, from listening to what they said and from paying attention to the way they operated.

"You made me an offer," she said. "A quarter of a million dollars. And in the next breath you advised me not to take it."

"Aren't you glad you didn't?"

"I wound up with almost five times as much."

"I thought you might."

"You're an honest man," she said, "and an ethical one, but I don't see why that should stop you from accepting a bonus. You have a daughter. You told me her name but I don't remember it."

"Jenny."

"I bet she's smart."

"Like her mother," he said.

"Oh, I think you probably deserve some of the credit. But she's college material, wouldn't you say?"

"Not for a few years now."

"That's just as well," she said, "because what I'm going to do is put a hundred thousand dollars into a trust fund to mature on her eighteenth birthday. It should appreciate considerably by then, and might even increase as much as the cost of a college education. You really can't object to this, Nicholas. It doesn't even concern you. It's between me and Jennifer."

"Jenny."

"Jenny, but isn't it Jennifer on her birth certificate?"

"No, just Jenny."

"And my husband's given name was Jeb, not short for Jebediah, as some people tended to assume. His full name was Jeb Stuart Soderling, though I've no idea why his father, a North Dakota Swede, would name his son after a Civil War general. And Jeb was an acronym to begin with, you know."

"It was J. E. B. Stuart, wasn't it? I don't remember what the initials stood for."

"James Ewell Brown Stuart. I would know, wouldn't I, having been married to his namesake. Well, that's a handful, isn't it? You can see why they went with Jeb. But won't it be awkward for your daughter? She'll spend half her life correcting people who assume her full name is Jennifer."

He'd had this conversation with Julia. "She can always change it," he said. "But for now it's Jenny. See, she was a breech birth."

"I beg your pardon?"

"A breech presentation. She was upside down in the birth canal, and——"

"I understand the term, Nicholas. What I don't begin to understand is why that would make her a Jenny instead of a Jennifer."

He reached for his cup, took a sip of coffee. "I'm not sure this will make any sense," he said, "but that's when we realized she wasn't going to be, you know, ordinary. And there were so many little girls named Jennifer, and we knew we weren't going to call her Jennifer anyway, so—well, that's why it says Jenny on her birth certificate."

"And it doesn't have to be short for Jennifer," Denia said. "Think of Pirate Jenny, in *The Threepenny Opera*. But your little pirate's name is Jenny Edwards. And does she have a middle name, Nicholas? Because I'm serious about putting that money in trust for her."

"It's Roussard," he said, and spelled it. "My wife's maiden name."

FORTY-SEVEN

Pirate Jenny," he said. "Maybe that's what you'll be next Halloween. We'll get you an eye patch, and your mother can make you a cutlass out of cardboard."

"Daddy home," said the future pirate, bouncing happily on his lap. "Daddy home!"

"Daddy's home," he agreed. "And in fifteen years or so, he'll be the one stuck at home while you toddle off to college."

"And it's all paid for," Julia said. "You really think she'll go through with it? Set up our little bundle of joy with a six-figure trust fund?"

"Well, you never know," he said. "It was her idea, and I couldn't talk her out of it. She could change her mind, but I don't think she will."

"And where will the pirate go to college, do you suppose? She could follow in her mommy's footsteps and go to Sophie

Newcomb, but they went and merged my old school into Tulane. I'm not sure it would be the same. With all that money she could go someplace fancy. All New England preppy. Where would you want her to go?"

"Nowhere, for the time being. Fifteen years from now? I don't know. Some school where there aren't any boys, how's that?"

"Aren't you the dreamer. How about Sweet Briar, in Virginia? I knew a girl who went there, and don't you know she got to keep her own horse there."

"Right in the dormitory?"

"In the stable, you idiot. Jenny, you'll be a pirate on horseback. How does that sound?"

"Daddy home," Jenny said.

"Well, you know what's important, don't you? Yes, Daddy's home. Aren't we lucky?"

After they'd put Jenny to bed and then gone to bed themselves, after the lovemaking and the easy shared silence that followed the lovemaking, she said she didn't think she'd ever known anyone named Gardenia.

"I gather no one ever calls her that," he said. "I believe she said she'd had it changed legally."

"Better than changing it illegally. Jeb, Jenny, Denia—all of y'all have got names that are short for something, except they're not."

"That's true, isn't it?"

"I guess. Is she pretty?"

"Denia Soderling? She's an attractive woman."

"Why didn't you sleep with her? Or did you? No, you didn't. What stopped you?"

"Huh?" He doubled up his pillow, propped himself up

with it. "Where did this come from? Why would that even be a possibility?"

"Oh, come on," she said. "A beautiful lonely widow? A handsome mysterious stranger? 'Stay in my guest room, it'll be so much more comfortable than that nasty old motel.' She didn't offer you the guest room in the hope that you'd stay in it."

"I guess she may have been interested."

"And you weren't?"

He considered the question. "The last night," he said, "when she wanted to set up a fund for Jenny's education, we talked about her name, and how it was just plain Jenny, and not short for anything."

"So they'd get it right on the paperwork."

"I suppose. I told her how Jenny was a breech presentation."

"And she got it right away? Or did you have to explain?"

What he could have told Denia Soderling:

"See, there's a very famous U.S. airmail stamp of 1918, Scott C3a. There were actually three stamps with the same design— a six-cent orange, a sixteen-cent green, and a twenty-four-cent carmine rose and blue. They all pictured a Curtiss biplane, called the Jenny because it was part of the company's JN series of aircraft.

"The high value, the twenty-four-cent stamp, was a bicolor, and that meant each pane of stamps had to make two passes through the printing process, once for each color. Only one sheet went through upside down, and as a result the stamps had what's called an inverted center.

"Now, this was an occasional consequence of bicolor printing. In some countries, where quality control wasn't a priority, or where enterprising employees had learned to make profitable mis-

takes, inverted centers turned up with some frequency. In 1901 the U.S. issued a stamp series to mark the Pan-American Exposition in Buffalo, the one where President McKinley was assassinated, and three of the six stamps could be found with their centers inverted. They all illustrated modes of transportation, so depending on the denomination, you'd have a steamship or a locomotive or an electric automobile, and it'd be upside down.

"Those three stamps were legitimate rarities, and nowadays bring substantial five-figure prices. But they didn't catch the imagination of the public the way that upside-down plane did. These were the first airmail stamps, and aviation was very new and very exciting, and here's this plane putting on an exhibition of philatelic stunt flying. You can buy a decent copy of the regular stamp, Scott C3, for around a hundred dollars. If you want the error, with the plane upside down, you'll probably have to spend over a million.

"Our Jenny was turned around in the birth canal, and they were going to do a caesarean because she was leading with her behind, and that makes for a difficult delivery. But the obstetrician managed to get her turned around some, so that she emerged feet first.

"We'd already decided that we both liked the name Jenny. It was high on our list. And then, when she flew into our lives upside down, well, that cinched it."

"She might have liked it," Julia said. "Don't you think? Her husband was a collector, and she had a million new reasons to like the whole idea of stamps."

"I figured it would take a long time to explain. It was nothing she needed to know, and I didn't feel like going through it."

"So you didn't sleep with her, and you didn't tell her how your daughter got her name. You're some houseguest. Glad to be home?"

"Very."

"And you're exhausted, aren't you? You can tell me the rest tomorrow. And I guess you've got stamps to put in."

"Magic beans," he said.

"I won't even ask what that means," she said. "Good night, my sweet."

But she asked him the following afternoon. He'd caught up with the mail by then, and driven to Slidell to pick up the envelope that was waiting for him at a Mail Boxes Etc. office. Cash, his share of the money Joanne Hudepohl had wired to Dot in Flagstaff.

Back home, he stashed the money, then went to work on his stamps. His office was not nearly so grand as Jeb Soderling's beautifully appointed stamp room, but it suited him just fine. His chair was comfortable, his desk the right size and height, and the light fell on his books and stamps without getting in his eyes.

Jenny took her usual perch on the chair beside his, and he kept up a running commentary while she watched every move he made. He was still hard at it when nap time came around, and Julia led Jenny away and came back to take her place at the stamp table.

"Stamps are educational," she said, "even when it's your father who collects them. I'll bet there's not a kid in her whole day care center who knows a damn thing about the Turco-Italian War and the Treaty of Roseanne."

"Lausanne."

"I was close. Lausanne's in Switzerland, isn't it? Or am I thinking of Lucerne?"

"They're both in Switzerland."

"Both of them? That's confusing, isn't it? Which one is full of magic beans? You don't have any idea what I'm talking about, do you? Well, that makes us even. Those were the last two words you said last night, right before you dropped off to sleep. Or maybe you were already asleep. Are you going to tell me about the magic beans?"

It took him a minute. Then he remembered and recounted his dreamy conversation with his dead mother.

"Magic beans," Julia said. "Well, your mother might not agree, but I think taking your commission in stamps makes perfect sense. What do you figure they're worth?"

"The Scott value's a little over a hundred thousand. On this sort of material, figure retail at somewhere between sixty and seventy-five percent of catalog. I couldn't get that for them, but that's what I'd have had to pay."

"But you didn't have to pay anything. That's nice."

"Very. You know, I don't think it cost her anything, either. I can't believe anybody's bid would have been higher if the stamps I took were still in their albums."

"So everybody wins?"

"Denia wins," he said, "and so do I. Would Talleyrand Stamp and Coin net a few dollars more if these stamps were included in what they bought? I suppose so, but they'll make out fine as it is."

"And they'll never miss what they never knew was there. And you're better off getting paid in stamps, because you'd have spent the money on stamps anyway. So you did fine with the magic beans, and that was only part of your compensation. The next time you talk with your mother you can let her know you picked up some cash while you were at it."

"That'll be a load off her mind."

"Do you want to tell me about that part of it? Jenny's good for another half hour minimum, if you feel like talking about what you did in Denver."

FORTY-EIGHT

I got in a twist over the GPS," he told her. "I'd programmed it with two addresses where things happened."

"The house that burned and where else? Oh, of course. The loft where you wrapped things up."

"And anything digital lasts forever."

"And of course you'd rented the car under your own name."

"I did everything under my own name, including the car rental. So I hatched one brilliant idea after another. I could pull the GPS, smash it with a hammer, drop it off a bridge, and report it as stolen."

"That would work, wouldn't it?"

"You'd think so," he said, "but suppose it's got some kind of cyberconnection to a computer somewhere? Then making it disappear just might lead somebody to check with the mother ship and find out where it had been before it got lost. So I thought of opening it up and messing with its insides."

"To reprogram it? You could do that?"

"Not in a million years. But I could probably find some way to make it stop working. I wouldn't mention it, and nobody would notice until the next person to rent it couldn't get it to work. If he even bothered to try."

"Is that what you did?"

He shook his head. "I just left it alone and gave the car back to them. I decided it was nothing to worry about. If they have reason to suspect me, they won't need GPS records. If they don't, they won't check them. And why should they? As far as they're concerned, the case is closed. Richard Hudepohl is dead as a result of a fire set by the former lover of his jilted girlfriend."

"All of which is true."

"Well, almost true, and there's nobody around to argue otherwise. Trish Heaney and Tyler Crowe are both dead. If the lab crew from *CSI* got on the case, they'd probably spot a few inconsistencies in the murder-suicide scenario, but real-life cops are in more of a hurry than the ones on TV. The case is closed, and the closest thing to a loose end is Joanne, and even if she's crazy enough to tell someone, what can she say? She's got the number of an unregistered phone that no longer exists, and she wired some money to a person who never existed in the first place."

"So it's all over. And yet you seem…"

"What?"

"I don't know. Moody? Dissatisfied?"

"Maybe."

"Did you do that memory exercise? Making the mental picture smaller and bleaching the color out of it?"

He shook his head. "I probably should," he said. "I've spent so little time thinking about them that I didn't even remember to fade them out of my memory. I can barely remember what they look like, Trish and Tyler. Very distinctive in appearance, both of them, and yet it's hard for me to picture them."

"I wonder why."

Later he said, "It was peripheral, all of it. What I was most interested in was getting the best possible price for the Soderling collection. The job in Denver was something to shunt aside and take care of in my spare time."

"When it was supposed to be the other way around."

"I was all involved with the stamps," he said, "and it took me a couple of days to go have a look at the house on Otis Drive. If I'd made it my first priority, there never would have been a fire. Hudepohl would have been a soft target, he wouldn't have had his guard up, so how hard could it have been?"

"For a man of your talents."

"Well," he said. "The point is, by the time I managed to go see where he lived, there was no house there. And then there was nothing to do, so I headed north and went back to work on selling the stamps."

"Which was what you were really interested in anyway."

"Right. And when Dot went proactive and got in touch with Mrs. Hudepohl, I wondered why she couldn't leave well enough alone."

"Because you already had half the money without doing anything."

"And now I'd have to do something. And I did, and it went smoothly enough, but it was a little like watching a movie."

"You weren't really involved."

"I managed to stay in the moment," he said, "because you have to. And I didn't get thrown off at the prospect of making bad things happen to good people."

"Because they weren't good people."

"They weren't just the kind of people you see on *Cops*. They were the kind who call up their friends to make sure they tune in and watch. She was a tramp and he was a glassy-eyed pyromaniac. And they smelled."

"Oh?"

"I don't think he bathed much. Maybe he resented water because people put out fires with it, but you could tell he gave it a wide berth. And she was wearing this overpowering perfume, with a trace of body odor under it."

"Charming."

"I smelled it again a few hours ago, when I made their images get fainter and smaller. I got rid of their faces, but I couldn't get rid of the perfume. Jesus, I'll bet that's what it was."

"What?"

"Jungle Gardenia. It's not as though I recognized it, because I don't believe I'd ever smelled it before, but I mentioned it, didn't I?"

"It's how your girlfriend got her name."

"Her mother wore it," he remembered, "and it evidently drove her father mad with desire."

"But it just made you want to get back to your stamps."

"It made me want to get out of there," he said. "I wish there was a way to get the smell out of my memory. If I can do it with a visual image, why can't I do it with an aroma?"

"Maybe you'll figure out something."

"Or maybe it'll go away on its own. It doesn't matter. The point is my work didn't have my full attention, and I think there's a lesson there."

"Don't try to do two things at once?"

"That's part of it," he allowed, "but there's more. The other thing, the Denver assignment. I don't think I can do that anymore."

"Maybe it's time to let go of it."

"That's what I've been thinking. I thought I was done with it before, when Donny and I were doing okay rehabbing houses. And then I had a reason to go back to it, or thought I did, and it's very seductive."

"Easy money," she said.

"Plus it's easy to get involved. It's problem solving, and you get caught up in it, and there's a good feeling when it works out. Well, there can be a bad feeling, too, but you push that part aside. Except this time I didn't get caught up in it, not really, and the good feeling didn't amount to much. And there wasn't exactly a bad feeling, but there was a bad smell."

"And it's still around."

"I'll tell Dot I'm done. We'll still be friends, but she can call me on the regular line. We won't need Pablo."

"Pablo?"

"It's not important. We've got plenty of money, and I think I can make money in the stamp business, even if that's not the original reason I got into it. And I just realized something else."

"Oh?"

"The real reason I didn't explain Jenny's name to Denia Soderling. It's the same reason I didn't sleep with her."

"It would be long and drawn out and she might not get it?"

"It would be bringing somebody else into something that's just for you and me. I didn't think of it in those terms, I just knew I didn't want to do it. Sleep with her or explain to her.

But that's why." He drew a breath. "I suppose that sounds pretty silly."

"No," she said. "Not to me."

"I'll call Dot."

She put her hand on his arm. "There's no rush," she said. "Call her in a little while."

KELLER'S
OBLIGATION

FORTY-NINE

Well, I guess you could walk there," the bellman said. His tone and expression suggested that the whole idea of walking anywhere struck him as outlandish. "It's not very far," he went on, warming to the notion. "You go out the door, you take a left, you go one, two, three blocks to Allen Street, turn right, and once you cross Pearl Street you're pretty much there. You can't miss it, really."

Keller repeated the directions and the bellman hung on every word, as if he were the one who wanted to get to the Y. "That's it," he said, when Keller had finished. "There's one-way streets involved, but you don't have to pay any attention to that, not if you're going on foot."

That, Keller agreed, was the beauty of walking, along with not needing a quarter for the parking meter. How would he know the building?

"You can't miss it," the bellman said again. "It's three or four stories tall, and it's got a big red *A* on the top of it."

Keller had read *The Scarlet Letter* in high school. Or at least he thought he had, but he might have scraped by with the *Classic Comic Book* version. A couple of years ago he'd read *Adventures of Huckleberry Finn,* which he'd always thought he'd read in school, but the book turned out to be much richer and fuller than what he remembered, and he had a strong visual memory of Huck and Jim on the raft, and decided it owed less to Mark Twain's description than to the broader strokes of a comic book artist. So maybe he'd read Hawthorne and maybe he hadn't, but either way he recalled the woman's name—Hester Prynne, nobody'd ever forget a name like that. And he knew the significance of the title. The scarlet letter was an *A,* and she'd been branded with it to indicate that she was an adulteress.

And the building, the YMCA, was one he couldn't miss. Because it had an *A* on its top.

The bellman's directions turned out to be right on the money, and Keller had no trouble spotting the building, four stories tall, with a classic limestone facade and, no question, the letter *A* mounted on its top, glowing like an ember to tell the whole world what poor Hester Prynne had done. Keller posted himself diagonally across the street and kept an eye on the entrance, then gave it up when he realized he didn't know who or what he was looking for. He crossed the street and mounted a few steps and went inside, and a pleasantly plump woman with a kind face told him he'd find the stamp club on the third floor. "It's to the left when you get off the elevator," she said, "or to the right if you take the stairs."

"One if by land," Keller said.

"And two if by sea, and I on the opposite shore will be, and I forget what comes next. Ready to ride and spread the alarm through every Middlesex village and farm."

"I thought you forgot."

"It came back to me. Why Middlesex? What does a county in England have to do with Paul Revere? Well, let's find out, shall we?"

She tapped away at her keyboard, squinted at her computer terminal. "Ah," she said. "Middlesex is the most populous county in Massachusetts, and was first designated a county in 1643. There's a list of towns, and Concord is one of them."

"Where the embattled farmers stood," Keller heard himself say.

She beamed. "And fired the shot heard round the world, and we've gone from Longfellow to Ralph Waldo Emerson, haven't we? Now *this* is interesting. Since 1997, Middlesex has been a county in name only. The state took over all the government functions. They seem to have done that with all the counties. That's not really terribly interesting after all, is it? I wonder why I thought it was." She sighed. "Between Google and Wikipedia," she said, "you can learn almost anything, and some of it may even be accurate. I'm keeping you from your meeting."

"That's all right."

"This thing," she said, waving a hand at the computer terminal, "is either the greatest time-saver ever invented, or the greatest waste of time. Do you know how long it would have taken me to learn about Middlesex County without it?"

"Ages."

"And then some. I'd have had to go to the library, I'd have had to pull heavy books off high shelves, and in the end I might still not have found what I wanted to know. On the other hand, I wouldn't have bothered. 'Why Middlesex?' I'd have mused, and then I'd have thought of something else, and that would have been the end of it. A time-saver *and* a waste of time. But if you've got a question, the silly thing can give you the answer."

He took the stairs, climbed two flights of them, and turned right, and a sign on an easel pointed him to the stamp club meeting place halfway down the hall. Inside, five men and a woman sat behind tables, while another dozen men and women perched on modular white plastic chairs, the kind you could stack when the meeting was over. The ones at the tables would be dealers, he knew. Vest-pocket dealers, part-timers who helped finance their hobby by selling what they could at local shows and club meetings. The ones in the chairs would be collectors, but some of them might do a little dealing now and then, just as most of the dealers were more interested in their own collections than the few dollars they might make tonight.

Everyone was watching the screen at the front of the room, where a man with a wispy mustache was guiding the audience through a PowerPoint presentation on the various post–World War I plebiscite issues. This surprised Keller; the topic was one that actually interested him.

In the aftermath of the First World War, the victors had redrawn the map of Europe, in accordance with the principle of self-determination of nations as voiced by Woodrow Wilson. Plebiscites were scheduled for disputed regions, and the residents could cast ballots to determine which country they would be a part of.

Until then, each plebiscite region had its own administration, and its own stamps, and they were interesting in themselves, and so was their history. One such district in East

Prussia, Allenstein to the Germans and Olsztyn to the Poles, issued two series of fourteen stamps each in 1920, both consisting of overprinted German issues. Keller owned both complete sets—they weren't expensive, or difficult to find—but an Allenstein collection wasn't limited to those twenty-eight stamps as listed in the Scott catalog. There were color varieties, shades, several of them Scott-listed, some noted in the German-language Michel catalog. And there were other German stamps, five in the first series and one in the second, which had been overprinted, as the rest had been, but had never seen postal service. These unissued varieties were noted in the Scott catalog, with a value given to them, and Keller owned a couple of them and would have been glad for the chance to acquire the others.

And if he did, he might find himself with another specialty—Allenstein, specifically, or plebiscite issues in general. Then he'd find himself seeking out shades, which he didn't ordinarily bother with, and adding items of postal history, such as envelopes mailed to and from Allenstein and Memel and Schleswig and Marienwerder and both Upper and Eastern Silesia.

That seemed to be how it worked. Keller's main specialty was Martinique, the French island in the Caribbean. Keller had never been there, and had no particular desire to visit the place. He'd collected its stamps as he collected those of every other country, and without making any particular effort he'd reached a point where he owned examples of all of Martinique's stamps, except for two high-priced rarities. Then, when both stamps came up in an auction just after he'd had a nice windfall, he'd been high bidder on both lots and his collection of Martinique was complete.

Except it wasn't, because the next thing he knew he was

seeking out additional items, like doubled and inverted over-prints. Scott 33, a common one-centime stamp from 1892, bore the island's name in red, but there was a variety—number 33a—with the word *Martinique* in blue. It cataloged at $650, and Keller would have paid twice that for a decent example, but so far he'd had no luck in finding one. And there were other minor varieties, some of which he owned and others he was still looking for, and then there were the covers, envelopes bearing Martinique's stamps. You could go on amassing covers forever, because in a sense every last one was unique, mailed on a certain date, bearing certain stamps, sent from this person to that person, from this place to that place, and carrying the postmarks and stickers and imprints attesting to its peregrinations.

He wasn't sure he wanted to get into all that with Allenstein, let alone Memel and the rest. But he wasn't ready to rule it out, either, and he sat there and paid close attention to what the earnest gentleman with the tentative mustache had to say.

The presentation ran a little under half an hour, and ended with the speaker inviting questions. The first hand raised was that of an older man who wanted to know why the plebiscites almost invariably ended with a decisive vote in favor of the territory's being returned to Germany. The speaker didn't know, and another man suggested that the inhabitants wanted to avoid the harsh Polish winters.

Then a boy raised his hand. There were two boys in the room, both about fourteen, and they were seated side by side, and Keller had been glancing their way from time to time. It was the smaller of the two who raised his hand, and the speaker knew him. "Yes, Mark," the man said. "Do you have a question?"

"There's something I was wondering about the unissued Allenstein overprints," he said. "Two of them are on German stamps with shade varieties. The German five-pfennig stamp can be brown or dark brown, and the twenty-pfennig green also comes in yellow-green and blue-green. Are there shade varieties in the unissued overprints?"

Keller was impressed. Mark had asked a remarkably sophisticated question. Keller didn't know the answer, and neither, apparently, did the speaker, who said he didn't know of any such varieties, and would guess there weren't because so few of the unissued overprints had been produced. But, he added, he couldn't absolutely rule out the possibility, and why had Mark raised the point? Did he have an example of what he thought might be a shade variety?

"I wish," Mark said. "No, I was just wondering."

FIFTY

He'd been at his desk, working on his own stamp collection, when the phone rang. If Julia had been home he'd have left it for her to answer, but she was at the playground with Jenny, letting her polish her social skills even as she refined her sandbox technique. He debated letting the machine answer it, then picked it up in the middle of the third ring.

"*Lo siento mucho,*" said a familiar voice in an unconvincing accent. "*Quiero hablar a Pablo, pero yo tengo el número wrongo.*"

Oh?

His caller hung up before he could respond.

"I was beginning to wonder," Dot said. "All you said was 'Hello,' and it sounded like you, but what if I really did dial a wrong number? An hour went by and nothing happened. I figured I'd give you another ten minutes, and here you are. What happened? You couldn't find the phone?"

"I had to recharge it."

"Now why the hell didn't that occur to me? It should have, because I had to charge my own Pablo phone, which I haven't used since you got back from Denver and said *no más*. That's Spanish, it means—"

"I know what it means. It's about as hard to translate as *el número wrongo*."

"I looked it up," she said, "and what I should have said is *el número equivocado*. But I figured you'd know what I meant. Look, I know you're not doing this anymore."

"Right."

"And I think that's fine. Nobody should stay too long at the fair, and maybe the stamp business will work out for you, and if it doesn't, well, sooner or later construction will be good again, won't it?"

"Probably."

"While I, on the other hand, can't claim a huge interest in either stamps or houses. So I get my hair done and I have lunch with my girlfriends, and when a job comes in I find somebody to do it. And then this one came in, and I decided to call you, and all you have to do is tell me to forget it."

"And you'll find somebody else."

"Nope. I'll forget it."

Well, she had his interest. "Why's that?"

"A child."

"Fourteen years old, and either I saw an old photograph or he looks young for his years."

"Before all this," he said, "that was a line I always drew. I

325

didn't care who the targets were, and the less I knew about them, the better. But no kids."

"It rarely came up," she said. "And when it did, I turned the job down. I didn't always tell you. I just turned it down and that was that."

"So why is this different? Is this kid some kind of bad seed out of a horror movie?"

"I think he's a perfectly nice little boy."

"Then I don't get it."

"Pablo," she said, "the phone rang, and the assignment came, and I drove to Flagstaff to pick up the first payment and the instructions. And there's this photo straight out of *Leave It to Beaver,* and a name and address, and so on. And I thought, well, it's good I didn't have the money in my hand for very long, because that makes it a little easier to send it back."

"But you didn't."

"I was about to," she said, "but then I asked myself a question. You know what the question was?"

"What?"

"'Now what happens?'"

"Oh."

"Right. I don't know why that never occurred to me in the past, when somebody wanted us to hit a kid and I told them thanks but no thanks. But it dawned on me this time that what I was really saying was you'll have to find somebody else, and of course that's exactly what would happen. They'd find somebody else, and the kid would still be dead, even if we didn't wind up with blood on our hands."

"What I always used to tell myself," he said, "was that any job I drew, the guy was dead whether I did it or not. Because somebody wanted him dead badly enough to pay the money, and if I didn't do it somebody else would."

"All of which is true."

"But just because we wouldn't do a kid, that doesn't mean somebody else wouldn't take the job."

"Your average sociopath," she said, "would probably prefer a kid, the same way a mugger would prefer a frail old lady."

"Safer and simpler."

"So let me ask you this, Pablo. What do you figure became of the handful of kids I thought I was saving?"

"Jesus. Not much fun to think about that."

"Not much fun at all. Here's the thing, though. If the voice on the phone had let me know he was talking about a kid, my thinking never would have gotten that far. I'd have turned the job down, and I'd have felt good about it, as if I'd just sent in a big donation to Father Flanagan's Boys Town. Let's hear it for Wilma-Known-as-Dot, who just saved a child's life. And then I'd have gone off to get my hair done."

"How often do you do that?"

"Once a week, whether it needs it or not. But there I was, looking at a picture of the kid, and I know I don't want any part of this one, but if I turn down the job it's the same as killing him myself."

"Not exactly."

"He's just as dead."

"Well, I guess that's true."

"And if I did it myself at least I'd make it as painless as I could. But I wouldn't do it at all, and neither would you, Pablo, and the kind of person who would, well, maybe he's the type who enjoys it. There are people like that in the world, you know."

"Lots of them."

"Even in our line of work, you get the occasional nut job."

He nodded. "By and large," he said, "they don't last long."

"But they get a lot done in their brief careers, don't they? That type of person enjoys his work, takes his time, gets all he can out of it. That's disgusting enough with any target, but when it's a kid—"

He got the point. He said, "What was it that general said? Or maybe it was somebody in the Defense Department. 'We had to destroy the village in order to save it.'"

"Rings a muted bell. But we don't have to kill the kid in order to save him. All we have to do is take the job."

"And not carry it out."

"Have to be a little more proactive than that, don't you think?"

"Carry it out," he said, "but not on the kid."

"Right. On the person who ordered the hit."

"Do we know who that is?"

"No."

"Do we know how to find out?"

"Same answer. We don't."

"Can't you get somebody else?"

"The others," she said, "are just voices on the phone, as far as I'm concerned, and that's all I am to them. If I even broached the subject they'd figure I was going soft in the head. 'Somebody wants a kid hit? So I'll hit him, ma'am. What's the problem?'"

"They call you ma'am?"

She sighed. "What you probably ought to do," she said, "is turn me down. Then you can go play with your stamps and I can send the money back and wash my hands of the whole thing. Isn't that what whatsisname did?"

"Who?"

"In the Bible. The guy who washed his hands. He was famous for it. Never mind. Did I mention where the boy lives? Well, it's Buffalo. I don't even know if you've been there."

"Not in years. I can't remember a thing about it, except for Niagara Falls."

"You went to Niagara Falls?"

"No," he said. "But I could have."

FIFTY-ONE

You know," Keller said, "I own a couple of the unissued overprints, though I couldn't tell you offhand if I've got the five-pfennig brown or the twenty-pfennig green. Those were the ones you mentioned, weren't they?"

The boy nodded. "Some of the issued stamps come in shades, and sometimes there's a big price difference. A dollar for the common shade and twenty or thirty dollars for the variety. And in both sets, for the two-and-a-half-mark lilac rose, the Scott listing just says 'shades.' I guess that means that the stamp comes in brown lilac and magenta as well, like the German stamp, and that they're all equally common and low-priced."

Keller said that struck him as a reasonable guess. "You know a lot about Allenstein," he said.

"Not that much. I know it was founded by the Teutonic

Knights, which is kind of interesting, but I'm not too clear on who they were."

"I never even heard of them. Was that in Scott?"

"Wikipedia. I actually own one of the minor varieties, Scott 11a, the one-and-a-quarter-mark in blue-green. It's nine dollars, which is no fortune, but it's scarcer than the common green."

"It sounds as though you specialize in Allenstein."

"More like the whole German area," the boy said, and talked about the albums that housed his collection, and how they'd been a present—"Several presents, really"—from his grandmother. "I'm Mark, by the way, but I guess you know that, because Mr. Hasselbend said my name when he called on me. Not that you'd necessarily remember that."

Keller remembered, and hadn't needed to hear Hasselbend, either. "I'm Nick Edwards," he said.

"And what do you collect, Mr. Edwards?"

"You can call me Nick," Keller said, and told him what he collected, and about his Martinique specialty.

"That's one you'll never complete," Mark said. "There are a couple of super-expensive rarities, aren't there? Or am I thinking of Guadeloupe?"

"Either one," Keller said. "There's a Guadeloupe postage-due that's unknown in mint condition, and extremely rare used. And with Martinique you've got Scott 11 and 17, both with five-figure price tags, and that's if you can find them."

Keller could find them. All he had to do was look in his album. He'd bought both at the same auction, after a nice windfall. But that didn't strike him as something he needed to share with Mark.

They chatted, and then Mark excused himself to trade duplicates with a motherly woman who could have been the sister of the Google fan on the desk downstairs. Each had brought a small stock book and a pair of stamp tongs, and they sat side by side at a table and haggled amiably, like Levantine merchants.

"You can still go," Dot said. "Last I heard, the Falls was still up and running. If you fly up to Buffalo on Sunday, you could fit in a day at the Falls."

"I think I'll stay home."

"I figured you'd say that. And I can't say I blame you."

"Why would anyone want to kill a kid? To go and pay money to have him killed?"

"His grandmother died," she said, "and left all her money in trust for him. He gets it when he turns twenty-one."

"*If* he turns twenty-one."

"There you go. So in a sense you've got seven years to do the job, but the client doesn't want to wait that long."

He thought about it. "Shouldn't be too hard to work out who the client is. Who gets the money if the kid's out of the picture?"

"It gets divided up. Three main beneficiaries, so the odds are that one of them's our client."

"Or they're all in it together, like something on *Masterpiece Theatre*. Dot, it's not really my problem."

"I know."

"For all we know, he could be a mean little bastard. Starts fires, tortures animals, wets the bed."

"And whoever kills him will be doing the world a favor."

"For all we know. Why would I fly up there on a Sunday? What happens on Monday?"

"That's when he's easy to find," she said, "because every

Monday after dinner he gets on the bus and goes downtown to his stamp club meeting."

Keller checked out the offerings of some of the vest-pocket dealers, but didn't see anything he could use. He fell into a couple of conversations, none of them as absorbing as the one he'd had with the boy. At an adjacent table, he overheard the other lad, taller and heavier than Mark, contemplating the purchase of a set of World Cup stamps from Transnistria, the breakaway province of Moldova, which itself had broken away from the Soviet Union. Transnistria, its autonomy recognized only by Russia, didn't field a World Cup team, and Keller wasn't sure the inhabitants cared much about soccer, but that didn't keep them from issuing stamps, and selling them to collectors.

The meeting ended with an auction—a handful of members' lots, with listless bidding and the highest sale price under $10. And then there was a raffle, and Mark's trading partner won a souvenir sheet from Saint Vincent and the Grenadines, donated by one of the dealers.

And that was that. Keller took his chair to the back of the room, where some men were stacking them, and Mark made a point of coming over and extending his hand. "I enjoyed talking with you, Nick," he said. "Will you be coming again next week?"

"I'm afraid not. I'm just in town on business."

"Next time bring your duplicates. Maybe we can trade."

"I'll do that," Keller said. "You spend a lot of time on stamps?"

"As much as I can. I do okay in school, so homework doesn't take much time, and I'm hopeless in sports, so that doesn't take any time at all."

"I see your friend collects World Cup issues."

"He likes soccer. He even likes to play it."

"But you don't."

"I like to sit at my desk and work on my stamps. Pretty boring, most people would say."

"Not in this room."

"Well, that's true," the boy agreed. "When I come here I don't feel like a misfit. I don't even feel like a kid." He grinned. "In here," he said, "I'm just another philatelist."

Downstairs, Keller found himself pausing at the desk on his way to the door. The same woman, who did in fact strongly resemble young Mark's trading partner, smiled brightly. Keller said, "Why an *A?*"

She didn't hesitate. Because she could read his mind? No, more likely he was not the first person to ask. Possibly not even the first person that day.

"It used to say YMCA," she said.

"Before the tornado struck?"

"Only metaphorically. YMCA stands for Young Men's Christian Association."

"And?"

"And gradually one word after another became problematic. 'Christian'? That might put off potential Jewish or Muslim members, and irritate atheists. Not to mention the Druids."

"I never mention the Druids."

"Then came 'Men's.' There was a YWCA as well, but the two merged a while back, to eliminate sexism, and cut costs in the bargain. So what's left? 'Young Association'? In addition to sounding stupid, and vaguely ageist, it was just plain inaccurate. This place is more of a senior center than a young association. So all the letters came down."

"Except for the *A*. Is that what they call it now? The *A*?"

"No, of course not," she said. "Everybody calls it the Y, the same as they always did. Don't you love it? And aren't you glad you asked? But not so glad as I. Because now I feel useful, having just supplied some information you probably couldn't have found on Google."

Keller walked back to his hotel, went up to his room, turned on the TV. He found a Spanish-language channel showing a soccer game, and turned it off when he realized he wasn't paying it the slightest bit of attention. The only part he was enjoying, in a sort of subliminal way, was the audio, and that was because he couldn't understand it.

He called home, spoke to Julia. "I was hoping I wouldn't like him," he said, "but he's a very nice boy. And serious about his stamps."

"So I guess you'll be a few days."

"I could turn around and come home," he said, "except I can't."

He switched phones, called Dot. "Well, I'm in," he told her. "I got here, and I met him, and I'm in."

"I figured the stamps would cinch it."

"I was probably in anyway. What choice do I have? It's an obligation."

"That's just waiting to be turned into a joke," she said, "but I'm not going to touch it. Where do the two of us get off talking about moral obligations? But there's no getting around it. That's what it is."

He thought for a moment. "There are three people who collect if the kid doesn't, right?"

"Two aunts and an uncle. They each get a fourth, and that's a lot, because Grandma was a wealthy lady."

"That's three people each getting a fourth."

"The boy's mother would get the last share, but—"

"But it's probably not her."

"Unless we're back to *Masterpiece Theatre,* and she's the classic Least Likely Suspect."

"If I brace them in turn, I should be able to pick a winner. I guess I'll start with the uncle."

He took a shower, turned the TV on, turned it off again. Instead of arriving on Sunday, he'd flown in that very morning. So he hadn't been to the Falls, and probably wouldn't get there, either. If he hadn't been working, he'd have brought Julia and Jenny along, and all three of them could have made the trip. Put on those yellow slickers, rode the *Maid of the Mist* right under the Falls, did all the tourist things.

But if he hadn't been working, how likely was it that he'd have come to Buffalo at all?

Two aunts and an uncle. He could hang around for a week, then go home. Maybe the client would change his mind, maybe the broker would tell him to look elsewhere. Maybe it would take seven years before the uncle (or the aunt, or the other aunt) found somebody to do the job, and by then there'd be no job to do.

Maybe what he himself ought to do was take out all three of them, the uncle and both aunts. The odds were they all three had it coming. If one of them happened to be the client, that was just because he (or she or she) thought of it first, or knew a number to call.

He'd thought he was done with all of this crap. And all it took to draw him back in was a kid with a pair of tongs and a magnifier, a kid who knew a lot of useless information about Allenstein. (And wasn't that redundant? Was it possible to know any *useful* information about Allenstein?)

Was he going to be doing this sort of thing for the rest of his life? Couldn't he just pack up his things and go home?

Evidently not. And Mark was a nice young man, with a keen interest in his hobby, and philately needed a next generation. The torch had to be passed, and every issue of *Linn's* held a lament for the paucity of future torchbearers.

Not to worry, Keller told himself. He'd think of something.